Advance in the Treatment
of Pediatric Leukemia

Advance in the Treatment of Pediatric Leukemia

Editor

Rupert Handgretinger

MDPI • Basel • Beijing • Wuhan • Barcelona • Belgrade • Manchester • Tokyo • Cluj • Tianjin

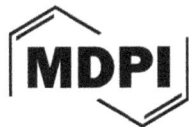

Editor
Rupert Handgretinger
University Hospital Tübingen
Germany
Abu Dhabi Stem Cell Center
United Arab Emirates

Editorial Office
MDPI
St. Alban-Anlage 66
4052 Basel, Switzerland

This is a reprint of articles from the Special Issue published online in the open access journal *Journal of Clinical Medicine* (ISSN 2077-0383) (available at: https://www.mdpi.com/journal/jcm/special_issues/Pediatric_Leukemia).

For citation purposes, cite each article independently as indicated on the article page online and as indicated below:

LastName, A.A.; LastName, B.B.; LastName, C.C. Article Title. *Journal Name* **Year**, *Volume Number*, Page Range.

ISBN 978-3-0365-4167-9 (Hbk)
ISBN 978-3-0365-4168-6 (PDF)

© 2022 by the authors. Articles in this book are Open Access and distributed under the Creative Commons Attribution (CC BY) license, which allows users to download, copy and build upon published articles, as long as the author and publisher are properly credited, which ensures maximum dissemination and a wider impact of our publications.

The book as a whole is distributed by MDPI under the terms and conditions of the Creative Commons license CC BY-NC-ND.

Contents

About the Editor vii

Preface to "Advance in the Treatment of Pediatric Leukemia" ix

Rupert Handgretinger
Editorial to: Advance in the Treatment of Pediatric Leukemia
Reprinted from: *J. Clin. Med.* 2022, *11*, 2361, doi:10.3390/jcm11092361 1

Hiroto Inaba and Ching-Hon Pui
Advances in the Diagnosis and Treatment of Pediatric Acute Lymphoblastic Leukemia
Reprinted from: *J. Clin. Med.* 2021, *10*, 1926, doi:10.3390/jcm10091926 7

Ilaria Iacobucci, Shunsuke Kimura and Charles G. Mullighan
Biologic and Therapeutic Implications of Genomic Alterations in Acute Lymphoblastic Leukemia
Reprinted from: *J. Clin. Med.* 2021, *10*, 3792, doi:10.3390/jcm10173792 31

Andrej Lissat, Claudia van Schewick, Ingo G. Steffen, Ayumu Arakawa, Jean-Pierre Bourquin, Birgit Burkhardt, Guenter Henze, Georg Mann, Christina Peters, Lucie Sramkova, Cornelia Eckert, Arend von Stackelberg and Christiane Chen-Santel
Other (Non-CNS/Testicular) Extramedullary Localizations of Childhood Relapsed Acute Lymphoblastic Leukemia and Lymphoblastic Lymphoma—A Report from the ALL-REZ Study Group
Reprinted from: *J. Clin. Med.* 2021, *10*, 5292, doi:10.3390/jcm10225292 55

Thies Bartram, Peter Schütte, Anja Möricke, Richard S. Houlston, Eva Ellinghaus, Martin Zimmermann, Anke Bergmann, Britt-Sabina Löscher, Norman Klein, Laura Hinze, Stefanie V. Junk, Michael Forster, Claus R. Bartram, Rolf Köhler, Andre Franke, Martin Schrappe, Christian P. Kratz, Gunnar Cario and Martin Stanulla
Genetic Variation in *ABCC4* and *CFTR* and Acute Pancreatitis during Treatment of Pediatric Acute Lymphoblastic Leukemia
Reprinted from: *J. Clin. Med.* 2021, *10*, 4815, doi:10.3390/jcm10214815 77

Manon Queudeville and Martin Ebinger
Blinatumomab in Pediatric Acute Lymphoblastic Leukemia—From Salvage to First Line Therapy (A Systematic Review)
Reprinted from: *J. Clin. Med.* 2021, *10*, 2544, doi:10.3390/jcm10122544 95

Michael Boettcher, Alexander Joechner, Ziduo Li, Sile Fiona Yang and Patrick Schlegel
Development of CAR T Cell Therapy in Children—A Comprehensive Overview
Reprinted from: *J. Clin. Med.* 2022, *11*, 2158, doi:10.3390/jcm11082158 111

Dorothee Winterberg, Lennart Lenk, Maren Oßwald, Fotini Vogiatzi, Carina Lynn Gehlert, Fabian-Simon Frielitz, Katja Klausz, Thies Rösner, Thomas Valerius, Anna Trauzold, Matthias Peipp, Christian Kellner and Denis Martin Schewe
Engineering of CD19 Antibodies: A CD19-TRAIL Fusion Construct Specifically Induces Apoptosis in B-Cell Precursor Acute Lymphoblastic Leukemia (BCP-ALL) Cells In Vivo
Reprinted from: *J. Clin. Med.* 2021, *10*, 2634, doi:10.3390/jcm10122634 155

Jamie L. Stokke and Deepa Bhojwani
Antibody–Drug Conjugates for the Treatment of Acute Pediatric Leukemia
Reprinted from: *J. Clin. Med.* 2021, *10*, 3556, doi:10.3390/jcm10163556 173

Bernice L. Z. Oh, Shawn H. R. Lee and Allen E. J. Yeoh
Curing the Curable: Managing Low-Risk Acute Lymphoblastic Leukemia in Resource Limited Countries
Reprinted from: *J. Clin. Med.* **2021**, *10*, 4728, doi:10.3390/jcm10204728 189

Dirk Reinhardt, Evangelia Antoniou and Katharina Waack
Pediatric Acute Myeloid Leukemia—Past, Present, and Future
Reprinted from: *J. Clin. Med.* **2022**, *11*, 504, doi:10.3390/jcm11030504 211

Christina Mayerhofer, Charlotte M. Niemeyer and Christian Flotho
Current Treatment of Juvenile Myelomonocytic Leukemia
Reprinted from: *J. Clin. Med.* **2021**, *10*, 3084, doi:10.3390/jcm10143084 227

Meinolf Suttorp, Andrea Webster Carrion and Nobuko Hijiya
Chronic Myeloid Leukemia in Children: Immune Function and Vaccinations
Reprinted from: *J. Clin. Med.* **2021**, *10*, 4056, doi:10.3390/jcm10184056 245

Mattia Algeri, Pietro Merli, Franco Locatelli and Daria Pagliara
The Role of Allogeneic Hematopoietic Stem Cell Transplantation in Pediatric Leukemia
Reprinted from: *J. Clin. Med.* **2021**, *10*, 3790, doi:10.3390/jcm10173790 259

About the Editor

Rupert Handgretinger

Rupert Handgretinger, M.D., is Emeritus Professor at the University of Tuebingen, Germany. From 2000 to 2005, he was the director of the division of stem cell transplantation at the St.Jude Children's Research Hospital in Memphis, USA. From 2005 to 2021, he was the department chair of Hematology/Oncology at the Children's University Hospital in Tuebingen, Germany, from where he retired in 2021. He is currently working as a consultant at the Yas Clinic Khalifa City and Abu Dhabi Stem Cell Center in Abu Dhabi, UAE. Prof. Handgretinger was one of the first to introduce CD34+ positive selection in haploidentical transplantation and, together with other researchers, developed methods for the ex vivo negative depletion of T-cells from mobilized peripheral blood from matched unrelated and haploidentical donors. The more recently developed depletion of $\alpha\beta$+ T-lymphocytes is now widely used in pediatric haploidentical transplantation. His other research interests have been the development of novel approaches of humoral and cellular immunotherapies for various forms of cancer. He was the first in 2008 to use the bispecific T-cell Engager (BiTE) Blinatumomab in children with refractory pre-B leukemia and was the first in 1989 to use the murine anti-GD2 antibody 14.G2a in children with refractory neuroblastoma. More recently. Prof. Handgretinger's team is focusing on the generation of new chimeric antigen receptor (CAR) constructs, and one of them is the development of an unique adapter CAR approach directed against hematological and solid tumors. Prof. Handgretinger has authored and co-authored >500 papers in peer-reviewed journals and contributed to various textbooks dealing with stem cell transplantation and immunotherapy. He is a member of the German academy of science Leopoldina and associate editor of the journal *Bone Marrow Transplantation*. In 2021, he was awarded the Life Time Achievement Award from the Pediatric Transplantation and Cellular Therapy Consortium (PTCTC).

Preface to "Advance in the Treatment of Pediatric Leukemia"

Since the first mention of childhood leukemia in 1860, tremendous progress has been made in understanding its biology and treatment. This book brings together leading experts in the field aiming to further improve pediatric leukemia outcomes through research and international collaboration. This book is dedicated to Prof. Hans-Jörg Riehm and the late Dr. Donald Pinkel, who, firmly believing that childhood leukemia is a curable disease, began the clinical trials for pediatric ALL that paved the way for today's high survival rates.

Rupert Handgretinger
Editor

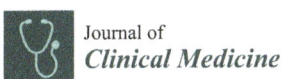

Editorial

Editorial to: Advance in the Treatment of Pediatric Leukemia

Rupert Handgretinger [1,2]

1. Department I–General Pediatrics, Hematology/Oncology, Children's Hospital, University Hospital Tübingen, 72076 Tübingen, Germany; rupert.handgretinger@med.uni-tuebingen.de
2. Abu Dhabi Stem Cell Center, Abu Dhabi, United Arab Emirates

Citation: Handgretinger, R. Editorial to: Advance in the Treatment of Pediatric Leukemia. *J. Clin. Med.* 2022, *11*, 2361. https://doi.org/10.3390/jcm11092361

Received: 18 April 2022
Accepted: 19 April 2022
Published: 22 April 2022

Publisher's Note: MDPI stays neutral with regard to jurisdictional claims in published maps and institutional affiliations.

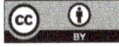

Copyright: © 2022 by the author. Licensee MDPI, Basel, Switzerland. This article is an open access article distributed under the terms and conditions of the Creative Commons Attribution (CC BY) license (https:// creativecommons.org/licenses/by/ 4.0/).

The history of leukemia goes back many years and John Bennet, a Scottish physician, described in 1845 a 28-year old patient with swelling of the spleen who then developed fever, bleeding and increasing swellings in his neck, groin and armpits. The patient finally succumbed to this unknown disease. At autopsy, Bennet found a massive increase of white blood cells, which he interpreted as pus. However, he did not find a source of the pus, but nevertheless he called it a suppuration of blood. A few months later, the German pathologist Rudolf Virchow published a case report describing a patient in her mid-fifties whose white blood cells had overgrown her blood, and at autopsy, a milky white layer of white blood cells was seen without a microscope. Virchow knew of Bennet's case, but did not agree with Bennet's interpretation of the suppuration of blood, but rather wondered whether this was a disease of the blood itself. He named it in German "weisses Blut" (white blood) but later changed it to the more academic-sounding word "Leukemia" from leukos and haima, which means white and blood in Greek, respectively. In 1860, the first case of childhood leukemia was described by Biermer, a student of Virchow. A 5-year old girl became increasingly lethargic and developed skin bruises. Biermer found a high number of leukemic cells in her blood and the girl died within 3 days after Biermer's diagnosis. In the next 100 years, no therapy was available for the affected children, and the mortality was 100%. When antifolates became available in the 1940ies, it was Sydney Farber who treated the first children with acute lymphoblastic leukemia (ALL) in 1947 with the antifolate aminopterin, with which he could induce at least temporary remissions [1]. In 1962, Danny Thomas founded the St. Jude Children Research Hospital in Memphis, USA, and the focus of the hospital at that time was the treatment of mainly lymphoblastic leukemia. Dr. Donald Pinkel, who was the first director of the hospital, initiated several consecutive clinical trials with modified regimes as new cytotoxic drugs became increasingly available. Given the combination of the different drugs, Dr. Pinkel called his studies "Total Therapy", and in 1971, Pinkel and his colleagues published the first results of the total therapy [2]. Of 31 treated patients, 27 achieved remission, and the time to relapse was almost 5 years compared to the few months achieved by Farber. More importantly, 13 patients never experienced a relapse and in 1979, the St. Jude group reported on 639 patients treated in 8 consecutive total therapy studies, of which 278 patients had all treatment stopped after 2 1/2 years of complete remission. Fifty-five of the 278 patients relapsed, mainly in the bone marrow. None of the 79 patients who remained in complete remission for at least 4 years off therapy have relapsed and ALL appeared curable in over one third of newly diagnosed patients who receive treatment for approximately 2 1/2 years [3]. Dr. Pinkel stated in 1979 that ALL in children cannot be considered any more as an incurable disease and that palliation is no longer an acceptable approach to its initial treatment [4]. In parallel in 1969, Prof. Hans-Jörg Riehm and his colleagues in Germany initiated the West-Berlin Therapy study of ALL in which 8 drugs including Prednison, Vincristine, Daunorubicin, L-Asparaginase, Cyclophosphamide, Cytarabine, Methotrexate and prophylactic central nervous system (CNS) irradiation were applied until the patients' tolerance limits. In 1977, Riehm et al. reported the 6-year experience of this approach on 73 children and adolescents. Six children died from therapy-related toxicity, 17 out of the 67 patients relapsed and 50 out of the 67 patients were in remission [5]. Based on these promising data, Prof. Riehm then introduced the concept of re-intensification in high risk patients and initiated the first cooperative ALL-BFM 76/79 studies in Germany, which initially comprised 3 centers (Berlin, Frankfurt, Münster) [6]. Currently, 115 German and international centers are participating in the most recent AIEOP-BFM ALL 2017 study. Through the cooperative trials in the US, Europe and many other countries, the cure rate of patients with ALL has increased with a 5-year overall survival (OS) rate exceeding 90% in high income countries. Based on the experience of the cooperative trials in ALL, similar trials were also initiated for the treatment of pediatric AML, JMML, and CML in children.

Since most of the children suffer from ALL, the focus of this special edition is mainly but not only on the advances in diagnosis, therapy, risk classification, clinical features, pharmacogenomics and new immunological approaches to the treatment of ALL, and new approaches to the therapy of AML, JMML and CML are also discussed. Finally, the indications for allogeneic transplantation and new transplantation approaches are presented.

Inaba and Pui start with advances in the diagnosis and treatment of pediatric acute leukemia. They describe the dramatic increase of the OS in the total therapy studies beginning with Total I-IV with an OS of 10% to 94% in the last Total XVI study. They describe in detail the cytotoxic drugs currently used and the medications used for molecular targeted therapy and for immunotherapy and discuss the classification of risk groups and the therapeutic approaches for the various genetic subtypes for acute pre-B- as well as for T-lymphoblastic leukemia. The authors emphasize the very important role of minimal residual disease (MRD), which has a major prognostic and therapeutic impact, and they point out that MRD levels, genetic classifications and clinical factors should be considered for risk stratification [7].

The biological and therapeutic implications of genomic alterations in ALL are discussed by Iacobucci, Kimura and Mullighan. They describe subtypes of ALL according to their specific genetic alterations, among them gross chromosomal abnormalities, transcription factor rearrangements and kinase alterations. They discuss in detail the gene expression signature for Ph-Like ALL, which comprises 10–15% in children. The correct diagnosis of Ph-Like ALL is important, since these patients may have targetable kinase alterations. In addition, they give a comprehensive genomic overview of T-ALL and its implication for diagnosis and treatment. The authors further discuss the value of the clinical implementation of high-throughput sequencing, including WTS (whole transcriptome sequencing, RNAseq), WGS (whole genome sequencing), WES (whole exome sequencing) and targeted DNA or RNA sequencing) for the detection of difficult subtypes of B- and T-ALL [8].

Although the cure rate is high, relapse of ALL is still the major reason for therapy failure. Most relapses occur in the bone marrow but can also occur in the CNS and testis, which are both considered to be sanctuary sites where chemotherapy is not effective. While in CNS and testes relapses, a specific local treatment together with systemic chemotherapy including irradiation, intrathecal therapy and orchiectomy and even allogeneic hematopoietic stem cell transplantation (HSCT) in high risk disease is necessary to induce long-term remission, much less is known on the outcome of children who have an non-CNS, non-testicular extramedullary relapse (other extramedullary relapse, OEMR). Lissat and colleagues have analyzed patients with OEMR who were treated in the multicenter ALL-REZ BFM trials between 1983 and 2015. Among 2323 patients, they identified 132 patients (5.6%) with OEMR. They describe in detail the different features and organ sites where the OEMR occurred and have classified OEMR into 5 subgroups. OEMR is more often seen in T-ALL compared to B-ALL, which is of prognostic relevance. The authors also give some guidance regarding the therapy of these patients, but also emphasize that based on the rareness of OEMR, international collaborations are necessary to prospectively evaluate the biology and treatment of his specific feature of ALL [9].

The intensive chemotherapy of ALL can come with severe organ toxicity, which can be life-threatening. In the beginning of the total therapies at Stjude, the patients often suffered from severe side effects, so that the fellows caring for the patients at that time called the total therapy among them "total hell" (R. Handgretinger, own observation). However, tremendous progress has been made over the years in supportive therapies, but drug-specific toxicities still occur during therapy, including methotrexate-related encephalopathy, steroid-induced avascular bone necrosis, topoisomerase-II-associated secondary AML, and acute pancreatitis (AP) developing during treatment with L-Asparaginase. The important role of pharmacogenomic studies is demonstrated by Bartram and colleagues in AP, which is induced by L-Asparaginase. They conducted a genome-wide association (GWAS) study in 51 patients with AP and in 1388 patients without AP. They found single-nucleotide variants (SNVs) within the ABCC4 gene, which is an ABC transporter mediating the efflux of drugs and also is involved in the development of drug resistance. These findings emphasize the increasingly important role of pharmacogenomics, which might help in the future to identify patients at risk before they receive the therapy. The authors also emphasize that international joint efforts are needed to better assess genetic risks for AP and other rare toxicities based on GWAS studies [10].

Until more recently, chemotherapy and irradiation were the major pillars of the treatment of ALL. When patients became therapy-resistant, no other therapies were available, and most patients succumbed to their disease. With the introduction of the bispecific T-cell engaging (BiTE) antibody a decade ago, an immunotherapy became available which induced complete and MRD-negative remissions in chemoresistant patients. This new drug, now called Blinatumomab, activates T-lymphocytes which then attack and kill CD19-positive ALL blasts. Queudeville and Ebinger describe the introduction of Blinatumomab from the beginning until its approval by the authorities. They give a comprehensive review and summarize the various studies which have been and are currently being performed. They show that Blinatumab is finding more and more its way in frontline therapies rather than being used late in chemo-refractory patients. It is hoped that Blinatumomab might be able to replace some of the cytotoxic chemotherapy without compromising the OS and EFS. Therefore, the authors stress the fact that many questions are still open, such as the need for HSCT after remission induction by Blinatumomab, and that future clinical trials should reveal the role of Blinatumomab in frontline and relapse therapy [11].

Another way to activate T-cells against ALL blasts is the construction of artificial T-cell receptors. This technique uses the antigen-binding part of an antibody directed against targets on the ALL blasts in combination with additional costimulatory factors. T-cells are then genetically modified so that they express the antigen-binding part of the antibody on their surface, which makes them Chimeric Antigen Receptor (CAR) T-cells. Especially CAR T-cells directed against the CD19 antigen (CART19) have induced complete remissions in chemorefractory patients. Boettcher and colleagues present a very comprehensive overview on the development and biology of CAR T-cells for the treatment mainly but not only for ALL. They also discuss the side effects of CAR T-cell therapy, such as the Cytokine Release Syndrome (CRS) and the immune effector cell-associated neurotoxicity syndrome (ICANS), and point out new CAR constructs to improve the efficacy while reducing the side effects. The difference between Blinatumomab and CARs is the penetration of the CARs into the CNS and the long persistence in the patients, which is associated with a lower rate of relapse as long as the CAR T-cells are persisting. However, relapses can still occur, especially when the blasts lose the antigen, as it has been seen with CARs directed against the CD19 antigen. The authors review all current studies for the treatment of leukemia and also for solid pediatric tumors and discuss ways how to circumvent the antigen-negative relapses [12].

As in Blinatumomab and for CART19 cells, the CD19 antigen has been identified as an optimal target for immunotherapy of ALL with engineered anti-CD19 antibodies by Winterberg and colleagues. They developed an antibody fused to a single chain tumor necrosis factor (TNF)-related apoptosis-inducing ligand (TRAIL) domain. TRAIL was chosen because it induces apoptosis in malignant but not healthy cells. Indeed, the authors could demonstrate that this new antibody construct binds to ALL blasts and induces pronounced apoptosis in vitro and prolonged survival in mice transplanted with patients' derived blasts. Interestingly, the combination of this construct with Venetoclax, which is an inhibitor of the anti-apoptotic protein BCL-2, induced synergistic apoptosis in vitro and in vivo in the mice models. These promising preclinical results warrant future preclinical and clinical studies [13].

The clinical outcome of other antibody conjugates is presented by Stokke and Bhojwani. For the treatment of ALL, the conjugate is composed of an antibody directed against CD22, which is, as CD19, almost universally expressed on ALL blasts. The antibody is conjugated to calicheamicin, a cytotoxic drug known as Inotuzumab ozogamicin. It has shown complete remission rates of 60–80% in patients with relapsed/refractory ALL. A similar construct comprised of an anti-CD33 antibody linked to calicheamicin (Gemtuzumab ozogamicin) is currently used for the treatment of AML. In addition, the authors give a comprehensive overview of other antibody/drug conjugates which are currently being studied in clinical trials for the treatment of ALL and AML and point out that the identification of optimal combinations with standard chemotherapy requires more clinical studies [14].

The current 5-year survival rates using intensive chemotherapy and also the new immunotherapies have only been achieved in high-income countries, and there is a great global disparity in treatment outcomes of ALL. Oh, Lee and Yeoh address this problem and show ways how to cure the curable patients with low-toxicity therapies in resource-limited countries (low-middle income countries, LMIC). They present data that for risk stratification, National Cancer Institute (NCI) standard risk criteria (age 1–10 years, WBC < 50,000 µL) are simple and effective. Depending on the available resources, other factors can be added. In LMIC, supportive care is also often limited, and the treatment-related morbidity and mortality can be more critical than relapses. Therefore, low-toxicity regimens should lead to improved OS. Since 80% of childhood ALL occurs in LMIC, the authors discuss the first steps to cure ALL in LMIC with less intensive therapy and less toxicity and with a better outcome, which could have a major impact on the 80% of children with ALL living in LMIC [15].

Progress has also been made in the treatment of patients with pediatric AML, which accounts for 15–20% of the pediatric leukemias with an incidence of approximately seven per million. Reinhardt, Antoniou and Waak give an overview of the past, present, and future and show the impressive progress, which has been made over the years. They discuss that this progress has been achieved by risk classification, CNS prophylaxis, introduction of MRD diagnostics, and the use of HSCT in high-risk patients. They also discuss the current cooperative trials and give an outlook on new therapies with targeted therapies and immunotherapies, including CAR T-cells [16].

Juvenile Myelomonocytic Leukemia (JMML) is a rare pediatric leukemia with shared features of myelodysplastic and myeloproliferative neoplasms. A common feature is the deregulation of the intracellular Ras signal transduction pathway. Mayerhofer, Niemeyer and Flotho present an overview of current treatment strategies. While HSCT is the only curative option for most patients, the authors describe a smaller proportion of children who survive long-term without transplantation. They review in detail the clinical and molecular risk factors which will give guidance to the therapy of this rare disease. The authors also point out experimental agents and targeted therapies, which might help to further improve the prognosis of patients with JMML [17].

Chronic Myeloid Leukemia (CML) is a clonal malignant disease characterized by the detection of the BCR-ABL1 fusion gene as a consequence of the t(9;22) reciprocal chromosomal translocation. Suttorp, Carrion and Hijiya give an overview of current treatment strategies. Since the current standard of care is the indefinite treatment with tyrosine kinase inhibitors (TKI), the humoral and cellular immune function might be reduced, and questions regarding the use of vaccines, including COVID-19 vaccines arise. The authors discuss the implication of TKI therapy for immunizations and for surveillance strategies and give guidance for the long-term care of these patients [18].

Finally, Algeri and colleagues discuss the role of HSCT in pediatric leukemia. Despite the remarkable achievements obtained with frontline therapies, transplantation is still for a number of patients the only curative approach. The authors discuss in detail the indications for HSCT for patients with ALL in first or second remission. In addition to some genetic factors, the MRD response has become an important indication for HSCT in first remission and in patients with late relapse. They then discuss the indication for HSCT in AML. Once again, genetic risk factors and well as MRD response will help to decide whether a patient needs an HSCT in first remission. All patients with a relapse of AML will have an indication for HSCT. The authors also discuss in detail the choice of the conditioning regimen and discuss the advantages and disadvantages of the various regimens. The detection of MRD pre-and/or post-transplant has become very important, and the authors discuss strategies for interventions using immunotherapy. Since not all patients will have a compatible donor, the authors also present data on alternative donors, including haploidentical donors. They stress the fact that, based on current outcome data, every patient in need of a transplant will have a donor. However, given the transplant-associated late effects, the determination of the appropriate role of HSCT in childhood leukemia remains a challenge [19].

Funding: This research received no external funding.

Conflicts of Interest: The author declares no conflict of interest.

References

1. Farber, S.; Diamond, L.K. Temporary remissions in acute leukemia in children produced by folic acid antagonist, 4-aminopteroyl-glutamic acid. *N. Engl. J. Med.* **1948**, *238*, 787–793. [CrossRef] [PubMed]
2. Pinkel, D. Five-year follow-up of "total therapy" of childhood lymphocytic leukemia. *JAMA* **1971**, *216*, 648–652. [CrossRef] [PubMed]
3. George, S.L.; Aur, R.J.; Mauer, A.M.; Simone, J.V. A reappraisal of the results of stopping therapy in childhood leukemia. *N. Engl. J. Med.* **1979**, *300*, 269–273. [CrossRef] [PubMed]
4. Pinkel, D. Treatment of childhood acute lymphocytic leukemia. *Haematol. Blood Transfus.* **1979**, *23*, 25–33. [PubMed]
5. Riehm, H.; Gadner, H.; Welte, K. The west-berlin therapy study of acute lymphoblastic leukemia in childhood–report after 6 years (author's transl). *Klin. Padiatr.* **1977**, *189*, 89–102. [PubMed]
6. Henze, G.; Langermann, H.J.; Brämswig, J.; Breu, H.; Gadner, H.; Schellong, G.; Welte, K.; Riehm, H. The BFM 76/79 acute lymphoblastic leukemia therapy study (author's transl). *Klin. Padiatr.* **1981**, *193*, 145–154. [CrossRef] [PubMed]
7. Inaba, H.; Pui, C.H. Advances in the Diagnosis and Treatment of Pediatric Acute Lymphoblastic Leukemia. *J. Clin. Med.* **2021**, *10*, 1926. [CrossRef] [PubMed]
8. Iacobucci, I.; Kimura, S.; Mullighan, C.G. Biologic and Therapeutic Implications of Genomic Alterations in Acute Lymphoblastic Leukemia. *J. Clin. Med.* **2021**, *10*, 3792. [CrossRef] [PubMed]
9. Lissat, A.; van Schewick, C.; Steffen, I.G.; Arakawa, A.; Bourquin, J.P.; Burkhardt, B.; Henze, G.; Mann, G.; Peters, C.; Sramkova, L.; et al. Other (Non-CNS/Testicular) Extramedullary Localizations of Childhood Relapsed Acute Lymphoblastic Leukemia and Lymphoblastic Lymphoma-A Report from the ALL-REZ Study Group. *J. Clin. Med.* **2021**, *10*, 5292. [CrossRef]
10. Bartram, T.; Schütte, P.; Möricke, A.; Houlston, R.S.; Ellinghaus, E.; Zimmermann, M.; Bergmann, A.; Löscher, B.S.; Klein, N.; Hinze, L.; et al. Genetic Variation in ABCC4 and CFTR and Acute Pancreatitis during Treatment of Pediatric Acute Lymphoblastic Leukemia. *J. Clin. Med.* **2021**, *10*, 4815. [CrossRef]
11. Queudeville, M.; Ebinger, M. Blinatumomab in Pediatric Acute Lymphoblastic Leukemia-From Salvage to First Line Therapy (A Systematic Review). *J. Clin. Med.* **2021**, *10*, 2544. [CrossRef]
12. Boettcher, M.; Joechner, A.; Li, Z.; Yang, S.F.; Schlegel, P. Development of CAR T Cell Therapy in Children—A Comprehensive Overview. *J. Clin. Med.* **2022**, *11*, 2158. [CrossRef]
13. Winterberg, D.; Lenk, L.; Oßwald, M.; Vogiatzi, F.; Gehlert, C.L.; Frielitz, F.S.; Klausz, K.; Rösner, T.; Valerius, T.; Trauzold, A.; et al. Engineering of CD19 Antibodies: A CD19-TRAIL Fusion Construct Specifically Induces Apoptosis in B-Cell Precursor Acute Lymphoblastic Leukemia (BCP-ALL) Cells In Vivo. *J. Clin. Med.* **2021**, *10*, 2634. [CrossRef] [PubMed]
14. Stokke, J.L.; Bhojwani, D. Antibody-Drug Conjugates for the Treatment of Acute Pediatric Leukemia. *J. Clin. Med.* **2021**, *10*, 3556. [CrossRef] [PubMed]
15. Oh, B.L.Z.; Lee, S.H.R.; Yeoh, A.E.J. Curing the Curable: Managing Low-Risk Acute Lymphoblastic Leukemia in Resource Limited Countries. *J. Clin. Med.* **2021**, *10*, 4728. [CrossRef] [PubMed]
16. Reinhardt, D.; Antoniou, E.; Waack, K. Pediatric Acute Myeloid Leukemia-Past, Present, and Future. *J. Clin. Med.* **2022**, *11*, 504. [CrossRef] [PubMed]
17. Mayerhofer, C.; Niemeyer, C.M.; Flotho, C. Current Treatment of Juvenile Myelomonocytic Leukemia. *J. Clin. Med.* **2021**, *10*, 3084. [CrossRef] [PubMed]

18. Suttorp, M.; Webster Carrion, A.; Hijiya, N. Chronic Myeloid Leukemia in Children: Immune Function and Vaccinations. *J. Clin. Med.* **2021**, *10*, 4056. [CrossRef] [PubMed]
19. Algeri, M.; Merli, P.; Locatelli, F.; Pagliara, D. The Role of Allogeneic Hematopoietic Stem Cell Transplantation in Pediatric Leukemia. *J. Clin. Med.* **2021**, *10*, 3790. [CrossRef] [PubMed]

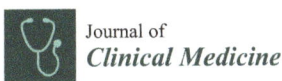

Review

Advances in the Diagnosis and Treatment of Pediatric Acute Lymphoblastic Leukemia

Hiroto Inaba [1,2,*] and Ching-Hon Pui [1,2]

[1] Department of Oncology, St. Jude Children's Research Hospital, Memphis, TN 38105, USA; ching-hon.pui@stjude.org

[2] Department of Pediatrics, University of Tennessee Health Science Center, Memphis, TN 38163, USA

* Correspondence: hiroto.inaba@stjude.org; Tel.: +1-901-595-3300; Fax: +1-901-521-9005

Abstract: The outcomes of pediatric acute lymphoblastic leukemia (ALL) have improved remarkably during the last five decades. Such improvements were made possible by the incorporation of new diagnostic technologies, the effective administration of conventional chemotherapeutic agents, and the provision of better supportive care. With the 5-year survival rates now exceeding 90% in high-income countries, the goal for the next decade is to improve survival further toward 100% and to minimize treatment-related adverse effects. Based on genome-wide analyses, especially RNA-sequencing analyses, ALL can be classified into more than 20 B-lineage subtypes and more than 10 T-lineage subtypes with prognostic and therapeutic implications. Response to treatment is another critical prognostic factor, and detailed analysis of minimal residual disease can detect levels as low as one ALL cell among 1 million total cells. Such detailed analysis can facilitate the rational use of molecular targeted therapy and immunotherapy, which have emerged as new treatment strategies that can replace or reduce the use of conventional chemotherapy.

Keywords: acute lymphoblastic leukemia; pediatric; advances; diagnosis; treatment

1. Introduction

Approximately 6000 new cases of acute lymphoblastic leukemia (ALL) are diagnosed in the United States annually [1–4]. ALL is the most common pediatric cancer (representing approximately 25% of cancer diagnoses), and approximately 60% of all cases occur in children and adolescents younger than 20 years, with an annual incidence of 36.2 per 1 million persons and a peak age of incidence of two to five years (at which there are >90 cases per 1 million persons) [5]. ALL is diagnosed more frequently in boys than in girls, with a ratio of approximately 1.3:1. The annual incidence of ALL differs markedly according to race and ethnic group; there are 40.9 cases per million in the Hispanic population, 35.6 cases per million in the white population, and 14.8 cases per million in the black population [6]. ALL cases are broadly classified as B-ALL or T-ALL based on immunophenotyping, with B-ALL comprising approximately 85% of cases, although this percentage can differ depending on age at diagnosis, race, or ethnicity.

Currently, the survival of pediatric patients with ALL treated in high-income countries exceeds 90% (Figure 1) [1–4]. Chemotherapy is given in four important phases: remission induction, consolidation, reinduction (delayed intensification), and continuation (maintenance). Chemotherapy is administered based on stratified risk classification, as determined by clinical factors (e.g., age (1–9.9 years vs. <1 or ≥10 years) and white blood cell (WBC) counts (<50 × 10^9/L vs. ≥50 × 10^9/L) at diagnosis), cytogenetic and genomic analysis of ALL cells, and response evaluation with a minimal residual disease (MRD) assay. Dosage adjustment based on pharmacodynamic and pharmacogenomic studies and supportive care (e.g., prevention and treatment of infection) have also contributed substantially to improved outcomes. Therefore, current dosages/schedules for "conventional" chemotherapy have been truly optimized.

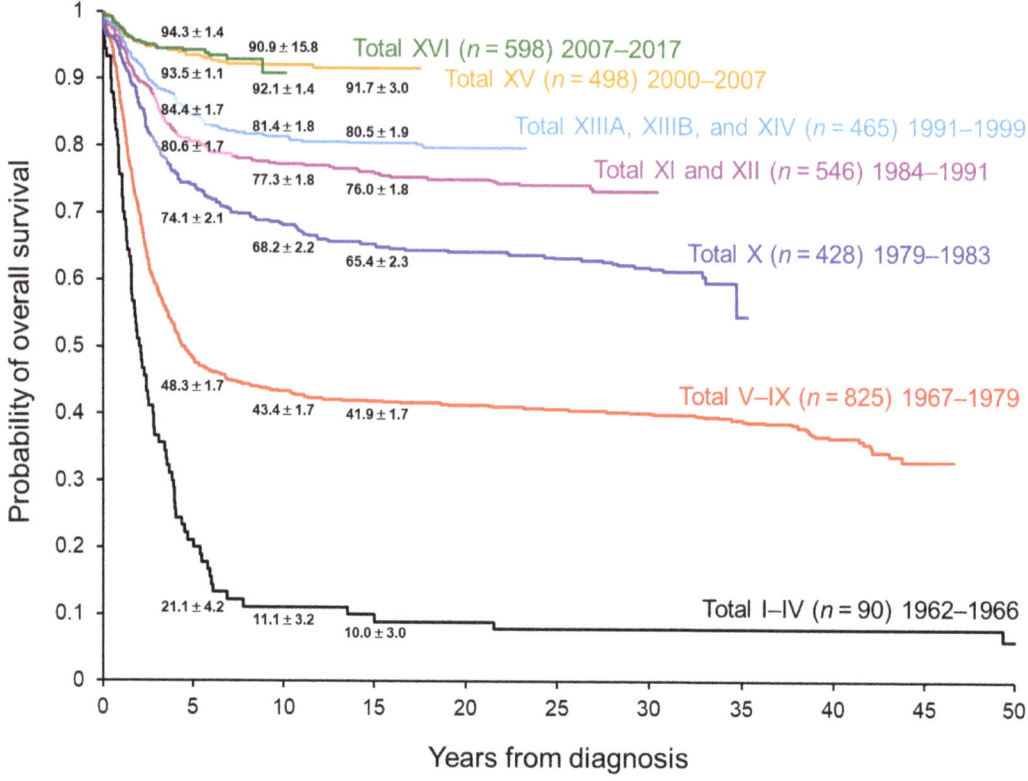

Figure 1. Overall survival of pediatric patients with acute lymphoblastic leukemia treated in the St. Jude Total Therapy studies.

With the current high rate of survival, further improvement in outcomes with conventional chemotherapy is challenging. In fact, there was very little improvement in 5-year overall survival (OS) between our two recent frontline ALL trials, St. Jude Total Therapy XV (5-year OS: 93.5%) and XVI (5-year OS: 94.3%) (Figure 1) [7,8]. Most of the conventional chemotherapy agents were approved by the US Food and Drug Administration before 1980 (Table 1), and their therapeutic intensity has been pushed to the limit of tolerance. Accordingly, further intensification of conventional chemotherapy could lead to only minimal improvement in overall outcomes while increasing adverse effects.

Recently, several molecular targeted agents and immunotherapy approaches have been introduced, and they promise to improve outcomes. For these agents to be used optimally, detailed genetic characterization of leukemia cells and response evaluation by MRD in individual patients are critical. In this review, we will review the genetic subgroups of ALL, the evaluation of MRD, and newer treatment strategies.

Table 1. Representative medications used in the treatment of patients with acute lymphoblastic leukemia and the year of US Food and Drug Administration approval.

Drugs	Year Approved in the US *
Conventional chemotherapy	
Mercaptopurine	1953
Methotrexate	1953
Prednisone	1955
Dexamethasone	1958
Cyclophosphamide	1959
Vincristine	1963
Thioguanine	1966
Cytarabine	1969
Doxorubicin	1974
L-Asparaginase	1978
Daunorubicin	1979
New formulations or agents	
Pegaspargase	1994
Nelarabine	2005
Erwinase	2011
Vincristine sulfate liposome injection	2012
Calaspargase	2018
Molecular targeted therapy	
ABL1 inhibitors	
Imatinib	2001
Dasatinib	2006
Nilotinib	2007
Ponatinib	2012
JAK inhibitor	
Ruxolitinib	2011
BCL-2 and BCL-X_L inhibitors	
Venotoclax	2016
Navitoclax	NA
Proteasome inhibitors	
Bortezomib	2003
Carfilzomib	2012
Ixazomib	2015
mTOR inhibitors	
Sirolimus	1999
Temsirolimus	2007
Everolimus	2009
DNA methyltransferase inhibitors	
Azacitidine	2004
Decitabine	2006
Histone deacetylase inhibitors	
Vorinostat	2006
Panobinostat	2015
Bromodomain inhibitor	
JQ1	NA
DOT1 inhibitor	
Pinometostat	NA
Menin inhibitor	
SNDX-5613	NA

Table 1. Cont.

Drugs	Year Approved in the US *
Immunotherapy	
Unconjugated antibodies	
Rituximab (CD20)	1997
Ofatumumab (CD20)	2009
Epratuzumab (CD22)	NA
Daratumumab (CD38)	2015
Alemtuzumab (CD52)	2001
Bispecific antibody	
Blinatumomab (CD19)	2014
Chimeric antigen receptor (CAR) T cells	
Tisagenlecleucel (CD19)	2017
Antibody–drug conjugate	
Inotuzumab ozogamicin (CD22)	2017

* Approval by the US Food and Drug Administration is not limited to indications for pediatric acute lymphoblastic leukemia. Abbreviation: NA, not approved.

2. Genetic Characterization of Acute Lymphoblastic Leukemia

The revolutionized approach to genomic analysis subdivides pediatric ALL into more than 30 genetic subgroups [9–11]. In B-ALL, recurrent genomic subtypes are characterized by chromosomal aneuploidy, i.e., hyperdiploidy (>50 chromosomes) or hypodiploidy (<44 chromosomes), and by rearrangements: *ETV6/RUNX1* fusion, *TCF3/PBX1* fusion, *BCR/ABL1* fusion, and *KMT2A* (*MLL*) rearrangement (Figure 2 and Table 2). Genetic abnormalities newly identified by comprehensive genomic analyses include *BCR/ABL1*-like ALL (Ph-like ALL), intrachromosomal amplification of chromosome 21 (iAMP21), *DUX4*-rearranged ALL, *ZNF384*-rearranged ALL, *MEF2D*-rearranged ALL, *PAX5*-altered (PAX5alt) ALL, *NUTM1*-rearranged ALL, and *ETV6/RUNX1*-like ALL. Characterization of genetic abnormalities in ALL cells is important in order to identify unfavorable genetic abnormalities and to incorporate molecular targeted therapy to reduce the risk of relapse.

Table 2. Genetic subtypes and treatment approach.

Category	Characteristics	Therapeutic Approach
B-lymphoblastic leukemia		
Low-risk genetics		
ETV6/RUNX1	Excellent prognosis	Reduction of intensity, MRD based
Hyperdiploidy	Excellent prognosis	Reduction of intensity, MRD based
DUX4-rearranged	Most have focal *ERG* deletions and favorable outcome despite *IKZF1* alterations	Standard dose intensity, MRD based
Intermediate-risk genetics		
TCF3/PBX1	Higher incidence in African Americans, cytoplasmic μ-chain	Standard dose intensity, MRD based, intensive intrathecal therapy
PAX5alt	*PAX5* fusions, mutation, or amplifications	Standard dose intensity, MRD based
PAX5 p.Pro80Arg	Frequent signaling pathway alterations	Standard dose intensity, MRD based, JAK inhibitors
ZNF384-rearranged	Peak age and prognosis vary by fusion partner, expression of myeloid markers	Standard dose intensity, MRD based

Table 2. Cont.

Category	Characteristics	Therapeutic Approach
B-lymphoblastic leukemia		
iAMP21	Additional copies of chromosome 21, worse outcome with low-intensity therapy	Intensification of therapy
NUTM1-rearranged *	Rare; more common in infants, excellent prognosis	Standard dose intensity, MRD based
High-risk genetics		
Near-haploid	24–31 chromosomes, Ras-activating mutations, inactivation of IKZF3	Intensification of therapy, MRD based, BCL-2 inhibitors
Low-hypodiploid	32–39 chromosomes, TP53 mutations (somatic and germline)	Intensification of therapy, MRD based, BCL-2 inhibitors
BCR/ABL1	Prognosis improved with ABL1 inhibitors, common deletions of IKZF1	ABL1 inhibitors, BCL-2 inhibitors
BCR/ABL1-like; JAK-STAT activating mutation	CRLF2 rearranged (IGH-CRLF2, P2RY8-CRLF2), JAK1/2, EPOR, IL7R, SH2B3 mutation	JAK inhibitors, BCL-2 inhibitors
BCR/ABL1-like; ABL1-class	Kinase-activating lesions, potentially amenable to kinase inhibition	ABL1 inhibitors, BCL-2 inhibitors
KMT2A (MLL)-rearranged	Common in infant ALL, few cooperating mutations	DOT1L inhibitors, menin inhibitors, proteasome inhibitors, histone deacetylase inhibitors, BCL-2 inhibitors
MEF2D-rearranged	Mature B cell leukemia morphology, cytoplasmic μ-chain	Histone deacetylase inhibitors, proteasome inhibitors
TCF3-HLF	Rare; dismal prognosis	BCL-2 inhibitors
ETV6/RUNX1-like *	Similar gene expression profile to ETV6-RUNX1 but lacks fusion	Intensification of therapy, MRD based
T-lymphoblastic leukemia		
Non-early T-cell precursor	Deregulation of TAL1, TAL2, LYL1, LMO1, LMO2, TLX1 (HOX11), TLX3 (HOX11L2), and HOXA; NOTCH1 activating mutation	Standard dose intensity, MRD based, nelarabine, BCL-2 inhibitors
JAK-STAT activating mutation	Approximately 25% of patients with T-ALL	Standard dose intensity, MRD based, nelarabine, JAK inhibitors, BCL-2 inhibitors
ABL1 fusions (e.g., NUP214-ABL1)	Fusion with BCR and NUP214, potentially amenable to tyrosine kinase inhibition	Standard dose intensity, MRD based, ABL1 inhibitors, nelarabine, BCL-2 inhibitors
Early T-cell precursor ALL	Mutations in transcriptional regulators, JAK-STAT and Ras signaling, and epigenetic modifiers	Standard dose intensity, MRD based, JAK inhibitors, BCL-2 inhibitors

* Newly identified subgroups, necessary to confirm their prognosis in a larger number of patients. Abbreviations: MRD, minimal residual disease; iAMP21, intrachromosomal amplification of chromosome 21; ALL, acute lymphoblastic leukemia.

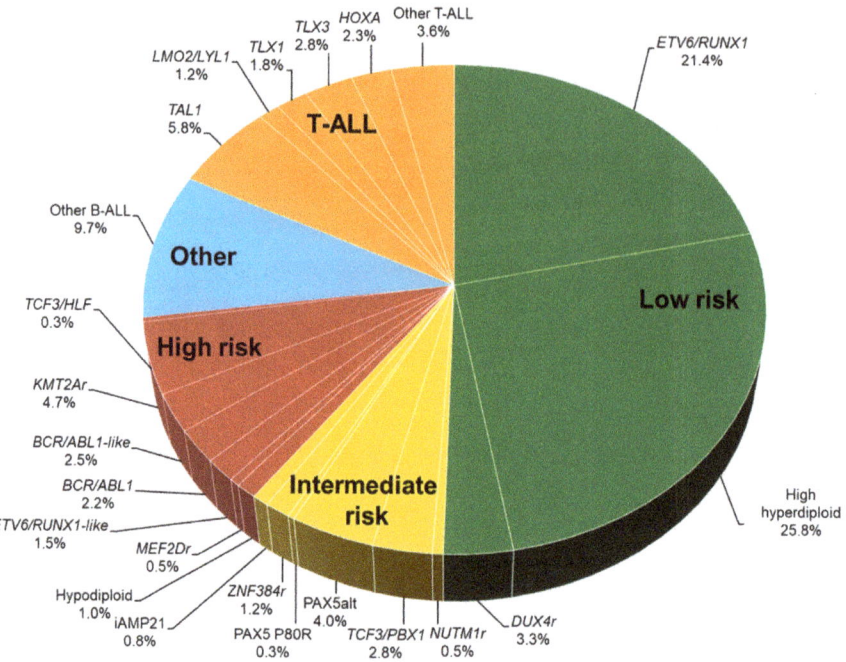

Figure 2. Distribution of genetic subtypes Genetic subgroups are listed based on the patients treated in St. Jude Total Therapy Study XVI and on patients with T-ALL who were treated in Children's Oncology Group studies and evaluated for genetics as part of the Therapeutically Applicable Research to Generate Effective Treatments initiative [11,12]. Percentages are the approximate incidence in pediatric ALL. B-ALL is categorized as low-, intermediate-, or high-risk disease. For T-ALL, no genetic subtypes are clearly associated with outcomes, but the group as a whole is considered an intermediate-risk group. Abbreviations: ALL, acute lymphoblastic leukemia.

3. Low-Risk Genetic Subgroups

3.1. ETV6/RUNX1-Rearranged ALL

ETV6/RUNX1-rearranged ALL represents approximately 20% of pediatric ALL and is associated with excellent outcomes [13]. Up to 5% of normal newborns carry the ETV6/RUNX1 fusion at birth [14], and post-natal environmental or spontaneous oncogenic second hits are required to induce overt leukemia [15,16]. Patients with the ETV6/RUNX1 fusion are good candidates for reductions in the intensity of chemotherapy if their initial MRD responses are good [17,18]. A randomized study of patients with standard-risk ALL enrolled on the Associazione Italiana di Ematologia e Oncologia Pediatrica–Berlin-Frankfurt–Münster (AIEOP–BFM) ALL 2000 protocol tested whether dose reductions by 30% for dexamethasone and by 50% for vincristine, doxorubicin, and cyclophosphamide during the delayed intensification phase resulted in outcomes comparable to those in the historical arm [19]. Although this study led to worse outcomes for the dose-reduction arm as a whole, outcomes in patients with ETV6/RUNX1 fusion and in those aged 1 to 6 years were equivalent for the two arms. Furthermore, in the Tokyo Children's Cancer Study Group L92-13 study, which featured only 1 year of intensive chemotherapy, only two-thirds of the enrolled patients experienced continuous remission, but those with ETV6/RUNX1 and TCF3/PBX1 rearrangements had excellent outcomes with this abbreviated therapy [20]. Notably, patients with high hyperdiploidy fared poorly in this study.

3.2. Hyperdiploid ALL

Hyperdiploid ALL is the most common subtype of ALL, accounting for up to 25% of pediatric ALL. Different study groups have variously identified this subtype as having a DNA index of 1.16 or higher [21], a chromosome number of 51 to 67 [22], or trisomy of chromosomes 4 and 10 (double trisomy) [23]. Non-random gains of chromosome 4, 10, 14, 17, and 21 are common. Methotrexate is particularly useful for treating this subtype of ALL, and the disease response is influenced by the intracellular accumulation of active methotrexate polyglutamate metabolites (MTXPGs), which is higher in hyperdiploid ALL than in *ETV6/RUNX1* ALL, *TCF3/PBX1* ALL, or T-ALL [24–26]. This is partly due to the higher expression of the gene encoding the folate influx transporter *SLC19A1* in hyperdiploid ALL, resulting in the presence of a somatically acquired additional chromosome 21 on which this gene is located. Therefore, among patients with induction failure, those with hyperdiploid ALL had better outcomes than did those in other subgroups because they responded well to high-dose methotrexate, which is typically given as post-induction therapy, and these patients can be salvaged even without a hematopoietic cell transplant (HCT) [27].

Patients with *ETV6/RUNX1* fusion and hyperdiploidy and negative MRD on day 15 (as in St. Jude Total Therapy XVI) or day 19 (as in Total Therapy XV) and at the end of induction therapy have an excellent prognosis [11,17,18]. In St. Jude Total Therapy studies, patients with *ETV6/RUNX1* fusion and hyperdiploidy are provisionally treated in the low-risk (National Cancer Institute [NCI] standard-risk) arm regardless of their age or WBC count at diagnosis, but those patients with high MRD levels on day 15 ($\geq 1\%$) or at the end of induction therapy ($\geq 0.01\%$) or with extramedullary (central nervous system or testis) involvement are subsequently treated in the standard-risk (NCI high-risk) arm. This approach has been successful, with excellent outcomes for both subgroups [11,13,17].

3.3. DUX4-Rearranged ALL

DUX4-rearranged ALL is a newly identified subtype seen in 3% to 5% of pediatric ALL cases. The rearrangement occurs most commonly in the immunoglobulin heavy-chain locus (*IGH*) and results in the expression of DUX4 protein with a truncated C-terminus [28–30]. This truncated form binds an intragenic region of the ETS-family transcription factor *ERG* (ETS-related gene) and commonly results in the expression of a C-terminal ERG protein fragment that is a dominant-negative inhibitor of wild-type ERG function. *DUX4*-rearranged B-ALL has a unique immunophenotype (CD2 and CD371 positive), and a favorable outcome can be obtained, even with the deletion of *IKZF1*, by adjusting the intensity of the chemotherapy based on the MRD [31,32].

4. High-Risk Genetic Subgroups in B-ALL

4.1. Hypodiploid ALL

Hypodiploid ALL, which is defined by there being fewer than 44 chromosomes or a DNA index of less than 0.81, accounts for 1% to 2% of pediatric ALL. It is associated with poor outcomes, with reported EFS of 50% to 55% [33,34]. It can be classified into three distinct subtypes: near haploid (24 to 31 chromosomes), low hypodiploid (32 to 39 chromosomes), and high hypodiploid (40 to 43 chromosomes). Near-haploid ALL is associated with Ras pathway mutations (particularly in *NF1*) and *IKZF3* deletion [35]. Low-hypodiploid ALL is characterized by *TP53* mutations in the leukemia cells in more than 90% of cases and also in the germline in approximately 50% of patients, in addition to the somatic alterations in *IKZF2* and *RB1*. Therefore, patients with low-hypodiploid ALL should undergo germline testing for *TP53* germline pathogenic variants (i.e., Li–Fraumeni syndrome) to enable treatment modification to avoid the use of carcinogenic agents and for genetic consultation purposes [36]. It is important to distinguish "masked" hypodiploid ALL, in which the hypodiploid clone is duplicated, from true hyperdiploid ALL, considering the possible germline *TP53* mutations and the poor prognosis of hypodiploid ALL [37]. Recently, two multicenter studies demonstrated that HCT confers no benefit in hypodiploid

ALL, particularly for patients who are MRD negative after remission-induction therapy, for whom EFS was approximately 70% [33,34]. Therefore, patients with persistently positive MRD can be considered for treatment with molecular targeted agents such as BCL-2 inhibitors and PI3K inhibitors or with immunotherapy such as bispecific antibody therapy or chimeric antigen receptor (CAR) T-cell therapy [35,38,39].

4.2. BCR/ABL1 (Philadelphia Chromosome)-Positive ALL

BCR/ABL1-positive ALL accounts for approximately 2% to 3% of pediatric ALL [40]. Before tyrosine kinase inhibitors (TKIs) became available, the survival of patients who were treated only with conventional chemotherapy was dismal, and HCT from a matched related donor or an unrelated donor during the first remission provided a cure in only approximately 50% of children [41]. The combination of the TKI imatinib with multi-agent chemotherapy significantly improved outcomes, with 5-year disease-free survival increasing to 70% in the Children's Oncology Group AALL0031 study [42]. A second-generation TKI, dasatinib, targets both the ABL1 and SRC kinases, has activity against BCR/ABL1 that is approximately 300 times more potent than that of imatinib, and can cross the blood–brain barrier [40]. The Children's Oncology Group AALL0622 study, in which dasatinib was used at 60 mg/m^2/day, showed no improvement in outcomes relative to those in the preceding AALL0031 study, in which imatinib (340 mg/m^2/day) was given with the same chemotherapy backbone [43]. However, the Chinese Children's Cancer Group has shown that patients who received dasatinib (80 mg/m^2/day) had significantly better EFS and OS and a lower relapse rate when compared with those who received imatinib (300 mg/m^2/day) in a randomized study [44]. Ponatinib is one of a newer generation of TKIs and has potent activity in both wild-type BCR/ABL1-positive ALL and mutant forms (e.g., with the gatekeeper mutation ABL1 T315I) [40]. Treatment with ponatinib in combination with hyperfractionated cyclophosphamide, vincristine, doxorubicin, and dexamethasone (hyper-CVAD), alternating with high-dose methotrexate and cytarabine, resulted in excellent 2-year EFS in adults with newly diagnosed BCR/ABL1-positive ALL [45]. Using ponatinib in combination with a pediatric regimen that includes asparaginase and glucocorticoids can be difficult as ponatinib is also associated with an increased risk of thrombosis and pancreatitis. In adult patients with BCR/ABL1-positive ALL, a chemotherapy-free regimen with glucocorticoid and dasatinib followed by blinatumomab and dasatinib was associated with a high molecular response and high survival rates with few adverse effects [46]. Nevertheless, the results of a recent preclinical study suggest that dasatinib may adversely affect the efficacy of blinatumomab [47]; additional studies are needed to determine whether these two agents should be used separately.

4.3. BCR/ABL1 (Philadelphia Chromosome)-Like ALL

BCR/ABL1 (Philadelphia chromosome)-like ALL was initially identified as a subgroup of leukemias with a leukemic cell gene expression profile similar to that of BCR/ABL1-positive ALL and frequent IKZF1 alterations but without the BCR/ABL1 fusion [48,49]. Although the percentage can vary depending on the ethnicity of the patients, this variant occurs in approximately 3% of pediatric ALL cases and is associated with worse outcomes. It is commonly seen in patients with NCI high-risk disease; however, BCR/ABL1-like ALL is also seen in patients with NCI standard-risk disease, and the outcome is associated with the MRD levels during and at the end of induction [50,51]. Many study groups have identified the genetic lesions associated with BCR/ABL1-like ALL, and these are classified in three main groups: JAK-STAT signaling activating mutations, ABL1-class fusions, and alterations that are less common and that involve other kinases [52,53].

JAK-STAT signaling activating mutations constitute the largest group and are genetically more diverse [52,53]. CRLF2 rearrangements (P2RY8/CRLF2 and IGH/CRLF2) and mutations (CRLF2 F232C) lead to CRLF2 overexpression, which may be detected by flow cytometry, and these mutations are present in approximately half of BCR/ABL1-like ALL cases, being more commonly seen in patients with Native American ancestry. Most of the

JAK1 and *JAK2* mutations are seen in this group. Other JAK-STAT signaling activating mutations are present in approximately 10% of *BCR/ABL1*-like ALL cases and include *JAK2* fusions (translocations or interstitial deletions) that retain the tyrosine kinase domain, *EPOR* truncating rearrangements (e.g., with *IGH*, *IGK*, and *LAIR1*), *IL7R* insertion/deletions in the transmembrane domain, and deletions or mutations of *SH2B3* (a negative regulator of JAK-STAT signaling, the mutation of which augments JAK-STAT signaling). A JAK inhibitor, ruxolitinib, is currently being tested in clinical trials [53].

ABL1-class fusions involve *ABL1*, *ABL2*, *CSF1R*, *PDGFRB*, and, rarely, *PDGFRA* and *LYN* and are seen in 15% to 20% of *BCR/ABL1*-like ALL cases [52,53]. Pediatric patients with *ABL1*-class fusions have poor outcomes when treated with regimens that do not contain a TKI, even when they receive a high-risk chemotherapy regimen and/or HCT [54]. As seen in *JAK2* fusions, these are chimeric in-frame fusions that preserve the tyrosine kinase domain and are, therefore, sensitive to treatment with ABL1 inhibitors such as imatinib and dasatinib [52,55].

Other rare kinase-activating alterations include those in *NTRK3*, *FLT3*, *PTK2B*, and *TYK2*, and preclinical studies have shown the efficacy of treatment of these variants with a TRK inhibitor, an FLT3 inhibitor, an FAK inhibitor, and a TYK2 inhibitor, respectively [52,53].

4.4. KMT2A-Rearranged ALL

The *KMT2A* (*MLL*) gene is located on chromosome 11q23 and can be rearranged with more than 80 different partner genes, which are seen in both lymphoid and myeloid leukemia [56]. *KMT2A*-rearranged ALL is characterized by the CD10-negative pro-B cell phenotype with co-expression of myeloid markers. It accounts for approximately 5% of pediatric ALL and 75% of infant ALL. In infant ALL, *KMT2A* rearrangement is acquired in utero and is associated with dismal outcomes, especially in infants younger than 6 months at diagnosis with a presenting WBC count of $\geq 300 \times 10^9$/L or with a poor prednisone response [56]. Although two international randomized studies were performed to examine standard vs. more intensive therapy before maintenance therapy (the Interfant-99 study) and myeloid- vs. lymphoid-type consolidation therapy (the Interfant-06 study), there were no significant differences in outcomes between interventions or studies [57,58]. *KMT2A* rearrangement results in the assembly of a unique multi-protein complex with DOT1L, BRD4, and menin [59]. Therefore, there is great potential for molecular targeted therapy with inhibitors of DOT1L, bromodomain, menin, and BCL-2. Immunotherapy with blinatumomab and autologous or allogeneic CAR T cells can be considered, although there is a possibility of a lineage switch to acute myeloid leukemia (AML) [56].

4.5. MEF2D-Rearranged ALL

MEF2D-rearranged ALL is seen in approximately 1% of pediatric ALL cases. The *MEF2D* gene can rearrange with several partner genes: *BCL9* (the most common partner), *CSF1R*, *DAZAP1*, *HNRNPUL1*, *SS18*, and *FOXJ2* [9,10]. *MEF2D*-rearranged ALL is characterized by older age at diagnosis (median, 14 years), mature B-cell leukemia morphology (large, densely basophilic, and heavily vacuolated leukemic blasts), a unique immunophenotype (weak or absent expression of CD10, high expression of CD38, and cytoplasmic immunoglobulin μ-chain), and poor outcome due to early relapse [60–62]. Exogenous expression of *MEF2D/BCL9* in a B-ALL cell line promoted cell growth, increased the expression of HDAC9 (a known *MEF2D* target), and induced resistance to dexamethasone [60]. Patient-derived leukemia cells were sensitive to histone deacetylase inhibitors (vorinostat and panobinostat) and to a proteasome inhibitor (bortezomib) in vitro and in xenograft models. *MEF2D/CSF1R* can be targeted by ABL1 inhibitors.

4.6. TCF3/HLF-Rearranged ALL

TCF3/HLF-rearranged ALL is a rare (representing <0.5% of cases) but very aggressive subtype of ALL. It is mostly resistant to conventional chemotherapy and has extremely poor outcomes even with intensified chemotherapy and HCT [63]. *TCF3/HLF*-rearranged

ALL is characterized by enrichment of stem cell and myeloid gene signatures, *PAX5* and *VPREB1* deletions, and Ras pathway gene mutations. *TCF3/HLF*-rearrangement plays a role as a pioneer transcription factor in recruiting EP300 to drive MYC, and EP300 inhibition reduces *TCF3/HLF*-dependent gene expression and ALL growth [64]. Drug activity profiling and preclinical studies have shown striking activity of a BCL-2 inhibitor, venetoclax [63]. Furthermore, all of nine patients with *TCF3/HLF*-rearranged ALL experienced molecular remission after being treated with blinatumomab, and four of them are in long-term remission after HCT, suggesting that an immunotherapy approach can overcome the chemotherapy resistance [65].

5. Intermediate-Risk Genetic Subtypes in B-ALL

5.1. TCF3/PBX1-Rearranged ALL

TCF3/PBX1-rearranged ALL is generated with the t(1;19)(q23;p13) translocation and is present in approximately 2% to 5% of pediatric ALL cases, commonly expressing cytoplasmic μ chain (a pre-B phenotype) [66]. As with *ETV6/RUNX1*-rearranged ALL, the preleukemic *TCF/PBX1* gene fusion is present in approximately 0.6% of healthy newborns [67]. The incidence of this leukemia variant is higher in African Americans [68], and a genome-wide association study identified a germline risk locus in an intergenic region between *BCL11A* and *PAPOLG*: rs2665658 [69]. In the St. Jude Total XV study, which eliminated cranial irradiation, *TCF/PBX1*-rearranged ALL was associated with a higher incidence of CNS relapse but a lower incidence of hematologic relapse compared to other forms of B-ALL [7,66]. In patients treated in the Total XVI study, the incidence of CNS relapse was reduced as a result of the increased frequency of early intrathecal treatments [8]. In the TCCSG L92-13 study, *TCF3/PBX1*-rearranged ALL had excellent outcomes with 1 year of intensive chemotherapy from diagnosis [20].

5.2. Intrachromosomal Amplification of Chromosome 21 (iAMP21)

Intrachromosomal amplification of chromosome 21 (iAMP21) ALL is characterized by the presence of additional copies of a region of chromosome 21 that includes *RUNX1* (five or more copies per cell), and it can be associated with the germline Robertsonian translocation rob(15;21) [70,71]. iAMP21 ALL is seen in approximately 1% to 2% of pediatric ALL cases and is associated with older age (median, 9 years) and low WBC counts. Secondary cytogenetic and genetic changes include the gain of chromosome X, the loss or deletion of chromosome 7, *ETV6* and *RB1* deletions, and *SH2B2* inactivation through copy number-neutral loss of heterozygosity of chromosome 12q [72,73]. Patients with iAMP21 had dismal outcomes when treated with a low-intensity NCI standard-risk regimen [74,75]. Although intensified treatment has significantly improved the outcomes for these patients, their EFS remains inadequate at approximately 70%. Therefore, they can also be considered candidates for recently introduced novel therapies.

5.3. PAX5-Driven Subtypes: PAX5alt and PAX5 p.Pro80Arg

PAX5 is the B-lymphoid transcription factor that is essential for early stages of B-cell development [76,77]. Germline alterations of the *PAX5* gene predispose patients to ALL, and somatic alterations of *PAX5* are commonly seen in pediatric ALL (e.g., *PAX5* focal deletions are present in approximately 30% of *ETV6/RUNX1*-rearranged ALL) [77]. The two distinct disease-initiating alterations of *PAX5* that result in PAX5alt and PAX5 p.Pro80Arg ALL account for approximately 3% to 5% and less than 1% of childhood ALL, respectively [9,10]. PAX5alt B-ALL is characterized by diverse *PAX5* alterations, including rearrangements (most commonly with *ETV6* or *NOL4L*), sequence mutations, and intragenic amplification. PAX5 p.Pro80Arg is characterized by universal p.Pro80Arg mutation with deletion or mutation of the remaining allele and alterations in Ras and JAK-STAT pathway genes. Patients with PAX5alt or PAX5 p.Pro80Arg B-ALL have an intermediate prognosis [9,10].

5.4. ZNF384-Rearranged ALL

ZNF384-rearrangement is seen in approximately 1% to 2% of childhood ALL cases and in half of B/myeloid mixed-phenotype acute leukemia (MPAL) cases in children. This rearrangement has more than 10 partner genes, such as *EP300*, *TCF3*, *TAF15*, and *CREBBP* [62,78,79]. In B-ALL, the age of onset and the prognosis differ according to the fusion partner: with the *EP300/ZNF384* fusion, the median age of onset is 11 years and outcomes are excellent, whereas with the *TCF3/ZNF384* fusion, the median age of onset is 5 years and there are occasional late relapses [78,80]. The immunophenotype of *ZNF384*-rearranged B-ALL is characterized by negative or weak expression of CD10 and aberrant expression of CD13 and/or CD33 [78,80]. As with *ETV6/RUNX1*-rearranged and *TCF3/PBX1*-rearranged B-ALL, a study in monozygotic twins showed that *TCF3/ZNF384* fusion can occur in utero, suggesting that a fetal hematopoietic progenitor is the cell of origin in this ALL subgroup [81]. Importantly, the secondary genomic alterations and gene expression profiles for *ZNF384*-rearranged B-ALL and B/myeloid MPAL cases are essentially indistinguishable, which suggests that ALL-directed therapy should be initiated for patients with newly diagnosed B/myeloid MPAL [79]. Due to its inherent lineage plasticity, *ZNF384*-rearranged leukemia may develop a lineage switch at relapse (from ALL to AML or vice versa) under the selective pressure of conventional chemotherapy or immunotherapy.

6. Other Newly Identified B-ALL Subtypes

6.1. ETV6/RUNX1-Like ALL

ETV6/RUNX1-like ALL is seen in 1% to 3% of pediatric ALL cases and is particularly common in younger children [9,10,30]. It has a similar gene expression profile and immunophenotype to *ETV6/RUNX1*-rearranged ALL but lacks the *ETV6/RUNX1* fusion. Within this group, alterations in *ETV6*, *IKZF1*, and *TCF3* have been reported. As the number of patients identified to date is small and several relapses have been reported, it is important to evaluate the actual outcomes of patients in this group, which appear to be worse than those of patients with *ETV6/RUNX1*-rearranged ALL.

6.2. NUTM1-Rearranged ALL

NUTM1-rearranged ALL is seen in 5% to 7% of all infants with ALL and represents 21.7% of non-*KMT2A*-rearranged infant ALL, but it is very rare in children (accounting for less than 1% in that population) [9,10,82,83]. Partner genes include *ACIN1*, *CUX1*, *BRD9*, and *ZNF618*. In an international study, the 4-year OS in 45 infants and 36 children was 100%, which is indicative of a favorable genetic subtype, although further studies are required to confirm this finding and to determine whether a reduction in treatment intensity is possible [82].

7. T-Acute Lymphoblastic Leukemia

T-ALL represents approximately 12% to 15% of pediatric ALL and is characterized by having an incidence in boys that is two to three times that in girls; a higher proportion of patients with African ancestry, in whom the rate is twice that in patients of European ancestry; high initial WBC counts; and higher frequencies of mediastinal mass and CNS involvement [12,84]. The higher incidence in boys can be partly explained by inactivating mutations or deletions of the tumor suppressor gene *PHF6* on chromosome X, which are seen in 16% of pediatric T-ALL cases [85]. The genetic alterations in T-ALL are diverse, and no clear associations with outcomes have yet been identified. Hence, unlike B-ALL, T-ALL lacks a consensus genetic classification with prognostic implications. In most cases of T-ALL, there is aberrant expression of transcription factors and oncogenes, including *TAL1*, *TAL2*, *LYL1*, *LMO1*, *LMO2*, *TLX1* (*HOX11*), *TLX3* (*HOX11L2*), and *HOXA* [86]. *NOTCH1* activating mutations and alterations in *CDKN2A/CDKN2B* are seen in more than 70% of cases, and *MLLT10* and *KMT2A* rearrangements are each seen in 5% of cases. Approximately 25% of patients have JAK-STAT activating mutations, and *ABL1* fusions with *BCR* and *NUP214* are occasionally detected [86]. These patients are candidates for treatment with JAK inhibitors and ABL1 inhibitors, respectively.

In most studies, the survival of patients with T-ALL is 5% to 10% worse than that of patients with B-ALL [12]. With regard to conventional chemotherapy, the treatment component of the BFM IB phase that includes cyclophosphamide, cytarabine, and mercaptopurine is of greater importance for T-ALL than for B-ALL [87]. In one study, patients with T-ALL who received nelarabine had significantly fewer incidences of CNS relapse (isolated and combined) when compared to patients who did not receive nelarabine [88]. However, approximately 90% of the total patients and all of the nelarabine-treated patients received cranial irradiation in this randomized study; therefore, the efficacy of nelarabine should be confirmed in patients whose disease is managed with intrathecal therapy only. The results of the recent randomized study of bortezomib are described below [89].

Early T-Cell Precursor ALL

Early T-cell precursor (ETP) ALL accounts for 10% to 15% of T-ALL, having a specific immunophenotype of early T-cell development (cytoplasmic CD3+, CD5weak, CD8−, CD1a−) with aberrant expression of myeloid and/or early progenitor cell markers [90]. The genetic features of this subtype are similar to those of hematopoietic stem cells; it is characterized by alterations in transcriptional regulators, epigenetic regulation, and JAK-STAT and Ras pathway genes [86,91]. Furthermore, ETP ALL shares genomic features with T/myeloid MPAL, with frequent biallelic *WT1* alterations and signaling pathway mutations (e.g., in the JAK-STAT and *FLT3* pathways) [79]. ETP-ALL is usually glucocorticoid resistant, has a higher incidence of induction failure, especially after the BFM IA phase [92,93], and is historically associated with worse outcomes [90,94]. However, ETP-ALL responds to a regimen that includes cyclophosphamide, cytarabine, and mercaptopurine (e.g., the BFM IB phase), and its outcomes are approaching those of non-ETP T-ALL [92,93,95]. The results of a preliminary study suggested that patients with ETP-ALL would benefit from treatment with venetoclax, a BCL-2 inhibitor [96].

8. Minimal Residual Disease

Although genetic subclassification is essential for risk stratification, MRD has equally important prognostic and therapeutic impact [97–99]. MRD has been quantified by multiparametric flow cytometry or by allele-specific oligonucleotide PCR analysis. The flow cytometric assay uses the leukemia-specific aberrant immunophenotype, has a typical sensitivity of 0.01%, and can be applied to almost all cases of ALL [98,99]. It is rapid, enables accurate quantification of ALL cells, and provides an overview of the hematopoietic cell population status. However, it can be difficult to achieve sensitivity better than 0.01%, and the assay may fail to detect an ALL population that has undergone a phenotypic change, especially after immunotherapy targeting CD19 and/or CD22. The PCR assay amplifies leukemia-specific fusion transcripts (available for approximately 40% of ALL cases) or immunoglobulin (Ig) or T-cell receptor (TCR) genes (available for approximately 90% of ALL cases) with a sensitivity of 0.001%, 10 times that of the flow cytometry assay [98,99]. In RT-PCR analysis of fusion transcripts, there is a possibility of RNA degradation or cross-contamination from other samples. For Ig and TCR DNA, tailor-made primers are needed for each patient. Furthermore, ALL can be oligoclonal and may escape detection by clonal evolution during treatment. Recently, next-generation sequencing (NGS) of Ig or TCR genes has been applied for MRD detection (NGS MRD) with sensitivity as low as 0.0001% (equivalent to detecting one ALL cell among 1 million total cells) [100,101]. The use of universal primers enables the detection of clonal evolution and can also detect the background repertoire of normal B and T cells. With this technology, negative NGS MRD at the end of induction has been associated with 100% OS among NCI standard-risk patients [102]. In pediatric patients with ALL who received HCT, negative pre-HCT MRD and post-HCT MRD were associated with significantly fewer relapses and better survival [103]. The NGS MRD assay might not be affected by phenotypic changes after immunotherapy, and negative NGS MRD after CAR T-cell therapy was also associated with better outcomes as compared with those in patients with positive NGS MRD among the patients with negative flow MRD [104]. These clinical benefits will result in expanded use of NGS MRD in contemporary protocols.

When considering risk stratification, clinicians should consider MRD levels in combination with genetic classification and clinical factors (e.g., age, WBC counts at diagnosis, and lineage) [17,18,97,105]. Patients with favorable genetic features clear MRD faster than do those with unfavorable genetics or T-ALL. Furthermore, as seen in *ETV6/RUNX1*-rearranged and hyperdiploid ALL, some patients with favorable genetics but slow MRD clearance can be cured by intensifying their post-remission chemotherapy [11,17,27]. Conversely, patients with high-risk genetics have inferior outcomes even when they have undetectable MRD at the end of induction therapy [11,17,18]. It is also important to evaluate whether more sensitive NGS MRD can identify patients with better outcomes among those patients with high-risk genetic features. Furthermore, patients with T-ALL who had negative MRD ($<10^3$) on day 78 had a cumulative risk of relapse similar to that of patients who had negative MRD on day 33 [87]. In such patients, the MRD level on day 33 was not relevant, suggesting that the MRD response to the BFM IB phase (two courses of cyclophosphamide, cytarabine, and mercaptopurine) is critical in T-ALL.

9. Emerging Therapy: Molecular Targeted Therapy

9.1. Tyrosine Kinase Inhibitors

Tyrosine kinase inhibitors have been employed in combination with standard chemotherapy to improve its efficacy (Table 1). As described earlier, ABL1 inhibitors (e.g., imatinib, dasatinib, nilotinib, and ponatinib) are used to treat patients with *BCR/ABL*-positive ALL and *ABL1*-class fusions that occasionally occur in *BCR/ABL*-like ALL and T-ALL [40,53,55]. Ruxolitinib is being tested in clinical trials for patients with JAK-STAT activating mutations as seen in *BCR/ABL*-like ALL and T-ALL (including ETP-ALL) [53]. Currently, however, this targeted approach is limited to less than 10% of pediatric ALL cases. Further identification of ALL driving mutations and their targets will expand the use of TKIs. In this regard, ex vivo leukemia drug-sensitivity profiling identified that 44.4% of childhood T-ALL samples and 16.7% of adult T-ALL samples as being sensitive to dasatinib through the inhibition of preTCR-LCK signaling [106].

9.2. BCL-2 and BCL-X_L Inhibitors

Members of the B-cell lymphoma 2 (BCL-2) protein family play critical roles in the intrinsic mitochondrial apoptosis pathway through interactions between pro- and anti-apoptotic proteins (Table 1) [107]. Venetoclax is a selective inhibitor of BCL-2 and displaces the pro-apoptotic proteins BIM and BAX, which leads to mitochondrial outer membrane permeabilization, cytochrome c release, and the activation of intracellular caspases, resulting in apoptosis. Preclinical studies have shown that venetoclax is active for leukemias in the high-risk genetic group, such as *KMT2A*-rearranged ALL [108], hypodiploid ALL [38], *BCR/ABL*-positive ALL [109], *TCF3/HLF*-rearranged ALL [63], and T-ALL (including ETP-ALL) [110,111]. Low expression of *CELSR2* is associated with the overexpression of *BCL2* and glucocorticoid resistance in ALL cells [112]. Venetoclax mitigated glucocorticoid resistance and had synergistic effects with prednisolone and dexamethasone.

Phase I studies of venetoclax in combination with chemotherapy in pediatric and young adult patients with ALL have shown the regimen to be well tolerated with preliminary efficacies [113]. As the results of a preclinical study suggested that ALL cells were dependent on both BCL-2 and BCL-X_L, navitoclax (a BCL-2 and BCL-X_L inhibitor) was tested in combination with venetoclax and chemotherapy for pediatric and adult patients with relapsed/refractory ALL or lymphoblastic lymphoma [114]. Among 47 heavily pre-treated patients, the complete remission rate was 60%, showing the regimen to have promising efficacy.

9.3. Proteasome Inhibitors

Proteasome inhibitors have shown efficacy in ALL and work synergistically with chemotherapy agents such as corticosteroids and doxorubicin (Table 1) [115]. In 22 children with relapsed ALL treated with bortezomib in combination with vincristine, dexamethasone, pegaspargase, and doxorubicin, the overall response rate was 73% [116]. In a randomized study of patients with newly diagnosed T-ALL or T-lymphoblastic lymphoma (T-LLy), adding bortezomib to the induction and delayed intensification phases was associated with better outcomes, as compared to those in patients who did not receive bortezomib, in patients with standard-risk and intermediate-risk T-ALL, as well as in those with T-LLy [89]. However, addition of bortezomib was associated with worse outcomes in patients with high-risk T-ALL. Newer proteasome inhibitors (carfilzomib and ixazomib) are under investigation.

9.4. Other Molecular Targeted Therapies

Dysregulation of the PI3K/AKT/mTOR pathway is frequently observed in ALL and is associated with resistance to chemotherapy [117,118]. mTOR inhibitors have been shown to inhibit ALL growth and reverse glucocorticoid resistance and to work synergistically with other chemotherapeutic agents, such as dexamethasone, vincristine, and doxorubicin (Table 1) [119–121]. A phase I study of everolimus with vincristine, prednisone, pegaspargase, and doxorubicin in children and adolescents with ALL in first marrow relapse occurring more than 18 months after first complete remission showed that the regimen was tolerable [122]. Nineteen (86%) of 22 enrolled patients had a second complete remission, and 13 (68%) of them had negative MRD.

Epigenetic modification, the biochemical alteration of chromatin, has been implicated in the pathogenesis of cancer [123]. Instead of changes in the nucleotide sequence, epigenetic modifications involve DNA methylation and histone modification, which affect the activity of genes and their cellular expression. These modifications can silence tumor suppressor genes or activate oncogenes. They are prevalent in ALL and are associated with chemotherapy resistance and relapse [124]. Epigenetic modifications may be reversible with targeted agents such as DNA methyltransferase inhibitors and histone deacetylase inhibitors (Table 1). In a phase 1 study of decitabine and vorinostat in combination with vincristine, dexamethasone, mitoxantrone, and pegaspargase, 22 children and adolescents with relapsed or refractory ALL were treated [125]. Although this regimen was associated with a high incidence of infectious complications, nine patients (39%) had a complete response, and potent pharmacodynamic modulations of biological pathways associated with antileukemic effects were observed.

10. Emerging Therapy: Immunotherapy

Three major categories of immunotherapy are currently in use for pediatric ALL (Figure 3 and Table 1): bispecific antibodies (e.g., blinatumomab), CAR T cells, and antibody–drug conjugates (e.g., inotuzumab) [126]. Immunotherapy has been used mostly for B-ALL because the surface markers CD19, CD20, and CD22 are expressed only on B cells and not on hematopoietic stem cells or other tissues. Such therapy can eradicate not only B-ALL but also normal B cells, thereby causing hypogammaglobulinemia, which can be managed by intravenous or subcutaneous immunoglobulin administration. For T-ALL, antibody therapy (e.g., with daratumumab against CD38) and CAR T cells (e.g., anti-CD1a, CD5, and CD7) are under investigation (Figure 3).

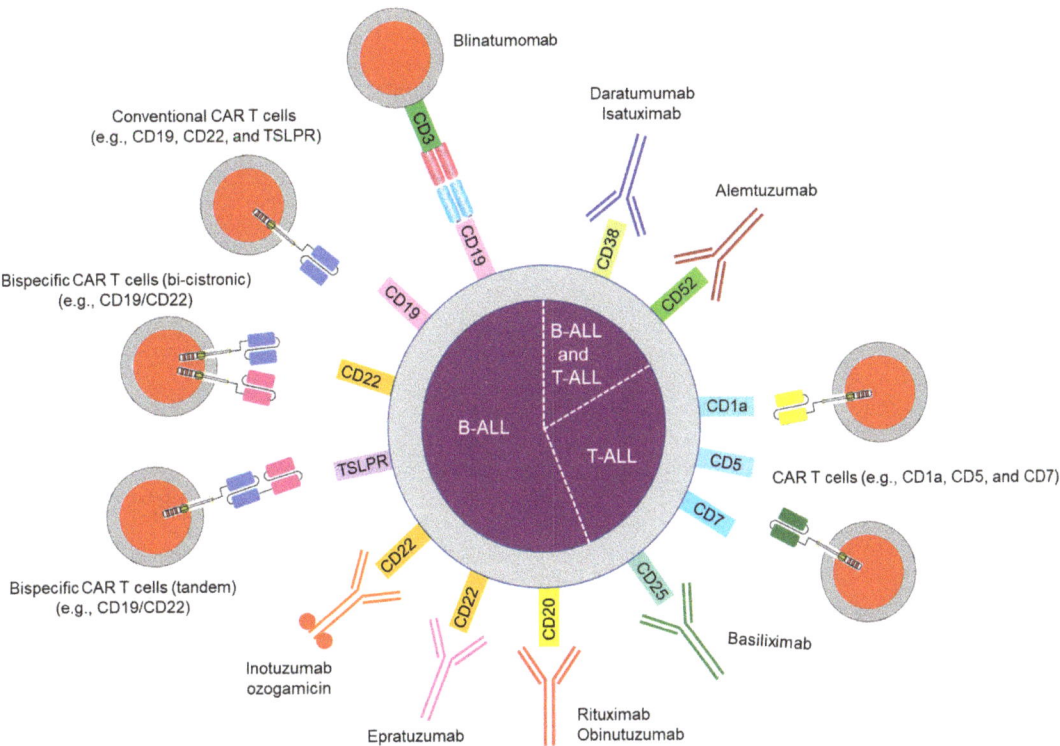

Figure 3. Immunotherapy in acute lymphoblastic leukemia. Abbreviations: ALL, acute lymphoblastic leukemia; CAR, chimeric antigen receptor; TSLPR, thymic stromal lymphopoietin receptor.

10.1. Bispecific Antibody Therapy

Blinatumomab has bispecific single-chain Fv fragments that link CD3+ T cells to CD19+ leukemia cells and cause a cytotoxic immune response (Figure 3 and Table 1) [127,128]. It is approved for use in pediatric and adult relapsed/refractory and MRD-positive B-ALL by the US Food and Drug Administration. The main adverse effects are cytokine release syndrome and neurotoxicity, which coincide with T cell activation. Two randomized studies in children, adolescents, and young adults with intermediate-risk or high-risk relapsed/refractory B-ALL showed blinatumomab to have benefits over intensive consolidation chemotherapy [129,130]. The loss of CD19 expression is a major mechanism of resistance to blinatumomab treatment and is also observed with CAR T cell therapy. Acquired genetic mutations in *CD19* exons 2–5 or alternative splicing at exon 2 produce a truncated protein with a nonfunctional or absent transmembrane domain and/or no antibody binding site [131,132]. Sustained CD19-antibody pressure can result in lineage switches as described in *KMT2A*- and *ZNF384*-rearranged B-ALL [133,134]. An alteration in CD81, which is a chaperone protein for the maturation and trafficking of the CD19 molecule from the Golgi apparatus to the cell surface, has been also reported [135].

10.2. Chimeric Antigen Receptor (CAR) T Cells

CAR T cells express single-chain Fv fragments against B-lineage markers (e.g., CD19, CD22, or both) with intracellular signaling domains such as 4-1BB or CD28 with CD3ζ [136]. A phase 2 international study of anti-CD19 CAR T cells (tisagenlecleucel) in pediatric and young adult patients with relapsed/refractory B-ALL showed a complete remission rate of 81% at 3 months and EFS and OS of 73% and 90%, respectively, at 6 months [137]. Currently, tisagenlecleucel is approved for patients up to 25 years of age with B-ALL that is refractory or in a second or later relapse. Several groups consider CAR T cells to be curative therapy, although others view them as a bridging therapy to HCT. As with blinatumomab, cytokine release syndrome and neurotoxicity are commonly seen with CAR T-cell therapy [138]. Preemptive administration of tocilizumab (an anti-IL-6 receptor antibody) decrease the incidence of severe cytokine release syndrome without compromising the efficacy of CAR T cells [139]. CAR T-cell recipients are also at high risk for infection, and they should be considered for bacterial and fungal prophylaxis until their neutropenia resolves, in addition to immunoglobulin supplement and *Pneumocystis jirovecii* pneumonia prophylaxis [140].

Mechanisms of resistance to CAR T-cell therapy include the loss of CAR T-cell persistence and B-cell aplasia and antigen loss on ALL cells [141,142]. In the former scenario, the type of co-stimulatory molecule (e.g., 4-1BB vs. CD28), rejection due to the murine component in tisagenlecleucel, and T-cell exhaustion are considered important factors. The use of two co-stimulatory molecules or new types of co-stimulatory molecule; humanized CAR T cells; in vivo stimulation with a CD19 vaccine, cytokines, or check point inhibitors; or early collection of T cells during treatment for high-risk patients may overcome this issue. With regard to target antigen loss, CAR T cells that can target other antigens (e.g., CD22 or the thymic stromal lymphopoietin receptor) or that can simultaneously target dual antigens (e.g., CD19/CD22) and the administration of two independent CAR T cells that target different antigens are being investigated [143–147].

For extramedullary relapse (e.g., in the CNS and testes), CAR T cells can migrate and show anti-leukemia effects; therefore, they can be considered not only for isolated bone marrow relapses but also for isolated or combined extramedullary relapses, thereby avoiding radiation therapy [148,149].

10.3. Antibody-Drug Conjugates

Inotuzumab ozogamicin is an anti-CD22 antibody that is linked to calicheamicin, a cytotoxic antitumor antibiotic that causes double-strand DNA breaks [150]. Inotuzumab is currently approved for use in adult patients with relapsed/refractory B-ALL. It is associated with sinusoidal obstruction syndrome, especially after HCT [150]. Fractionated weekly dosing of inotuzumab at the dose lower than a single dose given every 3–4 weeks and a longer interval between inotuzumab administration and HCT (i.e., 2 months or more) can reduce the incidence of this syndrome [151]. Additionally, it is recommended to use prophylactic pharmacologic agents (e.g., ursodiol), to limit the inotuzumab use to two cycles if HCT is planned, and to avoid HCT conditioning regimens that contain dual alkylating agents (e.g., thiotepa and melphalan) and concomitant hepatotoxic drugs (e.g., azoles) [152]. In a pediatric phase I study that used fractionated weekly dosing for relapsed/refractory B-ALL, complete remission was seen in 80% of the patients and 84% of those with available flow cytometry data had negative MRD [153].

11. Conclusions

The diagnosis of ALL, the treatment of patients, and the evaluation of the treatment response have undergone remarkable improvement. The detailed genetic characterization of ALL cells, functional genomics and proteomics, and drug sensitivity assays with ex vivo and patient-derived xenograft (PDX) models for molecular targeted agents and immunotherapy will lead to new therapeutic strategies. Furthermore, the evaluation of germline genetics can lead to an understanding of leukemogenesis, cancer predisposition, and the differences in drug response and metabolism (pharmacogenomics). Basic, translational, and clinical research on ALL will not end until all patients can be cured without acute complications or late sequelae.

Author Contributions: Conceptualization, H.I. and C.-H.P.; data curation, H.I.; writing—original draft preparation, H.I.; writing—review and editing, H.I. and C.-H.P.; funding acquisition, H.I. and C.-H.P. All authors have read and agreed to the published version of the manuscript.

Funding: Supported in part by Cancer Center Core Grant CA21765 from the National Institutes of Health and by the American Lebanese Syrian Associated Charities (ALSAC). The funding organizations had no role in the design and conduct of the review; the collection, management, analysis, and interpretation of the data; the preparation, review, or approval of the manuscript; or the decision to submit the manuscript for publication. The content is solely the responsibility of the authors and does not necessarily represent the official views of the National Institutes of Health.

Institutional Review Board Statement: Not applicable.

Informed Consent Statement: Not applicable.

Data Availability Statement: Data sharing not applicable.

Acknowledgments: The authors thank Keith A. Laycock for scientific editing of the manuscript.

Conflicts of Interest: The authors have no conflict of interest, including specific financial interests, relationships, or affiliations relevant to the subject of this manuscript.

References

1. Hunger, S.P.; Mullighan, C.G. Acute Lymphoblastic Leukemia in Children. *N. Engl. J. Med.* **2015**, *373*, 1541–1552. [CrossRef] [PubMed]
2. Inaba, H.; Greaves, M.; Mullighan, C.G. Acute lymphoblastic leukaemia. *Lancet* **2013**, *381*, 1943–1955. [CrossRef]
3. Pui, C.H.; Nichols, K.E.; Yang, J.J. Somatic and germline genomics in paediatric acute lymphoblastic leukaemia. *Nat. Rev. Clin. Oncol.* **2019**, *16*, 227–240. [CrossRef]
4. Malard, F.; Mohty, M. Acute lymphoblastic leukaemia. *Lancet* **2020**, *395*, 1146–1162. [CrossRef]
5. National Cancer Institute. Age-Adjusted and Age-Specific SEER Cancer Incidence Rates, 2014–2018. Available online: https://seer.cancer.gov/csr/1975_2018/results_merged/sect_02_childhood_cancer_iccc.pdf (accessed on 18 April 2021).
6. Lim, J.Y.; Bhatia, S.; Robison, L.L.; Yang, J.J. Genomics of racial and ethnic disparities in childhood acute lymphoblastic leukaemia. *Cancer* **2014**, *120*, 955–962. [CrossRef]
7. Pui, C.H.; Campana, D.; Pei, D.; Bowman, W.P.; Sandlund, J.T.; Kaste, S.C.; Ribeiro, R.C.; Rubnitz, J.E.; Raimondi, S.C.; Onciu, M.; et al. Treating childhood acute lymphoblastic leukemia without cranial irradiation. *N. Engl. J. Med.* **2009**, *360*, 2730–2741. [CrossRef]
8. Jeha, S.; Pei, D.; Choi, J.; Cheng, C.; Sandlund, J.T.; Coustan-Smith, E.; Campana, D.; Inaba, H.; Rubnitz, J.E.; Ribeiro, R.C.; et al. Improved CNS control of childhood acute lymphoblastic leukemia without cranial irradiation: St Jude Total Therapy Study 16. *J. Clin. Oncol.* **2019**, *37*, 3377–3391. [CrossRef]
9. Gu, Z.; Churchman, M.L.; Roberts, K.G.; Moore, I.; Zhou, X.; Nakitandwe, J.; Hagiwara, K.; Pelletier, S.; Gingras, S.; Berns, H.; et al. *PAX5*-driven subtypes of B-progenitor acute lymphoblastic leukemia. *Nat. Genet.* **2019**, *51*, 296–307. [CrossRef]
10. Li, J.F.; Dai, Y.T.; Lilljebjörn, H.; Shen, S.H.; Cui, B.W.; Bai, L.; Liu, Y.F.; Qian, M.X.; Kubota, Y.; Kiyoi, H.; et al. Transcriptional landscape of B cell precursor acute lymphoblastic leukemia based on an international study of 1223 cases. *Proc. Natl. Acad. Sci. USA* **2018**, *115*, E11711–E11720. [CrossRef]
11. Jeha, S.; Choi, J.; Roberts, K.G.; Pei, D.; Coustan-Smith, E.; Inaba, H.; Rubnitz, J.E.; Ribeiro, R.C.; Gruber, T.A.; Raimondi, S.C.; et al. Clinical significance of novel subtypes of acute lymphoblastic leukemia in the context of minimal residual disease-directed therapy. *Blood Cancer Discov.* **2021**, in press. [CrossRef]
12. Teachey, D.T.; Pui, C.H. Comparative features and outcomes between paediatric T-cell and B-cell acute lymphoblastic leukaemia. *Lancet Oncol.* **2019**, *20*, e142–e154. [CrossRef]
13. Bhojwani, D.; Pei, D.; Sandlund, J.T.; Jeha, S.; Ribeiro, R.C.; Rubnitz, J.E.; Raimondi, S.C.; Shurtleff, S.; Onciu, M.; Cheng, C.; et al. *ETV6-RUNX1*-positive childhood acute lymphoblastic leukemia: Improved outcome with contemporary therapy. *Leukemia* **2012**, *26*, 265–270. [CrossRef] [PubMed]
14. Schäfer, D.; Olsen, M.; Lähnemann, D.; Stanulla, M.; Slany, R.; Schmiegelow, K.; Borkhardt, A.; Fischer, U. Five percent of healthy newborns have an *ETV6-RUNX1* fusion as revealed by DNA-based GIPFEL screening. *Blood* **2018**, *131*, 821–826. [CrossRef] [PubMed]
15. Alpar, D.; Wren, D.; Ermini, L.; Mansur, M.B.; van Delft, F.W.; Bateman, C.M.; Titley, I.; Kearney, L.; Szczepanski, T.; Gonzalez, D.; et al. Clonal origins of *ETV6-RUNX1*+ acute lymphoblastic leukemia: Studies in monozygotic twins. *Leukemia* **2015**, *29*, 839–846. [CrossRef] [PubMed]
16. Rodríguez-Hernández, G.; Hauer, J.; Martín-Lorenzo, A.; Schäfer, D.; Bartenhagen, C.; García-Ramírez, I.; Auer, F.; González-Herrero, I.; Ruiz-Roca, L.; Gombert, M.; et al. Infection exposure promotes *ETV6-RUNX1* precursor B-cell leukemia via impaired H3K4 demethylases. *Cancer Res.* **2017**, *77*, 4365–4377. [CrossRef]
17. Pui, C.H.; Pei, D.; Raimondi, S.C.; Coustan-Smith, E.; Jeha, S.; Cheng, C.; Bowman, W.P.; Sandlund, J.T.; Ribeiro, R.C.; Rubnitz, J.E.; et al. Clinical impact of minimal residual disease in children with different subtypes of acute lymphoblastic leukemia treated with Response-Adapted therapy. *Leukemia* **2017**, *31*, 333–339. [CrossRef]

18. O'Connor, D.; Enshaei, A.; Bartram, J.; Hancock, J.; Harrison, C.J.; Hough, R.; Samarasinghe, S.; Schwab, C.; Vora, A.; Wade, R.; et al. Genotype-specific minimal residual disease interpretation improves stratification in pediatric acute lymphoblastic leukemia. *J. Clin. Oncol.* **2018**, *36*, 34–43. [CrossRef] [PubMed]
19. Schrappe, M.; Bleckmann, K.; Zimmermann, M.; Biondi, A.; Möricke, A.; Locatelli, F.; Cario, G.; Rizzari, C.; Attarbaschi, A.; Valsecchi, M.G.; et al. Reduced-intensity delayed intensification in standard-risk pediatric acute lymphoblastic leukemia defined by undetectable minimal residual disease: Results of an international randomized trial (AIEOP-BFM ALL 2000). *J. Clin. Oncol.* **2018**, *36*, 244–253. [CrossRef]
20. Kato, M.; Ishimaru, S.; Seki, M.; Yoshida, K.; Shiraishi, Y.; Chiba, K.; Kakiuchi, N.; Sato, Y.; Ueno, H.; Tanaka, H.; et al. Long-term outcome of 6-month maintenance chemotherapy for acute lymphoblastic leukemia in children. *Leukemia* **2017**, *31*, 580–584. [CrossRef]
21. Look, A.T.; Roberson, P.K.; Williams, D.L.; Rivera, G.; Bowman, W.P.; Pui, C.H.; Ochs, J.; Abromowitch, M.; Kalwinsky, D.; Dahl, G.V.; et al. Prognostic importance of blast cell DNA content in childhood acute lymphoblastic leukemia. *Blood* **1985**, *65*, 1079–1086. [CrossRef] [PubMed]
22. Williams, D.L.; Tsiatis, A.; Brodeur, G.M.; Look, A.T.; Melvin, S.L.; Bowman, W.P.; Kalwinsky, D.K.; Rivera, G.; Dahl, G.V. Prognostic importance of chromosome number in 136 untreated children with acute lymphoblastic leukemia. *Blood* **1982**, *60*, 864–871. [CrossRef] [PubMed]
23. Harris, M.B.; Shuster, J.J.; Carroll, A.; Look, A.T.; Borowitz, M.J.; Crist, W.M.; Nitschke, R.; Pullen, J.; Steuber, C.P.; Land, V.J. Trisomy of leukemic cell chromosomes 4 and 10 identifies children with B-progenitor cell acute lymphoblastic leukemia with a very low risk of treatment failure: A Pediatric Oncology Group study. *Blood* **1992**, *79*, 3316–3324. [CrossRef]
24. Whitehead, V.M.; Vuchich, M.J.; Lauer, S.J.; Mahoney, D.; Carroll, A.J.; Shuster, J.J.; Esseltine, D.W.; Payment, C.; Look, A.T.; Akabutu, J.; et al. Accumulation of high levels of methotrexate polyglutamates in lymphoblasts from children with hyperdiploid (greater than 50 chromosomes) B-lineage acute lymphoblastic leukemia: A Pediatric Oncology Group study. *Blood* **1992**, *80*, 1316–1323. [CrossRef] [PubMed]
25. Kager, L.; Cheok, M.; Yang, W.; Zaza, G.; Cheng, Q.; Panetta, J.C.; Pui, C.H.; Downing, J.R.; Relling, M.V.; Evans, W.E. Folate pathway gene expression differs in subtypes of acute lymphoblastic leukemia and influences methotrexate pharmacodynamics. *J. Clin. Investig.* **2005**, *115*, 110–117. [CrossRef] [PubMed]
26. Lopez-Lopez, E.; Autry, R.J.; Smith, C.; Yang, W.; Paugh, S.W.; Panetta, J.C.; Crews, K.R.; Bonten, E.J.; Smart, B.; Pei, D.; et al. Pharmacogenomics of intracellular methotrexate polyglutamates in patients' leukemia cells in vivo. *J. Clin. Investig.* **2020**, *130*, 6600–6615. [CrossRef] [PubMed]
27. Schrappe, M.; Hunger, S.P.; Pui, C.H.; Saha, V.; Gaynon, P.S.; Baruchel, A.; Conter, V.; Otten, J.; Ohara, A.; Versluys, A.B.; et al. Outcomes after induction failure in childhood acute lymphoblastic leukemia. *N. Engl. J. Med.* **2012**, *366*, 1371–1381. [CrossRef] [PubMed]
28. Yasuda, T.; Tsuzuki, S.; Kawazu, M.; Hayakawa, F.; Kojima, S.; Ueno, T.; Imoto, N.; Kohsaka, S.; Kunita, A.; Doi, K.; et al. Recurrent *DUX4* fusions in B cell acute lymphoblastic leukemia of adolescents and young adults. *Nat. Genet.* **2016**, *48*, 569–574. [CrossRef]
29. Zhang, J.; McCastlain, K.; Yoshihara, H.; Xu, B.; Chang, Y.; Churchman, M.L.; Wu, G.; Li, Y.; Wei, L.; Iacobucci, I.; et al. Deregulation of *DUX4* and *ERG* in acute lymphoblastic leukemia. *Nat. Genet.* **2016**, *48*, 1481–1489. [CrossRef]
30. Lilljebjörn, H.; Henningsson, R.; Hyrenius-Wittsten, A.; Olsson, L.; Orsmark-Pietras, C.; von Palffy, S.; Askmyr, M.; Rissler, M.; Schrappe, M.; Cario, G.; et al. Identification of *ETV6-RUNX1*-like and *DUX4*-rearranged subtypes in paediatric B-cell precursor acute lymphoblastic leukaemia. *Nat. Commun.* **2016**, *7*, 11790. [CrossRef]
31. Schinnerl, D.; Mejstrikova, E.; Schumich, A.; Zaliova, M.; Fortschegger, K.; Nebral, K.; Attarbaschi, A.; Fiser, K.; Kauer, M.O.; Popitsch, N.; et al. CD371 cell surface expression: A unique feature of *DUX4*-rearranged acute lymphoblastic leukemia. *Haematologica* **2019**, *104*, e352–e355. [CrossRef]
32. Stanulla, M.; Dagdan, E.; Zaliova, M.; Möricke, A.; Palmi, C.; Cazzaniga, G.; Eckert, C.; Te Kronnie, G.; Bourquin, J.P.; Bornhauser, B.; et al. *IKZF1*^{plus} defines a new minimal residual disease-dependent very-poor prognostic profile in pediatric B-cell precursor acute lymphoblastic leukemia. *J. Clin. Oncol.* **2018**, *36*, 1240–1249. [CrossRef]
33. Pui, C.H.; Rebora, P.; Schrappe, M.; Attarbaschi, A.; Baruchel, A.; Basso, G.; Cave, H.; Elitzur, S.; Koh, K.; Liu, H.C.; et al. Outcome of children with hypodiploid acute lymphoblastic leukemia: A retrospective multinational study. *J. Clin. Oncol.* **2019**, *37*, 770–779. [CrossRef] [PubMed]
34. McNeer, J.L.; Devidas, M.; Dai, Y.; Carroll, A.J.; Heerema, N.A.; Gastier-Foster, J.M.; Kahwash, S.B.; Borowitz, M.J.; Wood, B.L.; Larsen, E.; et al. Hematopoietic stem-cell transplantation does not improve the poor outcome of children with hypodiploid acute lymphoblastic leukemia: A report from Children's Oncology Group. *J. Clin. Oncol.* **2019**, *37*, 780–789. [CrossRef]
35. Holmfeldt, L.; Wei, L.; Diaz-Flores, E.; Walsh, M.; Zhang, J.; Ding, L.; Payne-Turner, D.; Churchman, M.; Andersson, A.; Chen, S.C.; et al. The genomic landscape of hypodiploid acute lymphoblastic leukemia. *Nat. Genet.* **2013**, *45*, 242–252. [CrossRef]
36. Qian, M.; Cao, X.; Devidas, M.; Yang, W.; Cheng, C.; Dai, Y.; Carroll, A.; Heerema, N.A.; Zhang, H.; Moriyama, T.; et al. *TP53* germline variations influence the predisposition and prognosis of B-cell acute lymphoblastic leukemia in children. *J. Clin. Oncol.* **2018**, *36*, 591–599. [CrossRef] [PubMed]
37. Safavi, S.; Paulsson, K. Near-haploid and low-hypodiploid acute lymphoblastic leukemia: Two distinct subtypes with consistently poor prognosis. *Blood* **2017**, *129*, 420–423. [CrossRef]

38. Diaz-Flores, E.; Comeaux, E.Q.; Kim, K.L.; Melnik, E.; Beckman, K.; Davis, K.L.; Wu, K.; Akutagawa, J.; Bridges, O.; Marino, R.; et al. Bcl-2 is a therapeutic target for hypodiploid B-lineage acute lymphoblastic leukemia. *Cancer Res.* **2019**, *79*, 2339–2351. [CrossRef] [PubMed]
39. Talleur, A.C.; Maude, S.L. What is the role for HSCT or immunotherapy in pediatric hypodiploid B-cell acute lymphoblastic leukemia? *Hematol. Am. Soc. Hematol. Educ. Program.* **2020**, *2020*, 508–511. [CrossRef]
40. Slayton, W.B.; Schultz, K.R.; Silverman, L.B.; Hunger, S.P. How we approach Philadelphia chromosome-positive acute lymphoblastic leukemia in children and young adults. *Pediatr. Blood Cancer* **2020**, *67*, e28543. [CrossRef]
41. Aricò, M.; Schrappe, M.; Hunger, S.P.; Carroll, W.L.; Conter, V.; Galimberti, S.; Manabe, A.; Saha, V.; Baruchel, A.; Vettenranta, K.; et al. Clinical outcome of children with newly diagnosed Philadelphia chromosome-positive acute lymphoblastic leukemia treated between 1995 and 2005. *J. Clin. Oncol.* **2010**, *28*, 4755–4761. [CrossRef]
42. Schultz, K.R.; Carroll, A.; Heerema, N.A.; Bowman, W.P.; Aledo, A.; Slayton, W.B.; Sather, H.; Devidas, M.; Zheng, H.W.; Davies, S.M.; et al. Long-term follow-up of imatinib in pediatric Philadelphia chromosome-positive acute lymphoblastic leukemia: Children's Oncology Group study AALL0031. *Leukemia* **2014**, *28*, 1467–1471. [CrossRef]
43. Slayton, W.B.; Schultz, K.R.; Kairalla, J.A.; Devidas, M.; Mi, X.; Pulsipher, M.A.; Chang, B.H.; Mullighan, C.; Iacobucci, I.; Silverman, L.B.; et al. Dasatinib plus intensive chemotherapy in children, adolescents, and young adults with Philadelphia chromosome-positive acute lymphoblastic leukemia: Results of Children's Oncology Group trial AALL0622. *J. Clin. Oncol.* **2018**, *36*, 2306–2314. [CrossRef]
44. Shen, S.; Chen, X.; Cai, J.; Yu, J.; Gao, J.; Hu, S.; Zhai, X.; Liang, C.; Ju, X.; Jiang, H.; et al. Effect of dasatinib vs. imatinib in the treatment of pediatric philadelphia chromosome-positive acute lymphoblastic leukemia: A randomized clinical trial. *JAMA Oncol.* **2020**, *6*, 358–366. [CrossRef] [PubMed]
45. Jabbour, E.; Kantarjian, H.; Ravandi, F.; Thomas, D.; Huang, X.; Faderl, S.; Pemmaraju, N.; Daver, N.; Garcia-Manero, G.; Sasaki, K.; et al. Combination of hyper-CVAD with ponatinib as first-line therapy for patients with Philadelphia chromosome-positive acute lymphoblastic leukaemia: A single-centre, phase 2 study. *Lancet Oncol.* **2015**, *16*, 1547–1555. [CrossRef]
46. Foà, R.; Bassan, R.; Vitale, A.; Elia, L.; Piciocchi, A.; Puzzolo, M.C.; Canichella, M.; Viero, P.; Ferrara, F.; Lunghi, M.; et al. Dasatinib–blinatumomab for Ph-positive acute lymphoblastic leukemia in adults. *N. Engl. J. Med.* **2020**, *383*, 1613–1623. [CrossRef] [PubMed]
47. Leonard, J.T.; Kosaka, Y.; Malla, P.; LaTocha, D.; Lamble, A.; Hayes-Lattin, B.; Byrd, K.; Druker, B.J.; Tyner, J.W.; Chang, B.H.; et al. Concomitant use of a dual Src/ABL kinase inhibitor eliminates the in vitro efficacy of blinatumomab against Ph+ ALL. *Blood* **2021**, *137*, 939–944. [CrossRef] [PubMed]
48. Mullighan, C.G.; Su, X.; Zhang, J.; Radtke, I.; Phillips, L.A.; Miller, C.B.; Ma, J.; Liu, W.; Cheng, C.; Schulman, B.A.; et al. Deletion of *IKZF1* and prognosis in acute lymphoblastic leukemia. *N. Engl. J. Med.* **2009**, *360*, 470–480. [CrossRef]
49. Den Boer, M.L.; van Slegtenhorst, M.; de Menezes, R.X.; Cheok, M.H.; Buijs-Gladdines, J.G.; Peters, S.T.; van Zutven, L.J.; Beverloo, H.B.; van der Spek, P.J.; Escherich, G.; et al. A subtype of childhood acute lymphoblastic leukaemia with poor treatment outcome: A genome-wide classification study. *Lancet Oncol.* **2009**, *10*, 125–134. [CrossRef]
50. Roberts, K.G.; Pei, D.; Campana, D.; Payne-Turner, D.; Li, Y.; Cheng, C.; Sandlund, J.T.; Jeha, S.; Easton, J.; Becksfort, J.; et al. Outcomes of children with *BCR-ABL1*-like acute lymphoblastic leukemia treated with risk-directed therapy based on the levels of minimal residual disease. *J. Clin. Oncol.* **2014**, *32*, 3012–3020. [CrossRef]
51. Roberts, K.G.; Reshmi, S.C.; Harvey, R.C.; Chen, I.M.; Patel, K.; Stonerock, E.; Jenkins, H.; Dai, Y.; Valentine, M.; Gu, Z.; et al. Genomic and outcome analyses of Ph-like ALL in NCI standard-risk patients: A report from the Children's Oncology Group. *Blood* **2018**, *132*, 815–824. [CrossRef]
52. Roberts, K.G.; Li, Y.; Payne-Turner, D.; Harvey, R.C.; Yang, Y.L.; Pei, D.; McCastlain, K.; Ding, L.; Lu, C.; Song, G.; et al. Targetable kinase-activating lesions in Ph-like acute lymphoblastic leukemia. *N. Engl. J. Med.* **2014**, *371*, 1005–1015. [CrossRef] [PubMed]
53. Tasian, S.K.; Loh, M.L.; Hunger, S.P. Philadelphia chromosome-like acute lymphoblastic leukemia. *Blood* **2017**, *130*, 2064–2072. [CrossRef] [PubMed]
54. Den Boer, M.L.; Cario, G.; Moorman, A.V.; Boer, J.M.; de Groot-Kruseman, H.A.; Fiocco, M.; Escherich, G.; Imamura, T.; Yeoh, A.; Sutton, R.; et al. Outcomes of paediatric patients with B-cell acute lymphocytic leukaemia with ABL-class fusion in the pre-tyrosine-kinase inhibitor era: A multicentre, retrospective, cohort study. *Lancet Haematol.* **2021**, *8*, e55–e66. [CrossRef]
55. Tanasi, I.; Ba, I.; Sirvent, N.; Braun, T.; Cuccuini, W.; Ballerini, P.; Duployez, N.; Tanguy-Schmidt, A.; Tamburini, J.; Maury, S.; et al. Efficacy of tyrosine kinase inhibitors in Ph-like acute lymphoblastic leukemia harboring ABL-class rearrangements. *Blood* **2019**, *134*, 1351–1355. [CrossRef] [PubMed]
56. Brown, P.; Pieters, R.; Biondi, A. How I treat infant leukemia. *Blood* **2019**, *133*, 205–214. [CrossRef] [PubMed]
57. Pieters, R.; Schrappe, M.; De Lorenzo, P.; Hann, I.; De Rossi, G.; Felice, M.; Hovi, L.; LeBlanc, T.; Szczepanski, T.; Ferster, A.; et al. A treatment protocol for infants younger than 1 year with acute lymphoblastic leukaemia (Interfant-99): An observational study and a multicentre randomised trial. *Lancet* **2007**, *370*, 240–250. [CrossRef]
58. Pieters, R.; De Lorenzo, P.; Ancliffe, P.; Aversa, L.A.; Brethon, B.; Biondi, A.; Campbell, M.; Escherich, G.; Ferster, A.; Gardner, R.A.; et al. Outcome of infants younger than 1 year with acute lymphoblastic leukemia treated with the Interfant-06 protocol: Results from an international phase III randomized study. *J. Clin. Oncol.* **2019**, *37*, 2246–2256. [CrossRef] [PubMed]
59. Neff, T.; Armstrong, S.A. Recent progress toward epigenetic therapies: The example of mixed lineage leukemia. *Blood* **2013**, *121*, 4847–4853. [CrossRef] [PubMed]

60. Suzuki, K.; Okuno, Y.; Kawashima, N.; Muramatsu, H.; Okuno, T.; Wang, X.; Kataoka, S.; Sekiya, Y.; Hamada, M.; Murakami, N.; et al. *MEF2D-BCL9* fusion gene is associated with high-risk acute B-cell precursor lymphoblastic leukemia in adolescents. *J. Clin. Oncol.* **2016**, *34*, 3451–3459. [CrossRef]
61. Ohki, K.; Kiyokawa, N.; Saito, Y.; Hirabayashi, S.; Nakabayashi, K.; Ichikawa, H.; Momozawa, Y.; Okamura, K.; Yoshimi, A.; Ogata-Kawata, H.; et al. Clinical and molecular characteristics of *MEF2D* fusion-positive B-cell precursor acute lymphoblastic leukemia in childhood, including a novel translocation resulting in *MEF2D-HNRNPH1* gene fusion. *Haematologica* **2019**, *104*, 128–137. [CrossRef]
62. Liu, Y.F.; Wang, B.Y.; Zhang, W.N.; Huang, J.Y.; Li, B.S.; Zhang, M.; Jiang, L.; Li, J.F.; Wang, M.J.; Dai, Y.J.; et al. Genomic profiling of adult and pediatric B-cell acute lymphoblastic leukemia. *EBioMedicine* **2016**, *8*, 173–183. [CrossRef] [PubMed]
63. Fischer, U.; Forster, M.; Rinaldi, A.; Risch, T.; Sungalee, S.; Warnatz, H.J.; Bornhauser, B.; Gombert, M.; Kratsch, C.; Stütz, A.M.; et al. Genomics and drug profiling of fatal *TCF3-HLF*-positive acute lymphoblastic leukemia identifies recurrent mutation patterns and therapeutic options. *Nat. Genet.* **2015**, *47*, 1020–1029. [CrossRef]
64. Huang, Y.; Mouttet, B.; Warnatz, H.J.; Risch, T.; Rietmann, F.; Frommelt, F.; Ngo, Q.A.; Dobay, M.P.; Marovca, B.; Jenni, S.; et al. The leukemogenic TCF3-HLF complex rewires enhancers driving cellular identity and self-renewal conferring EP300 vulnerability. *Cancer Cell* **2019**, *36*, 630–644.e639. [CrossRef]
65. Mouttet, B.; Vinti, L.; Ancliff, P.; Bodmer, N.; Brethon, B.; Cario, G.; Chen-Santel, C.; Elitzur, S.; Hazar, V.; Kunz, J.; et al. Durable remissions in *TCF3-HLF* positive acute lymphoblastic leukemia with blinatumomab and stem cell transplantation. *Haematologica* **2019**, *104*, e244–e247. [CrossRef]
66. Jeha, S.; Pei, D.; Raimondi, S.C.; Onciu, M.; Campana, D.; Cheng, C.; Sandlund, J.T.; Ribeiro, R.C.; Rubnitz, J.E.; Howard, S.C.; et al. Increased risk for CNS relapse in pre-B cell leukemia with the t(1;19)/*TCF3-PBX1*. *Leukemia* **2009**, *23*, 1406–1409. [CrossRef] [PubMed]
67. Hein, D.; Dreisig, K.; Metzler, M.; Izraeli, S.; Schmiegelow, K.; Borkhardt, A.; Fischer, U. The preleukemic *TCF3-PBX1* gene fusion can be generated in utero and is present in ≈0.6% of healthy newborns. *Blood* **2019**, *134*, 1355–1358. [CrossRef]
68. Pui, C.H.; Sandlund, J.T.; Pei, D.; Rivera, G.K.; Howard, S.C.; Ribeiro, R.C.; Rubnitz, J.E.; Razzouk, B.I.; Hudson, M.M.; Cheng, C.; et al. Results of therapy for acute lymphoblastic leukemia in black and white children. *JAMA* **2003**, *290*, 2001–2007. [CrossRef] [PubMed]
69. Lee, S.H.R.; Qian, M.; Yang, W.; Diedrich, J.D.; Raetz, E.; Yang, W.; Dong, Q.; Devidas, M.; Pei, D.; Yeoh, A.; et al. Genome-wide association study of susceptibility loci for *TCF3-PBX1* acute lymphoblastic leukemia in children. *J. Natl. Cancer Inst.* **2020**. [CrossRef]
70. Harrison, C.J. Blood Spotlight on iAMP21 acute lymphoblastic leukemia (ALL), a high-risk pediatric disease. *Blood* **2015**, *125*, 1383–1386. [CrossRef]
71. Li, Y.; Schwab, C.; Ryan, S.; Papaemmanuil, E.; Robinson, H.M.; Jacobs, P.; Moorman, A.V.; Dyer, S.; Borrow, J.; Griffiths, M.; et al. Constitutional and somatic rearrangement of chromosome 21 in acute lymphoblastic leukaemia. *Nature* **2014**, *508*, 98–102. [CrossRef]
72. Harrison, C.J.; Moorman, A.V.; Schwab, C.; Carroll, A.J.; Raetz, E.A.; Devidas, M.; Strehl, S.; Nebral, K.; Harbott, J.; Teigler-Schlegel, A.; et al. An international study of intrachromosomal amplification of chromosome 21 (iAMP21): Cytogenetic characterization and outcome. *Leukemia* **2014**, *28*, 1015–1021. [CrossRef] [PubMed]
73. Sinclair, P.B.; Ryan, S.; Bashton, M.; Hollern, S.; Hanna, R.; Case, M.; Schwalbe, E.C.; Schwab, C.J.; Cranston, R.E.; Young, B.D.; et al. SH2B3 inactivation through CN-LOH 12q is uniquely associated with B-cell precursor ALL with iAMP21 or other chromosome 21 gain. *Leukemia* **2019**, *33*, 1881–1894. [CrossRef]
74. Heerema, N.A.; Carroll, A.J.; Devidas, M.; Loh, M.L.; Borowitz, M.J.; Gastier-Foster, J.M.; Larsen, E.C.; Mattano, L.A., Jr.; Maloney, K.W.; Willman, C.L.; et al. Intrachromosomal amplification of chromosome 21 is associated with inferior outcomes in children with acute lymphoblastic leukemia treated in contemporary standard-risk Children's Oncology Group studies: A report from the Children's Oncology Group. *J. Clin. Oncol.* **2013**, *31*, 3397–3402. [CrossRef] [PubMed]
75. Moorman, A.V.; Robinson, H.; Schwab, C.; Richards, S.M.; Hancock, J.; Mitchell, C.D.; Goulden, N.; Vora, A.; Harrison, C.J. Risk-directed treatment intensification significantly reduces the risk of relapse among children and adolescents with acute lymphoblastic leukemia and intrachromosomal amplification of chromosome 21: A comparison of the MRC ALL97/99 and UKALL2003 trials. *J. Clin. Oncol.* **2013**, *31*, 3389–3396. [CrossRef] [PubMed]
76. Cobaleda, C.; Schebesta, A.; Delogu, A.; Busslinger, M. Pax5: The guardian of B cell identity and function. *Nat. Immunol.* **2007**, *8*, 463–470. [CrossRef] [PubMed]
77. Mullighan, C.G.; Goorha, S.; Radtke, I.; Miller, C.B.; Coustan-Smith, E.; Dalton, J.D.; Girtman, K.; Mathew, S.; Ma, J.; Pounds, S.B.; et al. Genome-wide analysis of genetic alterations in acute lymphoblastic leukaemia. *Nature* **2007**, *446*, 758–764. [CrossRef]
78. Hirabayashi, S.; Butler, E.R.; Ohki, K.; Kiyokawa, N.; Bergmann, A.K.; Möricke, A.; Boer, J.M.; Cavé, H.; Cazzaniga, G.; Yeoh, A.E.J.; et al. Clinical characteristics and outcomes of B-ALL with *ZNF384* rearrangements: A retrospective analysis by the Ponte di Legno Childhood ALL Working Group. *Leukemia* **2021**. [CrossRef]
79. Alexander, T.B.; Gu, Z.; Iacobucci, I.; Dickerson, K.; Choi, J.K.; Xu, B.; Payne-Turner, D.; Yoshihara, H.; Loh, M.L.; Horan, J.; et al. The genetic basis and cell of origin of mixed phenotype acute leukaemia. *Nature* **2018**, *562*, 373–379. [CrossRef]

80. Hirabayashi, S.; Ohki, K.; Nakabayashi, K.; Ichikawa, H.; Momozawa, Y.; Okamura, K.; Yaguchi, A.; Terada, K.; Saito, Y.; Yoshimi, A.; et al. ZNF384-related fusion genes define a subgroup of childhood B-cell precursor acute lymphoblastic leukemia with a characteristic immunotype. *Haematologica* **2017**, *102*, 118–129. [CrossRef]
81. Bueno, C.; Tejedor, J.R.; Bashford-Rogers, R.; González-Silva, L.; Valdés-Mas, R.; Agraz-Doblás, A.; Díaz de la Guardia, R.; Ribera, J.; Zamora, L.; Bilhou-Nabera, C.; et al. Natural history and cell of origin of TCF3-ZNF384 and PTPN11 mutations in monozygotic twins with concordant BCP-ALL. *Blood* **2019**, *134*, 900–905. [CrossRef]
82. Boer, J.; Valsecchi, M.; Hormann, F.; Antic, Z.; Zaliova, M.; Schwab, C.; Cazzaniga, G.; Arfeuille, C.; Cavé, H.; Attarbaschi, A.; et al. NUTM1-rearranged infant and pediatric B cell precursor acute lymphoblastic leukemia: A good prognostic subtype identified in a collaborative international study. *Blood* **2020**, *136*, 25–26. [CrossRef]
83. Hormann, F.M.; Hoogkamer, A.Q.; Beverloo, H.B.; Boeree, A.; Dingjan, I.; Wattel, M.M.; Stam, R.W.; Escherich, G.; Pieters, R.; den Boer, M.L.; et al. NUTM1 is a recurrent fusion gene partner in B-cell precursor acute lymphoblastic leukemia associated with increased expression of genes on chromosome band 10p12.31-12.2. *Haematologica* **2019**, *104*, e455–e459. [CrossRef] [PubMed]
84. Cordo, V.; van der Zwet, J.; Canté-Barrett, K.; Pieters, R.; Meijerink, J. T-cell acute lymphoblastic leukemia: A roadmap to targeted therapies. *Blood Cancer Discov.* **2021**, *2*, 19–31. [CrossRef]
85. Van Vlierberghe, P.; Palomero, T.; Khiabanian, H.; van der Meulen, J.; Castillo, M.; van Roy, N.; de Moerloose, B.; Philippé, J.; González-García, S.; Toribio, M.L.; et al. PHF6 mutations in T-cell acute lymphoblastic leukemia. *Nat. Genet.* **2010**, *42*, 338–342. [CrossRef]
86. Liu, Y.; Easton, J.; Shao, Y.; Maciaszek, J.; Wang, Z.; Wilkinson, M.R.; McCastlain, K.; Edmonson, M.; Pounds, S.B.; Shi, L.; et al. The genomic landscape of pediatric and young adult T-lineage acute lymphoblastic leukemia. *Nat. Genet.* **2017**, *49*, 1211–1218. [CrossRef]
87. Schrappe, M.; Valsecchi, M.G.; Bartram, C.R.; Schrauder, A.; Panzer-Grümayer, R.; Möricke, A.; Parasole, R.; Zimmermann, M.; Dworzak, M.; Buldini, B.; et al. Late MRD response determines relapse risk overall and in subsets of childhood T-cell ALL: Results of the AIEOP-BFM-ALL 2000 study. *Blood* **2011**, *118*, 2077–2084. [CrossRef]
88. Salzer, W.L.; Burke, M.J.; Devidas, M.; Dai, Y.; Hardy, K.K.; Kairalla, J.A.; Gore, L.; Hilden, J.M.; Larsen, E.; Rabin, K.R.; et al. Impact of intrathecal triple therapy versus intrathecal methotrexate on disease-free survival for high-risk B-lymphoblastic leukemia: Children's Oncology Group Study AALL1131. *J. Clin. Oncol.* **2020**, *38*, 2628–2638. [CrossRef]
89. Teachey, D.T.; Devidas, M.; Wood, B.L.; Chen, Z.; Hayashi, R.J.; Annett, R.D.; Asselin, B.L.; August, K.J.; Cho, S.Y.; Dunsmore, K.P.; et al. Cranial radiation can be eliminated in most children with T-cell acute lymphoblastic leukemia (T-ALL) and bortezomib potentially improves survival in children with T-cell lymphoblastic lymphoma (T-LL): Results of Children's Oncology Group (COG) trial AALL1231. *Blood* **2020**, *136*, 11–12. [CrossRef]
90. Coustan-Smith, E.; Mullighan, C.G.; Onciu, M.; Behm, F.G.; Raimondi, S.C.; Pei, D.; Cheng, C.; Su, X.; Rubnitz, J.E.; Basso, G.; et al. Early T-cell precursor leukaemia: A subtype of very high-risk acute lymphoblastic leukaemia. *Lancet Oncol.* **2009**, *10*, 147–156. [CrossRef]
91. Zhang, J.; Ding, L.; Holmfeldt, L.; Wu, G.; Heatley, S.L.; Payne-Turner, D.; Easton, J.; Chen, X.; Wang, J.; Rusch, M.; et al. The genetic basis of early T-cell precursor acute lymphoblastic leukaemia. *Nature* **2012**, *481*, 157–163. [CrossRef]
92. Conter, V.; Valsecchi, M.G.; Buldini, B.; Parasole, R.; Locatelli, F.; Colombini, A.; Rizzari, C.; Putti, M.C.; Barisone, E.; Lo Nigro, L.; et al. Early T-cell precursor acute lymphoblastic leukaemia in children treated in AIEOP centres with AIEOP-BFM protocols: A retrospective analysis. *Lancet Haematol.* **2016**, *3*, e80–e86. [CrossRef]
93. Raetz, E.A.; Teachey, D.T. T-cell acute lymphoblastic leukemia. *Hematol. Am. Soc. Hematol. Educ. Program.* **2016**, *2016*, 580–588. [CrossRef] [PubMed]
94. Jain, N.; Lamb, A.V.; O'Brien, S.; Ravandi, F.; Konopleva, M.; Jabbour, E.; Zuo, Z.; Jorgensen, J.; Lin, P.; Pierce, S.; et al. Early T-cell precursor acute lymphoblastic leukemia/lymphoma (ETP-ALL/LBL) in adolescents and adults: A high-risk subtype. *Blood* **2016**, *127*, 1863–1869. [CrossRef]
95. Patrick, K.; Wade, R.; Goulden, N.; Mitchell, C.; Moorman, A.V.; Rowntree, C.; Jenkinson, S.; Hough, R.; Vora, A. Outcome for children and young people with Early T-cell precursor acute lymphoblastic leukaemia treated on a contemporary protocol, UKALL 2003. *Br. J. Haematol.* **2014**, *166*, 421–424. [CrossRef]
96. Richard-Carpentier, G.; Jabbour, E.; Short, N.J.; Rausch, C.R.; Savoy, J.M.; Bose, P.; Yilmaz, M.; Jain, N.; Borthakur, G.; Ohanian, M.; et al. Clinical experience with venetoclax combined with chemotherapy for relapsed or refractory T-cell acute lymphoblastic leukemia. *Clin. Lymphoma Myeloma Leuk.* **2020**, *20*, 212–218. [CrossRef] [PubMed]
97. Campana, D.; Pui, C.H. Minimal residual disease-guided therapy in childhood acute lymphoblastic leukemia. *Blood* **2017**, *129*, 1913–1918. [CrossRef] [PubMed]
98. Van Dongen, J.J.; van der Velden, V.H.; Bruggemann, M.; Orfao, A. Minimal residual disease diagnostics in acute lymphoblastic leukemia: Need for sensitive, fast, and standardized technologies. *Blood* **2015**, *125*, 3996–4009. [CrossRef]
99. Della Starza, I.; Chiaretti, S.; de Propris, M.S.; Elia, L.; Cavalli, M.; de Novi, L.A.; Soscia, R.; Messina, M.; Vitale, A.; Guarini, A.; et al. Minimal residual disease in acute lymphoblastic leukemia: Technical and clinical advances. *Front. Oncol.* **2019**, *9*, 726. [CrossRef]
100. Faham, M.; Zheng, J.; Moorhead, M.; Carlton, V.E.; Stow, P.; Coustan-Smith, E.; Pui, C.H.; Campana, D. Deep-sequencing approach for minimal residual disease detection in acute lymphoblastic leukemia. *Blood* **2012**, *120*, 5173–5180. [CrossRef] [PubMed]

101. Wu, D.; Emerson, R.O.; Sherwood, A.; Loh, M.L.; Angiolillo, A.; Howie, B.; Vogt, J.; Rieder, M.; Kirsch, I.; Carlson, C.; et al. Detection of minimal residual disease in B lymphoblastic leukemia by high-throughput sequencing of IGH. *Clin. Cancer Res.* **2014**, *20*, 4540–4548. [CrossRef] [PubMed]
102. Wood, B.; Wu, D.; Crossley, B.; Dai, Y.; Williamson, D.; Gawad, C.; Borowitz, M.J.; Devidas, M.; Maloney, K.W.; Larsen, E.; et al. Measurable residual disease detection by high-throughput sequencing improves risk stratification for pediatric B-ALL. *Blood* **2018**, *131*, 1350–1359. [CrossRef] [PubMed]
103. Pulsipher, M.A.; Carlson, C.; Langholz, B.; Wall, D.A.; Schultz, K.R.; Bunin, N.; Kirsch, I.; Gastier-Foster, J.M.; Borowitz, M.; Desmarais, C.; et al. IgH-V(D)J NGS-MRD measurement pre- and early post-allotransplant defines very low- and very high-risk ALL patients. *Blood* **2015**, *125*, 3501–3508. [CrossRef] [PubMed]
104. Hay, K.A.; Gauthier, J.; Hirayama, A.V.; Voutsinas, J.M.; Wu, Q.; Li, D.; Gooley, T.A.; Cherian, S.; Chen, X.; Pender, B.S.; et al. Factors associated with durable EFS in adult B-cell ALL patients achieving MRD-negative CR after CD19 CAR T-cell therapy. *Blood* **2019**, *133*, 1652–1663. [CrossRef]
105. Enshaei, A.; O'Connor, D.; Bartram, J.; Hancock, J.; Harrison, C.J.; Hough, R.; Samarasinghe, S.; den Boer, M.L.; Boer, J.M.; de Groot-Kruseman, H.A.; et al. A validated novel continuous prognostic index to deliver stratified medicine in pediatric acute lymphoblastic leukemia. *Blood* **2020**, *135*, 1438–1446. [CrossRef] [PubMed]
106. Gocho, Y.; Liu, J.; Hu, J.; Yang, W.; Dharia, N.V.; Zhang, J.; Shi, H.; Du, G.; John, A.; Lin, T.-N.; et al. Network-based systems pharmacology reveals heterogeneity in LCK and BCL2 signaling and therapeutic sensitivity of T-cell acute lymphoblastic leukemia. *Nat. Cancer* **2021**, *2*, 284–299. [CrossRef]
107. Kapoor, I.; Bodo, J.; Hill, B.T.; Hsi, E.D.; Almasan, A. Targeting BCL-2 in B-cell malignancies and overcoming therapeutic resistance. *Cell Death Dis.* **2020**, *11*, 941. [CrossRef]
108. Khaw, S.L.; Suryani, S.; Evans, K.; Richmond, J.; Robbins, A.; Kurmasheva, R.T.; Billups, C.A.; Erickson, S.W.; Guo, Y.; Houghton, P.J.; et al. Venetoclax responses of pediatric ALL xenografts reveal sensitivity of MLL-rearranged leukemia. *Blood* **2016**, *128*, 1382–1395. [CrossRef]
109. Scherr, M.; Elder, A.; Battmer, K.; Barzan, D.; Bomken, S.; Ricke-Hoch, M.; Schröder, A.; Venturini, L.; Blair, H.J.; Vormoor, J.; et al. Differential expression of miR-17~92 identifies BCL2 as a therapeutic target in BCR-ABL-positive B-lineage acute lymphoblastic leukemia. *Leukemia* **2014**, *28*, 554–565. [CrossRef]
110. Peirs, S.; Matthijssens, F.; Goossens, S.; van de Walle, I.; Ruggero, K.; de Bock, C.E.; Degryse, S.; Canté-Barrett, K.; Briot, D.; Clappier, E.; et al. ABT-199 mediated inhibition of BCL-2 as a novel therapeutic strategy in T-cell acute lymphoblastic leukemia. *Blood* **2014**, *124*, 3738–3747. [CrossRef] [PubMed]
111. Chonghaile, T.N.; Roderick, J.E.; Glenfield, C.; Ryan, J.; Sallan, S.E.; Silverman, L.B.; Loh, M.L.; Hunger, S.P.; Wood, B.; DeAngelo, D.J.; et al. Maturation stage of T-cell acute lymphoblastic leukemia determines BCL-2 versus BCL-XL dependence and sensitivity to ABT-199. *Cancer Discov.* **2014**, *4*, 1074–1087. [CrossRef] [PubMed]
112. Autry, R.J.; Paugh, S.W.; Carter, R.; Shi, L.; Liu, J.; Ferguson, D.C.; Lau, C.E.; Bonten, E.J.; Yang, W.; McCorkle, J.R.; et al. Integrative genomic analyses reveal mechanisms of glucocorticoid resistance in acute lymphoblastic leukemia. *Nat. Cancer* **2020**, *1*, 329–344. [CrossRef]
113. Karol, S.E.; Cooper, T.M.; Bittencourt, H.; Gore, L.; O'Brien, M.M.; Fraser, C.; Gambart, M.; Cario, G.; Zwaan, C.M.; Bourquin, J.-P.; et al. Safety, efficacy, and PK of the BCL2 inhibitor venetoclax in combination with chemotherapy in pediatric and young adult patients with relapsed/refractory acute myeloid leukemia and acute lymphoblastic leukemia: Phase 1 study. *Blood* **2019**, *134*, 2649. [CrossRef]
114. Pullarkat, V.A.; Lacayo, N.J.; Jabbour, E.; Rubnitz, J.E.; Bajel, A.; Laetsch, T.W.; Leonard, J.; Colace, S.I.; Khaw, S.L.; Fleming, S.A.; et al. Venetoclax and navitoclax in combination with chemotherapy in patients with relapsed or refractory acute lymphoblastic leukemia and lymphoblastic lymphoma. *Cancer Discov.* **2021**. [CrossRef]
115. Horton, T.M.; Gannavarapu, A.; Blaney, S.M.; D'Argenio, D.Z.; Plon, S.E.; Berg, S.L. Bortezomib interactions with chemotherapy agents in acute leukemia in vitro. *Cancer Chemother. Pharmacol.* **2006**, *58*, 13–23. [CrossRef] [PubMed]
116. Messinger, Y.H.; Gaynon, P.S.; Sposto, R.; van der Giessen, J.; Eckroth, E.; Malvar, J.; Bostrom, B.C.; Therapeutic Advances in Childhood Leukemia & Lymphoma (TACL) Consortium. Bortezomib with chemotherapy is highly active in advanced B-precursor acute lymphoblastic leukemia: Therapeutic Advances in Childhood Leukemia & Lymphoma (TACL) Study. *Blood* **2012**, *120*, 285–290. [CrossRef] [PubMed]
117. Gutierrez, A.; Sanda, T.; Grebliunaite, R.; Carracedo, A.; Salmena, L.; Ahn, Y.; Dahlberg, S.; Neuberg, D.; Moreau, L.A.; Winter, S.S.; et al. High frequency of PTEN, PI3K, and AKT abnormalities in T-cell acute lymphoblastic leukemia. *Blood* **2009**, *114*, 647–650. [CrossRef] [PubMed]
118. Teachey, D.T.; Obzut, D.A.; Cooperman, J.; Fang, J.; Carroll, M.; Choi, J.K.; Houghton, P.J.; Brown, V.I.; Grupp, S.A. The mTOR inhibitor CCI-779 induces apoptosis and inhibits growth in preclinical models of primary adult human ALL. *Blood* **2006**, *107*, 1149–1155. [CrossRef]
119. Wei, G.; Twomey, D.; Lamb, J.; Schlis, K.; Agarwal, V.; Stam, R.W.; Opferman, J.T.; Sallan, S.E.; den Boer, M.L.; Pieters, R.; et al. Gene expression-based chemical genomics identifies rapamycin as a modulator of MCL1 and glucocorticoid resistance. *Cancer Cell* **2006**, *10*, 331–342. [CrossRef] [PubMed]
120. Crazzolara, R.; Cisterne, A.; Thien, M.; Hewson, J.; Baraz, R.; Bradstock, K.F.; Bendall, L.J. Potentiating effects of RAD001 (Everolimus) on vincristine therapy in childhood acute lymphoblastic leukemia. *Blood* **2009**, *113*, 3297–3306. [CrossRef] [PubMed]

121. Avellino, R.; Romano, S.; Parasole, R.; Bisogni, R.; Lamberti, A.; Poggi, V.; Venuta, S.; Romano, M.F. Rapamycin stimulates apoptosis of childhood acute lymphoblastic leukemia cells. *Blood* **2005**, *106*, 1400–1406. [CrossRef]
122. Place, A.E.; Pikman, Y.; Stevenson, K.E.; Harris, M.H.; Pauly, M.; Sulis, M.L.; Hijiya, N.; Gore, L.; Cooper, T.M.; Loh, M.L.; et al. Phase I trial of the mTOR inhibitor everolimus in combination with multi-agent chemotherapy in relapsed childhood acute lymphoblastic leukemia. *Pediatr. Blood Cancer* **2018**, *65*, e27062. [CrossRef] [PubMed]
123. Sandoval, J.; Esteller, M. Cancer epigenomics: Beyond genomics. *Curr. Opin. Genet. Dev.* **2012**, *22*, 50–55. [CrossRef] [PubMed]
124. Garcia-Manero, G.; Bueso-Ramos, C.; Daniel, J.; Williamson, J.; Kantarjian, H.M.; Issa, J.P. DNA methylation patterns at relapse in adult acute lymphocytic leukemia. *Clin. Cancer Res.* **2002**, *8*, 1897–1903. [PubMed]
125. Burke, M.J.; Kostadinov, R.; Sposto, R.; Gore, L.; Kelley, S.M.; Rabik, C.; Trepel, J.B.; Lee, M.J.; Yuno, A.; Lee, S.; et al. Decitabine and Vorinostat with Chemotherapy in Relapsed Pediatric Acute Lymphoblastic Leukemia: A TACL Pilot Study. *Clin. Cancer Res.* **2020**, *26*, 2297–2307. [CrossRef]
126. Inaba, H.; Pui, C.H. Immunotherapy in pediatric acute lymphoblastic leukemia. *Cancer Metastasis Rev.* **2019**, *38*, 595–610. [CrossRef]
127. Kantarjian, H.; Stein, A.; Gökbuget, N.; Fielding, A.K.; Schuh, A.C.; Ribera, J.M.; Wei, A.; Dombret, H.; Foà, R.; Bassan, R.; et al. Blinatumomab versus chemotherapy for advanced acute lymphoblastic leukemia. *N. Engl. J. Med.* **2017**, *376*, 836–847. [CrossRef]
128. Gökbuget, N.; Dombret, H.; Bonifacio, M.; Reichle, A.; Graux, C.; Faul, C.; Diedrich, H.; Topp, M.S.; Bruggemann, M.; Horst, H.A.; et al. Blinatumomab for minimal residual disease in adults with B-cell precursor acute lymphoblastic leukemia. *Blood* **2018**, *131*, 1522–1531. [CrossRef]
129. Brown, P.A.; Ji, L.; Xu, X.; Devidas, M.; Hogan, L.E.; Borowitz, M.J.; Raetz, E.A.; Zugmaier, G.; Sharon, E.; Bernhardt, M.B.; et al. Effect of postreinduction therapy consolidation with blinatumomab vs. chemotherapy on disease-free survival in children, adolescents, and young adults with first relapse of B-cell acute lymphoblastic leukemia: A randomized clinical trial. *JAMA* **2021**, *325*, 833–842. [CrossRef]
130. Locatelli, F.; Zugmaier, G.; Rizzari, C.; Morris, J.D.; Gruhn, B.; Klingebiel, T.; Parasole, R.; Linderkamp, C.; Flotho, C.; Petit, A.; et al. Effect of blinatumomab vs. chemotherapy on event-free survival among children with high-risk first-relapse B-cell acute lymphoblastic leukemia: A randomized clinical trial. *JAMA* **2021**, *325*, 843–854. [CrossRef]
131. Orlando, E.J.; Han, X.; Tribouley, C.; Wood, P.A.; Leary, R.J.; Riester, M.; Levine, J.E.; Qayed, M.; Grupp, S.A.; Boyer, M.; et al. Genetic mechanisms of target antigen loss in CAR19 therapy of acute lymphoblastic leukemia. *Nat. Med.* **2018**, *24*, 1504–1506. [CrossRef]
132. Sotillo, E.; Barrett, D.M.; Black, K.L.; Bagashev, A.; Oldridge, D.; Wu, G.; Sussman, R.; Lanauze, C.; Ruella, M.; Gazzara, M.R.; et al. Convergence of acquired mutations and alternative splicing of CD19 enables resistance to CART-19 immunotherapy. *Cancer Discov.* **2015**, *5*, 1282–1295. [CrossRef] [PubMed]
133. Jacoby, E.; Nguyen, S.M.; Fountaine, T.J.; Welp, K.; Gryder, B.; Qin, H.; Yang, Y.; Chien, C.D.; Seif, A.E.; Lei, H.; et al. CD19 CAR immune pressure induces B-precursor acute lymphoblastic leukaemia lineage switch exposing inherent leukaemic plasticity. *Nat. Commun.* **2016**, *7*, 12320. [CrossRef] [PubMed]
134. Oberley, M.J.; Gaynon, P.S.; Bhojwani, D.; Pulsipher, M.A.; Gardner, R.A.; Hiemenz, M.C.; Ji, J.; Han, J.; O'Gorman, M.R.G.; Wayne, A.S.; et al. Myeloid lineage switch following chimeric antigen receptor T-cell therapy in a patient with TCF3-ZNF384 fusion-positive B-lymphoblastic leukemia. *Pediatr. Blood Cancer* **2018**, *65*, e27265. [CrossRef] [PubMed]
135. Braig, F.; Brandt, A.; Goebeler, M.; Tony, H.P.; Kurze, A.K.; Nollau, P.; Bumm, T.; Bottcher, S.; Bargou, R.C.; Binder, M. Resistance to anti-CD19/CD3 BiTE in acute lymphoblastic leukemia may be mediated by disrupted CD19 membrane trafficking. *Blood* **2017**, *129*, 100–104. [CrossRef]
136. Maude, S.L.; Teachey, D.T.; Porter, D.L.; Grupp, S.A. CD19-targeted chimeric antigen receptor T-cell therapy for acute lymphoblastic leukemia. *Blood* **2015**, *125*, 4017–4023. [CrossRef] [PubMed]
137. Maude, S.L.; Laetsch, T.W.; Buechner, J.; Rives, S.; Boyer, M.; Bittencourt, H.; Bader, P.; Verneris, M.R.; Stefanski, H.E.; Myers, G.D.; et al. Tisagenlecleucel in children and young adults with B-cell lymphoblastic leukemia. *N. Engl. J. Med.* **2018**, *378*, 439–448. [CrossRef] [PubMed]
138. Maude, S.L.; Frey, N.; Shaw, P.A.; Aplenc, R.; Barrett, D.M.; Bunin, N.J.; Chew, A.; Gonzalez, V.E.; Zheng, Z.; Lacey, S.F.; et al. Chimeric antigen receptor T cells for sustained remissions in leukemia. *N. Engl. J. Med.* **2014**, *371*, 1507–1517. [CrossRef]
139. Kadauke, S.; Myers, R.M.; Li, Y.; Aplenc, R.; Baniewicz, D.; Barrett, D.M.; Barz Leahy, A.; Callahan, C.; Dolan, J.G.; Fitzgerald, J.C.; et al. Risk-adapted preemptive tocilizumab to prevent severe cytokine release syndrome after CTL019 for pediatric B-cell acute lymphoblastic leukemia: A prospective clinical trial. *J. Clin. Oncol.* **2021**, *39*, 920–930. [CrossRef]
140. Hill, J.A.; Seo, S.K. How I prevent infections in patients receiving CD19-targeted chimeric antigen receptor T cells for B-cell malignancies. *Blood* **2020**, *136*, 925–935. [CrossRef]
141. Shah, N.N.; Fry, T.J. Mechanisms of resistance to CAR T cell therapy. *Nat. Rev. Clin. Oncol.* **2019**, *16*, 372–385. [CrossRef]
142. Majzner, R.G.; Mackall, C.L. Tumor antigen escape from CAR T-cell therapy. *Cancer Discov.* **2018**, *8*, 1219–1226. [CrossRef]
143. Fry, T.J.; Shah, N.N.; Orentas, R.J.; Stetler-Stevenson, M.; Yuan, C.M.; Ramakrishna, S.; Wolters, P.; Martin, S.; Delbrook, C.; Yates, B.; et al. CD22-targeted CAR T cells induce remission in B-ALL that is naive or resistant to CD19-targeted CAR immunotherapy. *Nat. Med.* **2018**, *24*, 20–28. [CrossRef] [PubMed]

144. Qin, H.; Cho, M.; Haso, W.; Zhang, L.; Tasian, S.K.; Oo, H.Z.; Negri, G.L.; Lin, Y.; Zou, J.; Mallon, B.S.; et al. Eradication of B-ALL using chimeric antigen receptor-expressing T cells targeting the TSLPR oncoprotein. *Blood* **2015**, *126*, 629–639. [CrossRef] [PubMed]
145. Schultz, L.M.; Muffly, L.S.; Spiegel, J.Y.; Ramakrishna, S.; Hossain, N.; Baggott, C.; Sahaf, B.; Patel, S.; Craig, J.; Yoon, J.; et al. Phase I trial using CD19/CD22 bispecific CAR T cells in pediatric and adult acute lymphoblastic leukemia (ALL). *Blood* **2019**, *134*, 744. [CrossRef]
146. Wang, N.; Hu, X.; Cao, W.; Li, C.; Xiao, Y.; Cao, Y.; Gu, C.; Zhang, S.; Chen, L.; Cheng, J.; et al. Efficacy and safety of CAR19/22 T-cell cocktail therapy in patients with refractory/relapsed B-cell malignancies. *Blood* **2020**, *135*, 17–27. [CrossRef] [PubMed]
147. Pan, J.; Zuo, S.; Deng, B.; Xu, X.; Li, C.; Zheng, Q.; Ling, Z.; Song, W.; Xu, J.; Duan, J.; et al. Sequential CD19-22 CAR T therapy induces sustained remission in children with r/r B-ALL. *Blood* **2020**, *135*, 387–391. [CrossRef]
148. He, X.; Xiao, X.; Li, Q.; Jiang, Y.; Cao, Y.; Sun, R.; Jin, X.; Yuan, T.; Meng, J.; Ma, L.; et al. Anti-CD19 CAR-T as a feasible and safe treatment against central nervous system leukemia after intrathecal chemotherapy in adults with relapsed or refractory B-ALL. *Leukemia* **2019**, *33*, 2102–2104. [CrossRef]
149. Chen, X.; Wang, Y.; Ruan, M.; Li, J.; Zhong, M.; Li, Z.; Liu, F.; Wang, S.; Chen, Y.; Liu, L.; et al. Treatment of testicular relapse of B-cell acute lymphoblastic leukemia with CD19-specific chimeric antigen receptor T cells. *Clin. Lymphoma Myeloma Leuk.* **2019**, *20*, 366–370. [CrossRef]
150. Kantarjian, H.M.; DeAngelo, D.J.; Stelljes, M.; Martinelli, G.; Liedtke, M.; Stock, W.; Gökbuget, N.; O'Brien, S.; Wang, K.; Wang, T.; et al. Inotuzumab ozogamicin versus standard therapy for acute lymphoblastic leukemia. *N. Engl. J. Med.* **2016**, *375*, 740–753. [CrossRef]
151. Jabbour, E.; Ravandi, F.; Kebriaei, P.; Huang, X.; Short, N.J.; Thomas, D.; Sasaki, K.; Rytting, M.; Jain, N.; Konopleva, M.; et al. Salvage Chemoimmunotherapy With Inotuzumab Ozogamicin Combined with Mini-Hyper-CVD for Patients With Relapsed or Refractory Philadelphia Chromosome-Negative Acute Lymphoblastic Leukemia: A Phase 2 Clinical Trial. *JAMA Oncol.* **2018**, *4*, 230–234. [CrossRef]
152. Kebriaei, P.; Cutler, C.; de Lima, M.; Giralt, S.; Lee, S.J.; Marks, D.; Merchant, A.; Stock, W.; van Besien, K.; Stelljes, M. Management of important adverse events associated with inotuzumab ozogamicin: Expert panel review. *Bone Marrow Transpl.* **2018**, *53*, 449–456. [CrossRef] [PubMed]
153. Brivio, E.; Locatelli, F.; Lopez-Yurda, M.; Malone, A.; Díaz-de-Heredia, C.; Bielorai, B.; Rossig, C.; van der Velden, V.H.J.; Ammerlaan, A.C.; Thano, A.; et al. A Phase I study of inotuzumab ozogamicin in pediatric relapsed/refractory acute lymphoblastic leukemia (ITCC-059 study). *Blood* **2021**, *137*, 1582–1590. [CrossRef] [PubMed]

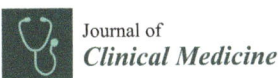

Review

Biologic and Therapeutic Implications of Genomic Alterations in Acute Lymphoblastic Leukemia

Ilaria Iacobucci [1,*], Shunsuke Kimura [1] and Charles G. Mullighan [1,2,*]

1. Department of Pathology, St. Jude Children's Research Hospital, 262 Danny Thomas Place, Memphis, TN 38105, USA; shunsuke.kimura@stjude.org
2. Comprehensive Cancer Center, Hematological Malignancies Program, St. Jude Children's Research Hospital, 262 Danny Thomas Place, Memphis, TN 38105, USA
* Correspondence: ilaria.iacobucci@stjude.org (I.I.); charles.mullighan@stjude.org (C.G.M.)

Abstract: Acute lymphoblastic leukemia (ALL) is the most successful paradigm of how risk-adapted therapy and detailed understanding of the genetic alterations driving leukemogenesis and therapeutic response may dramatically improve treatment outcomes, with cure rates now exceeding 90% in children. However, ALL still represents a leading cause of cancer-related death in the young, and the outcome for older adolescents and young adults with ALL remains poor. In the past decade, next generation sequencing has enabled critical advances in our understanding of leukemogenesis. These include the identification of risk-associated ALL subtypes (e.g., those with rearrangements of *MEF2D*, *DUX4*, *NUTM1*, *ZNF384* and *BCL11B*; the PAX5 P80R and IKZF1 N159Y mutations; and genomic phenocopies such as Ph-like ALL) and the genomic basis of disease evolution. These advances have been complemented by the development of novel therapeutic approaches, including those that are of mutation-specific, such as tyrosine kinase inhibitors, and those that are mutation-agnostic, including antibody and cellular immunotherapies, and protein degradation strategies such as proteolysis-targeting chimeras. Herein, we review the genetic taxonomy of ALL with a focus on clinical implications and the implementation of genomic diagnostic approaches.

Keywords: B-ALL; *DUX4*; *IKZF1*; *PAX5*; Ph-like; *ZNF384*; *NUTM1*; T-ALL; *NOTCH1*; *BCL11B*; transcriptome; genome

1. Introduction

Acute lymphoblastic leukemia (ALL) is the most frequent childhood tumor and despite cure rates now exceeding 90% in children, outcomes for older children and adults remain poor with cure rates below 40% in those over the age of 40 [1–3], despite pediatric-inspired chemotherapy regimens [4]. This discrepancy is in part attributable to the different prevalence of genetic alterations across age. ALL may be of B- (B-ALL) or T-lymphoid (T-ALL) lineage, and comprises over thirty distinct subtypes characterized by germline and somatic genetic alterations that converge on distinct gene expression profiles [5–12]. These subtypes are defined by disease-initiating recurrent chromosomal gains and losses (hyper- and hypodiploidy, and complex intrachromosomal amplification of chromosome 21); chromosomal rearrangements that deregulate oncogenes or encode chimeric fusion oncoproteins, importantly often including cryptic rearrangements not identifiable by conventional cytogenetic approaches, such as *DUX4* and *EPOR* rearrangements; subtypes defined by single point mutations (e.g., PAX5 P80R or IKZF1 N159Y); subtypes defined by enhancer hijacking (e.g., *BCL11B*-rearrangements in T-ALL and lineage ambiguous leukemia) [5]; and subtypes that "phenocopy" established subtypes, with similar gene expression profile but different founding alterations (e.g., *BCR-ABL1*-like ALL and *ETV6-RUNX1*-like ALL) [7,13–15]. Secondary somatic DNA copy number alterations and sequence mutations are also important in leukemogenesis and treatment response, and their nature and

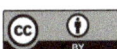

prevalence vary according to the ALL subtype [6]. Multiple genes are associated with predisposition to ALL, including polymorphic variants in *ARID5B, BAK1, CDKN2A, CDKN2B, CEBPE, ELK3, ERG, GATA3, IGF2BP1, IKZF1, IKZF3, LHPP, MYC, PTPRJ, TP63* and the *BMI1-PIP4K2A* locus or rare mutations in *PAX5, TP53, IKZF1* and *ETV6* [16]. Several are associated with ALL subtype, for example, variants in *GATA3* have been associated with an increased risk of Philadelphia- like (Ph-like) ALL in patients of Hispanic ancestry [17], variants in *TP63* and *PTPRJ* with *ETV6-RUNX1* ALL [18] and in *ERG* with *TCF3-PBX1* ALL and African American ancestry [19,20]. A variant in the deubiquitinase gene *USP7* has been instead associated with risk of T-lineage ALL [19].

Accurate identification of the genetic abnormalities that drive ALL is important to risk stratify disease, and to guide the incorporation of molecular targeted therapeutic approaches to reduce the risk of relapse. This has been previously relied upon conventional karyotyping, fluorescence in situ hybridization (FISH) and targeted-molecular analyses. However, studies from this past decade have highlighted the importance of next generation sequencing (NGS) approaches to identify cryptic genetic rearrangements, structural DNA variation and gene expression signatures otherwise not identifiable that demand a revision of diagnostic approaches. This review describes the current genomic landscape of B- and T-ALL, highlighting their genetic characterization and diagnostic classification, clinical features, and therapeutic implications.

2. B-Cell Precursor Acute Lymphoblastic Leukemia

2.1. Previously Established Subtypes with Recurring Chromosomal Abnormalities

Prior the advent of NGS, classification of ALL has been relied on conventional karyotyping, FISH and targeted-molecular analyses for the identification of recurring chromosomal abnormalities including aneuploidy, chromosomal rearrangements and/or known gene fusions (Figure 1).

2.1.1. Subtypes with Chromosomal Aneuploidy

Chromosomal aneuploidies [21], such as hyperdiploidy and hypodiploidy, are generally early initiating events acquired prenatally during fetal hematopoiesis and likely require secondary cooperating oncogenic insults to promote leukemia development [22].

High hyperdiploidy (modal number of 51–67 chromosomes, with nonrandom gains most commonly of chromosomes X, 4, 6, 10, 14, 17, 18, and 21) is present in 25–30% of ALL in children and is associated with young age (3–5 years) at diagnosis and favorable outcome [23,24]. Mutations of genes encoding mediators of Ras signaling (*KRAS, NRAS, FLT3, PTPN11*) and regulators of chromatin state (e.g., the histone 3 lysine 18 and 27 acetylase and transcriptional coregulator *CREBBP*, and the H3K36 methylase *WHSC1*) are frequent concomitant genetic events in high hyperdiploid ALL [23]. *CREBBP* mutations are enriched in the histone acetyl transferase domain and are selected during disease evolution [25]. As a potential mechanism for the generation of aneuploidy, hyperdiploid ALL blasts show a delay in early mitosis at prometaphase associated with defects in chromosome alignment, which lead to chromosome-segregation defects and nonmodal karyotypes [26]. Moreover, condensin complex activity is impaired, leading to chromosome hypocondensation, loss of centromere stiffness, and mislocalization of the chromosome passenger complex proteins Aurora B kinase (AURKB) and BIRC5 (survivin) in early mitosis [26]. Notwithstanding the favorable outcome of this subtype, condensin impairment suggests novel molecular targets (condensin-complex members, AURKB, or the spindle assembly checkpoint) for potential pharmacological intervention.

Hypodiploid ALL includes near haploid (24–31 chromosomes) and low hypodiploid (32–39 chromosomes) subtypes [27]. Near haploidy is present in ~2% of childhood ALL and is associated with Ras mutations (particularly *NF1*) and deletion/mutation of *IKZF3*. The gene expression profile and patterns of co-mutation (e.g., *CREBBP* and the Ras signaling pathway) are similar to high hyperdiploid ALL, suggesting a potential common origin of these two forms of leukemia. Low hypodiploidy instead is uncommon in children (~1%) but present in >10% of adults, and is characterized by deletion of *IKZF2*, *RB1*, *CDKN2A/CDKN2B* and near-universal mutations of *TP53* mutations, which are inherited in approximately half of cases and indicate that low hypodiploid ALL is a manifestation of Li-Fraumeni syndrome [28]. Duplication of the aneuploid genome, resulting in clones with 50 to 78 chromosomes, is common, with duplicated subclones present in the majority of cases. Predominance of the duplicated clone, known as masked hypodiploidy, may be misdiagnosed as high hyperdiploidy [29]. However, these states may usually be distinguished as the duplicated hypodiploid genome typically exhibits diploid and tetraploid chromosomes; in contrast high hyperdiploidy is characterized by a mixture of triploid and some tetraploid chromosomes (e.g., chromosomes 21, X). Moreover, the pattern of chromosomal losses in hypodiploid ALL is not random and chromosome 21 is never lost indicating a central role in leukemic cell fitness [27]. Hypodiploid ALL is associated with unfavorable outcome, although this is mitigated by minimal residual disease (MRD) risk-stratified therapy in several studies [30]. Moreover, for patients who achieve MRD-negative status after induction, allogeneic transplantation has been shown to be not successful in improving overall survival [31,32]. Although MRD-oriented protocols, older adults and elderly patients with low hypodiploidy do fairly poor with higher five-year cumulative incidence of relapse compared to high hypodiploid cases [33], making them candidates for different treatment approaches (e.g., immunotherapy and targeted therapies). Among those, preclinical studies have shown that hypodiploid ALL cells are sensitive to Phosphoinositide 3-kinase (PI3K) and BCL2 Apoptosis Regulator (BCL2) inhibitors [27,34].

2.1.2. iAMP21

Intrachromosomal amplification of chromosome 21 (iAMP21) accounts for 1% of childhood ALL and is associated with older children (median age at diagnosis 9 years) and a low white cell count. Behind the formation of this chromosomal abnormality there is a characteristic mechanism of breakage–fusion–bridge cycles followed by chromothripsis and other complex structural rearrangements of chromosome 21 [35]. Two germline genomic alterations are associated with a markedly elevated risk of iAMP21. These are a germline Robertsonian translocation rob (15;21) and a germline ring chromosome 21 [36]. The presence of iAMP21 is associated with poor prognosis in most studies, although this has been improved with intensive treatment [37].

2.1.3. Subtypes with Recurrent Chromosomal Translocations and/or Gene Fusions

The t(12;21)(p13;q22) translocation with the *ETV6-RUNX1* (*TEL-AML1*) fusion is the most common alteration in childhood B-ALL occurring in 20–25% of cases [38–40]. The *ETV6-RUNX1* fusion is considered to be a leukemia-initiating alteration which arises in utero, as demonstrated by the identification in umbilical cord blood [39] and by the prenatal monoclonal origin in identical twins [41]. The typically prolonged latency from birth to clinically manifest leukemia indicates that *ETV6-RUNX1* alone requires cooperating genetic events to induce leukemia, including deletion of the non-rearranged *ETV6* allele, focal deletion of *PAX5* and mutation of *WHSC1* [39,42–44].

The t(1;19)(q23;p13) translocation encoding *TCF3-PBX1* defines a subtype of 5–6% of pediatric B-ALL but only 1% of adult cases. This fusion is associated with a pre-B immunophenotype and expression of cytoplasmic immunoglobulin heavy chain and with higher peripheral blood white cell count at diagnosis [6,7,45]. Current intensive treatment has changed the historically high risk of *TCF3-PBX1* childhood ALL that was in part ascribed to central nervous system (CNS) involvement and relapse in favorable and intermediate risk cases [46,47]. *TCF3-PBX1* leukemic cells may be amenable to inhibition of pre-BCR signaling by dasatinib and ponatinib [48,49]. This approach may lead to compensatory upregulation of *ROR1* expression, and thus, concomitant inhibition of ROR1 could enhance the sensitivity of dasatinib [50]. *TCF3* and *TCF4* are also rearranged to *HLF*, and define a rare subtype of ALL (<1%) associated with an extremely poor prognosis [3,7]. *TCF3-PBX1* and *TCF3-HLF* ALL have distinct gene expression profiles and mutational landscapes [7,51]. *TCF3-HLF* ALL is associated with expression of stem cell and myeloid markers, alterations of *PAX5* (deletions) and the Ras signaling pathway [7,51] and sensitivity to therapies inhibiting BCL2 and the pre-B cell receptor [52,53], immunologic therapies [54], and to Aurora A kinase inhibitors [55].

Rearrangements of the mixed-lineage leukemia 1 (*MLL1*) gene (now renamed Lysine [K]-specific methyl transferase 2A or *KMT2A*) on chromosome 11q23 to over 80 different partner genes define a subtype of leukemia with lymphoid and myeloid features and poor prognosis [12,56]. It occurs predominantly in infants (~80%), with a second peak of onset in adulthood where the most common partner of rearrangement is *AFF1* [57]. It is typically associated with pro-B (CD10-) immunophenotype, and expression of myeloid markers. Irrespective of fusion partner or lineage phenotype this subtype shows a distinct gene expression signature with overexpression of *HOX* cluster genes and the HOX cofactor *MEIS1* [58,59]. In infant *KMT2A*-rearranged ALL, the PI3K and Ras pathways are commonly altered [7,60,61]. *KMT2A* rearrangement is associated with altered chromatin patterning including H3K79 methylation, which has stimulated development of novel therapeutic approaches including inhibition of DOT1L [62], bromodomain, Menin, and the polycomb repressive complex [57,63,64]. The lineage plasticity characteristic of *KMT2A*-rearranged ALL is important in the context of immunotherapy, as this may facilitate loss of expression of CD19 and escape from CD19 Chimeric antigen receptor T cell (CAR-T) therapy [65].

The frequency of patients with *BCR-ABL1* (Philadelphia chromosome) arising from the t(9;22)(q34;q11) translocation increases with age with 2–5% in childhood, 6% in adolescents and young adults (AYA), and more than 25% in adults [66,67]. Although historically considered a high-risk subtype, the incorporation of tyrosine kinase inhibitors (TKIs) into the standard treatment regimen for *BCR-ABL1*-positive ALL significantly improved clinical outcomes [68–70]. Secondary cooperative mutations are *IKZF1*, *PAX5* and *CDKN2A/B* deletions [42,69,71,72]. *IKZF1* alterations (most commonly deletions) have been associated with unfavorable outcome irrespective of TKI exposure [68,73], especially when co-occurring with (*CDKN2A* or *CDKN2B*, *PAX5*, or both: *IKZF1*^{plus}) [68,69].

2.2. Emerging B-ALL Subtypes Defined by Genome Sequencing Studies

NGS approaches, particularly whole transcriptome sequencing (WTS), have enabled several research groups the identification of a large number of novel genetic alterations. These include cryptic rearrangements not identifiable by conventional approaches; novel subtypes that "phenocopy" established subtypes sharing similar gene expression profile but having different founding alterations; and subtypes defined by a single point mutation.

2.2.1. *DUX4*, *MEF2D*, *ZNF384* and *NUTM1* Gene Fusions

Translocation of *DUX4* to the immunoglobulin heavy chain locus (*IGH*) is a cytogenetically cryptic alteration occurring in 5–10% of B-ALL and resulting in overexpression of a 3′ truncated DUX4 protein [7,13,74–77]. *DUX4* is located within the D4Z4 subtelomeric repeat element on chromosome 4q/10q and encodes a double homeobox transcription factor that activates expression of large number of genes in early developing embryos, but it is thereafter silenced in most somatic cells [78]. Aberrant *DUX4* expression is associated with facioscapulohumeral dystrophy (FSHD) [79], while *DUX4* rearrangements have been also identified in Ewing-like sarcoma [80] and rhabdomyosarcoma [81]. In B-ALL, truncated DUX4 protein binds to an intragenic region of *ERG* resulting in transcriptional deregulation, and commonly, expression of a C-terminal ERG protein fragment, and/or *ERG* deletion. This subtype has a very distinctive gene expression profile and immunophenotype (CD2 and CD371 positive), common deletions of *IKZF1* (40%) and despite this, excellent outcome [76,77,82,83]. Accurate identification of all cases of *DUX4*-rearranged ALL requires direct identification of rearrangement (e.g., by WTS), or alternatively, gene expression-based clustering or high *DUX4* expression. The detection of strong CD371 cell surface expression by flow cytometry is a promising surrogate marker for this subtype [84].

Although *ERG* deletion is common in, and largely restricted to *DUX4*-rearranged ALL, these deletions are secondary events, commonly subclonal, and not present in all cases. Thus, the use of *ERG* deletion as a surrogate for identification of *DUX4*-rearranged ALL is suboptimal and should be avoided.

MEF2D (myocyte enhancer factor 2D) rearrangements occur in ~4% of childhood and 10% adult B-ALL cases. This subtype shows a distinct immunophenotype with low/absent expression of CD10, and positivity for CD38 and cytoplasmic µ chain, and distinct expression profiles [7,85–88]. *MEF2D* is the 5′ partner in all described fusions, whereas B-cell CLL/lymphoma (*BCL*) 9 and heterogeneous nuclear ribonucleoprotein U-like 1 (*HNRNPUL1*) are the two most recurrent 3′ partners. The rearrangements result in enhanced MEF2D transcriptional activity, increased *HDAC9* expression and sensitivity to histone deacetylase inhibitors, such as panobinostat [85]. MEF2D has also been implicated in a core transcription factor regulatory circuit involving SREBF1 that regulates pre-BCR and lipid metabolism, that are therapeutic vulnerabilities [89]. Sensitivity to staurosporine and venetoclax has been also described [90]. *MEF2D*-rearranged ALL shows high levels of minimal residual disease and is considered to be an unfavorable subtype because of its poor event-free survival rates [82,83].

ZNF384-, or less commonly, *ZNF362*-rearranged acute leukemia is a biologically and clinically distinct leukemic subtype present in ~6% of childhood, 7.3% of adult, and 15% of AYA B-ALL, and in 48% of B/myeloid mixed phenotype acute leukemia (MPAL) [7,13,91–93]. These cases show a characteristic immunophenotype with weak CD10 and aberrant expression of the myeloid markers, CD13, and/or CD33 [92,94]. Expression of myeloperoxidase (MPO) is often the only feature distinguishing cases diagnosed as B-ALL (MPO−) or B/myeloid MPAL (MPO+). Different fusion partners, usually transcription factor (e.g., *TAF15* and *TCF3*) or chromatin modifiers (e.g., *CREBBP*, *EP300*, *SMARCA2*, and *ARID1B*) have been identified for ZNF384, with EP300 being the most common. In all rearrangements the zinc-finger domains of the C2H2-type zinc-finger transcription factors ZNF384/ZNF362 are retained [7,13,91,92,95]. The same cooperating genetic alterations and transcriptional profile is observed in *ZNF384*-rearranged B-ALL and MPAL, and both exhibit lineage plasticity during disease progression (e.g., with shift in immunophenotype from lymphoid to myeloid from diagnosis to relapse). *ZNF384* rearrangements are acquired in a subset of hematopoietic stem cells and prime leukemia cells for lineage plasticity [92]. A report of *ZNF384*-rearranged ALL in twins implicated a fetal hematopoietic progenitor as the cell of origin confirming that these rearrangements are founder alterations [96]. Prognosis varies by fusion partner: the *EP300-ZNF384* fusion is associated with favorable outcome while the *TCF3-ZNF384* fusion is frequently associated with late relapses and a poor prognosis [92,93]. However, overexpression of *FLT3*, characteristic of this subtype, makes this leukemia amenable to FLT3 inhibition [97].

NUTM1 (nuclear protein in testis midline carcinoma family 1) rearrangements (<2% of childhood B-ALL and mostly infant without *KMT2A*-rearrangements) [7,13,88,98–100] are characterized by fusion of *NUTM1* to different partners, including transcription factors and epigenetic regulators (e.g., *ACIN1*, *AFF1*, *ATAD5*, *BRD9*, *CHD4*, *CUX1*, *IKZF1*, *RUNX1*, *SLC12A6*, and *ZNF618*), that drive aberrant *NUTM1* expression [7,13]. In all fusions, the NUT domain is retained, and this is hypothesized to lead to global changes in chromatin acetylation [101] and to sensitivity to histone deacetylase inhibitors or bromodomain inhibitors in case of fusions with BRD9. *NUTM1* rearrangements confer an excellent prognosis to current therapeutic approaches [82,83,98]. Since not all *NUTM1* fusions are detectable by karyotyping either break-apart FISH or, preferably, WTS are the best approaches for diagnosis. In addition, the finding that both RNA expression of the 3′ exons and protein expression are highly specific for this subtype may help in diagnosis.

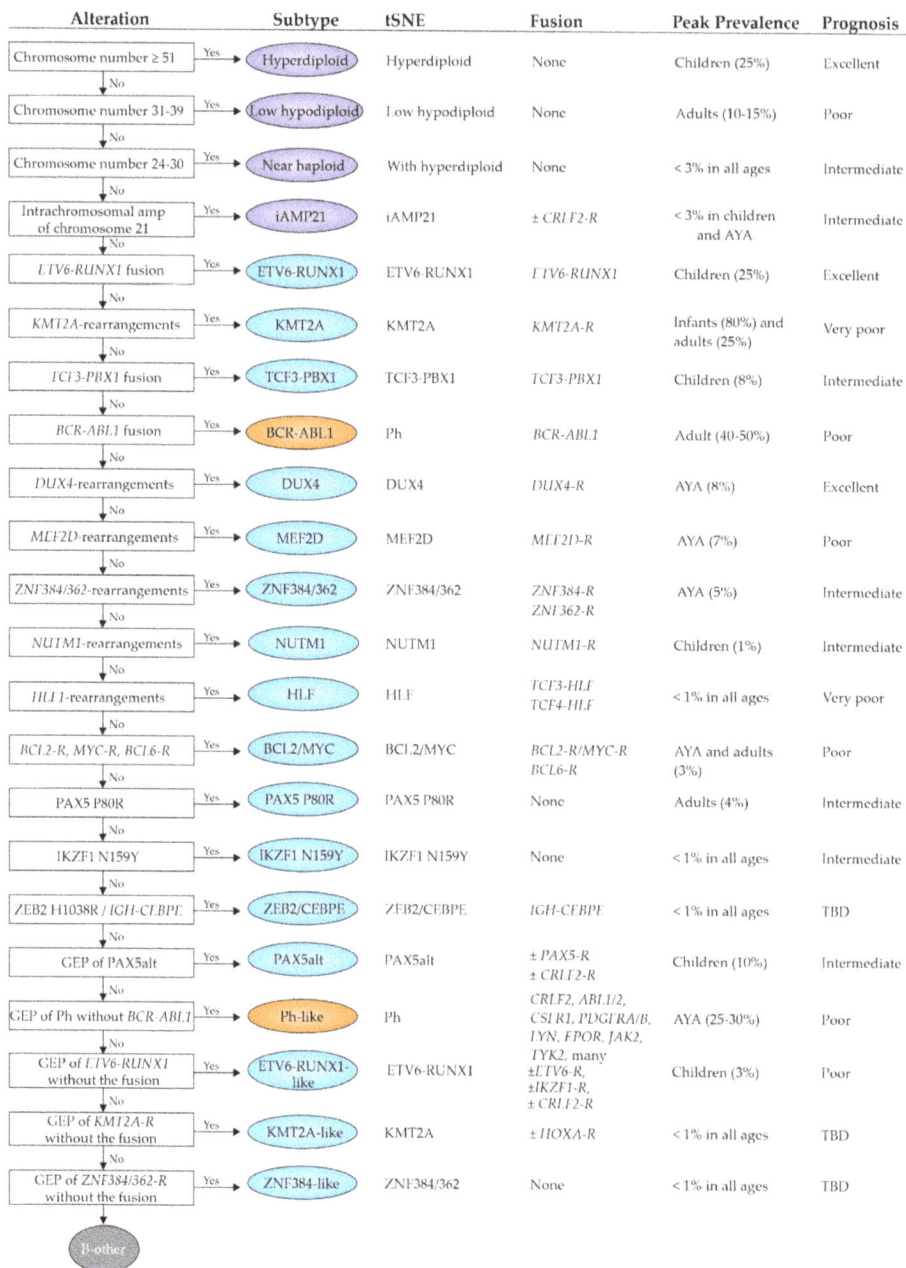

Figure 1. This schematic algorithm for B-ALL subtyping was modified from the figure originally published in Paietta E. et al. Molecular Classification Improves Risk Assessment in Adult BCR-ABL1-negative B-ALL. Blood Prepublished Apr 25 2021; doi:10.1182/blood.2020010144 [83]. This figure describes each B-ALL subtype according to the specific genetic alterations and gene expression profile. Moreover, for each subtype peak prevalence and prognosis are shown. Subtypes are colored according to defining genetic alteration: gross chromosomal abnormalities (purple), transcription factor rearrangements (blue), other transcription factor alterations (blue), and kinase alterations (orange). Abbreviations: AYA, adolescent and young adult; tSNE, t-distributed stochastic neighbor embedding; TBD: to be defined; -R: rearranged.

2.2.2. Subtypes That Phenocopy Established Subtypes

Ph-Like ALL

Ph-like or *BCR-ABL1*-like ALL is characterized by a gene expression signature similar to that of Ph-positive ALL but lacking the pathognomonic BCR-ABL1 oncoprotein of Ph+ ALL [15,66,102–110]. Its incidence ranges from ~10–15% in children to ~20% in older adults, with a peak (25–30%) in the AYA ALL population. Similar to patients with Ph+ ALL, patients with Ph-like ALL often exhibit adverse clinical features and poor outcome and frequently harbor alterations of *IKZF1* or other B-lymphoid transcription factor genes. Over 60 heterogenous genetic alterations in kinases and cytokine receptors drive constitutively active kinase or cytokine receptor signaling, many of which have been shown to be druggable with a variety of kinase inhibitors. The most commonly mutated pathways are the ABL and JAK-STAT pathways with multiple rearrangements and lesions that converge on downstream ABL/JAK-STAT signaling. Founder alterations may be grouped into three broad types: (i) JAK/STAT alterations including: mutations activating cytokine receptors (e.g., *CRLF2* and *IL7R*); enhancer hijacking gene rearrangements deregulating cytokine receptor expression (e.g., *IGH-CRLF2* and *P2RY8–CRLF2*) [111–114]; gene fusions and/or mutations activating kinases (e.g., *JAK1, JAK2, JAK3, TYK2*); and rearrangements hijacking and truncating cytokine receptor expression (e.g., cryptic *EPOR* rearrangements) [115]; (ii) fusions involving ABL-class genes (*ABL1, ABL2, CSF1R, LYN, PDGFRA, PDGFRB*); and (iii) less common fusions (*FLT3, FGFR1, NTRK3, PTK2B*) [109] whose number is growing with increasing sequencing studies of different cohorts. Among these, alterations of *CRLF2* are present in approximately half of Ph-like ALL in AYAs and adults. *CRLF2* is located in the pseudoautosomal region of the sex chromosomes (*PAR1*) at Xp22.3/Yp11.3, and its alterations include: (1) a cryptic rearrangement that juxtaposes *CRLF2* to the IGH locus; (2) a focal deletion in the pseudoautosomal region of the sex chromosomes resulting in P2Y receptor family member 8 (*P2RY8*)-*CRLF2* fusion that positions *CRLF2* under the control of the *P2RY8* promoter; and less frequently by (3) an activating *CRLF2* point mutation, F232C. PAR1 deletions, as a surrogate for rearrangement of *CRLF2*, have been incorporated into the criteria for "*IKZF1*^{plus}", a designation based on DNA copy number profiling, commonly by single nucleotide polymorphism (SNP) or multiplex ligation-dependent probe amplification (MLPA) arrays. In some studies, *IKZF1*^{plus} has been associated with a higher risk of relapse defined by co-occurrence of the *IKZF1* deletion with deletion of *CDKN2A, CDKN2B, PAX5*, and/or PAR1 region in the absence of *ERG* deletion [116]. Notably, however, the *IKZF1*^{plus} designation typically does not consider cases with *IGH-CRLF2* due to the inability of these platforms to detect this alteration.

The heterogeneous genomic landscape and often cytogenetically cryptic alterations identified in Ph-like ALL may make diagnosis of this entity and its driver alterations challenging, but several tractable diagnostic approaches are available, depending on technical capability of a laboratory, and the desired clinical/diagnostic endpoint (e.g., identification of the gene expression profile of Ph-like ALL c.f. identification of the most common driver kinase alterations). Comprehensive clinical NGS, including WTS, is the best approach to identify Ph-like ALL patients with targetable kinase alterations, as it enables analysis of gene expression, fusions, aneuploidy and sequence mutations. Selective/capture-based sequencing approaches (e.g., Archer FusionPlex, and FoundationOne Heme) also identify the majority of kinase-deregulating rearrangements in Ph-like ALL. If genomic approaches are not available, a more targeted screening approach using routine diagnostics, including flow cytometry (especially for *CRLF2*, for which positivity on flow cytometry is strongly correlated with rearrangement) and FISH for the most common kinase targets of rearrangement, is still effective for swift identification of Ph-like ALL [104]. The identification of specific genetic lesions is important for guiding targeted therapeutic intervention as a proportion of kinase-activating alterations in Ph-like ALL can, at least based on in vitro and preclinical models, be targeted by FDA-approved TKIs: JAK-STAT signaling (JAK inhibition); ABL-class fusions (ABL inhibitor); FLT3 and NTRK3 fusions (FLT3 and NTRK3 inhibitor) [104]. Several recent studies have described the efficacy of

ABL1 and NTRK inhibitors in the treatment of Ph-like ALL cases with rearrangement of these genes [117,118]. Combinatorial use of kinase inhibitors against multiple signaling has shown synergism in patient-derived xenograft (PDX) models of CRLF2/JAK mutant (JAK and PI3K/mTOR inhibitors), ABL/PDGFR mutant (dasatinib and PI3K/mTOR inhibitor) and EPOR-rearranged (ponatinib and ruxolitinib) [119]. Moreover, recently dual JAK/GSPT1-degrading proteolysis-targeting chimeras PROTACs have been developed and showed efficacy in Ph-like B-ALL kinase-driven PDX models which were otherwise unresponsive to type I JAK inhibitors [120]. Lastly, the use of immunotherapeutic agents, such as blinatumomab, inotuzumab, and CAR-T cells (including those targeting CRLF2 [121], represents a promising alternative approach for this subtype which is irrespective of a specific genetic alteration or response to prior chemotherapies [104]).

ETV6-RUNX1-like ALL

ETV6-RUNX1-like ALL is characterized by a gene expression profile and immunophenotype (CD27 positive, CD44 low to negative) similar to *ETV6-RUNX1* ALL, but lacking the *ETV6-RUNX1* fusion [122] and favorable prognosis [7,13,75,122,123]. These cases harbor alternate gene fusions or copy number alterations in ETS family transcription factors (*ETV6, ERG, FLI1*), *IKZF1* or *TCF3*. *ETV6-RUNX1*-like ALL develops in children harboring germline *ETV6* mutations with subsequent somatic alterations of the second *ETV6* allele, consistent with the notion that biallelic alteration of *ETV6* is central in leukemogenesis [124]. It is more common children (~3%) and confers an unfavorable prognosis in children due to high levels of MRD and worst event-free survival rates [82].

2.2.3. Subtypes Defined by a Single Point Mutation
PAX5 P80R and PAX5alt

The PAX5 P80R subtype (~3% of B-ALL cases) is characterized by the presence of a hot spot mutation at amino acid 80 in the DNA binding domain of the paired box DNA-binding transcription factor PAX5 [7,13,125,126]. B-ALL cases with PAX5 P80R show a distinct gene expression profile with the majority of cases having either hemizygous or homozygous mutation, caused by deletion of the wild-type *PAX5* allele or copy-neutral loss of heterozygosity. In a subset of cases, in addition to PAX5 P80R there is a second frameshift, nonsense or deleterious missense *PAX5* mutation. Thus, biallelic *PAX5* alterations—with mutation of one allele and loss of activity of the second allele—are a hallmark of this subtype [7,125]. In support of the role of biallelic alteration of *PAX5* in the pathogenesis of this subtype, knock-in mouse models of germline *Pax5* mutations have shown that heterozygous Pax5$^{P80R/+}$ knock-in mice develop transplantable B-ALL, with genetic inactivation of the wildtype *Pax5* allele [7]. In contrast, Pax5$^{G183S/+}$ knock in mice (modeling the germline PAX5 G183S mutation observed in familial ALL) show a low penetrance of ALL [127], supporting its role as a haploinsufficient tumor suppressor. Additional important cooperating lesions include *CDKN2A* loss and signaling pathway mutations, most commonly in Ras signaling genes or in the JAK/STAT pathway [7,125].

PAX5alt comprises about 7% cases with diverse *PAX5* alterations, including rearrangements, sequence mutations and focal intragenic amplifications [7]. Over 20 different partner genes have been identified with *PAX5-ETV6* being the most common. Children in this subtype are more commonly classified as high risk rather than standard risk (according to National Cancer Institute (NCI) criteria). In addition to *PAX5* alterations, recurrent genetic lesions observed in these cases include copy number losses affecting cell-cycle regulation genes such as *CDKN2A, RB1* and *BTG1*, B-cell development genes, transcriptional regulators and/or epigenetic modifiers (for example, *KDM6A, KMT2A* and *ATRX*) [7]. Both PAX5 P80R and PAX5alt subtypes are associated with intermediate to favorable prognosis [7,82,83,126].

IKZF1 N159Y

IKZF1 encodes the transcription factor IKAROS, which is a member of the family of zinc finger DNA-binding proteins required for lymphoid lineage ontogeny and homeostasis [128,129]. The most common type of *IKZF1* alteration is a focal deletion occurring in 15% of ALL cases and in >50% of high risk ALL [42,72,103]. Deletions result in loss-of-function or in the dominant negative IK6 isoform and are associated with poor outcome [73,103]. In addition to deletions, missense, frameshift and nonsense mutations have been also described in pediatric high-risk B-ALL patients. Among those the missense p.Asn159Tyr mutation defines a subtype (<1% of B-ALL) with a distinct gene expression profile characterized by upregulation of genes with roles in oncogenesis (the IKZF1-interacting gene *YAP1*), chromatin remodeling (*SALL1*), and signaling (*ARHGEF28*) that are not deregulated in other subgroups of *IKZF1*-altered ALL [7,74]. In contrast to PAX5 P80R ALL, the nonmutated wild-type allele of the mutated transcription factor (here *IKZF1*) is retained [72]. As for most other missense mutations observed in IKZF1 zinc fingers, IKZF1 N159Y induces misregulation of IKZF1 transcriptional activation, in part through distinctive nuclear mislocalization and enhanced intercellular adhesion [130].

ZEB2 H1038R and IGH-CEBPE

In unsupervised clustering of leukemic cell gene expression, cases with the H1038R mutation in *ZEB2* phenocopy the translocation t(14;14)(q11;q32) [13], which results in IGH-CEBPE fusion, suggesting a common activated pathway of leukemogenesis and defining a rare B-ALL subtype (<1%). This is associated with *NRAS* sequence mutations (>50% of cases), upregulation of *LMO1* and downregulation of *SMAD1* and *BMP2* [10]. However, neither the *IGH* or *ZEB2* mutations are unique to this group, nor do they explain all cases in this distinct gene expression and experimental validation is required to demonstrate their role as leukemogenic drivers. B-ALL with *ZEB2* mutation is associated with poor event-free survival and high relapse [131].

2.3. Prognostic Implications

The frequent and wide use of genomics to profile the landscape of ALL has allowed a tailored refinement of risk in association with standard criteria, such as MRD levels [82] (Figure 1). In childhood B-ALL, *ETV6-RUNX1*, high-hyperdiploid, and *DUX4*-rearranged B-ALL are categorized as favorable due the highest overall survival rates and the lowest relapse rates, despite elevated early MRD in *DUX4*-rearranged cases. *BCR-ABL1*, *BCR-ABL1*-like, *ETV6-RUNX1*-like, *KMT2A*-rearranged, and *MEF2D*-rearranged ALL show high levels of MRD and the worst event-free survival rates and thus are categorized as unfavorable subtypes. The remaining subtypes including *TCF3-PBX1*, *PAX5*alt, iAMP21, hypodiploid, *ZNF384*-rearranged, *NUTM1*-rearranged, and *PAX5* P80R ALL have intermediate risk [81]. These prognostic groups have been mostly confirmed in a historic, non-MRD risk adapted trial (UKALLXII/ECOG-ACRIN E2993, NCT00002514) in adolescents and adult B-ALL cases [83] according to the following risk assignment: standard risk genotypes: *DUX4*-rearranged, *ETV6-RUNX1*/-like, *TCF3-PBX1*, PAX5 P80R, high-hyperdiploid; high-risk genotypes: Ph-like, *KMT2A-AFF1*, low-hypodiploid/near-haploid, BCL2/MYC-rearranged; and intermediate-risk genotypes: *PAX5*alt, *ZNF384*/-like, and *MEF2D*-rearranged.

3. T-Cell Acute Lymphoblastic Leukemia (T-ALL)

3.1. Genomic Overview of T-ALL

T-ALL leukemic cells express a subset of T-cell makers (CD3, cyCD3, CD2, CD5, CD7, CD8) and arises from immature T-cell progenitors [132,133]. Pediatric T-ALL accounts for 10–15% of newly diagnosed pediatric ALL and is characterized by higher incidence in boys, high initial white blood cell counts, mediastinal mass, CNS infiltration, and slightly worse prognosis compared to B-ALL [134]. The majority of T-ALL cases may be subclassified into subtypes according to the aberrant expression and dysregulated pathways of transcription factors and oncogenes induced by leukemia-initiating alterations involving basic helix–loop–helix (bHLH) factors (*TAL1, TAL2, LYL1*), homeobox genes (*TLX1* (*HOX11*), *TLX3* (*HOX11L2*), *NKX2-1, NKX2-5, HOXA*), *LMO1, LMO2, MYB, BCL11B* and *SPI1* (Figure 2) [5,135,136]. These subtypes are defined with expression profiles by WTS or microarray, however, almost half of these leukemia-initiating alterations in T-ALL show intergenic breakpoints that can be missed by WTS but rescued by whole genome sequencing (WGS) [135,136]. Epigenomic analyses have also identified novel leukemia-initiating alterations in non-coding regions [5,137,138].

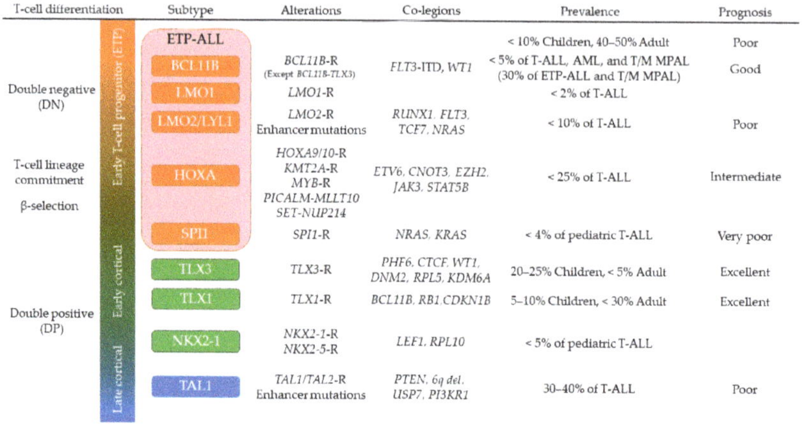

T-cell differentiation		Subtype	Alterations	Co-legions	Prevalence	Prognosis
Double negative (DN)	Early T-cell progenitor (ETP)	ETP-ALL			< 10% Children, 40–50% Adult	Poor
		BCL11B	BCL11B-R (Except BCL11B-TLX3)	FLT3-ITD, WT1	< 5% of T-ALL, AML, and T/M MPAL (30% of ETP-ALL and T/M MPAL)	Good
		LMO1	LMO1-R		< 2% of T-ALL	
T-cell lineage commitment		LMO2/LYL1	LMO2-R Enhancer mutations	RUNX1, FLT3, TCF7, NRAS	< 10% of T-ALL	Poor
β-selection		HOXA	HOXA9/10-R KMT2A-R MYB-R PICALM-MLLT10 SET-NUP214	ETV6, CNOT3, EZH2, JAK3, STAT5B	< 25% of T-ALL	Intermediate
		SPI1	SPI1-R	NRAS, KRAS	< 4% of pediatric T-ALL	Very poor
Double positive (DP)	Early cortical	TLX3	TLX3-R	PHF6, CTCF, WT1, DNM2, RPL5, KDM6A	20–25% Children, < 5% Adult	Excellent
		TLX1	TLX1-R	BCL11B, RB1, CDKN1B	5–10% Children, < 30% Adult	Excellent
		NKX2-1	NKX2-1-R NKX2-5-R	LEF1, RPL10	< 5% of pediatric T-ALL	
	Late cortical	TAL1	TAL1/TAL2-R Enhancer mutations	PTEN, 6q del, USP7, PI3KR1	30–40% of T-ALL	Poor

Figure 2. T-cell differentiation and T-ALL subtyping. This schema describes differentiation stages of each T-ALL subtype according to the specific genetic alterations leading to aberrant expression of rearranged or mutated genes. Prevalence and prognosis of each subtype are shown. Subtypes are colored according to corresponding normal T-cell differentiation stage: early T-cell precursor (ETP, red and orange), early stages of cortical thymocytes maturation (green), and late stages of cortical thymocytes maturation (blue). Abbreviations: T-ALL: T-cell acute lymphoblastic leukemia; T/M MPAL: T/myeloid mixed phenotype acute leukemia; -R: rearranged.

NOTCH1 activating mutations and deletion of *CDKN2A*/*CDKN2B* loci (9p21) are found in over 70% of T-ALL cases and considered as secondary but core events in leukemogenesis [135,136,139]. Concurrent somatic mutations and copy number alterations are frequently observed in T-ALL leading to dysregulation of several cellular pathways, including JAK-STAT signaling (*IL7R, JAK1, JAK3, DNM2*), Ras signaling (*NRAS, KRAS,* and *NF1*), PI3K-AKT signaling (*PTEN, AKT1, PIK3CA PIK3CD*), epigenetic regulation (*PHF6, SUZ12, EZH2, KDM6A*), transcription factors and regulators (*ETV6, GATA3, RUNX1, LEF1, WT1, BCL11B*), and translation regulators (*CNOT3, RPL5, RPL10*) [135,136,140,141]. Accumulation of these aberrant expression and dysregulated pathways disrupt the normal T-cell differentiation, proliferation, and survival, and results in T-ALL with unique gene expression signatures reflecting the point of differentiation arrest during T-cell development [133,140]. In addition to expression profiles, DNA methylation signatures are also associated with immunophenotypic profiles and normal T-cell development differentiation stage [142,143].

3.2. T-ALL in Early Stages of Cortical Thymocyte Maturation

T-ALL with CD1a$^+$, CD4$^+$, and CD8$^+$ immunophenotype includes several subgroups, such as rearrangements of *TLX1, TLX3, NKX2-1*, reflecting a differentiation arrest in early stages of cortical thymocyte maturation and confers a relatively favorable prognosis [144,145]. These subgroups almost commonly harbor *NOTCH1* and *CDKN2A* alterations. Dysregulated expression of HOX transcription factor genes is mostly induced by chromosomal translocations and inversions that juxtapose these genes to enhancers in the *TCR* and

BCL11B regulatory regions [135,146]. Importantly, BCL11B rearrangements (BCL11B-TLX3) in this subgroup are mechanistically distinct from those identified in BCL11B-rearranged lineage ambiguous leukemias, in that in the BCL11B-TLX3 leukemia, the BCL11B enhancer is used for aberrant expression of TLX3 at the cost of the loss of expression of BCL11B, leading to complete difference in expression profiles [5,146,147]. Instead, TLX3 rearranged T-ALL (including BCL11B-TLX3) shares gene expression signatures, DNA methylation profiles, somatic mutations (BCL11B, WT1, PHF6, DNM2), and downstream targets (JAK-STAT, epigenetic regulators) with TLX1 rearranged T-ALL [135,136,142,143,145]. Some of overlapping genomic features with TLX1/TLX3 rearranged T-ALL, including NUP214-ABL1 (TKIs) and JAK-STAT pathway (ruxolitinib, a JAK-STAT inhibitor), can be targetable and have been incorporated into ongoing clinical trials [148].

3.3. TAL1-Driven T-ALL with Late Stages of Cortical Thymocyte Maturation

Deregulation of the TAL1 oncogene is a feature of T-ALL that typically exhibits a late cortical thymocyte immunophenotype (CD4$^+$, CD8$^+$, CD3$^+$) and comprises approximately 40% of T-ALL [135,136]. This T-ALL subtype includes TAL1 and TAL2 rearranged cases and is further classified into two subgroups by expression profiles whose one expresses PTCRA (pre-TCR) suggesting LCK activation that correlated with dasatinib sensitivity [136,145,149]. During normal T-cell differentiation, TAL1 expression is transcriptionally silenced along with T-cell lineage commitment to proceed appropriate TCR rearrangements and differentiation [133]. TAL1 overexpression is induced by several mechanisms: (1) chromosomal translocations with TCRA/D; (2) sub-microscopic interstitial deletion (STIL-TAL1); (3) disruption of insulated neighborhoods by losing CTCF binding sites [150]; and (4) somatic indels in a noncoding intergenic regulatory element upstream of TAL1 to generate aberrant MYB binding site (MuTE) [137]. The latter two mechanisms have benefited of NGS technologies for their identification. Dysregulated TAL1 expression inhibits the function of E-protein dimers by forming TAL1-E-protein heterodimer [151]. Furthermore, TAL1 forms the central node of the core regulatory circuit to coordinately regulate downstream target genes with several hematopoietic transcription factors including GATA3, RUNX1, MYB, and the ETS family genes, which is active in normal hematopoietic stem cell (HSC) and progenitor cells [152,153], and RUNX1 inhibition is reported to impair the growth of T-ALL but not normal hematopoietic cells [154]. However, although TAL1 functions as a master transcription factor related to T-cell differentiation and leukemogenesis of T-ALL, only 30% of transgenic mice develop T-ALL after a latent period, indicating that additional abnormalities are required for leukemogenesis [155]. Expression of Lmo2 accelerates the onset of leukemia in Tal1 transgenic mice, and LMO1/LMO2 are commonly expressed in human TAL1-driven T-ALL [156,157]. Other cooperative genes and noncoding RNAs in TAL1-driven T-ALL include ARID5B, ARIEL, and MYC, driving aberrant expression of TAL1 [158,159]. In addition, PI3K-AKT pathway genes including PTEN are frequently mutated in this subgroup [135,136], which associates with glucocorticoid resistance and can be reversed by the inhibition of this pathway [160]. Several cell cycle regulators including CDK6 and CCND3 are regulated by TAL1 complex [152] and may be potential targets of therapeutic intervention [161].

3.4. Early T-Cell Precursor (ETP) ALL and Mixed Phenotype Acute Leukemia

ETP-ALL is often referred to as a subtype of T-ALL as it exhibits an immunophenotype analogous to the earliest stages of T-cell development (cytoplasmic CD3$^+$, CD7$^+$; CD8$^-$, CD1a$^-$, CD5^{weak}), and with expression of myeloid and/or stem-cell markers [144,162]. However, the genomic alterations and gene expression profile of ETP-ALL are more similar to a hematopoietic stem cell than a T cell precursor, suggesting that ETP-ALL could be included in a subgroup of immature acute leukemias of ambiguous lineage (ALAL), originating from a hematopoietic progenitor at a maturational stage prior to initiation of a definitive program of T cell differentiation. Consistent with this, recent studies have defined a subgroup of BCL11B-deregulated ALAL, that includes one third of ETP-ALL and T/myeloid mixed phenotype acute leukemia (T/M MPAL) cases with a very distinct expression profile [5]. *BCL11B*-deregulated ALAL is characterized by structural variations of the region containing *BCL11B* at 14q32 including translocations and high-copy amplification generating a distal neo-enhancer, that each leads to aberrant expression of *BCL11B*, in the case of the rearrangements by hijacking super-enhancers active in CD34+ hematopoietic stem and progenitor cell (HSPCs) [5,147]. *FLT3* activating mutations were found in 80% of *BCL11B*-deregulated ALAL, and concurrent expression of *BCL11B* and FLT3-ITD on HSPC exhibited synergistic effects on activating T-cell directed differentiation to express cytoplasmic CD3 while blocking myeloid differentiation [5]. Other genomic features of ETP-ALL include a subgroup of aberrant expression of PU.1 (*SPI1* fusions), *HOXA* genes (rearrangements of *HOXA* genes, *KMT2A* rearrangements, *PICALM-MLLT10*, *SET-NUP214*) and mutations of multiple cellular pathways (Ras signaling, JAK-STAT signaling, and epigenetic regulators) and transcription factors related to T-cell development [135,136,163]. Especially, T-ALL with *SPI1* fusions represents unique expression profiles with high relapse rate [5,136]. Again, several of these genomic mutations were shared with T/M MPAL, including biallelic *WT1* alterations, mutations of hematopoietic transcription factors (*ETV6*, *RUNX1*, *CEBPA*) and activating mutations of signaling pathways (JAK-STAT, *FLT3*, Ras) [92,163], supporting that they are similar entities in the spectrum of immature leukemias and both might have sensitivity to FLT3 and/or JAK inhibition [164].

3.5. NOTCH1 Activating Mutations in T-ALL

NOTCH1 encodes a highly conserved ligand-dependent transcription factor. The NOTCH1 signaling pathway plays an important role in the commitment of T-cell lineage specification and for further T-cell development [133,165]. In T-ALL, NOTCH1 activating mutations are found in more than 70% of cases and is considered an oncogene involved in leukemogenesis [135,136]. Aberrant activation of NOTCH1 pathway in T-ALL is mostly induced by (1) ligand-independent activation (somatic mutations, indels and large deletions that disrupt the negative regulatory region), or (2) impairment of the proteasomal degradation of intracellular domain of NOTCH1 (truncation of the PEST domain, *NOTCH1* mutations in 3′ untranslated region, and *FBXW7* mutations) [166–171]. These two types of *NOTCH1* activating mutations have synergistic effects and more than 20% of T-ALL cases harbor both types of alterations [166]. However, most *NOTCH1* activating mutations found in human T-ALL are considered as a weak tumor initiator event. Co-existence of both types of *NOTCH1* mutations in hematopoietic progenitors tends to induce a transient preleukemic CD4$^+$/CD8$^+$ double positive cells and takes 10 to 15 weeks to fully transform into T-ALL, suggesting that they are alone incompletely leukemogenic [172–174]. In addition, more than 40% of T-ALL cases harbor subclonal *NOTCH1* activating mutations and their heterogeneity at diagnosis was reported by several studies [135,136,175]. Furthermore, *NOTCH1* activating mutations are considered to be acquired as a late secondary event in leukemogenesis [139,175,176].

A key target of NOTCH1 is the *MYC* oncogene that shares several overlapping target genes with NOTCH1 to promote cell proliferation and dysregulate anabolic pathways in T-ALL [174,177,178]. NOTCH1 controls T-cell-specific distal enhancer of *MYC* ("NMe"), resulting in the NOTCH1-MYC regulatory circuit [174,177,178]. In addition, pre-TCR signaling also correlates with NOTCH signaling, leading to LCK signaling and robust cell growth at DN3 stage in the T-cell development, which can be targetable by dasatinib [149,179].

Due to the high prevalence and importance of *NOTCH1* activating mutations in T-ALL, targeted therapy on NOTCH1 pathway has been a major interest. This includes γ-secretase inhibitors (GSIs), ADAM inhibitors, SERCA inhibitors, and monoclonal antibodies [180]. Among them, GSIs, that block the activation process of NOTCH receptors by inhibiting proteolytic cleavage, have been tested in preclinical and Phase 1 studies [181,182]. However, the usage of GSIs in T-ALL is still in a developing phase due to gastrointestinal toxicity and insufficient antitumor responses that mostly induce transient growth arrest rather than cell death [183,184]. To overcome these problems, combination with other agents have been explored including glucocorticoids that showed synergistic effects by reversing glucocorticoid resistance [185]. Inhibition of mTORC1 signaling and PKCδ signaling are also promising combination strategies to restore GSIs sensitivity in resistant cells [186,187].

4. Implications for Diagnosis

The revolution in genomic characterization of ALL has created important opportunities and challenges for the clinical implementation of sequencing-based approaches for diagnosis and management of ALL (Table 1). This is particularly true for B-ALL, where many of the recently identified subtypes are associated with prognosis (even in the context of MRD-based risk-adapted therapy) [82,83] and where molecular characterization is needed to identify patients suitable for targeted therapy (an exemplar being Ph-like ALL). This is currently less compelling for T-ALL where identification of founding lesions driving T-ALL subtypes are of biological and mechanistic interest but are not typically used to risk stratify or guide therapy, exceptions possibly being kinase inhibition for JAK-STAT alterations and *ABL1* rearrangements, identification of alterations in Ras, *PTEN*, *NOTCH1* and/or *FBXW7* that have been found to be associated with outcome in some studies [188], and LCK dependence for dasatinib therapy [149]. The challenge is clinical implementation of appropriately comprehensive diagnostic approaches to identify all key genomic features. Despite the mutationally sparse genome of ALL, there is striking diversity of the nature of underlying driver alterations, including sequence mutations, DNA copy number alterations, and structural variations, many of which may involve the non-coding genome. Accurate subtyping is also challenged by the inability of conventional cytogenetic and targeted molecular approaches to identify several types of driver (e.g., *DUX4*-rearrangement) and the importance of identifying phenocopies (e.g., *ETV6-RUNX1*-like, and Ph-like ALL). Thus, moving forward, optimal clinical diagnostics require genomic approaches. The choice of approach in part rests on how clinical information will be used. If comprehensive subtyping and identification of all potentially clinically relevant genomic alterations is desirable, a combination of DNA and RNA-based technologies is required. For example, the combination of WGS and WTS enables the identification of sequence mutations, DNA copy number alterations, aneuploidy and structural variants (from WGS) together with identification of fusion chimeras, mutant allele expression, and gene expression profiling (from WTS). The use of one or both approaches is becoming increasingly widely used, and at St Jude Children's Research Hospital, three platform sequencing (WGS, WTS and exome sequencing) is clinical standard of care, informs clinical decision making in ALL [148], and retrieves more actionable clinical information than any single platform alone [189]. WGS is offered using a paired non-tumor sample to aid identification of somatic variants and provides the opportunity to return clinically relevant germline findings. Moreover, this comprehensive approach enables a more streamlined workflow [190–192], provided the demands of analysis and interpretation can be met.

However, WGS is not yet widely used clinically, and many clinicians and providers seek alternative approaches to identify clinically relevant alterations. These fall into three main categories: single platform sequencing, sub-genomic sequencing, and targeted detection of genomic alterations. In the first category, single platform WTS provides near comprehensive characterization of clinically relevant alterations in ALL, particularly B-ALL: gene expression-based profiling to identify subgroups and phenocopies; fusion transcripts; and interrogation of specific sequence mutations (e.g., JAKs, PAX5 and IKZF1) [7,193]. Moreover, several methods are available that utilize expression and mutant allele fraction to robustly identify large scale chromosomal copy number changes, thus providing a surrogate for conventional cytogenetic identification of aneuploidy [7,194]. WTS as a single platform has limitations—it is challenging to identify all sequence variations although analytic platforms are improving, it cannot identify focal DNA copy number alterations that may impact targetable pathways (e.g., *SH2B3* deletions in JAK-STAT-driven Ph-like ALL) and does not identify rearrangements that may deregulate oncogenes without resulting in a RNA chimera—for example rearrangements of oncogenes in T-ALL such as *TLX3* and those involving TCR, where breakpoints are frequently intergenic [135], the diverse rearrangements in *BCL11B*-rearranged ALAL [5], or non-coding sequence mutations that drive oncogenes such as *TAL1* and *LMO1/2* [137,138].

Several platforms are available for targeted DNA and/or RNA sequencing, often using capture-based approaches. These including Foundation Medicine [195] and the FusionPlex ALL Kit (Invitae, previously ArcherDx). These have the advantage of being somewhat simpler to access or implement in routine diagnostic laboratories, and the ability to detect the majority of chimeric fusion events in B-ALL. Similar reservations to WTS apply regarding the limited ability of these platforms to detect intergenic rearrangements in ALL; moreover, these platforms either have limited (Foundation) or no (Archer) capability to detect DNA copy number alterations, particularly those that are single copy, and may have difficulty resolving complex rearrangements (e.g., truncating rearrangements of *EPOR* in Ph-like ALL) [115]. Capture based DNA sequencing for sequence mutations is widely used in hematological malignancies, but is not well suited to diagnosis of ALL due to the lack of detection of rearrangements and structural variations. As described above, the MLPA platform is widely used by several groups to identify focal DNA copy number alterations and the "*IKZF1*^{plus}" composite genotype, but this platform is not an adequate surrogate for sensitive detection of several key subtypes: e.g., *ERG* deletion in *DUX4*-rearranged ALL (only ~50% of cases have clonal *ERG* deletion), and PAR1 deletion in *CRLF2*-rearranged ALL (*IGH-CRLF2* is usually not accompanied by PAR1 deletion).

Table 1. Clinical implementation of high-throughput sequencing.

Platform	Capability	Cost	Detectable Subtypes	Difficult Subtypes
WTS (RNAseq)	Fusion chimeras Gene expression profiling Mutant allele expression Alternative splicing analysis (BCR/TCR rearrangements) (Sequence mutations) (Copy number analysis)	Moderate	B-ALL ETV6-RUNX1; KMT2A; TCF3-PBX1; BCR-ABL1; DUX4; MEF2D; ZNF384/362 NUTM1; HLF; BCL2/MYC; PAX5alt; ZEB2/CEBPE; -like subtypes	B-ALL Aneuploidies
			T-ALL HOXA (*KMT2A-R*, *PICALM-MLLT10*, *SET-NUP214*); SPI1; NKX2-1; TAL1 (*STIL-TAL1*)	T-ALL BCL11B; TLX1/3; LMO1/2; HOXA (others); TAL1 (others); T-other
WGS	Sequence mutations Structural variants Copy number analysis (BCR/TCR rearrangements) (GWAS)	High	B-ALL Aneuploidies; ETV6-RUNX1; KMT2A; TCF3-PBX1; BCR-ABL1; DUX4; MEF2D; ZNF384/362; NUTM1; HLF; BCL2/MYC; PAX5 P80R; IKZF1 N159Y; ZEB2/CEBPE; Sequence and structural alterations in Ph-like ALL	B-ALL -like subtypes; Part of PAX5alt
			T-ALL BCL11B; TLX1/3; LMO1/2; HOXA; SPI1; NKX2-1; TAL1	T-ALL T-other
WES	Sequence mutations (coding) Structural variants (coding) Copy number analysis	Moderate	B-ALL (Aneuploidies) PAX5 P80R IKZF1 N159Y Sequence mutations in Ph-like ALL (e.g., JAK1/2/3, Ras)	Most of other B-ALL and T-ALL subtypes
Targeted sequencing (DNA and/or RNA)	Fusion chimeras (targeted) Gene expression (targeted) Sequence mutations (targeted) Structural variants (targeted) (Copy number analysis)	Low	Targeted alterations	Non-targeted alterations

The parenthesis in "Capability" indicates analyses in development. Abbreviations: WTS: whole transcriptome sequencing; BCR: B-cell receptor; TCR: T-cell receptor; WGS: whole genome sequencing; GWAS: genome wide association study; WES: whole exome sequencing; -R: rearranged.

In the absence of sequencing-based approaches, several subtypes and drivers may be identified by flow cytometry, immunophenotypic and targeted molecular approaches. Flow cytometry may be used to detect CRLF2 rearrangements, that result in cell surface expression of *CRLF2*, as well as markers associated with distinct subtypes (e.g., CD371 in *DUX4*-rearranged ALL). FISH may be used to detect rearrangement of the most commonly rearranged genes in Ph-like ALL for which targeted therapies are currently available (e.g., *ABL*-family kinase genes, *CRLF2*, *NTRK3*) with caveats—for example, the focal insertions of *EPOR* into *IGH* and similar enhancer regions are not robustly detected by FISH due to the small size of the *EPOR* insertion. Specific subtype-defining rearrangements may be detected by conventional molecular approaches such as RT-PCR. Thus, these composite approaches may be suitable to detect many actionable alterations in ALL, but do not provide a pathway to comprehensive identification of all driver lesions of prognostic significance.

5. Conclusions

Large-scale integrative genome-wide sequencing studies have profoundly transformed the molecular taxonomy of ALL, resulting in the identification of new entities with prognostic and therapeutic significance. There are over 30 different B/T-ALL subtypes defined by distinct constellations of somatic and/or germline genetic alterations that converge on distinct gene expression patterns. The identification of these dysregulated pathways is crucial for clinical management of ALL patients and most importantly for guiding therapeutic intervention. The best example is provided by the constitutively active kinases in Ph-like which are druggable by a variety of single or combinatorial TKIs. Although the enormous clinical and genetic progress of the past decade, much work remains, as most studies have lacked NGS and have not validated the mechanisms by which fusions/mutations cooperate in leukemogenesis, and not fully defined potential for targeting. Due to the heterogeneity of genetic lesions, optimal clinical diagnosis of ALL requires genomic and/or transcriptomic sequencing in order to identify fusions, aneuploidy and sequence mutations required for disease stratification. The use of such approaches is becoming increasingly widespread. Recently, new immunotherapeutic agents (e.g., developed antibodies and CAR-T cells) have been efficacious in a proportion of patients, but failed in others. Thus, efforts should be focused in the future on defining subtype specific vulnerabilities to improve treatment strategy and outcome.

Author Contributions: Writing—original draft preparation, I.I., S.K. and C.G.M.; writing—review and editing, I.I., S.K. and C.G.M.; visualization, I.I. and S.K.; supervision, I.I. and C.G.M. All authors have read and agreed to the published version of the manuscript.

Funding: Work conducted by the authors described in this review was supported by the National Institutes of Health, including an NCI Outstanding Investigator Award R35 CA197697 (to C.G.M.), NCI Cancer Center Support Grant (CA021765) an St. Baldrick's Foundation Robert J. Arceci Innovation Award (to C.G.M.) and the Henry Schueler 41&9 Foundation (to C.G.M.); a Garwood Postdoctoral Fellowship of the Hematological Malignancies Program of the St Jude Children's Research Hospital Comprehensive Cancer Center (to S.K.); and the American Lebanese Syrian Associated Charities of St. Jude Children's Research Hospital.

Acknowledgments: The authors thank collaborators that have contributed patient samples, data, intellectual and technical expertise to the work described in this study, particularly the St. Jude Children's Research Hospital—Washington University Pediatric Cancer Genome Project, Children's Oncology Group Therapeutically Applicable Research to Generate Effective Treatments (TARGET) project (https://ocg.cancer.gov/programs/target/projects/acute-lymphoblastic-leukemia, accessed on 19 August 2021), the Eastern Cooperative Oncology Group—American College of Radiology Imaging Network (ECOG-ACRIN), The Alliance—Cancer and Leukemia Group B, and MD Anderson Cancer Center.

Conflicts of Interest: I.I. has received honoraria from Amgen and Mission Bio; S.K. declares no conflict of interest.; C.G.M. has received research funding from Loxo Oncology (relevant to the use of TRK inhibition in Ph-like ALL), AbbVie (venetoclax in ALL) and Pfizer; honoraria from Amgen and Illumina. These funders had no role in the writing of this manuscript.

References

1. Tran, T.H.; Hunger, S.P. The genomic landscape of pediatric acute lymphoblastic leukemia and precision medicine opportunities. *Semin. Cancer Biol.* **2020**. [CrossRef]
2. Pui, C.-H. Precision medicine in acute lymphoblastic leukemia. *Front. Med.* **2020**, *14*, 689–700. [CrossRef] [PubMed]
3. Inaba, H.; Mullighan, C.G. Pediatric acute lymphoblastic leukemia. *Haematologica* **2020**, *105*, 2524. [CrossRef] [PubMed]
4. Stock, W.; Luger, S.M.; Advani, A.S.; Yin, J.; Harvey, R.C.; Mullighan, C.G.; Willman, C.L.; Fulton, N.; Laumann, K.M.; Malnassy, G.; et al. A pediatric regimen for older adolescents and young adults with acute lymphoblastic leukemia: Results of CALGB 10403. *Blood* **2019**, *133*, 1548–1559. [CrossRef] [PubMed]
5. Montefiori, L.E.; Bendig, S.; Gu, Z.; Chen, X.; Polonen, P.; Ma, X.; Murison, A.; Zeng, A.; Garcia-Prat, L.; Dickerson, K.; et al. Enhancer hijacking drives oncogenic BCL11B expression in lineage ambiguous stem cell leukemia. *Cancer Discov.* **2021**. [CrossRef]
6. Iacobucci, I.; Mullighan, C.G. Genetic Basis of Acute Lymphoblastic Leukemia. *J. Clin. Oncol.* **2017**, *35*, 975–983. [CrossRef]
7. Gu, Z.; Churchman, M.L.; Roberts, K.G.; Moore, I.; Zhou, X.; Nakitandwe, J.; Hagiwara, K.; Pelletier, S.; Gingras, S.; Berns, H.; et al. PAX5-driven subtypes of B-progenitor acute lymphoblastic leukemia. *Nat. Genet.* **2019**, *51*, 296–307. [CrossRef]
8. Pui, C.-H.; Nichols, K.E.; Yang, J.J. Somatic and germline genomics in paediatric acute lymphoblastic leukaemia. *Nat. Rev. Clin. Oncol.* **2018**, *16*, 227–240. [CrossRef]
9. Schwab, C.; Harrison, C.J. Advances in B-cell Precursor Acute Lymphoblastic Leukemia Genomics. *HemaSphere* **2018**, *2*, e53. [CrossRef]
10. Li, J.; Dai, Y.; Wu, L.; Zhang, M.; Ouyang, W.; Huang, J.; Chen, S. Emerging molecular subtypes and therapeutic targets in B-cell precursor acute lymphoblastic leukemia. *Front. Med.* **2021**, *15*, 347–371. [CrossRef]
11. Mullighan, C.G. How advanced are we in targeting novel subtypes of ALL? *Best Pract. Res. Clin. Haematol.* **2019**, *32*, 101095. [CrossRef]
12. Kimura, S.; Mullighan, C.G. Molecular markers in ALL: Clinical implications. *Best Pract. Res. Clin. Haematol.* **2020**, *33*, 101193. [CrossRef] [PubMed]
13. Li, J.-F.; Dai, Y.-T.; Lilljebjörn, H.; Shen, S.-H.; Cui, B.-W.; Bai, L.; Liu, Y.-F.; Qian, M.-X.; Kubota, Y.; Kiyoi, H.; et al. Transcriptional landscape of B cell precursor acute lymphoblastic leukemia based on an international study of 1223 cases. *Proc. Natl. Acad. Sci. USA* **2018**, *115*, E11711–E11720. [CrossRef] [PubMed]
14. Roberts, K.G.; Morin, R.D.; Zhang, J.; Hirst, M.; Zhao, Y.; Su, X.; Chen, S.-C.; Payne-Turner, D.; Churchman, M.L.; Harvey, R.; et al. Genetic Alterations Activating Kinase and Cytokine Receptor Signaling in High-Risk Acute Lymphoblastic Leukemia. *Cancer Cell* **2012**, *22*, 153–166. [CrossRef]
15. Roberts, K.G.; Li, Y.; Payne-Turner, D.; Harvey, R.; Yang, Y.-L.; Pei, D.; McCastlain, K.; Ding, L.; Lu, C.; Song, G.; et al. Targetable Kinase-Activating Lesions in Ph-like Acute Lymphoblastic Leukemia. *N. Engl. J. Med.* **2014**, *371*, 1005–1015. [CrossRef]
16. Klco, J.M.; Mullighan, C.G. Advances in germline predisposition to acute leukaemias and myeloid neoplasms. *Nat. Rev. Cancer* **2020**, *21*, 122–137. [CrossRef]
17. Perez-Andreu, V.; Roberts, K.G.; Harvey, R.; Yang, W.; Cheng, C.; Pei, D.; Xu, H.; Gastier-Foster, J.; Lim, J.Y.-S.; Chen, I.-M.; et al. Inherited GATA3 variants are associated with Ph-like childhood acute lymphoblastic leukemia and risk of relapse. *Nat. Genet.* **2013**, *45*, 1494–1498. [CrossRef] [PubMed]
18. Ellinghaus, E.; Stanulla, M.; Richter, G.; Kronnie, G.T.; Cario, G.; Cazzaniga, G.; Horstmann, M.; Grümayer, R.P.; Cavé, H.; Trka, J.; et al. Identification of germline susceptibility loci in ETV6-RUNX1-rearranged childhood acute lymphoblastic leukemia. *Leukemia* **2011**, *26*, 902–909. [CrossRef] [PubMed]
19. Qian, M.; Zhao, X.; Devidas, M.; Yang, W.; Gocho, Y.; Smith, C.; Gastier-Foster, J.M.; Li, Y.; Xu, H.; Zhang, S.; et al. Genome-Wide Association Study of Susceptibility Loci for T-Cell Acute Lymphoblastic Leukemia in Children. *J. Natl. Cancer Inst.* **2019**, *111*, 1350–1357. [CrossRef]
20. Qian, M.; Xu, H.; Perez-Andreu, V.; Roberts, K.G.; Zhang, H.; Yang, W.; Zhang, S.; Zhao, X.; Smith, C.; Devidas, M.; et al. Novel susceptibility variants at the ERG locus for childhood acute lymphoblastic leukemia in Hispanics. *Blood* **2019**, *133*, 724–729. [CrossRef]
21. Molina, O.; Abad, M.A.; Solé, F.; Menéndez, P. Aneuploidy in Cancer: Lessons from Acute Lymphoblastic Leukemia. *Trends Cancer* **2020**, *7*, 37–47. [CrossRef]
22. Greaves, M. A causal mechanism for childhood acute lymphoblastic leukaemia. *Nat. Rev. Cancer* **2018**, *18*, 471–484. [CrossRef]
23. Paulsson, K.; Lilljebjörn, H.; Biloglav, A.; Olsson, L.; Rissler, M.; Castor, A.; Barbany, G.; Fogelstrand, L.; Nordgren, A.; Sjögren, H.; et al. The genomic landscape of high hyperdiploid childhood acute lymphoblastic leukemia. *Nat. Genet.* **2015**, *47*, 672–676. [CrossRef]
24. Paulsson, K.; Johansson, B. High hyperdiploid childhood acute lymphoblastic leukemia. *Genes Chromosom. Cancer* **2009**, *48*, 637–660. [CrossRef] [PubMed]
25. Mullighan, C.G.; Zhang, J.; Kasper, L.H.; Lerach, S.; Payne-Turner, D.; Phillips, L.A.; Heatley, S.; Holmfeldt, L.; Collins-Underwood, J.R.; Ma, J.; et al. CREBBP mutations in relapsed acute lymphoblastic leukaemia. *Nature* **2011**, *471*, 235–239. [CrossRef] [PubMed]
26. Molina, O.; Vinyoles, M.; Granada, I.; Roca-Ho, H.; Gutierrez-Agüera, F.; Valledor, L.; López, C.M.L.; Rodríguez-González, P.; Trincado, J.L.; Tirados-Menéndez, S.; et al. Impaired Condensin Complex and Aurora B kinase underlie mitotic and chromosomal defects in hyperdiploid B-cell ALL. *Blood* **2020**, *136*, 313–327. [CrossRef]

27. Holmfeldt, L.; Wei, L.; Diaz-Flores, E.; Walsh, M.; Zhang, J.; Ding, L.; Payne-Turner, D.; Churchman, M.; Hagström-Andersson, A.; Chen, S.-C.; et al. The genomic landscape of hypodiploid acute lymphoblastic leukemia. *Nat. Genet.* **2013**, *45*, 242–252. [CrossRef] [PubMed]
28. Comeaux, E.Q.; Mullighan, C.G. TP53Mutations in Hypodiploid Acute Lymphoblastic Leukemia. *Cold Spring Harb. Perspect. Med.* **2016**, *7*, a026286. [CrossRef] [PubMed]
29. Carroll, A.J.; Shago, M.; Mikhail, F.M.; Raimondi, S.C.; Hirsch, B.A.; Loh, M.L.; Raetz, E.A.; Borowitz, M.J.; Wood, B.L.; Maloney, K.W.; et al. Masked hypodiploidy: Hypodiploid acute lymphoblastic leukemia (ALL) mimicking hyperdiploid ALL in children: A report from the Children's Oncology Group. *Cancer Genet.* **2019**, *238*, 62–68. [CrossRef] [PubMed]
30. Mullighan, C.G.; Jeha, S.; Pei, D.; Payne-Turner, D.; Coustan-Smith, E.; Roberts, K.G.; Waanders, E.; Choi, J.K.; Ma, X.; Raimondi, S.C.; et al. Outcome of children with hypodiploid ALL treated with risk-directed therapy based on MRD levels. *Blood* **2015**, *126*, 2896–2899. [CrossRef] [PubMed]
31. Pui, C.-H.; Rebora, P.; Schrappe, M.; Attarbaschi, A.; Baruchel, A.; Basso, G.; Cavé, H.; Elitzur, S.; Koh, K.; Liu, H.-C.; et al. Outcome of Children with Hypodiploid Acute Lymphoblastic Leukemia: A Retrospective Multinational Study. *J. Clin. Oncol.* **2019**, *37*, 770–779. [CrossRef] [PubMed]
32. McNeer, J.L.; Devidas, M.; Dai, Y.; Carroll, A.J.; Heerema, N.A.; Gastier-Foster, J.M.; Kahwash, S.; Borowitz, M.J.; Wood, B.L.; Larsen, E.; et al. Hematopoietic Stem-Cell Transplantation Does Not Improve the Poor Outcome of Children with Hypodiploid Acute Lymphoblastic Leukemia: A Report From Children's Oncology Group. *J. Clin. Oncol.* **2019**, *37*, 780–789. [CrossRef] [PubMed]
33. Ribera, J.; Granada, I.; Morgades, M.; Vives, S.; Genescà, E.; González, C.; Nomdedeu, J.; Escoda, L.; Montesinos, P.; Mercadal, S.; et al. The poor prognosis of low hypodiploidy in adults with B-cell precursor acute lymphoblastic leukaemia is restricted to older adults and elderly patients. *Br. J. Haematol.* **2019**, *186*, 263–268. [CrossRef]
34. Diaz-Flores, E.; Comeaux, E.Q.; Kim, K.L.; Melnik, E.M.; Beckman, K.; Davis, K.L.; Wu, K.; Akutagawa, J.; Bridges, O.; Marino, R.; et al. Bcl-2 Is a Therapeutic Target for Hypodiploid B-Lineage Acute Lymphoblastic Leukemia. *Cancer Res.* **2019**, *79*, 2339–2351. [CrossRef] [PubMed]
35. Harrison, C.J. Blood Spotlight on iAMP21 acute lymphoblastic leukemia (ALL), a high-risk pediatric disease. *Blood* **2015**, *125*, 1383–1386. [CrossRef] [PubMed]
36. Harrison, C.J.; Schwab, C. Constitutional abnormalities of chromosome 21 predispose to iAMP21-acute lymphoblastic leukaemia. *Eur. J. Med. Genet.* **2016**, *59*, 162–165. [CrossRef]
37. Moorman, A.V.; Robinson, H.; Schwab, C.; Richards, S.M.; Hancock, J.; Mitchell, C.D.; Goulden, N.; Vora, A.; Harrison, C. Risk-Directed Treatment Intensification Significantly Reduces the Risk of Relapse among Children and Adolescents with Acute Lymphoblastic Leukemia and Intrachromosomal Amplification of Chromosome 21: A Comparison of the MRC ALL97/99 and UKALL2003 Trials. *J. Clin. Oncol.* **2013**, *31*, 3389–3396. [CrossRef]
38. Golub, T.; McLean, T.; Stegmaier, K.; Ritz, J.; Sallan, S.; Neuberg, D.; Gilliland, D.G. TEL-AML1: The most common gene rearrangement in childhood ALL. *Blood* **1995**, *86*, 2377.
39. Sundaresh, A.; Williams, O. Mechanism of ETV6-RUNX1 Leukemia. *Adv. Exp. Med. Biol.* **2017**, *962*, 201–216. [CrossRef]
40. Shurtleff, S.A.; Buijs, A.; Behm, F.G.; Rubnitz, J.; Raimondi, S.C.; Hancock, M.L.; Chan, G.C.F.; Pui, C.H.; Grosveld, G.; Downing, J.R. TEL/AML1 fusion resulting from a cryptic t(12;21) is the most common genetic lesion in pediatric ALL and defines a subgroup of patients with an excellent prognosis. *Leukemia* **1995**, *9*, 1985–1989.
41. Ford, A.M.; Greaves, M. ETV6-RUNX1 + Acute Lymphoblastic Leukaemia in Identical Twins. *Adv. Exp. Med. Biol.* **2017**, *962*, 217–228. [CrossRef] [PubMed]
42. Mullighan, C.; Goorha, S.; Radtke, I.; Miller, C.B.; Coustan-Smith, E.; Dalton, J.D.; Girtman, K.; Mathew, S.; Ma, J.; Pounds, S.; et al. Genome-wide analysis of genetic alterations in acute lymphoblastic leukaemia. *Nature* **2007**, *446*, 758–764. [CrossRef] [PubMed]
43. Kuiper, R.P.; Schoenmakers, E.F.P.M.; Van Reijmersdal, S.V.; Hehir-Kwa, J.Y.; Van Kessel, A.G.; van Leeuwen, F.N.; Hoogerbrugge, P.M. High-resolution genomic profiling of childhood ALL reveals novel recurrent genetic lesions affecting pathways involved in lymphocyte differentiation and cell cycle progression. *Leukemia* **2007**, *21*, 1258–1266. [CrossRef] [PubMed]
44. Papaemmanuil, E.; Rapado, I.; Li, Y.; Potter, N.E.; Wedge, D.; Tubio, J.; Alexandrov, L.B.; Van Loo, P.; Cooke, S.L.; Marshall, J.; et al. RAG-mediated recombination is the predominant driver of oncogenic rearrangement in ETV6-RUNX1 acute lymphoblastic leukemia. *Nat. Genet.* **2014**, *46*, 116–125. [CrossRef] [PubMed]
45. Burmeister, T.; Gökbuget, N.; Schwartz, S.; Fischer, L.; Hubert, D.; Sindram, A.; Hoelzer, D.; Thiel, E. Clinical features and prognostic implications of TCF3-PBX1 and ETV6-RUNX1 in adult acute lymphoblastic leukemia. *Haematologica* **2009**, *95*, 241–246. [CrossRef] [PubMed]
46. Jeha, S.; Pei, D.; Choi, J.; Cheng, C.; Sandlund, J.T.; Coustan-Smith, E.; Campana, D.; Inaba, H.; Rubnitz, J.E.; Ribeiro, R.C.; et al. Improved CNS Control of Childhood Acute Lymphoblastic Leukemia without Cranial Irradiation: St Jude Total Therapy Study 16. *J. Clin. Oncol.* **2019**, *37*, 3377–3391. [CrossRef]
47. Pui, C.-H.; Tang, J.-Y.; Yang, J.J.; Chen, S.-J.; Chen, Z. International Collaboration to Save Children with Acute Lymphoblastic Leukemia. *J. Glob. Oncol.* **2019**, *5*, 1–2. [CrossRef]
48. Buchner, M.; Müschen, M. Targeting the B-cell receptor signaling pathway in B lymphoid malignancies. *Curr. Opin. Hematol.* **2014**, *21*, 341–349. [CrossRef]

49. Van der Veer, A.; van der Velden, V.H.; Willemse, M.E.; Hoogeveen, P.G.; Petricoin, E.F.; Beverloo, H.B.; Escherich, G.; Horstmann, M.A.; Pieters, R.; den Boer, M.L. Interference with pre-B-cell receptor signaling offers a therapeutic option for TCF3-rearranged childhood acute lymphoblastic leukemia. *Blood Cancer J.* **2014**, *4*, e181. [CrossRef] [PubMed]
50. Bicocca, V.; Chang, B.; Masouleh, B.K.; Muschen, M.; Loriaux, M.M.; Druker, B.J.; Tyner, J.W. Crosstalk between ROR1 and the Pre-B Cell Receptor Promotes Survival of t(1;19) Acute Lymphoblastic Leukemia. *Cancer Cell* **2012**, *22*, 656–667. [CrossRef]
51. Fischer, U.; Forster, M.; Rinaldi, A.; Risch, T.; Sungalee, S.; Warnatz, H.-J.; Bornhauser, B.; Gombert, M.; Kratsch, C.; Stütz, A.M.; et al. Genomics and drug profiling of fatal TCF3-HLF–positive acute lymphoblastic leukemia identifies recurrent mutation patterns and therapeutic options. *Nat. Genet.* **2015**, *47*, 1020–1029. [CrossRef] [PubMed]
52. Frismantas, V.; Dobay, M.P.; Rinaldi, A.; Tchinda, J.; Dunn, S.H.; Kunz, J.; Richter-Pechanska, P.; Marovca, B.; Pail, O.; Jenni, S.; et al. Ex vivo drug response profiling detects recurrent sensitivity patterns in drug-resistant acute lymphoblastic leukemia. *Blood* **2017**, *129*, e26–e37. [CrossRef]
53. Glover, J.M.; Loriaux, M.; Tyner, J.; Druker, B.; Chang, B.H. In vitro sensitivity to dasatinib in lymphoblasts from a patient with t(17;19)(q22;p13) gene rearrangement pre-B acute lymphoblastic leukemia. *Pediatr. Blood Cancer* **2011**, *59*, 576–579. [CrossRef] [PubMed]
54. Mouttet, B.; Vinti, L.; Ancliff, P.; Bodmer, N.; Brethon, B.; Cario, G.; Chen-Santel, C.; Elitzur, S.; Hazar, V.; Kunz, J.; et al. Durable remissions in TCF3-HLF positive acute lymphoblastic leukemia with blinatumomab and stem cell transplantation. *Haematologica* **2019**, *104*, e244–e247. [CrossRef]
55. Leonard, J.; Wolf, J.S.; Degnin, M.; Eide, C.A.; LaTocha, D.; Lenz, K.; Wilmot, B.; Mullighan, C.G.; Loh, M.; Hunger, S.P.; et al. Aurora A kinase as a target for therapy in *TCF3-HLF* rearranged acute lymphoblastic leukemia. *Haematologica* **2021**. [CrossRef] [PubMed]
56. El Chaer, F.; Keng, M.; Ballen, K.K. MLL-Rearranged Acute Lymphoblastic Leukemia. *Curr. Hematol. Malig. Rep.* **2020**, *15*, 83–89. [CrossRef]
57. Winters, A.C.; Bernt, K.M. MLL-Rearranged Leukemias—An Update on Science and Clinical Approaches. *Front. Pediatr.* **2017**, *5*, 4. [CrossRef]
58. Armstrong, S.A.; Staunton, J.E.; Silverman, L.B.; Pieters, R.; Boer, M.D.; Minden, M.D.; Sallan, S.E.; Lander, E.S.; Golub, T.R.; Korsmeyer, S.J. MLL translocations specify a distinct gene expression profile that distinguishes a unique leukemia. *Nat. Genet.* **2001**, *30*, 41–47. [CrossRef] [PubMed]
59. Yeoh, E.-J.; Ross, M.E.; Shurtleff, S.A.; Williams, W.; Patel, D.; Mahfouz, R.; Behm, F.G.; Raimondi, S.C.; Relling, M.V.; Patel, A.; et al. Classification, subtype discovery, and prediction of outcome in pediatric acute lymphoblastic leukemia by gene expression profiling. *Cancer Cell* **2002**, *1*, 133–143. [CrossRef]
60. Andersson, A.K.; Ma, J.; Wang, J.; Chen, X.; Gedman, A.L.; Dang, J.; Nakitandwe, J.; Holmfeldt, L.; Parker, M.; Easton, J.; et al. The landscape of somatic mutations in infant MLL-rearranged acute lymphoblastic leukemias. *Nat. Genet.* **2015**, *47*, 330–337. [CrossRef]
61. Valentine, M.C.; Linabery, A.; Chasnoff, S.; Hughes, A.E.O.; Mallaney, C.; Sanchez, N.; Giacalone, J.; Heerema, N.A.; Hilden, J.M.; Spector, L.; et al. Excess congenital non-synonymous variation in leukemia-associated genes in MLL−infant leukemia: A Children's Oncology Group report. *Leukemia* **2013**, *28*, 1235–1241. [CrossRef]
62. Perner, F.; Gadrey, J.Y.; Xiong, Y.; Hatton, C.; Eschle, B.K.; Weiss, A.; Stauffer, F.; Gaul, C.; Tiedt, R.; Perry, J.A.; et al. Novel inhibitors of the histone methyltransferase DOT1L show potent antileukemic activity in patient-derived xenografts. *Blood* **2020**, *136*, 1983–1988. [CrossRef]
63. Chen, C.-W.; Koche, R.; Sinha, A.U.; Deshpande, A.J.; Zhu, N.; Eng, R.; Doench, J.; Xu, H.; Chu, S.H.; Qi, J.; et al. DOT1L inhibits SIRT1-mediated epigenetic silencing to maintain leukemic gene expression in MLL-rearranged leukemia. *Nat. Med.* **2015**, *21*, 335–343. [CrossRef]
64. Klossowski, S.; Miao, H.; Kempinska, K.; Wu, T.; Purohit, T.; Kim, E.; Linhares, B.M.; Chen, D.; Jih, G.; Perkey, E.; et al. Menin inhibitor MI-3454 induces remission in MLL1-rearranged and NPM1-mutated models of leukemia. *J. Clin. Investig.* **2019**, *130*, 981–997. [CrossRef] [PubMed]
65. Liao, W.; Kohler, M.E.; Fry, T.; Ernst, P. Does lineage plasticity enable escape from CAR-T cell therapy? Lessons from MLL-r leukemia. *Exp. Hematol.* **2021**, *100*, 1–11. [CrossRef] [PubMed]
66. Roberts, K.G.; Gu, Z.; Payne-Turner, D.; McCastlain, K.; Harvey, R.; Chen, I.-M.; Pei, D.; Iacobucci, I.; Valentine, M.; Pounds, S.B.; et al. High Frequency and Poor Outcome of Philadelphia Chromosome–Like Acute Lymphoblastic Leukemia in Adults. *J. Clin. Oncol.* **2017**, *35*, 394–401. [CrossRef]
67. Bernt, K.; Hunger, S.P.M. Current Concepts in Pediatric Philadelphia Chromosome-Positive Acute Lymphoblastic Leukemia. *Front. Oncol.* **2014**, *4*, 54. [CrossRef] [PubMed]
68. Slayton, W.B.; Schultz, K.R.; Kairalla, J.A.; Devidas, M.; Mi, X.; Pulsipher, M.A.; Chang, B.H.; Mullighan, C.; Iacobucci, I.; Silverman, L.B.; et al. Dasatinib Plus Intensive Chemotherapy in Children, Adolescents, and Young Adults with Philadelphia Chromosome–Positive Acute Lymphoblastic Leukemia: Results of Children's Oncology Group Trial AALL0622. *J. Clin. Oncol.* **2018**, *36*, 2306–2314. [CrossRef]
69. Foà, R.; Bassan, R.; Vitale, A.; Elia, L.; Piciocchi, A.; Puzzolo, M.-C.; Canichella, M.; Viero, P.; Ferrara, F.; Lunghi, M.; et al. Dasatinib–Blinatumomab for Ph-Positive Acute Lymphoblastic Leukemia in Adults. *N. Engl. J. Med.* **2020**, *383*, 1613–1623. [CrossRef]

70. Foà, R.; Vitale, A.; Vignetti, M.; Meloni, G.; Guarini, A.; De Propris, M.S.; Elia, L.; Paoloni, F.; Fazi, P.; Cimino, G.; et al. Dasatinib as first-line treatment for adult patients with Philadelphia chromosome–positive acute lymphoblastic leukemia. *Blood* **2011**, *118*, 6521–6528. [CrossRef]
71. Mullighan, C.; Miller, C.B.; Radtke, I.; Phillips, L.A.; Dalton, J.T.; Ma, J.; White, D.; Hughes, T.; Le Beau, M.M.; Pui, C.-H.; et al. BCR–ABL1 lymphoblastic leukaemia is characterized by the deletion of Ikaros. *Nature* **2008**, *453*, 110–114. [CrossRef]
72. Iacobucci, I.; Storlazzi, C.T.; Cilloni, D.; Lonetti, A.; Ottaviani, E.; Soverini, S.; Astolfi, A.; Chiaretti, S.; Vitale, A.; Messa, F.; et al. Identification and molecular characterization of recurrent genomic deletions on 7p12 in the IKZF1 gene in a large cohort of BCR-ABL1–positive acute lymphoblastic leukemia patients: On behalf of Gruppo Italiano Malattie Ematologiche dell'Adulto Acute Leukemia Working Party (GIMEMA AL WP). *Blood* **2009**, *114*, 2159–2167. [CrossRef] [PubMed]
73. Martinelli, G.; Iacobucci, I.; Storlazzi, C.T.; Vignetti, M.; Paoloni, F.; Cilloni, D.; Soverini, S.; Vitale, A.; Chiaretti, S.; Cimino, G.; et al. IKZF1 (Ikaros) Deletions in BCR-ABL1–Positive Acute Lymphoblastic Leukemia Are Associated with Short Disease-Free Survival and High Rate of Cumulative Incidence of Relapse: A GIMEMA AL WP Report. *J. Clin. Oncol.* **2009**, *27*, 5202–5207. [CrossRef]
74. Liu, Y.-F.; Wang, B.-Y.; Zhang, W.-N.; Huang, J.-Y.; Li, B.-S.; Zhang, M.; Jiang, L.; Li, J.-F.; Wang, M.-J.; Dai, Y.-J.; et al. Genomic Profiling of Adult and Pediatric B-cell Acute Lymphoblastic Leukemia. *EBioMedicine* **2016**, *8*, 173–183. [CrossRef] [PubMed]
75. Lilljebjörn, H.; Henningsson, R.; Wittsten, A.H.; Olsson, L.; Orsmark-Pietras, C.; Von Palffy, S.; Askmyr, M.; Rissler, M.; Schrappe, M.; Cario, M.S.G.; et al. Identification of ETV6-RUNX1-like and DUX4-rearranged subtypes in paediatric B-cell precursor acute lymphoblastic leukaemia. *Nat. Commun.* **2016**, *7*, 11790. [CrossRef] [PubMed]
76. Yasuda, T.; Tsuzuki, S.; Kawazu, M.; Hayakawa, F.; Kojima, S.; Ueno, T.; Imoto, N.; Kohsaka, S.; Kunita, A.; Doi, K.; et al. Recurrent DUX4 fusions in B cell acute lymphoblastic leukemia of adolescents and young adults. *Nat. Genet.* **2016**, *48*, 569–574. [CrossRef]
77. Zhang, J.; McCastlain, K.; Yoshihara, H.; Xu, B.; Chang, Y.; Churchman, M.L.; Wu, G.; Li, Y.; Wei, L.; Iacobucci, I.; et al. Deregulation of DUX4 and ERG in acute lymphoblastic leukemia. *Nat. Genet.* **2016**, *48*, 1481–1489. [CrossRef] [PubMed]
78. Dib, C.; Zakharova, V.; Popova, E.; Kiseleva, E.; Chernyak, B.; Lipinski, M.; Vassetzky, Y.S. DUX4 Pathological Expression: Causes and Consequences in Cancer. *Trends Cancer* **2019**, *5*, 268–271. [CrossRef]
79. Himeda, C.L.; Jones, P.L. The Genetics and Epigenetics of Facioscapulohumeral Muscular Dystrophy. *Annu. Rev. Genom. Hum. Genet.* **2019**, *20*, 265–291. [CrossRef]
80. Miettinen, M.; Felisiak-Golabek, A.; Contreras, A.L.; Glod, J.; Kaplan, R.N.; Killian, J.K.; Lasota, J. New fusion sarcomas: Histopathology and clinical significance of selected entities. *Hum. Pathol.* **2019**, *86*, 57–65. [CrossRef]
81. Sirvent, N.; Trassard, M.; Ebran, N.; Attias, R.; Pedeutour, F. Fusion of EWSR1 with the DUX4 facioscapulohumeral muscular dystrophy region resulting from t(4;22)(q35;q12) in a case of embryonal rhabdomyosarcoma. *Cancer Genet. Cytogenet.* **2009**, *195*, 12–18. [CrossRef]
82. Jeha, S.; Choi, J.; Roberts, K.G.; Pei, D.; Coustan-Smith, E.; Inaba, H.; Rubnitz, J.E.; Ribeiro, R.C.; Gruber, T.A.; Raimondi, S.C.; et al. Clinical Significance of Novel Subtypes of Acute Lymphoblastic Leukemia in the Context of Minimal Residual Disease–Directed Therapy. *Blood Cancer Discov.* **2021**, *2*, 326–337. [CrossRef]
83. Paietta, E.; Roberts, K.G.; Wang, V.; Gu, Z.; Buck, G.; Pei, D.; Cheng, C.; Levine, R.L.; Abdel-Wahab, O.; Cheng, Z.; et al. Molecular Classification Improves Risk Assessment in Adult BCR-ABL1-negative B-ALL. *Blood* **2021**. [CrossRef]
84. Schinnerl, D.; Mejstrikova, E.; Schumich, A.; Zaliova, M.; Fortschegger, K.; Nebral, K.; Attarbaschi, A.; Fiser, K.; Kauer, M.O.; Popitsch, N.; et al. CD371 cell surface expression: A unique feature of DUX4-rearranged acute lymphoblastic leukemia. *Haematologica* **2019**, *104*, e352–e355. [CrossRef]
85. Gu, Z.; Churchman, M.; Roberts, K.; Li, Y.; Liu, Y.; Harvey, R.C.; McCastlain, K.; Reshmi, S.C.; Payne-Turner, D.; Iacobucci, I.; et al. Genomic analyses identify recurrent MEF2D fusions in acute lymphoblastic leukaemia. *Nat. Commun.* **2016**, *7*, 13331. [CrossRef] [PubMed]
86. Suzuki, K.; Okuno, Y.; Kawashima, N.; Muramatsu, H.; Okuno, T.; Wang, X.; Kataoka, S.; Sekiya, Y.; Hamada, M.; Murakami, N.; et al. MEF2D-BCL9 Fusion Gene Is Associated With High-Risk Acute B-Cell Precursor Lymphoblastic Leukemia in Adolescents. *J. Clin. Oncol.* **2016**, *34*, 3451–3459. [CrossRef] [PubMed]
87. Ohki, K.; Kiyokawa, N.; Saito, Y.; Hirabayashi, S.; Nakabayashi, K.; Ichikawa, H.; Momozawa, Y.; Okamura, K.; Yoshimi, A.; Ogata-Kawata, H.; et al. Clinical and molecular characteristics of MEF2D fusion-positive B-cell precursor acute lymphoblastic leukemia in childhood, including a novel translocation resulting in MEF2D-HNRNPH1 gene fusion. *Haematologica* **2018**, *104*, 128–137. [CrossRef] [PubMed]
88. Ueno, H.; Yoshida, K.; Shiozawa, Y.; Nannya, Y.; Iijima-Yamashita, Y.; Kiyokawa, N.; Shiraishi, Y.; Chiba, K.; Tanaka, H.; Isobe, T.; et al. Landscape of driver mutations and their clinical impacts in pediatric B-cell precursor acute lymphoblastic leukemia. *Blood Adv.* **2020**, *4*, 5165–5173. [CrossRef] [PubMed]
89. Tsuzuki, S.; Yasuda, T.; Kojima, S.; Kawazu, M.; Akahane, K.; Inukai, T.; Imaizumi, M.; Morishita, T.; Miyamura, T.; Ueno, T.; et al. Targeting MEF2D-fusion Oncogenic Transcriptional Circuitries in B-cell Precursor Acute Lymphoblastic Leukemia. *Blood Cancer Discov.* **2020**, *1*, 82–95. [CrossRef]
90. Tange, N.; Hayakawa, F.; Yasuda, T.; Odaira, K.; Yamamoto, H.; Hirano, D.; Sakai, T.; Terakura, S.; Tsuzuki, S.; Kiyoi, H. Staurosporine and venetoclax induce the caspase-dependent proteolysis of MEF2D-fusion proteins and apoptosis in MEF2D-fusion (+) ALL cells. *Biomed. Pharmacother.* **2020**, *128*, 110330. [CrossRef]

91. Zaliova, M.; Stuchly, J.; Winkowska, L.; Musilova, A.; Fiser, K.; Slamova, M.; Starkova, J.; Vaskova, M.; Hrusak, O.; Sramkova, L.; et al. Genomic landscape of pediatric B-other acute lymphoblastic leukemia in a consecutive European cohort. *Haematologica* **2019**, *104*, 1396–1406. [CrossRef] [PubMed]
92. Alexander, T.B.; Gu, Z.; Iacobucci, I.; Dickerson, K.; Choi, J.K.; Xu, B.; Payne-Turner, D.; Yoshihara, H.; Loh, M.L.; Horan, J.; et al. The genetic basis and cell of origin of mixed phenotype acute leukaemia. *Nature* **2018**, *562*, 373–379. [CrossRef] [PubMed]
93. Hirabayashi, S.; Butler, E.R.; Ohki, K.; Kiyokawa, N.; Bergmann, A.K.; Möricke, A.; Boer, J.M.; Cavé, H.; Cazzaniga, G.; Yeoh, A.E.J.; et al. Clinical characteristics and outcomes of B-ALL with ZNF384 rearrangements: A retrospective analysis by the Ponte di Legno Childhood ALL Working Group. *Leukemia* **2021**, 1–6. [CrossRef]
94. Hirabayashi, S.; Ohki, K.; Nakabayashi, K.; Ichikawa, H.; Momozawa, Y.; Okamura, K.; Yaguchi, A.; Terada, K.; Saito, Y.; Yoshimi, A.; et al. ZNF384-related fusion genes define a subgroup of childhood B-cell precursor acute lymphoblastic leukemia with a characteristic immunotype. *Haematologica* **2016**, *102*, 118–129. [CrossRef]
95. Janet, N.B.; Kulkarni, U.; Arun, A.K.; Bensega, B.; Devasia, A.J.; Korula, A.; Abraham, A.; George, B.; Mathews, V.; Balasubramanian, P. Systematic application of fluorescence in situ hybridization and immunophenotype profile for the identification of ZNF384 gene rearrangements in B cell acute lymphoblastic leukemia. *Int. J. Lab. Hematol.* **2021**, *43*, 658–663. [CrossRef]
96. Bueno, C.; Tejedor, J.R.; Bashford-Rogers, R.; González-Silva, L.; Valdés-Mas, R.; Agraz-Doblás, A.; de la Guardia, R.D.; Ribera, J.; Zamora, L.; Bilhou-Nabera, C.; et al. Natural history and cell of origin of TCF3-ZNF384 and PTPN11 mutations in monozygotic twins with concordant BCP-ALL. *Blood* **2019**, *134*, 900–905. [CrossRef]
97. Griffith, M.; Griffith, O.L.; Krysiak, K.; Skidmore, Z.; Christopher, M.J.; Klco, J.; Ramu, A.; Lamprecht, T.L.; Wagner, A.H.; Campbell, K.; et al. Comprehensive genomic analysis reveals FLT3 activation and a therapeutic strategy for a patient with relapsed adult B-lymphoblastic leukemia. *Exp. Hematol.* **2016**, *44*, 603–613. [CrossRef]
98. Boer, J.M.; Valsecchi, M.G.; Hormann, F.M.; Antic, Z.; Zaliova, M.; Schwab, C.; Cazzaniga, G.; Arfeuille, C.; Cave, H.; Attarbaschi, A.; et al. Favorable outcome of NUTM1-rearranged infant and pediatric B cell precursor acute lymphoblastic leukemia in a collaborative international study. *Leukemia* **2021**, 1–5. [CrossRef]
99. Hormann, F.M.; Hoogkamer, A.Q.; Beverloo, H.B.; Boeree, A.; Dingjan, I.; Wattel, M.M.; Stam, R.W.; Escherich, G.; Pieters, R.; Boer, M.L.D.; et al. NUTM1 is a recurrent fusion gene partner in B-cell precursor acute lymphoblastic leukemia associated with increased expression of genes on chromosome band 10p12.31-12.2. *Haematologica* **2019**, *104*, e455–e459. [CrossRef]
100. McEvoy, C.R.; Fox, S.B.; Prall, O.W.J. Emerging entities in NUTM1-rearranged neoplasms. *Genes Chromosom. Cancer* **2020**, *59*, 375–385. [CrossRef]
101. French, C.A. NUT Carcinoma: Clinicopathologic features, pathogenesis, and treatment. *Pathol. Int.* **2018**, *68*, 583–595. [CrossRef]
102. Boer, M.L.D.; van Slegtenhorst, M.; De Menezes, R.X.; Cheok, M.; Buijs-Gladdines, J.G.; Peters, S.T.; Van Zutven, L.J.; Beverloo, H.B.; Van der Spek, P.J.; Escherich, G.; et al. A subtype of childhood acute lymphoblastic leukaemia with poor treatment outcome: A genome-wide classification study. *Lancet Oncol.* **2009**, *10*, 125–134. [CrossRef]
103. Mullighan, C.; Su, X.; Zhang, J.; Radtke, I.; Phillips, L.A.; Miller, C.B.; Ma, J.; Liu, W.; Cheng, C.; Schulman, B.A.; et al. Deletion of IKZF1and Prognosis in Acute Lymphoblastic Leukemia. *N. Engl. J. Med.* **2009**, *360*, 470–480. [CrossRef]
104. Iacobucci, I.; Roberts, K. Genetic Alterations and Therapeutic Targeting of Philadelphia-Like Acute Lymphoblastic Leukemia. *Genes* **2021**, *12*, 687. [CrossRef] [PubMed]
105. Roberts, K.G.; Reshmi, S.C.; Harvey, R.; Chen, I.-M.; Patel, K.; Stonerock, E.; Jenkins, H.; Dai, Y.; Valentine, M.; Gu, Z.; et al. Genomic and outcome analyses of Ph-like ALL in NCI standard-risk patients: A report from the Children's Oncology Group. *Blood* **2018**, *132*, 815–824. [CrossRef] [PubMed]
106. Reshmi, S.C.; Harvey, R.C.; Roberts, K.G.; Stonerock, E.; Smith, A.; Jenkins, H.; Chen, I.-M.; Valentine, M.; Liu, Y.; Li, Y.; et al. Targetable kinase gene fusions in high-risk B-ALL: A study from the Children's Oncology Group. *Blood* **2017**, *129*, 3352–3361. [CrossRef]
107. Tasian, S.K.; Hurtz, C.; Wertheim, G.B.; Bailey, N.; Lim, M.; Harvey, R.; Chen, I.-M.; Willman, C.L.; Astles, R.; Zebrowski, A.; et al. High incidence of Philadelphia chromosome-like acute lymphoblastic leukemia in older adults with B-ALL. *Leukemia* **2016**, *31*, 981–984. [CrossRef]
108. Jain, N.; Roberts, K.G.; Jabbour, E.; Patel, K.; Eterovic, A.K.; Chen, K.; Zweidler-McKay, P.; Lu, X.; Fawcett, G.; Wang, S.A.; et al. Ph-like acute lymphoblastic leukemia: A high-risk subtype in adults. *Blood* **2017**, *129*, 572–581. [CrossRef]
109. Roberts, K.G. The biology of Philadelphia chromosome-like ALL. *Best Pract. Res. Clin. Haematol.* **2017**, *30*, 212–221. [CrossRef]
110. Chiaretti, S.; Messina, M.; Foà, R. BCR/ABL1-like acute lymphoblastic leukemia: How to diagnose and treat? *Cancer* **2018**, *125*, 194–204. [CrossRef]
111. Mullighan, C.G.; Collins-Underwood, J.R.; Phillips, L.A.; Loudin, M.G.; Liu, W.; Zhang, J.; Ma, J.; Coustan-Smith, E.; Harvey, R.C.; Willman, C.L.; et al. Rearrangement of CRLF2 in B-progenitor–and Down syndrome–associated acute lymphoblastic leukemia. *Nat. Genet.* **2009**, *41*, 1243–1246. [CrossRef]
112. Yoda, A.; Yoda, Y.; Chiaretti, S.; Bar-Natan, M.; Mani, K.; Rodig, S.J.; West, N.; Xiao, Y.; Brown, J.R.; Mitsiades, C.; et al. Functional screening identifies CRLF2 in precursor B-cell acute lymphoblastic leukemia. *Proc. Natl. Acad. Sci. USA* **2009**, *107*, 252–257. [CrossRef] [PubMed]

113. Russell, L.J.; Jones, L.; Enshaei, A.; Tonin, S.; Ryan, S.L.; Eswaran, J.; Nakjang, S.; Papaemmanuil, E.; Tubio, J.M.C.; Fielding, A.K.; et al. Characterisation of the genomic landscape of CRLF2-rearranged acute lymphoblastic leukemia. *Genes Chromosom. Cancer* **2017**, *56*, 363–372. [CrossRef] [PubMed]
114. Hertzberg, L.; Vendramini, E.; Ganmore, I.; Cazzaniga, G.; Schmitz, M.; Chalker, J.; Shiloh, R.; Iacobucci, I.; Shochat, C.; Zeligson, S.; et al. Down syndrome acute lymphoblastic leukemia, a highly heterogeneous disease in which aberrant expression of CRLF2 is associated with mutated JAK2: A report from the International BFM Study Group. *Blood* **2010**, *115*, 1006–1017. [CrossRef] [PubMed]
115. Iacobucci, I.; Li, Y.; Roberts, K.G.; Dobson, S.M.; Kim, J.C.; Payne-Turner, D.; Harvey, R.C.; Valentine, M.; McCastlain, K.; Easton, J.; et al. Truncating Erythropoietin Receptor Rearrangements in Acute Lymphoblastic Leukemia. *Cancer Cell* **2016**, *29*, 186–200. [CrossRef]
116. Stanulla, M.; Dagdan, E.; Zaliova, M.; Möricke, A.; Palmi, C.; Cazzaniga, G.; Eckert, C.; Kronnie, G.T.; Bourquin, J.-P.; Bornhauser, B.; et al. IKZF1plus Defines a New Minimal Residual Disease–Dependent Very-Poor Prognostic Profile in Pediatric B-Cell Precursor Acute Lymphoblastic Leukemia. *J. Clin. Oncol.* **2018**, *36*, 1240–1249. [CrossRef]
117. Tanasi, I.; Ba, I.; Sirvent, N.; Braun, T.; Cuccuini, W.; Ballerini, P.; Duployez, N.; Tanguy-Schmidt, A.; Tamburini, J.; Maury, S.; et al. Efficacy of tyrosine kinase inhibitors in Ph-like acute lymphoblastic leukemia harboring ABL-class rearrangements. *Blood* **2019**, *134*, 1351–1355. [CrossRef]
118. Schewe, D.M.; Lenk, L.; Vogiatzi, F.; Winterberg, D.; Rademacher, A.V.; Buchmann, S.; Henry, D.; Bergmann, A.K.; Cario, G.; Cox, M.C. Larotrectinib in TRK fusion–positive pediatric B-cell acute lymphoblastic leukemia. *Blood Adv.* **2019**, *3*, 3499–3502. [CrossRef]
119. Niswander, L.M.; Loftus, J.P.; Lainey, E.; Caye-Eude, A.; Pondrom, M.; Hottman, D.A.; Iacobucci, I.; Mullighan, C.G.; Jain, N.; Konopleva, M.; et al. Therapeutic potential of ruxolitinib and ponatinib in patients with EPOR-rearranged Philadelphia chromosome-like acute lymphoblastic leukemia. *Haematologica* **2021**. [CrossRef] [PubMed]
120. Chang, Y.; Min, J.; Jarusiewicz, J.; Actis, M.; Bradford, S.Y.-C.; Mayasundari, A.; Yang, L.; Chepyala, D.; Alcock, L.J.; Roberts, K.G.; et al. Degradation of Janus kinases in CRLF2-rearranged acute lymphoblastic leukemia. *Blood* **2021**. [CrossRef]
121. Qin, H.; Cho, M.; Haso, W.; Zhang, L.; Tasian, S.K.; Oo, H.Z.; Negri, G.L.; Lin, Y.; Zou, J.; Mallon, B.S.; et al. Eradication of B-ALL using chimeric antigen receptor–expressing T cells targeting the TSLPR oncoprotein. *Blood* **2015**, *126*, 629–639. [CrossRef] [PubMed]
122. Zaliova, M.; Kotrová, M.; Bresolin, S.; Stuchly, J.; Stary, J.; Hrusak, O.; Kronnie, G.T.; Trka, J.; Zuna, J.; Vaskova, M. ETV6/RUNX1-like acute lymphoblastic leukemia: A novel B-cell precursor leukemia subtype associated with the CD27/CD44 immunophenotype. *Genes Chromosom. Cancer* **2017**, *56*, 608–616. [CrossRef]
123. Zaliova, M.; Moorman, A.V.; Cazzaniga, G.; Stanulla, M.; Harvey, R.C.; Roberts, K.G.; Heatley, S.L.; Loh, M.L.; Konopleva, M.; Chen, I.-M.; et al. Characterization of leukemias with ETV6-ABL1 fusion. *Haematologica* **2016**, *101*, 1082–1093. [CrossRef]
124. Nishii, R.; Baskin-Doerfler, R.; Yang, W.; Oak, N.; Zhao, X.; Yang, W.; Hoshitsuki, K.; Bloom, M.; Verbist, K.C.; Burns, M.A.; et al. Molecular basis of ETV6-mediated predisposition to childhood acute lymphoblastic leukemia. *Blood* **2021**, *137*, 364–373. [CrossRef]
125. Bastian, L.; Schroeder, M.P.; Eckert, C.; Schlee, C.; Tanchez, J.O.; Kämpf, S.; Wagner, D.L.; Schulze, V.; Isaakidis, K.; Lázaro-Navarro, J.; et al. PAX5 biallelic genomic alterations define a novel subgroup of B-cell precursor acute lymphoblastic leukemia. *Leukemia* **2019**, *33*, 1895–1909. [CrossRef]
126. Passet, M.; Boissel, N.; Sigaux, F.; Saillard, C.; Bargetzi, M.; Ba, I.; Thomas, X.; Graux, C.; Chalandon, Y.; Leguay, T.; et al. PAX5 P80R mutation identifies a novel subtype of B-cell precursor acute lymphoblastic leukemia with favorable outcome. *Blood* **2019**, *133*, 280–284. [CrossRef]
127. Shah, S.; Schrader, K.; Waanders, E.; Timms, A.E.; Vijai, J.; Miething, C.; Wechsler, J.; Yang, J.; Hayes, J.; Klein, R.; et al. A recurrent germline PAX5 mutation confers susceptibility to pre-B cell acute lymphoblastic leukemia. *Nat. Genet.* **2013**, *45*, 1226–1231. [CrossRef] [PubMed]
128. Vairy, S.; Tran, T.H. IKZF1 alterations in acute lymphoblastic leukemia: The good, the bad and the ugly. *Blood Rev.* **2020**, *44*, 100677. [CrossRef] [PubMed]
129. Churchman, M.L.; Mullighan, C.G. Ikaros: Exploiting and targeting the hematopoietic stem cell niche in B-progenitor acute lymphoblastic leukemia. *Exp. Hematol.* **2016**, *46*, 1–8. [CrossRef]
130. Churchman, M.L.; Low, J.; Qu, C.; Paietta, E.M.; Kasper, L.H.; Chang, Y.; Payne-Turner, D.; Althoff, M.J.; Song, G.; Chen, S.-C.; et al. Efficacy of Retinoids in IKZF1-Mutated BCR-ABL1 Acute Lymphoblastic Leukemia. *Cancer Cell* **2015**, *28*, 343–356. [CrossRef] [PubMed]
131. Zaliova, M.; Potuckova, E.; Lukes, J.; Winkowska, L.; Starkova, J.; Janotova, I.; Sramkova, L.; Stary, J.; Zuna, J.; Stanulla, M.; et al. Frequency and prognostic impact of ZEB2 H1038 and Q1072 mutations in childhood B-other acute lymphoblastic leukemia. *Haematologica* **2020**, *106*, 886–890. [CrossRef] [PubMed]
132. Aifantis, I.; Raetz, E.A.; Buonamici, S. Molecular pathogenesis of T-cell leukaemia and lymphoma. *Nat. Rev. Immunol.* **2008**, *8*, 380–390. [CrossRef] [PubMed]
133. Yui, M.; Rothenberg, E. Developmental gene networks: A triathlon on the course to T cell identity. *Nat. Rev. Immunol.* **2014**, *14*, 529–545. [CrossRef] [PubMed]
134. Teachey, D.T.; Pui, C.-H. Comparative features and outcomes between paediatric T-cell and B-cell acute lymphoblastic leukaemia. *Lancet Oncol.* **2019**, *20*, e142–e154. [CrossRef]

135. Liu, Y.; Easton, J.; Shao, Y.; Maciaszek, J.; Wang, Z.; Wilkinson, M.R.; McCastlain, K.; Edmonson, M.; Pounds, S.B.; Shi, L.; et al. The genomic landscape of pediatric and young adult T-lineage acute lymphoblastic leukemia. *Nat. Genet.* **2017**, *49*, 1211–1218. [CrossRef]
136. Seki, M.; Kimura, S.; Isobe, T.; Yoshida, K.; Ueno, H.; Nakajima-Takagi, Y.; Wang, C.; Lin, L.; Kon, A.; Suzuki, H.; et al. Recurrent SPI1 (PU.1) fusions in high-risk pediatric T cell acute lymphoblastic leukemia. *Nat. Genet.* **2017**, *49*, 1274–1281. [CrossRef]
137. Mansour, M.; Abraham, B.; Anders, L.; Berezovskaya, A.; Gutierrez, A.; Durbin, A.; Etchin, J.; Lawton, L.; Sallan, S.E.; Silverman, L.B.; et al. An oncogenic super-enhancer formed through somatic mutation of a noncoding intergenic element. *Science* **2014**, *346*, 1373–1377. [CrossRef]
138. Hu, S.; Qian, M.; Zhang, H.; Guo, Y.; Yang, J.; Zhao, X.; He, H.; Lu, J.; Pan, J.; Chang, M.; et al. Whole-genome noncoding sequence analysis in T-cell acute lymphoblastic leukemia identifies oncogene enhancer mutations. *Blood* **2017**, *129*, 3264–3268. [CrossRef] [PubMed]
139. Mansour, M.R.; Duke, V.; Foroni, L.; Patel, B.; Allen, C.; Ancliff, P.J.; Gale, R.E.; Linch, D.C. Notch-1 Mutations Are Secondary Events in Some Patients with T-Cell Acute Lymphoblastic Leukemia. *Clin. Cancer Res.* **2007**, *13*, 6964–6969. [CrossRef]
140. Gianni, F.; Belver, L.; Ferrando, A. The Genetics and Mechanisms of T-Cell Acute Lymphoblastic Leukemia. *Cold Spring Harb. Perspect. Med.* **2019**, *10*, a035246. [CrossRef]
141. Belver, L.; Ferrando, L.B.A. The genetics and mechanisms of T cell acute lymphoblastic leukaemia. *Nat. Rev. Cancer* **2016**, *16*, 494–507. [CrossRef]
142. Kimura, S.; Seki, M.; Kawai, T.; Goto, H.; Yoshida, K.; Isobe, T.; Sekiguchi, M.; Watanabe, K.; Kubota, Y.; Nannya, Y.; et al. DNA methylation-based classification reveals difference between pediatric T-cell acute lymphoblastic leukemia and normal thymocytes. *Leukemia* **2019**, *34*, 1163–1168. [CrossRef] [PubMed]
143. Roels, J.; Thénoz, M.; Szarzyńska, B.; Landfors, M.; De Coninck, S.; Demoen, L.; Provez, L.; Kuchmiy, A.; Strubbe, S.; Reunes, L.; et al. Aging of Preleukemic Thymocytes Drives CpG Island Hypermethylation in T-cell Acute Lymphoblastic Leukemia. *Blood Cancer Discov.* **2020**, *1*, 274–289. [CrossRef] [PubMed]
144. Ferrando, A.A.; Neuberg, D.S.; Staunton, J.; Loh, M.L.; Huard, C.; Raimondi, S.C.; Behm, F.G.; Pui, C.-H.; Downing, J.R.; Gilliland, D.; et al. Gene expression signatures define novel oncogenic pathways in T cell acute lymphoblastic leukemia. *Cancer Cell* **2002**, *1*, 75–87. [CrossRef]
145. Soulier, J.; Clappier, E.; Cayuela, J.-M.; Regnault, A.; García-Peydró, M.; Dombret, H.; Baruchel, A.; Toribio, M.L.; Sigaux, F. HOXA genes are included in genetic and biologic networks defining human acute T-cell leukemia (T-ALL). *Blood* **2005**, *106*, 274–286. [CrossRef] [PubMed]
146. Dadi, S.; Le Noir, S.; Bornet, D.P.; Lhermitte, L.; Zacarias-Cabeza, J.; Bergeron, J.; Villarèse, P.; Vachez, E.; Dik, W.A.; Millien, C.; et al. TLX Homeodomain Oncogenes Mediate T Cell Maturation Arrest in T-ALL via Interaction with ETS1 and Suppression of TCRα Gene Expression. *Cancer Cell* **2012**, *21*, 563–576. [CrossRef] [PubMed]
147. Di Giacomo, D.; La Starza, R.; Gorello, P.; Pellanera, F.; Atak, Z.K.; De Keersmaecker, K.; Pierini, V.; Harrison, C.J.; Arniani, S.; Moretti, M.; et al. 14q32 rearrangements deregulating BCL11B mark a distinct subgroup of T and myeloid immature acute leukemia. *Blood* **2021**. [CrossRef] [PubMed]
148. Inaba, H.; Azzato, E.M.; Mullighan, C.G. Integration of Next-Generation Sequencing to Treat Acute Lymphoblastic Leukemia with Targetable Lesions: The St. Jude Children's Research Hospital Approach. *Front. Pediatr.* **2017**, *5*, 258. [CrossRef]
149. Gocho, Y.; Liu, J.; Hu, J.; Yang, W.; Dharia, N.V.; Zhang, J.; Shi, H.; Du, G.; John, A.; Lin, T.-N.; et al. Network-based systems pharmacology reveals heterogeneity in LCK and BCL2 signaling and therapeutic sensitivity of T-cell acute lymphoblastic leukemia. *Nat. Rev. Cancer* **2021**, *2*, 1–16. [CrossRef]
150. Hnisz, D.; Weintraub, A.S.; Day, D.S.; Valton, A.-L.; Bak, R.; Li, C.; Goldmann, J.; Lajoie, B.R.; Fan, Z.P.; Sigova, A.A.; et al. Activation of proto-oncogenes by disruption of chromosome neighborhoods. *Science* **2016**, *351*, 1454–1458. [CrossRef]
151. Park, S.T.; Sun, X.-H. The Tal1 Oncoprotein Inhibits E47-mediated Transcription. *J. Biol. Chem.* **1998**, *273*, 7030–7037. [CrossRef]
152. Sanda, T.; Lawton, L.N.; Barrasa, M.I.; Fan, Z.P.; Kohlhammer, H.; Gutierrez, A.; Ma, W.; Tatarek, J.; Ahn, Y.; Kelliher, M.A.; et al. Core Transcriptional Regulatory Circuit Controlled by the TAL1 Complex in Human T Cell Acute Lymphoblastic Leukemia. *Cancer Cell* **2012**, *22*, 209–221. [CrossRef]
153. Nottingham, W.T.; Jarratt, A.; Burgess, M.; Speck, C.L.; Cheng, J.F.; Prabhakar, S.; Rubin, E.M.; Li, P.S.; Sloane-Stanley, J.; Kong, A.S.J.; et al. Runx1-mediated hematopoietic stem-cell emergence is controlled by a Gata/Ets/SCL-regulated enhancer. *Blood* **2007**, *110*, 4188–4197. [CrossRef]
154. Choi, A.; Illendula, A.; Pulikkan, J.A.; Roderick, J.E.; Tesell, J.; Yu, J.; Hermance, N.; Zhu, L.J.; Castilla, L.H.; Bushweller, J.H.; et al. RUNX1 is required for oncogenic Myb and Myc enhancer activity in T-cell acute lymphoblastic leukemia. *Blood* **2017**, *130*, 1722–1733. [CrossRef] [PubMed]
155. O'Neil, J.; Shank, J.; Cusson, N.; Murre, C.; Kelliher, M. TAL1/SCL induces leukemia by inhibiting the transcriptional activity of E47/HEB. *Cancer Cell* **2004**, *5*, 587–596. [CrossRef]
156. Draheim, K.M.; Hermance, N.; Yang, Y.; Arous, E.; Calvo, J.; Kelliher, M.A. A DNA-binding mutant of TAL1 cooperates with LMO2 to cause T cell leukemia in mice. *Oncogene* **2010**, *30*, 1252–1260. [CrossRef] [PubMed]
157. Ferrando, A.A.; Look, A.T. Gene expression profiling in T-cell acute lymphoblastic leukemia. *Semin. Hematol.* **2003**, *40*, 274–280. [CrossRef]

158. Leong, W.Z.; Tan, S.H.; Ngoc, P.C.T.; Amanda, S.; Yam, A.W.Y.; Liau, W.-S.; Gong, Z.; Lawton, L.N.; Tenen, D.G.; Sanda, T. ARID5B as a critical downstream target of the TAL1 complex that activates the oncogenic transcriptional program and promotes T-cell leukemogenesis. *Genes Dev.* **2017**, *31*, 2343–2360. [CrossRef]
159. Tan, S.H.; Leong, W.Z.; Ngoc, P.C.T.; Tan, T.K.; Bertulfo, F.C.; Lim, M.C.; An, O.; Li, Z.; Yeoh, A.E.J.; Fullwood, M.J.; et al. The enhancer RNA ARIEL activates the oncogenic transcriptional program in T-cell acute lymphoblastic leukemia. *Blood* **2019**, *134*, 239–251. [CrossRef] [PubMed]
160. Piovan, E.; Yu, J.; Tosello, V.; Herranz, D.; Ambesi-Impiombato, A.; Da Silva, A.C.; Sanchez-Martin, M.; Perez-Garcia, A.; Rigo, I.; Castillo, M.; et al. Direct Reversal of Glucocorticoid Resistance by AKT Inhibition in Acute Lymphoblastic Leukemia. *Cancer Cell* **2013**, *24*, 766–776. [CrossRef]
161. Jena, N.; Sheng, J.; Hu, J.K.; Li, W.; Zhou, W.; Lee, G.; Tsichlis, N.; Pathak, A.; Brown, N.; Deshpande, A.; et al. CDK6-mediated repression of CD25 is required for induction and maintenance of Notch1-induced T-cell acute lymphoblastic leukemia. *Leukemia* **2015**, *30*, 1033–1043. [CrossRef] [PubMed]
162. Coustan-Smith, E.; Mullighan, C.; Onciu, M.; Behm, F.G.; Raimondi, S.C.; Pei, D.; Cheng, C.; Su, X.; Rubnitz, J.; Basso, G.; et al. Early T-cell precursor leukaemia: A subtype of very high-risk acute lymphoblastic leukaemia. *Lancet Oncol.* **2009**, *10*, 147–156. [CrossRef]
163. Zhang, J.; Ding, L.; Holmfeldt, L.; Wu, G.; Heatley, S.; Payne-Turner, D.; Easton, J.; Chen, X.; Wang, J.; Rusch, M.; et al. The genetic basis of early T-cell precursor acute lymphoblastic leukaemia. *Nature* **2012**, *481*, 157–163. [CrossRef]
164. Maude, S.L.; Dolai, S.; Delgado-Martin, C.; Vincent, T.; Robbins, A.; Selvanathan, A.; Ryan, T.; Hall, J.; Wood, A.C.; Tasian, S.K.; et al. Efficacy of JAK/STAT pathway inhibition in murine xenograft models of early T-cell precursor (ETP) acute lymphoblastic leukemia. *Blood* **2015**, *125*, 1759–1767. [CrossRef]
165. McCarter, A.C.; Wang, Q.; Chiang, M. Notch in Leukemia. *Adv. Exp. Med. Biol.* **2018**, *1066*, 355–394. [CrossRef] [PubMed]
166. Weng, A.; Ferrando, A.A.; Lee, W.; Iv, J.P.M.; Silverman, L.B.; Sanchez-Irizarry, C.; Blacklow, S.C.; Look, A.T.; Aster, J.C. Activating Mutations of NOTCH1 in Human T Cell Acute Lymphoblastic Leukemia. *Science* **2004**, *306*, 269–271. [CrossRef]
167. Sulis, M.L.; Williams, O.; Palomero, T.; Tosello, V.; Pallikuppam, S.; Real, P.J.; Barnes, K.; Zuurbier, L.; Meijerink, J.P.; Ferrando, A.A. NOTCH1 extracellular juxtamembrane expansion mutations in T-ALL. *Blood* **2008**, *112*, 733–740. [CrossRef]
168. Haydu, J.E.; De Keersmaecker, K.; Duff, M.K.; Paietta, E.; Racevskis, J.; Wiernik, P.H.; Rowe, J.M.; Ferrando, A. An activating intragenic deletion in NOTCH1 in human T-ALL. *Blood* **2012**, *119*, 5211–5214. [CrossRef]
169. Thompson, B.J.; Buonamici, S.; Sulis, M.L.; Palomero, T.; Vilimas, T.; Basso, G.; Ferrando, A.; Aifantis, I. The SCFFBW7 ubiquitin ligase complex as a tumor suppressor in T cell leukemia. *J. Exp. Med.* **2007**, *204*, 1825–1835. [CrossRef]
170. O'Neil, J.; Grim, J.; Strack, P.; Rao, S.; Tibbitts, D.; Winter, C.; Hardwick, J.; Welcker, M.; Meijerink, J.; Pieters, R.; et al. FBW7 mutations in leukemic cells mediate NOTCH pathway activation and resistance to γ-secretase inhibitors. *J. Exp. Med.* **2007**, *204*, 1813–1824. [CrossRef]
171. Suarez-Puente, X.; Beà, S.; Valdés-Mas, R.; Villamor, N.; Gutiérrez-Abril, J.; Martin-Subero, J.I.; Munar, M.; Rubio-Perez, C.; Jares, P.; Aymerich, M.; et al. Non-coding recurrent mutations in chronic lymphocytic leukaemia. *Nature* **2015**, *526*, 519–524. [CrossRef]
172. Chiang, M.; Xu, L.; Shestova, O.; Histen, G.; L'Heureux, S.; Romany, C.; Childs, M.E.; Gimotty, P.A.; Aster, J.C.; Pear, W.S. Leukemia-associated NOTCH1 alleles are weak tumor initiators but accelerate K-ras–initiated leukemia. *J. Clin. Investig.* **2008**, *118*, 3181–3194. [CrossRef]
173. Wendorff, A.A.; Quinn, S.A.; Rashkovan, M.; Madubata, C.J.; Ambesi-Impiombato, A.; Litzow, M.R.; Tallman, M.S.; Paietta, E.; Paganin, M.; Basso, G.; et al. Phf6 Loss Enhances HSC Self-Renewal Driving Tumor Initiation and Leukemia Stem Cell Activity in T-ALL. *Cancer Discov.* **2018**, *9*, 436–451. [CrossRef]
174. Herranz, D.; Ambesi-Impiombato, A.; Palomero, T.; Schnell, S.A.; Belver, L.; Wendorff, A.A.; Xu, L.; Castillo-Martin, M.; Llobet-Navás, D.; Cordon-Cardo, C.; et al. A NOTCH1-driven MYC enhancer promotes T cell development, transformation and acute lymphoblastic leukemia. *Nat. Med.* **2014**, *20*, 1130–1137. [CrossRef]
175. Albertí-Servera, L.; Demeyer, S.; Govaerts, I.; Swings, T.; De Bie, J.; Gielen, O.; Brociner, M.; Michaux, L.; Maertens, J.; Uyttebroeck, A.; et al. Single-cell DNA amplicon sequencing reveals clonal heterogeneity and evolution in T-cell acute lymphoblastic leukemia. *Blood* **2021**, *137*, 801–811. [CrossRef]
176. De Bie, J.; Demeyer, S.; Alberti-Servera, L.; Geerdens, E.; Segers, H.; Broux, M.; De Keersmaecker, K.; Michaux, L.; Vandenberghe, P.; Voet, T.; et al. Single-cell sequencing reveals the origin and the order of mutation acquisition in T-cell acute lymphoblastic leukemia. *Leukemia* **2018**, *32*, 1358–1369. [CrossRef]
177. Yashiro-Ohtani, Y.; Wang, H.; Zang, C.; Arnett, K.L.; Bailis, W.; Ho, Y.; Knoechel, B.; Lanauze, C.; Louis, L.; Forsyth, K.; et al. Long-range enhancer activity determines Myc sensitivity to Notch inhibitors in T cell leukemia. *Proc. Natl. Acad. Sci. USA* **2014**, *111*, E4946–E4953. [CrossRef]
178. Sanchez-Martin, M.; Ferrando, A. The NOTCH1-MYC highway toward T-cell acute lymphoblastic leukemia. *Blood* **2017**, *129*, 1124–1133. [CrossRef]
179. Reizis, B. Direct induction of T lymphocyte-specific gene expression by the mammalian Notch signaling pathway. *Genes Dev.* **2002**, *16*, 295–300. [CrossRef]
180. Zheng, R.; Li, M.; Wang, S.; Liu, Y. Advances of target therapy on NOTCH1 signaling pathway in T-cell acute lymphoblastic leukemia. *Exp. Hematol. Oncol.* **2020**, *9*, 31. [CrossRef]

181. Papayannidis, C.; De Angelo, D.J.; Stock, W.; Huang, B.; Shaik, M.N.; Cesari, R.; Zheng, X.; Reynolds, J.M.; English, P.A.; Ozeck, M.; et al. A Phase 1 study of the novel gamma-secretase inhibitor PF-03084014 in patients with T-cell acute lymphoblastic leukemia and T-cell lymphoblastic lymphoma. *Blood Cancer J.* **2015**, *5*, e350. [CrossRef] [PubMed]
182. Gavai, A.V.; Quesnelle, C.A.; Norris, D.J.; Han, W.-C.; Gill, P.S.; Shan, W.; Balog, A.; Chen, K.; Tebben, A.J.; Rampulla, R.; et al. Discovery of Clinical Candidate BMS-906024: A Potent Pan-Notch Inhibitor for the Treatment of Leukemia and Solid Tumors. *ACS Med. Chem. Lett.* **2015**, *6*, 523–527. [CrossRef]
183. Sanchez-Martin, M.; Ambesi-Impiombato, A.; Qin, Y.; Herranz, D.; Bansal, M.; Girardi, T.; Paietta, E.; Tallman, M.S.; Rowe, J.M.; De Keersmaecker, K.; et al. Synergistic antileukemic therapies inNOTCH1-induced T-ALL. *Proc. Natl. Acad. Sci. USA* **2017**, *114*, 2006–2011. [CrossRef] [PubMed]
184. Wei, P.; Walls, M.; Qiu, M.; Ding, R.; Denlinger, R.H.; Wong, A.; Tsaparikos, K.; Jani, J.P.; Hosea, N.A.; Sands, M.; et al. Evaluation of Selective γ-Secretase Inhibitor PF-03084014 for Its Antitumor Efficacy and Gastrointestinal Safety to Guide Optimal Clinical Trial Design. *Mol. Cancer Ther.* **2010**, *9*, 1618–1628. [CrossRef]
185. Real, P.; Tosello, V.; Palomero, T.; Castillo, M.; Hernando, E.; De Stanchina, E.; Sulis, M.L.; Barnes, K.; Sawai, C.; Homminga, I.; et al. γ-secretase inhibitors reverse glucocorticoid resistance in T cell acute lymphoblastic leukemia. *Nat. Med.* **2008**, *15*, 50–58. [CrossRef]
186. Cullion, K.; Draheim, K.M.; Hermance, N.; Tammam, J.; Sharma, V.M.; Ware, C.; Nikov, G.; Krishnamoorthy, V.; Majumder, P.K.; Kelliher, M.A. Targeting the Notch1 and mTOR pathways in a mouse T-ALL model. *Blood* **2009**, *113*, 6172–6181. [CrossRef]
187. Franciosa, G.; Smits, J.G.A.; Minuzzo, S.; Martinez-Val, A.; Indraccolo, S.; Olsen, J.V. Proteomics of resistance to Notch1 inhibition in acute lymphoblastic leukemia reveals targetable kinase signatures. *Nat. Commun.* **2021**, *12*, 2507. [CrossRef]
188. Trinquand, A.; Tanguy-Schmidt, A.; Ben Abdelali, R.; Lambert, J.; Beldjord, K.; Lengliné, E.; De Gunzburg, N.; Bornet, D.P.; Lhermitte, L.; Mossafa, H.; et al. Toward a NOTCH1/FBXW7/RAS/PTEN–Based Oncogenetic Risk Classification of Adult T-Cell Acute Lymphoblastic Leukemia: A Group for Research in Adult Acute Lymphoblastic Leukemia Study. *J. Clin. Oncol.* **2013**, *31*, 4333–4342. [CrossRef] [PubMed]
189. Newman, S.; Nakitandwe, J.; Kesserwan, C.A.; Azzato, E.M.; Wheeler, D.A.; Rusch, M.; Shurtleff, S.; Hedges, D.J.; Hamilton, K.V.; Foy, S.G.; et al. Genomes for Kids: The scope of pathogenic mutations in pediatric cancer revealed by comprehensive DNA and RNA sequencing. *Cancer Discov.* **2021**. [CrossRef]
190. Jobanputra, V.; Wrzeszczynski, K.O.; Buttner, R.; Caldas, C.; Cuppen, E.; Grimmond, S.; Haferlach, T.; Mulligan, C.; Schuh, A.; Elemento, O. Clinical interpretation of whole-genome and whole-transcriptome sequencing for precision oncology. *Semin. Cancer Biol.* **2021**. [CrossRef]
191. Rosenquist, R.; Cuppen, E.; Buettner, R.; Caldas, C.; Dreau, H.; Elemento, O.; Frederix, G.; Grimmond, S.; Haferlach, T.; Jobanputra, V.; et al. Clinical utility of whole-genome sequencing in precision oncology. *Semin. Cancer Biol.* **2021**. [CrossRef] [PubMed]
192. Meggendorfer, M.; Jobanputra, V.; Wrzeszczynski, K.O.; Roepman, P.; de Bruijn, E.; Cuppen, E.; Buttner, R.; Caldas, C.; Grimmond, S.; Mulligan, C.G.; et al. Analytical demands to use whole-genome sequencing in precision oncology. *Semin. Cancer Biol.* **2021**. [CrossRef] [PubMed]
193. Walter, W.; Shahswar, R.; Stengel, A.; Meggendorfer, M.; Kern, W.; Haferlach, T.; Haferlach, C. Clinical application of whole transcriptome sequencing for the classification of patients with acute lymphoblastic leukemia. *BMC Cancer* **2021**, *21*, 1–11. [CrossRef] [PubMed]
194. Flensburg, C.; Oshlack, A.; Majewski, I.J. Detecting copy number alterations in RNA-Seq using SuperFreq. *Bioinformatics* **2021**. [CrossRef]
195. He, J.; Abdel-Wahab, O.; Nahas, M.K.; Wang, K.; Rampal, R.K.; Intlekofer, A.; Patel, J.; Krivstov, A.; Frampton, G.; Young, L.E.; et al. Integrated genomic DNA/RNA profiling of hematologic malignancies in the clinical setting. *Blood* **2016**, *127*, 3004–3014. [CrossRef]

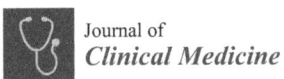

Article

Other (Non-CNS/Testicular) Extramedullary Localizations of Childhood Relapsed Acute Lymphoblastic Leukemia and Lymphoblastic Lymphoma—A Report from the ALL-REZ Study Group

Andrej Lissat [1,*,†], Claudia van Schewick [1,†], Ingo G. Steffen [1,†], Ayumu Arakawa [1], Jean-Pierre Bourquin [2], Birgit Burkhardt [3], Guenter Henze [1], Georg Mann [4], Christina Peters [4], Lucie Sramkova [5], Cornelia Eckert [1], Arend von Stackelberg [1] and Christiane Chen-Santel [1]

1. Department of Pediatric Hematology and Oncology, Charité-Universitätsmedizin Berlin, Augstenburger Platz 1, 13353 Berlin, Germany; Claudia.schewick@charite.de (C.v.S.); Ingo.steffen@charite.de (I.G.S.); aarakawa@ncc.go.jp (A.A.); guenter.henze@charite.de (G.H.); cornelia.eckert@charite.de (C.E.); arend.stackelberg@charite.de (A.v.S.); christiane.chen-santel@charite.de (C.C.-S.)
2. Eleonoren-Foundation, Pediatric Hematology Oncology Department, University Children's Hospital Zürich, Steinwiesstraße 75, CH-8032 Zürich, Switzerland; jean-pierre.bourquin@kispi.uzh.ch
3. Department of Pediatric Hematology and Oncology, Universitätsklinikum Münster, Albert-Schweitzer-Campus 1, Gebäude A1, 48149 Münster, Germany; birgit.burkhardt@ukmuenster.de
4. Department of Pediatric Hematology and Oncology, St. Anna Children's Hospital, Kinderspitalgasse 6, A-1090 Vienna, Austria; georg.mann@stanna.at (G.M.); christina.peters@stanna.at (C.P.)
5. Charles University 2nd Faculty of Medicine and UH Motol V Uvalu 84, Prague 5 15006, Czech Republic; Lucie.Sramkova@fnmotol.cz
* Correspondence: andrej.lissat@charite.de
† These authors contributed equally to this work.

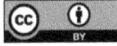

Abstract: Children with other extramedullary relapse of acute lymphoblastic leukemia are currently poorly characterized. We aim to assess the prevalence and the clinical, therapeutic and prognostic features of extramedullary localizations other than central nervous system or testis in children with relapse of acute lymphoblastic leukemia (ALL) and lymphoblastic lymphoma (LBL) treated on a relapsed ALL protocol. Patients and Methods: Patients with relapse of ALL and LBL, treated according to the multicentric ALL-REZ BFM trials between 1983 and 2015, were analyzed for other extramedullary relapse (OEMR) of the disease regarding clinical features, treatment and outcome. Local treatment/irradiation has been recommended on an individual basis and performed only in a minority of patients. Results: A total of 132 out of 2323 (5.6%) patients with ALL relapse presented with an OEMR (combined bone marrow relapse $n = 78$; isolated extramedullary relapse $n = 54$). Compared to the non-OEMR group, patients with OEMR had a higher rate of T-immunophenotype ($p < 0.001$), a higher rate of LBL ($p < 0.001$) and a significantly different distribution of time to relapse, i.e., more very early and late relapses compared to the non-OEMR group ($p = 0.01$). Ten-year probabilities of event-free survival (pEFS) and overall survival (pOS) in non-OEMR vs. OEMR were 0.38 ± 0.01 and 0.32 ± 0.04 ($p = 0.0204$) vs. 0.45 ± 0.01 and 0.37 ± 0.04 ($p = 0.0112$), respectively. OEMRs have been classified into five subgroups according to the main affected compartment: lymphatic organs ($n = 32$, 10y-pEFS 0.50 ± 0.09), mediastinum ($n = 35$, 10y-pEFS 0.11 ± 0.05), bone ($n = 12$, 0.17 ± 0.11), skin and glands ($n = 21$, 0.32 ± 0.11) and other localizations ($n = 32$, 0.41 ± 0.09). Patients with OEMR and T-lineage ALL/LBL showed a significantly worse 10y-pEFS (0.15 ± 0.04) than those with B-Precursor-ALL (0.49 ± 0.06, $p < 0.001$). Stratified into standard risk (SR) and high risk (HR) groups, pEFS and pOS of OEMR subgroups were in the expected range whereas the mediastinal subgroup had a significantly worse outcome. Subsequent relapses involved more frequently the bone marrow (58.4%) than isolated extramedullary compartments (41.7%). In multivariate Cox regression, OEMR confers an independent prognostic factor for inferior pEFS and pOS. Conclusion: OEMR is adversely related to prognosis. However, the established risk classification can be applied for all subgroups except mediastinal relapses requiring treatment intensification. Generally, isolated OEMR of T-cell-origin needs an intensified treatment including allogeneic stem cell transplantation (HSCT) as a curative approach independent from time to relapse. Local therapy such as surgery and irradiation may be of benefit in selected cases. The indication needs to be clarified in further investigations.

Keywords: other extramedullary relapse; pediatric; lymphoblastic leukemia

1. Introduction

Relapses in the central nervous system (CNS) and testis account for 87% of all extramedullary relapses in childhood ALL. These sites are considered sanctuary sites inhibiting the efficacy of systemic chemotherapy. In addition, interaction and biology of leukemic blast (sub)populations with the specific organ microenvironment can induce quiescence, prevent apoptosis and lead to treatment failure and relapse in these sanctuary sites (review in [1]). In CNS and testicular relapse, a specific local treatment (irradiation, intrathecal injections, orchiectomy) combined with systemic chemotherapy and in high-risk patients additional allogeneic hematopoietic stem cell transplantation (HSCT) is needed to induce long-term remission in patients suffering from relapse at these particular sites [2,3].

In contrast, ALL relapses in extramedullary compartments other than CNS or testis are poorly characterized and not addressed with specific treatment recommendations in current treatment protocols. Due to the relative rarity of these so-called other extramedullary relapses (OEMRs) and the large heterogeneity of organs involved, primarily case reports on single-center experience with unusual extramedullary localizations have been published so far [4–23]. Gunes and colleagues described other extramedullary relapses in 6 out of 51 adult and adolescent ALL patients following HSCT. OS after HSCT in all OEMR patients has not been significantly different compared to isolated BM relapses. The small patient number of OEMR precluded any statistical analysis [24]. Only a few analyses describing a cohort of more than 10 patients have been reported so far [25,26].

The lack of comprehensive clinical data and strong evidence impairs stratification of affected pediatric patients to systemic and local treatment. Clinical trial protocols of subsequent ALL—Relapse Berlin/Frankfurt/Muenster (ALL-REZ BFM) trials for childhood relapsed ALL recommend systemic chemotherapy for these patients without addition of local treatment. The latter is recommended only in case of tumor mass persistence after induction and consolidation verified by pathologic review and in sanctuary sites such as the eye. The reason for the current approach is based on the assumption that in OEMR no sanctuary mechanism such as the blood–brain barrier would prevent the efficacy of systemically administered chemotherapeutic drugs. However, it remains unclear whether risk group allocation, treatment intensity and strategy for local therapy in OEMR ALL are adequate for these patients and subgroups.

To improve treatment stratification by analysis of relapse patterns, response and survival in pediatric OEMR ALL patients, we summarized data of the entire cohort of patients enrolled into five consecutive ALL-REZ BFM trials conducted between 1983 and 2015. Herewith, we present the largest analysis of a pediatric cohort of OEMR ALL published so far, enabling us to better characterize its clinical and prognostic features as well as its therapeutic needs.

2. Materials and Methods

2.1. Patients

Between June 1983 and March 2015, 2323 children and adolescents with diagnosis of first relapsed ALL and LBL were enrolled into the randomized multicenter ALL—Relapse trials as well as registries of the ALL-REZ BFM study group. Of these, 132 were diagnosed with extramedullary relapse in compartments other than CNS or testis. Seventy-eight patients of this cohort presented with combined extramedullary and bone marrow relapse, and 54 were diagnosed with isolated extramedullary relapse. Written informed consent was obtained from patients and/or their guardians. Protocols of the trials ALL-REZ BFM 83, 85, 87, 96 and 2002 were approved by the institutional ethics committees of the participating institutions. The ALL-REZ BFM 2002 trial has been registered in the International Clinical Trials Registry Platform of the WHO (NCT00114348).

2.2. Definitions

Isolated extramedullary relapse has been defined as clinically overt relapse in an extramedullary compartment and less than 5% leukemic lymphoblasts in the bone marrow (BM). Combined extramedullary and BM relapse has been defined as extramedullary involvement and ≥5% BM blast infiltration. OEMR was diagnosed by biopsy in the majority of patients and by ultrasound, computer tomography, magnetic resonance imaging or scintigraphy.

Lymph node involvement was diagnosed in case of lymphatic mass beyond the usual lymphadenopathy with lymph node diameter > 2 cm assessed at the discretion of the treating PI. Biopsy was recommended in all isolated lymphatic organ relapse patients to secure diagnosis.

Time point of relapse has been defined as follows: very early, relapse within 18 months after diagnosis; early, relapse later than 18 months after diagnosis but less than 6 months after cessation of front-line treatment; late, relapse 6 months after end of front-line treatment.

Routine immunophenotyping and analyses for chromosomal translocations were performed as described elsewhere [27,28].

Risk stratification has been based on standard of care related to current definitions within the IntReALL protocol and ALL REZ clinical trials:

SR included: early isolated extramedullary (IEM) and combined bone marrow (CBM) BCP-ALL relapses; early IEM T-ALL relapses; late IEM, CBM and isolated bone marrow (IBM) BCP-ALL relapses; and late IEM T-ALL relapses.

HR included: all very early BCP- and T-ALL relapses, early IBM BCP-ALL and early CBM and IBM T-ALL relapses and late CBM and IBM T-ALL relapses.

S1 group: late IEM BCP- and T-ALL relapses, according to SR.

S2 group: early IEM and CBM and late IBM BCP-ALL relapses and early IEM T-ALL relapse, according to SR.

S3 group: early IBM BCP-ALL relapse, according to HR.

S4 group: all very early BCP- and T-ALL relapses excluding S1 and S2, according to HR.

Definition of nonresponse: in patients with BM involvement, absence of complete morphological remission (CMR) (<5% lymphoblasts) at the fifth therapy element (e.g., ALL-REZ BFM 2002: at day 29 Prot. II-IDA).

Likewise, in IEM relapse including OEMR no evidence of local disease was considered as complete remission and evidence of disease—in OEMR proven by biopsy—was assessed as nonresponse.

2.3. Treatment

All patients received either alternating courses of systemic and intrathecal chemotherapy (R1 and R2 blocks, since protocol ALL-REZ BFM 95 all groups started with F1- and F2-induction blocks) or continuous chemotherapy with lower dosage, but for a longer time period (protocol II-IDA) according to the ALL-REZ BFM protocols 85, 87 [29], 90 [30], 96 [31] and 2002 [32]. Cranial irradiation of 12 gray (Gy) was administered to all patients with CNS involvement. Treatment for OEMR did not differ from the approach for systemic relapse as has been published before [33]. As mentioned above, irradiation has not been recommended as standard of care in OEMR. Only 17 patients received additional local irradiation for the extramedullary compartment with the application of doses from 10 to 30 Gy based on individual choice and recommendation independent of response. Allogeneic HSCT was indicated in patients stratified into the high-risk group (S3/S4) with very early bone marrow involving relapse and since the trial ALL-REZ BFM 2002 in patients with minimal residual disease (MRD) poor response after induction chemotherapy or other high-risk features according to the ALL SZT-BFM 2003 trial and the international FORUM study which was initiated in 2012 [34]. HLA compatible siblings and if available unrelated donors have been considered as suitable stem-cell donors. In recent years, HLA mismatched family donors have also been used in high-risk patients. Conditioning regimen for children above 2 or recently above 4 years included total body irradiation with 12 Gy in the majority of the patients.

2.4. Statistical Methods

The association of categorical variables was analyzed using Pearson's chi-squared test and Fisher's exact test ($n \leq 5$/cell). EFS time was calculated from the date of relapse diagnosis to the date of an event (i.e., second relapse, therapy-related death and secondary malignancy) or the date of last follow-up. In case of nonresponse or death over the course of induction therapy, EFS time was set to zero. The probability of event-free survival (pEFS) and the probability of overall survival (pOS) were estimated by the Kaplan–Meier life-table method [34], and differences between groups were assessed by the log-rank test. The effect of prognostic factors on EFS and OS was analyzed using univariate and multivariate Cox proportional hazard regression model and the corresponding hazard ratios and their 95% confidence intervals (CIs). Akaike information criterion (AIC) minimization method was used to optimize the multivariate Cox regression model. All tests were two-sided and the significance level was set to $p < 0.05$. The software R 4.0.3 (R Foundation for Statistical Computing, Vienna, Austria), SAS 9.4 (SAS Institute, Cary, NC, USA) and SPSS 27.0 (IBM SPSS Statistics, Ehningen, Germany) were used for statistical analysis.

3. Results

3.1. Clinical Presentation of OEMR Differs Significantly from Non-OEMR Patients

One hundred thirty-two children with OEMR manifestations of ALL and LBL were included in the analysis. Involvement of 17 distinct extramedullary sites has been observed. The most frequent sites for OEMR were mediastinum ($n = 35$), lymph nodes ($n = 32$), skin ($n = 14$) and bone ($n = 12$). Localizations in organs such as the kidney ($n = 9$), eye/orbit ($n = 4$) or liver ($n = 3$) were rare (for a list of all sites and their distribution see Table 1 and Suppl. Figure S1).

We grouped OEMRs into five categories according to the main extramedullary compartment involved: "mediastinum" ($n = 35$), "lymphatic organs" ($n = 32$), a group named "other compartment" including all patients with localizations that did not fit in one of the other four groups ($n = 32$), "skin and glands" ($n = 21$) and "bone" ($n = 12$). In the case of more than one OEMR localization in one patient, only the main site as reported by the treating PI was considered for statistical analysis between the subgroups.

Compared with the entire non-OEMR cohort of 2191 first relapsed ALL patients, patients with OEMR presented more frequently a T-immunophenotype leukemia (OEMR 50.8%, $n = 67$, versus non-OEMR 11.0%, $n = 242$; $p \leq 0.001$; for complete analysis see Table 2). In addition, more patients in the OEMR group showed very early or late relapses, (31.8% and 49.2%, respectively) compared to the non-OEMR group (23.9% and 45.7%, respectively, $p = 0.01$). Significantly more patients in the OEMR group have been treated on T-LBL protocols during first-line therapy, 15.2% vs. 1.9% in the non-OEMR group ($p < 0.001$), most likely representing former T-LBL patients. Gender, age and the rate of HSCT in consolidation did not differ significantly in OEMR vs. non-OEMR subgroups.

Table 1. Distribution of other extramedullary relapses (OEMRs).

Site	Group	n	%
LN	Lymphat. organs	32	24.2
Skin	Skin/glands	14	10.6
Mediastinum/thymus	Mediastinum	35	26.5
Tonsils	Skin/glands	2	1.5
Female genital organs	Other	6	4.5
Eye/nervus opticus	Other	4	3.0
Bones	Bone	12	9.1
Paranasal sinuses/ENT	Other	2	1.5
Kidney	Other	9	6.8
Liver	Other	3	2.3
Pancreas	Other	1	0.8
Serosae (pleural/cardial/joints)	Skin/glands	1	0.8
Glands (mammae/g. parotis/g. lacrimae)	Skin/glands	4	3.0
Spleen	Other	1	0.8
Colon/intestine	Other	1	0.8
Epidural	Other	1	0.8
Abdomen	Other	2	1.5
Other	Other	2	1.5
Total		**132**	**100.0**

Legend to Table 1: ENT, ear nose throat; LN, lymph node; OEM, other extramedullary.

Table 2. Patient characteristics.

	ALL Relapse Trial Patients		Other Extramedullary Relapse Patients				Other Extramedullary Relapse Subgroups											
			No		Yes			Lymph. Organs		Mediast. Organs		Other Compartment		Skin/Glands		Bone		
	n	%	n	%	n	%	p**	n	%	n	%	n	%	n	%	n	%	p**
Total group	2323	100	2191	100	132	100		32	24.2	35	26.6	32	24.2	21	15.9	12	9.1	
Patient characteristics																		
Sex							0.37											0.71
Male	1474	63	1395	63.7	79	59.8		19	59.4	24	68.6	19	59.4	11	52.4	6	50	
Female	849	37	796	36.3	53	40.2		13	40.6	11	31.4	13	40.6	10	47.6	6	50	
Time point of relapse							0.01											0.04
Very early	565	24.3	523	23.9	42	31.9		11	34.4	15	42.9	5	15.6	6	28.6	5	41.7	
Early	691	29.8	666	30.4	25	18.9		5	15.6	11	31.4	5	15.6	2	7.1	2	16.6	
Late	1067	45.9	1002	45.7	65	49.2		16	50	9	25.7	22	68.8	13	46.4	5	41.7	
Age at relapse							0.38											0.25
≤5 years	386	16.6	369	16.8	17	12.9		4	12.5	5	14.3	2	6.3	2	9.5	4	33.3	
≥5 years and ≤10 years	1011	43.5	955	43.7	56	42.4		14	43.8	17	48.5	17	53.1	6	28.6	2	16.7	
>10 years and ≤15 years	648	27.9	610	27.8	38	28.8		9	28.1	10	28.6	9	28.1	6	28.6	4	33.3	
>15 years and <20 years	278	12.0	257	11.7	21	15.9		5	15.6	3	8.6	4	12.5	7	33.3	2	16.7	
Site of relapse							<0.001											0.32
Isolated BM	1439	62.0	1439	65.7	0	0												
Combined BM and EM	505	21.7	427	19.5	78	59.1		17	53.1	19	54.3	21	65.6	11	52.4	10	83.3	
Isolated extramedullary	379	16.3	325	14.8	54	40.9		15	46.9	16	45.7	11	34.4	10	47.6	2	16.7	
Immunophenotype							<0.001											<0.001
Precursor B cell	2014	86.7	1949	89	65	49.2		14	43.8	2	5.7	23	71.9	15	71.4	11	91.7	
T cell	309	13.3	242	11	67	50.8		18	56.2	33	94.3	9	28.1	6	28.6	1	8.3	
Therapy							0.29											0.23
Chemotherapy/radiotherapy exclusively	1550	66.7	1459	66.7	91	68.9		18	56.2	26	74.3	23	71.9	14	66.7	10	83.4	
Allogeneic SCT	664	28.6	632	28.8	32	24.2		12	37.5	7	20	5	15.6	7	33.3	1	8.3	
Autologous SCT	57	2.5	51	2.3	6	4.6		0	0	2	5.7	3	9.4	0	0	1	8.3	
No data	52	2.2	49	2.2	3	2.3		2	6.3	0	0	1	3.1	0	0	0	0	
NHL Therapy							<0.001											0.08
Other	2247	96.7	2135	97.4	112	84.8		25	78.1	26	74.3	30	93.8	20	95.2	11	91.7	
NHL-BFM	62	2.7	42	1.9	20	15.2		7	21.9	9	25.7	2	6.2	1	4.8	1	8.3	
No data	14	0.06	14	0.7	0	0												

Legend to Table 2: ** Pearson/chi-squared or Fisher's exact test, missing values excluded. Abbreviations: BCP, B-cell precursor; BM, bone marrow; EM, extramedullary; NHL-BFM, Non-Hodgkin's Lymphoma Berlin–Frankfurt–Munster protocol; SCT, stem cell transplantation; SE, standard error.

Molecular data on specific translocations (*BCR-ABL1*, *MLL-AF4* and *ETV6-RUNX1*) were available in 32.7% (n = 43) of OEMR patients. This lack of data was mainly caused by the long observation period covering early periods when genetic diagnostics had not been routinely performed, as well as the difficulty of performing genetic analyses in extramedullary material in general (Supplementary Table S1). One OEMR patient had evidence of a leukemia with TEL-AML fusion, and another patient was diagnosed with BCR-ABL fusion. The remaining 41 patients did not show any of the investigated genetic aberrations currently applied for risk stratification. Genetic characteristics were not recorded or reported in 67% of OEMR patients. This precludes any statement on the correlation of underlying genetic features with risk of OEMR or definition of new biomarkers which need to be established prospectively.

3.2. OEMR Subgroups Demonstrate Distinct Relapse Phenotypes

To improve treatment stratification, we analyzed high-risk patterns within OEMR subgroups (Table 2). T-immunophenotype was predominant in the mediastinal mass group and more frequent in the lymphatic organs group (94.3% ($n = 33$) and 56.2% ($n = 18$), respectively; $p < 0.001$). In the "skin/gland" and "other" OEMR subgroups, T-ALL subtype was diagnosed in a minority of patients (28.6%, $n = 6$; 28.1%, $n = 9$). In the "bone" OEMR subgroup, relapsed BCP-ALL subtype was far more frequent than T-ALL (91.7%, $n = 11$, vs. 8.3%, $n = 1$, respectively). In addition to phenotype, time to relapse differed significantly in the five OEMR subgroups ($p = 0.04$). Mediastinal and bone relapses occur more frequently in the very early (43%, 42%) and early (31%, 17%) relapse groups, whereas the subgroups "other", "skin/gland" and "lymphatic organs" occur predominantly as late relapses (69%, 62%, 50%; Table 2).

Since T-LBL and pB-LBL patients have been included in and treated according to clinical trial protocols for relapsed ALL in the past, our analysis included 43 patients who suffered from T-LBL and 19 patients who suffered from pB-LBL as primary disease and were treated according to NHL-BFM first-line protocols. Out of these 62 patients, 20 (32%) relapsed as lymphoblastic leukemia/lymphoma including an OEMR site (16 T-LBL and 4 pB-LBL). These 20 patients comprise 15% (20/132) of the OEMR cohort analyzed and are thus overrepresented as compared to the non-OEMR cohort ($p < 0.001$; Table 2). As expected, the "mediastinal" and "lymph node" OEMR subgroups comprise the majority—17—of these 20 LBL patients. Within these two subgroups, former LBL patients comprise 26% and 22% of patients, respectively. The vast majority of patients included in the OEMR analysis had been treated according to a first-line ALL protocol, i.e., 112 out of 132 patients. Sex, age and therapy did not show a significantly different distribution within the five OEMR cohorts.

3.3. OEMR Shows a Distinct Event Pattern Compared to Non-OEMR

Events are summarized in Table 3a. Relapse rate and complete continuous remission (CCR) did not differ significantly in OEMR vs. non-OEMR patients (Table 3a). We found significantly more deaths in induction and nonresponding patients in the OEMR group (non-OEMR vs. OEMR 3.7% vs. 8.3% ($p = 0.02$) and 9.8% vs. 15.9% ($p = 0.03$), respectively), which might be attributed to different risk patterns in both groups. Mediastinal and bone relapses were associated with "nonresponse to treatment/progressive disease" and "death in induction" (43% in the "mediastinal" and 42% in the "bone" vs. 14% in the remaining three OEMR subgroups). Fewer patients within the "mediastinal" and "bone" subgroups compared to the remaining three OEMR subgroups stayed in CCR, 11% and 17% vs. 42%, respectively. In contrast to that, in the group "lymphatic organs", more patients remained in CCR than any other subgroup (50%, $n = 16$).

Table 3. Events within the OEMR group.

(a) All Events

Event	OEM No n	OEM No %	OEM Yes n	OEM Yes %	p*	Lymphat. Organs n	Lymphat. Organs %	Skin/Glands n	Skin/Glands %	OEM Group Mediastinum n	OEM Group Mediastinum %	Bone n	Bone %	Other n	Other %	p*
Total	2191	100.0	132	100.0		32	100.0	21	100.0	35	100.0	12	100.0	32	100.0	0.025
Event in CCR	821	37.5	42	31.8	0.036	16	50.0	7	33.3	4	11.4	2	16.7	13	40.6	
Died in CR	138	6.3	7	5.3	0.23	1	3.1	2	9.5	3	8.6	1	8.3	.	.	
2nd malignoma	29	1.3	3	2.3	0.78	1	3.1	.	.	1	2.9	1	8.3	.	.	
Another relapse	889	40.6	48	36.4	0.60	9	28.1	11	52.4	12	34.3	3	25.0	13	40.6	
Nonresponder/progr. disease	215	9.8	21	15.9	0.39	4	12.5	.	.	11	31.4	2	16.7	4	12.5	
Death in induction	81	3.7	11	8.3	0.03	1	3.1	1	4.8	4	11.4	3	25.0	2	6.3	
Death of unknown origin	4	0.2	0	0	0.02	.	.	.	.	.	.	.	.	.	.	
					1											

(b) OEM Subsequent Relapse Sites

	OEM No n	OEM No %	OEM Yes n	OEM Yes %	p*	Lymphat. Organs n	Lymphat. Organs %	Skin/Glands n	Skin/Glands %	OEM Group Mediastinum n	OEM Group Mediastinum %	Bone n	Bone %	Other n	Other %
Subs. relapse	889	100.0	48	100.0	<0.001	9	100.0	11	100.0	12	100.0	3	100.0	13	100.0
Subseq_site															
IBM	680	76.5	20	41.7		4	44.4	5	45.5	6	50.0	1	33.3	4	30.8
CBM	94	10.6	8	16.7		1	11.1	2	18.2	2	16.7	2	66.7	1	7.7
IEM	115	12.9	20	41.7		4	44.4	4	36.4	4	33.3	.	.	8	61.5

Table 3. Cont.

(c) Subsequent Relapse Sites Compared to OEMR First Relapse Sites

OEM		Total	Subsequent OEMR	Subsequent Relapse CNS/Testis Only	Subsequent Relapse Site	n
LN	OEM group Lymphat. organs	32	5	0	LN	4
					Mediastinum	1
Skin	Skin/glands	14	3	3	LN	1
					glands	1
					skin	1
					CNS/testis	3
Mediastinum	Mediastinum	35	3	3	LN	3
					CNS/testis	3
Tonsils	Skin/glands	2	0	0		0
Female genital organs	Other	6	0	1	CNS/testis	1
Eye/nervus opticus	Other	4	0	0		0
Bones	Bone	12	1	1	Bones	1
					CNS/testis	1
Paranasal sinuses/ENT	Other	2	0	1	CNS/testis	1
Kidney	Other	9	1	1	Paranasal sinus	1
					CNS/testis	1
Liver	Other	3	1	0	Liver	1
Pancreas	Other	1	1	0	Pancreas	1
Serosae (pleural/cardial/joints)	Skin/glands	1	0	0		0
Glands (mammae/g. parotis/g. lacrimae)	Skin/glands	4	0	0		0
Spleen	Other	1	0	0		0
Colon/intestine	Other	1	1	0	Skin	1
Epidural	Other	1	1	0	Kidney	1
Abdomen	Other	2	0	0		0
Other	Other	2	1	0	Other	1
Total		132	18	10		28

Legend to Table 3: * Pearson/chi-squared including Yate's continuity correction; due to the exploratory character no correction for multiple testing has been performed. Missing values excluded. Abbreviations: BM, bone marrow; (C)CR, (continued) complete remission; IBM, isolated bone marrow; CBM, combined bone marrow; IEM, isolated extramedullary; LN, lymph node; CNS, central nervous system; OEM, other extramedullary; w/o, without.

To understand the relapse pattern of OEMR subgroups in detail and to improve recommendation on local therapy, we took a closer look at the site of the subsequent relapse (Table 3b,c). Out of 132 patients in the OEMR cohort, 48 experienced a subsequent relapse. Of these 48 patients, 28 (58%) relapsed as combined bone marrow ($n = 8$) or isolated extramedullary ($n = 20$) relapse, which differs significantly from non-OEMR patients, where only 23.5% relapsed as CBM or IEM ($p < 0.001$; Table 3b). Forty-two percent of observed subsequent relapses were isolated bone marrow relapses (20 patients). Within the "other" OEMR cohort, subsequent relapses occurred predominantly as isolated OEMR (62%; Table 3b). Only 9 out of 28 subsequent extramedullary relapses involved the initial relapse site. The majority of these relapses involved other EM sites including CNS and testis. Within the "other" OEMR subgroup, 3 out of 9 subsequent relapses involved the initial site (Table 3c).

As a consequence, we focused on the value of additional local irradiation on outcome in OEMR patients (Supplementary Table S2). In general, the ALL-REZ BFM protocols combine systemic and intrathecal chemotherapy as well as radiation in certain defined subgroups. However, since most of the OEM sites are not considered sanctuary sites, local radiation has not been recommended as standard of care. In general, out of 128 OEMR patients, on whom information on radiation was available, only a minority of 17 patients (13%) received local irradiation ($n = 15$) or local radiation combined with TBI ($n = 2$) whereas the majority did not (Supplementary Table S2). As an exception, relapses within the eye have been considered as specific local risk being potentially protected from chemotherapeutic agents by a blood–retina barrier [35]. Three out of four patients with ocular relapses received irradiation of the eye. No subsequent relapses were reported in these patients. Furthermore, 10 patients with mediastinal relapse (one patient in combination with TBI) and 5 patients belonging to the "other" subgroup (one patient in combination with TBI) underwent local radiotherapy. Final conclusions on the indication for specific local radiation therapy cannot be drawn. This needs to be addressed in further preferably prospective analyses. However, we would continue recommending local irradiation of sanctuary sites such as relapses within the eye.

Risk stratification and indication to undergo allogeneic HSCT in OEMR patients have been recommended based on established algorithms for all relapsed patients. However, detailed analysis revealed subtle differences in HSCT rate in non-OEMR vs. OEMR patients (Table 4a,b). Thirty-two patients (24%) with OEMR underwent an allogeneic HSCT. Nine of these belonged to the HR group (S4), and 23 belonged to the S1 and S2 group (SR), who are transplanted based on MRD response. Unfortunately, data on MRD response in the OEMR group were not available in the majority of patients, precluding a deeper insight into the indication of SCT and meeting criteria to perform the latter. Compared to non-OEMR patients, more patients in OEMR S1 underwent allogeneic HSCT (0% vs. 16.7%, respectively) and fewer patients in OEMR S4 underwent HSCT (32.0% vs. 20.9%, respectively). The latter could be partly attributed to overrepresentation of T-ALL and very early relapsed patients in the OEMR cohort, which both are associated with nonresponse to induction and refractoriness precluding HSCT.

Outcome following allogeneic HSCT in non-OEMR and OEMR patients did not show substantial differences. Due to selection biases and time dependency of HSCT, we did not perform statistical analysis on outcome after HSCT vs. chemotherapy alone in non-OEMR vs. OEMR patients (Table 4b). In general, OEMR patients who underwent HSCT experienced a considerable CCR rate of 44% (non-OEMR 53%). OEMR patients treated with chemotherapy alone experienced a CCR rate of 38% (non-OEMR 37%). The rate of subsequent relapses in the OEMR HSCT group was 38% (non-OEMR 28.7%) compared to 55% (non-OEMR 58%) in patients treated with chemotherapy only. The death-in-remission rate in the OEMR SCT group was 13% (non-OEMR 5%) (Table 4b). Based on these data, an HSCT stratification algorithm including HLA-mismatched donors for OEMR cannot be established, and recommendation for HSCT should be based on contemporary risk criteria.

Table 4. Events following HSCT.

(a) HSCT Performed Per Risk Group in OEMR and Non-OEMR Patients

	Total		S1		S2		HSCT—OEMR S4	
	n	%	n	%	n	%	n	%
Total *	132	100	30	100	59	100	43	100
No HSCT	91	68.9	20	66.6	39	66.1	32	74.5
Allogeneic HSCT	32	24.2	5	16.7	18	30.5	9	20.9
Autologous HSCT	6	4.5	3	10	2	3.4	1	2.3
Unknown	3	2.4	2	6.7			1	2.3

	Total		S1		S2		HSCT—Non-OEMR S3		S4	
	n	%	n	%	n	%	n	%	n	%
Total *	2190	100	71	100	1299	100	320	100	500	100
No HSCT	1459	66.7	67	94.3	915	70.4	162	50.6	315	63.0
Allogeneic HSCT	631	28.8	0	0	326	25.1	145	45.3	160	32.0
Autologous HSCT	51	2.3	1	1.4	26	2	9	2.8	15	3.0
Unknown	49	2.2	3	4.2	32	2.5	4	1.3	10	2.0

(b) HSCT, All Events in Non-OEMR and OEMR Groups

	Total Non-OEMR		Total OEMR		No HSCT Non-OEMR		No HSCT OEMR		HSCT—Events Allogeneic HSCT Non-OEMR		Allogeneic HSCT OEMR		Autologous Non-OEMR		Autologous OEMR		Unknown Non-OEMR		Unknown OEMR	
	n	%	n	%	n	%	n	%	n	%	n	%	n	%	n	%	n	%	n	%
Total **	1877	100	100	100	1150	100	60	100	628	100	32	100	51	100	6	100	48	100	2	100.0
Event in CCR	821	43.7	42	42.0	426	37	23	38.3	337	53.6	14	43.8	13	25.5	3	50	45	93.8	2	100.0
Died in CR	138	7.3	7	7.0	41	3.6	3	5.0	96	15.3	4	12.5	1	2						
2nd malignoma	29	1.5	3	3.0	13	1.1	1	1,7	15	2.4	2	6.3	1	2						
Subsequent relapse	889	47.3	48	48.0	670	58.3	33	55.0	180	28.7	12	37.5	36	70.5	3	50	3	6.2		

Legend to Table 4: * One patient excluded due to unknown risk group. ** Progressive disease, death in induction and death unknown excluded. Abbreviations: (C)CR, (continued) complete remission; HSCT, hematopoietic stem cell transplantation; OEM(R), other extramedullary (relapse); w/o, without.

3.4. OEMR Confers an Independent Risk Factor for Decreased Survival

The probability of 10-year event-free survival (10y-pEFS) and the probability of 10-year overall survival (10y-pOS) in comparison to the non-OEMR ALL cohort are shown in Figure 1 and Table 5. Patients suffering from OEMR had a significantly lower 10y-pEFS of 0.32 ± 0.04 vs. 0.38 ± 0.01, $p = 0.0204$, respectively. In addition, pOS was significantly inferior for OEMR patients compared to the whole cohort—0.37 ± 0.04 vs. 0.45 ± 0.01, $p = 0.0112$, respectively (Figure 1 and Table 5b). Ten-year pEFS and pOS in non-OEMR vs. OEMR differed based on established risk stratification and were correlated with outcome (Figure 2). Patients experienced a 10-year pEFS and pOS in non-OEMR SR vs. HR of 0.51 ± 0.01 vs. 0.20 ± 0.01 and 0.59 ± 0.01 vs. 0.24 ± 0.01, $p < 0.001$, respectively, and a 10-year pEFS and pOS in OEMR SR vs. HR of 0.48 ± 0.06 vs. 0.12 ± 0.04 and 0.54 ± 0.06 vs. 0.15 ± 0.05, $p < 0.001$, respectively (Figure 2).

We further focused on risk factors predicting inferior outcome within the OEMR subgroup. In that regard, immunophenotype and time to relapse were significantly associated with outcome. The 10y-pEFS and 10y-pOS of BCP-ALL OEMR patients were significantly superior to those of T-ALL OEMR patients (0.49 ± 0.06 vs. 0.15 ± 0.04 and 0.52 ± 0.06 vs. 0.22 ± 0.05, $p < 0.001$, respectively; Figure 3a; Supplementary Figure S2 and Table 5a,b). Time to first relapse confers an additional significant risk factor in the OEMR cohorts as described before for the entire relapsed ALL cohorts [36,37]. Very early OEMRs were found to have the worst prognosis compared to late OEMR: 10-year pEFS and 10-year pOS of 0.10 ± 0.05 vs. 0.47 ± 0.06, $p < 0.001$, and 0.14 ± 0.05 vs. 0.53 ± 0.06, $p < 0.001$, respectively (Figure 3b and Table 5a,b). Isolated OEMR has been associated with a superior prognosis compared to combined OEMR: 10-year pOS of 0.50 ± 0.07 vs. 0.27 ± 0.05, $p = 0.014$, respectively (Figure 3c and Table 5b). Age, previous protocol (Figure 3d) and gender do not confer an additional risk factor in the OEMR cohort.

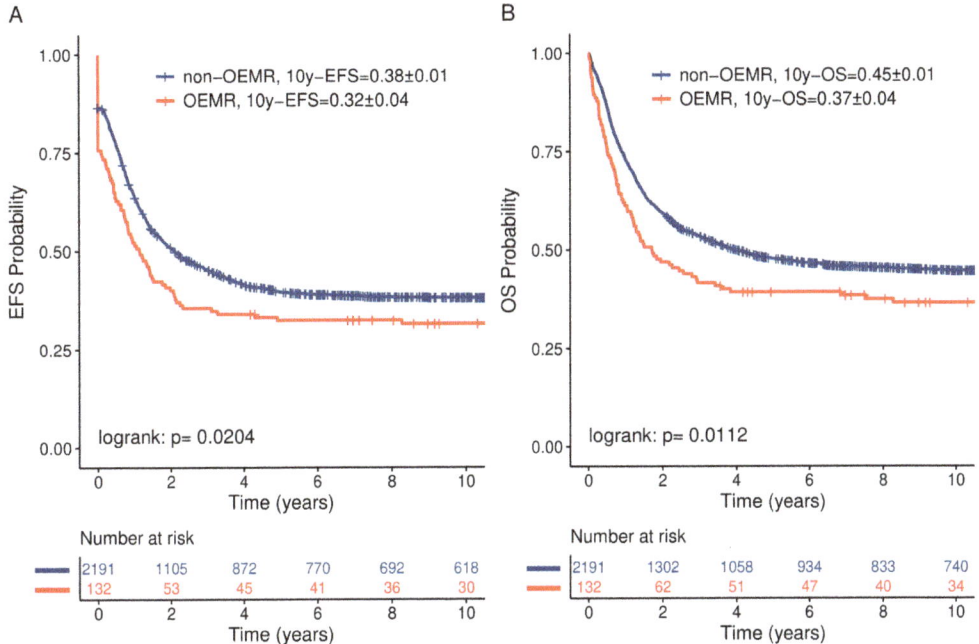

Figure 1. Ten-year pEFS (**A**) and pOS (**B**) of relapsed ALL patients differ significantly in OEMR vs. non-OEMR patients. The graphs have been calculated based on Kaplan–Meier analysis. $p < 0.05$.

Table 5. pEFS and pOS in non-OEMR, all OEMR and OEMR subgroups.

	(a) pEFS			
	\multicolumn{4}{c}{OEMR}			
	No—2191		Yes—132	
	pEFS ± SE (10 Years)	p *	pEFS ± SE (10 Years)	p *
Total group	0.38 ± 0.01		0.32 ± 0.04	0.0204
Patient characteristics				
Sex		0.49		0.18
Male	0.38 ± 0.01		0.28 ± 0.05	
Female	0.39 ± 0.02		0.38 ± 0.07	
Time point of relapse		<0.001		<0.001
Very early	0.20 ± 0.02		0.10 ± 0.05	
Early	0.29 ± 0.02		0.28 ± 0.09	
Late	0.54 ± 0.02		0.47 ± 0.06	
Age at relapse		<0.001		0.60
≤5 years	0.31 ± 0.02		0.29 ± 0.11	
≥5 years and ≤10 years	0.42 ± 0.02		0.37 ± 0.07	
>10 years and ≤15 years	0.37 ± 0.02		0.24 ± 0.07	
>15 years and <20 years	0.38 ± 0.03		0.33 ± 0.10	
Site of relapse		<0.001		0.093
Isolated BM	0.34 ± 0.01		–	
Combined BM and EM	0.45 ± 0.02		0.26 ± 0.05	
Isolated extramedullary	0.49 ± 0.03		0.39 ± 0.07	
Immunophenotype		<0.001		<0.001
Precursor B cell	0.40 ± 0.01		0.49 ± 0.06	
T cell	0.20 ± 0.03		0.15 ± 0.04	
Therapy		<0.001		0.010
Chemotherapy/radiotherapy only	0.30 ± 0.01		0.25 ± 0.05	
Allogeneic SCT	0.54 ± 0.02		0.42 ± 0.09	
Autologous SCT	0.25 ± 0.06		0.50 ± 0.20	
No data	0.92 ± 0.04		0.67 ± 27	
NHL Therapy		0.0043		0.76
Other	0.38 ± 0.01		0.33 ± 0.04	
NHL-BFM	0.26 ± 0.07		0.25 ± 0.10	

Table 5. Cont.

	(b) pOS			
	OEMR			
	No—2191		Yes—132	
	pOS ± SE (10 years)	$p\ *$	pOS ± SE (10 years)	$p\ *$
Total group	0.45 ± 0.01		0.37 ± 0.04	0.0112
Patient characteristics				
Sex		0.888		0.114
Male	0.45 ± 0.01		0.31 ± 0.0	
Female	0.44 ± 0.02		0.45 ± 0.02	
Time point of relapse		<0.001		<.001
Very early	0.23 ± 0.02		0.14 ± 0.05	
Early	0.34 ± 0.02		0.32 ± 0.09	
Late	0.63 ± 0.02		0.53 ± 0.06	
Age at relapse		<0.001		0.656
≤5 years	0.37 ± 0.03		0.35 ± 0.12	
≥5 years and ≤10 years	0.50 ± 0.02		0.42 ± 0.07	
>10 years and ≤15 years	0.43 ± 0.02		0.29 ± 0.07	
>15 years and <20 years	0.41 ± 0.03		0.37 ± 0.11	
Site of relapse		<0.001		0.014
Isolated BM	0.41 ± 0.01		–	
Combined BM and EM	0.49 ± 0.02		0.27 ± 0.05	
Isolated extramedullary	0.56 ± 0.03		0.50 ± 0.07	
Immunophenotype		<0.001		<0.001
Precursor B cell	0.47 ± 0.01		0.52 ± 0.06	
T cell	0.23 ± 0.03		0.22 ± 0.05	
Therapy		<.001		0.0055
Chemotherapy/radiotherapy exclusively	0.38 ± 0.01		0.30 ± 0.05	
Allogeneić SCT	0.59 ± 0.02		0.47 ± 0.09	
Autologous SCT	0.33 ± 0.07		0.50 ± 0.20	
No data	096 ± 0.03		0.67 ± 0.27	
NHL Therapy		0.0069		0.7645
Other	0.45 ± 0.01		0.36 ± 0.05	
NHL-BFM	0.31 ± 0.07		0.40 ± 0.11	

(c) pEFS and pOS in OEMR Subgroups					
		OEMR Subgroups			
	n	pEFS ± SE (10 years)	$p\ *$	pOS ± SE (10 years)	$p\ *$
			<0.001		<0.001
Lymph. organs	32	0.50 ± 0.09		0.62 ± 0.09	
SR	18	0.67 ± 0.11	0.005	0.77 ± 0.10	0.015
HR	14	0.29 ± 12		0.43 ± 0.13	
Mediast. organs	35	0.11 ± 0.05		0.14 ± 0.06	
SR	10	0.20 ± 0.13	0.113	0.30 ± 0.14	0.117
HR	25	0.08 ± 0.05		0.08 ± 0.05	
Other compartment	32	0.41 ± 0.09		0.47 ± 0.09	
SR	26	0.50 ± 0.10	<0.001	0.57 ± 0.10	<0.001
HR	6	**		**	
Skin/glands	21	0.32 ± 0.11		0.32 ± 0.11	
SR	12	0.47 ± 0.15	0.010	0.47 ± 0.15	0.01
HR	9	0.11 ± 0.10		0.11 ± 0.10	
Bone	12	0.17 ± 0.11		0.17 ± 0.11	
SR	7	0.29 ± 0.17	0.01	0.29 ± 0.17	0.035
HR	5	**		**	

Legend to Table 5: * Log-rank test and pairwise log-rank test, missing values excluded. ** Ten-year pEFS and pOS not reached. Abbreviations: BM, bone marrow; EM, extramedullary; HR, high risk; NHL-BFM, Non-Hodgkin's Lymphoma Berlin–Frankfurt–Munster protocol; OEM(R), other extramedullary (relapse); pEFS, probability of event-free survival; pOS probability of overall survival; SCT, stem cell transplantation; SE, standard error; SR, standard risk.

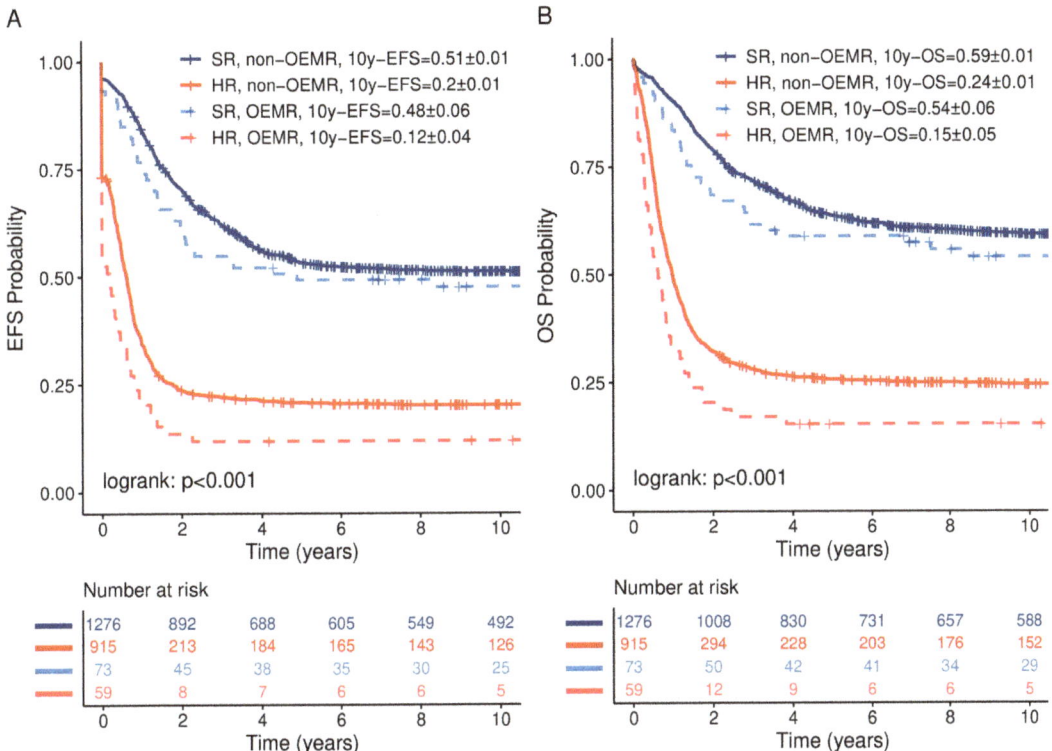

Figure 2. Ten-year pEFS (**A**) and pOS (**B**) of SR vs. HR patients differ significantly in OEMR and non-OEMR patients. The graphs have been calculated based on Kaplan–Meier analysis. Pairwise log-rank test applied in subgroup analysis. $p < 0.001$.

Analyzing 10y-pEFS amongst the OEMR subgroups revealed significant differences in outcomes (Figure 4 and Table 5c): "lymphatic organs", "other" and "skin and glands" OEMR groups had comparably better 10y-pEFS of 0.50 ± 0.09, 0.41 ± 0.09 and 0.32 ± 0.11, $p < 0.001$, respectively. Mediastinal relapse was found to be associated with a very low 10y-pEFS of 0.11 ± 0.05. Consequently, mediastinal relapses most likely contributed to the lower pEFS of the entire OEMR patient cohort. The 12 patients suffering from OEMR of "bone" experienced a similarly dismal 10-year pEFS of only 0.17 ± 0.11. In contrast to "mediastinal" OEMR, "bone" OEMR comprised predominantly BCP-ALL patients relapsing very early and early (11 out of 12 patients demonstrated BCP-ALL phenotype, 92%; Table 2). Limiting the analysis to isolated OEMR, event-free survival of patients with isolated "mediastinal" relapse remained very poor (10y-pEFS 0.12 ± 0.08). On the other hand, the isolated "skin and gland" relapse group showed an excellent 10y-pEFS of 0.60 ± 0.15 (Figure 4).

In addition to EFS, pOS differed significantly within the various OEMR subgroups (Figure 5 and Table 5b). Patients suffering from "mediastinal" OEMR were found to have a dismal prognosis with a pOS of only 0.14 ± 0.06 compared to patients who suffer an OEMR in "lymph nodes" who can expect a 10-year pOS of 0.62 ± 0.09. Interestingly, pOS within the isolated OEMR was excellent in the "other" group, i.e., 0.73 ± 0.13.

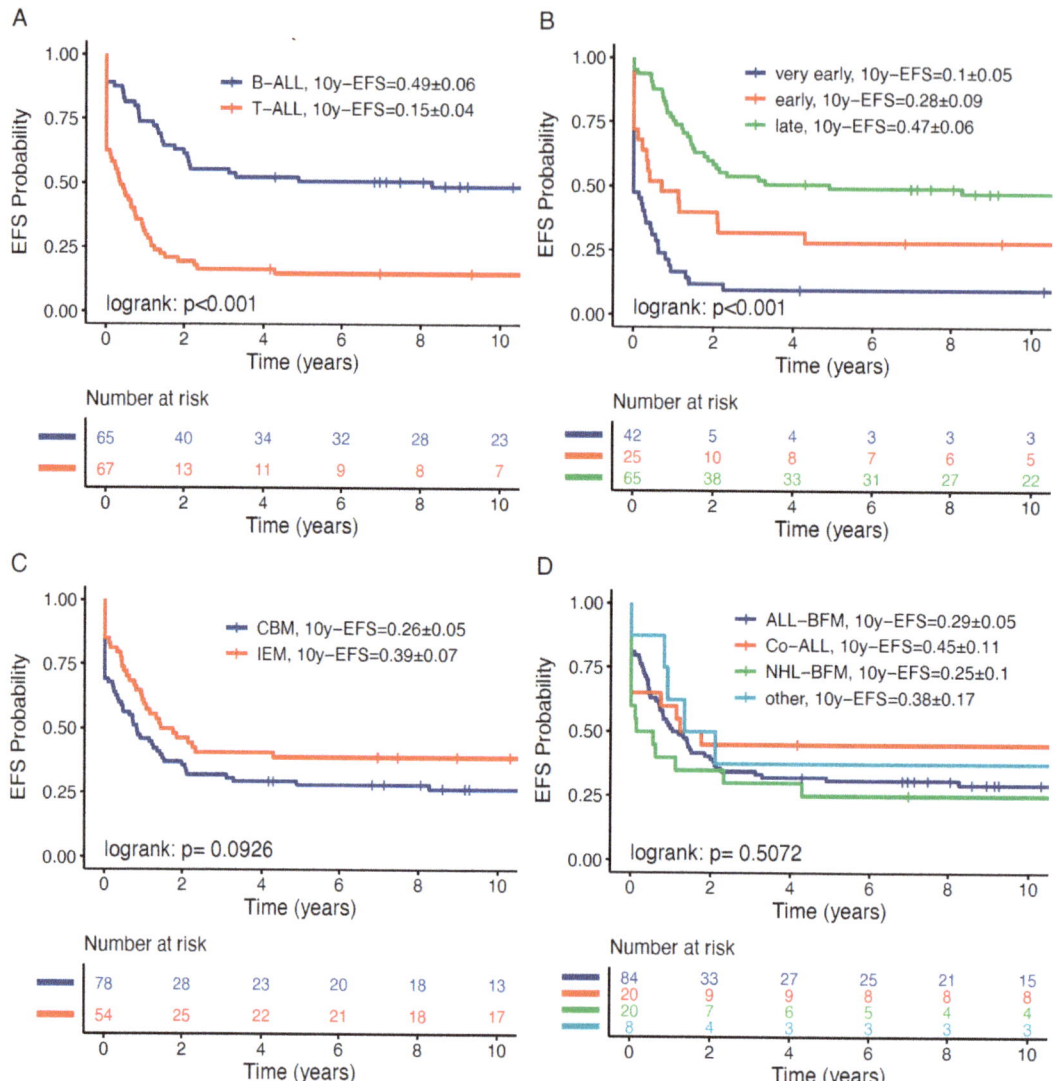

Figure 3. Ten-year pEFS (**A–D**) of OEMR patients in defined demographic subgroups. (**A**) T-ALL, (**B**) very early relapse and (**C**) combined BM relapse are correlated with significantly decreased 10-year pEFS. (**D**) Previous treatment protocol is not associated with outcome in OEMR patients. Calculation based on Kaplan–Meier analysis. $p < 0.05$.

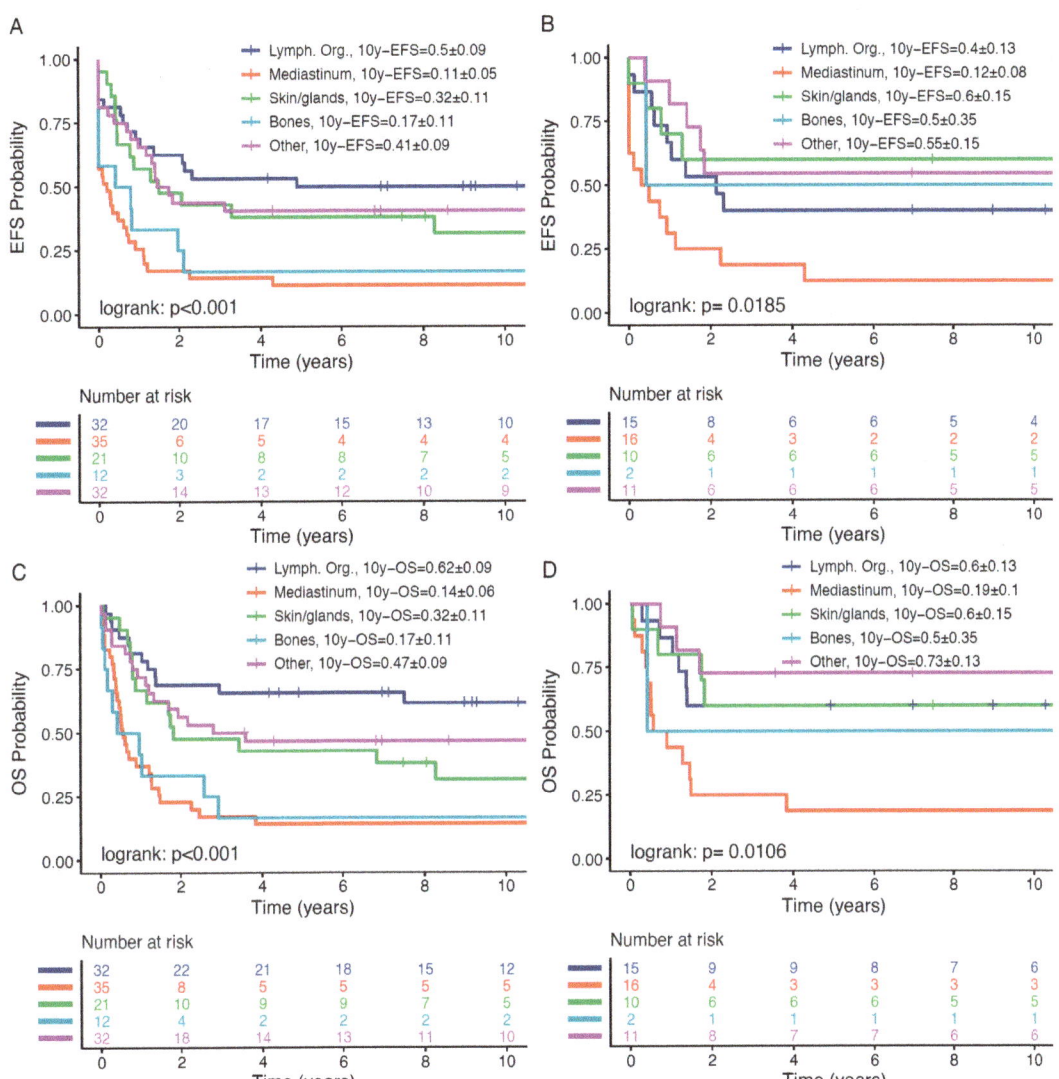

Figure 4. Ten-year pEFS (**A**,**B**) and pOS (**C**,**D**) of OEMR subgroups; (**A**,**C**): pEFS and pOS of combined bone marrow and isolated OEMR; (**B**,**D**): pEFS and pOS of isolated OEMR. Mediastinal and bone OEMR demonstrate inferior outcome compared to all other subgroups. Calculation based on Kaplan–Meier analysis. $p < 0.05$.

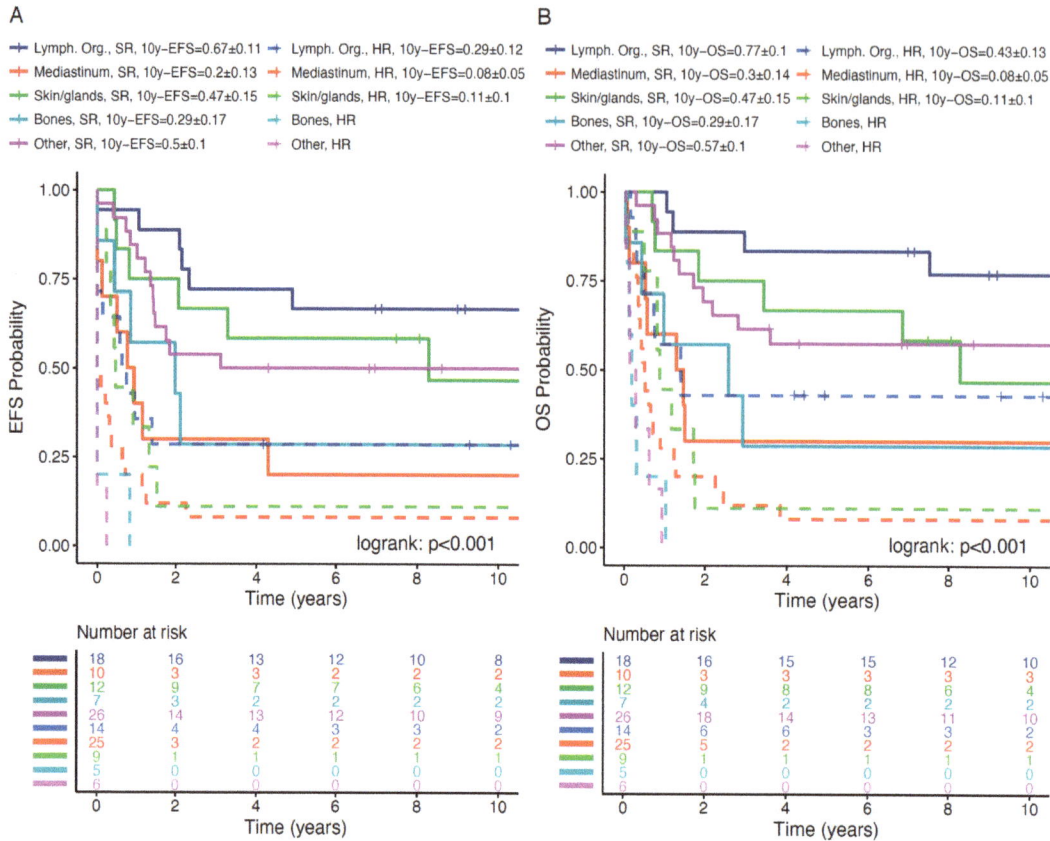

Figure 5. Ten-year pEFS (**A**) and pOS (**B**) of OEMR subgroups stratified by HR and SR criteria. HR OEMR is associated with significantly decreased 10-year pEFS and pOS except in mediastinal subgroup. Calculation based on Kaplan–Meier analysis. Pairwise log-rank applied in subgroup analysis. $p < 0.05$.

We further focused on outcome in OEMR SR vs. HR groups (for definitions please refer to Section 2). SR and HR stratification in OEMR revealed pEFS and pOS in the expected range in all but the mediastinal subgroup (Figure 5 and Table 5c). As in non-OEMR, T-ALL is associated with inferior outcome independent from other risk factors (Supplementary Figure S1) and should be treated according to the HR group with HSCT indication for all patients.

In multivariate Cox regression analysis on EFS and OS, the established risk factors age, time to relapse, site of relapse and immunophenotype were revealed to be independent prognostic factors. In addition, OEMR conferred an independent risk for inferior EFS and OS (hazard ratio 1.7 and 1.7, respectively; $p < 0.001$, Table 6). Excluding T-LBL treated on a former NHL regimen from multivariate Cox regression analysis revealed an independent correlation of OEMR with EFS and OS (hazard ratio 1.66 and 1.72, respectively, $p < 0.001$). Excluding all relapsed T-ALL and T-LBL patients from the Cox regression analysis demonstrated OEMR as an independent risk factor for OS in relapsed BCP-ALL/LBL patients (hazard ratio 1.48, $p = 0.038$).

Table 6. Cox regression; multivariate analysis.

(a) EFS; Cox Regression; Multivariate Analysis						
	Univariate Analysis			Mulitvariate Analysis		
	HR	95% CI	p (chi)	HR	95% CI	p (chi)
Gender: ref. male						
female	0.95	0.85–1.06	0.33			
Age: ref. < 5 years						
age > 5 to ≤ 10 years	0.7	0.6–0.8	0.009	1.13	0.97–1.31	0.13
age > 10 to ≤ 15 years	0.81	0.7–0.95	0.03	1.33	1.13–1.56	<0.001
age > 15 years	0.81	0.67–0.98	0.017	1.24	1.02–1.52	0.03
OEM: ref. no OEMR						
OEMR	1.30	1.05–1.06	<0.001	1.76	1.39–2.23	<0.001
Time: ref. very early						
early	0.57	0.5–0.64	<0.001	0.65	0.57–0.075	<0.001
late	0.26	0.23–0.29	<0.001	0.24	0.21–0.028	<0.001
Site: ref. IBM						
CBM	0.81	0.71–0.92	<0.001	0.68	.059–0.78	<0.001
IEM	0.67	0.57–0.78	<0.001	0.40	0.34–0.47	<0.001
Phenotype: ref. BCP						
T-ALL	2.37	2.06–2.72	<0.001	1.61	1.38–1.88	<0.001
NHL protocol: ref. no						
NHL-BFM	1.68	1.25–2.23	<0.001	1.25	0.92–1.70	0.80
(b) OS; Cox Regression; Multivariate Analysis						
	Univariable Analysis			Mulitvariable Analysis		
	HR	95% CI	p (chi)	HR	95% CI	p (chi)
Gender: ref. male						
female	0.99	0.88–1.11	0.821			
Age: ref. < 5 years						
age > 5 to ≤ 10 years	0.66	0.57–0.77	<0.001	1.08	0.92–1.27	0.33
age > 10 to ≤ 15 years	0.82	0.69–0.96	0.013	1.33	1.12–1.57	<0.001
age > 15 years	0.88	0.72–1.07	0.205	1.41	1.15–1.73	<0.001
OEM: ref. no OEMR						
OEMR	1.33	1.07–1.66	0.011	1.71	1.33–1.29	<0.001
Time: ref. very early						
early	0.57	0.5–0.65	<0.001	0.65	0.57–0.75	<0.001
late	0.24	0.21–0.27	<0.001	0.22	0.19–0.75	<0.001
Site: ref. IBM						
CBM	0.87	0.76–0.99	0.042	0.72	0.62–0.84	<0.001
IEM	0.63	0.54–0.75	<0.001	0.38	0.32–0.45	<0.001
Phenotype: ref. BCP						
T-ALL	2.41	2.09–2.78	<0.001	1.62	1.38–1.89	<0.001
NHL protocol: ref. no						
NHL-BFM	1.56	1.14–2.13	0.005	1.21	0.88–1.70	0.82

Legend to Table 6: Abbreviations: BCP, B-cell precursor; chi, chi-squared test; CBM, combined bone marrow relapse; CI, confidence interval; HR, hazard ratio; IEM, isolated bone marrow relapse; NHL-BFM, Non-Hodgkin's Lymphoma Berlin–Frankfurt–Munster protocol; OEMR, other extramedullary relapse.

4. Discussion

With this report, we present retrospective data covering a period of 32 years on outcome of 132 children with extramedullary ALL relapse other than CNS or testis summarizing those enrolled into five consecutive ALL relapse trials (ALL-REZ BFM) and/or the disease-specific registries in Germany, Austria and Switzerland and single centers in the Czech Republic and Canada. OEMR is a rare event and represents only 5.7% of ALL relapses registered in that period. Patients with relapse of lymphoblastic lymphoma have been treated within trials of the ALL-REZ BFM study group and represent 15% of the

OEMR group. Involved OEM localizations most often include lymph node or mediastinum as extramedullary compartment but also include a variety of rare manifestations.

The complete OEM relapse group showed inferior prognosis compared to non-OEMR patients mainly due to poor outcome of mediastinal and bone OEMR. Whereas most patients with OEMR were adequately stratified into a risk group according to established factors such as time to relapse, immunophenotype and site of relapse, defined subgroups of patients seemingly require treatment intensification: patients with late T-ALL isolated mediastinal or lymphatic organ relapse formerly stratified into a standard risk group have poor outcome and need to receive allogeneic HSCT and possibly additional local irradiation.

In our analysis, the subgroups "lymphatic organs" and "skin and glands" had relatively good outcomes. Both seem to be compartments where systemic chemotherapy can act without major obstacles. Considering the favorable 10y-pEFS of "skin and glands" relapse patients treated exclusively with chemotherapy, this location does not need any additional local therapy. In contrast, the subgroup "bone relapse" showed a very poor outcome. It was characterized by a high proportion of B-precursor cell immunophenotype (77%) and combined bone marrow relapses (77%). We hypothesize that particularly aggressive cells that infiltrate the surrounding bone tissue from the adjacent bone marrow might be responsible for that observation. Biopsy including deep molecular characterization, comparison to molecular features of previous lines of disease and deconvolution of clonal evolution could enable deeper insights into the biology of these very rare and aggressive relapse types. In addition, this subgroup might probably benefit from treatment intensification with irradiation and/or allogeneic HSCT. However, due to the limited number of reports on bone relapses and only 12 patients being diagnosed with bone relapses in the current analysis, explicit conclusions are cannot be driven and the indication for radiotherapy needs to be made on an individual basis [4,5].

In addition, the subgroup "other compartment" included extremely heterogeneous localizations. Thus, it was difficult to evaluate these as a single group. We tried to focus on some of these unusual locations of relapse. There were four relapses of the orbit, eyes or optic nerve. Three of these underwent radiotherapy and all of them survived in complete remission. Orbital relapses are considered sanctuary sites [38], and as reported in the past, radiotherapy might be beneficial for this site [6–8].

Based on the treating physician's discretion, individual relapsed patients with T-LBL and pB-LBL have been included in ALL relapsed protocols. The mediastinal relapse group showed a high proportion of primary T-cell LBL and a very dismal prognosis without significant differences in 10y-pEFS between the whole group (10y-pEFS 0.11 ± 0.05) and isolated mediastinal relapses (10y-pEFS 0.12 ± 0.08). Most patients died within 10 years. According to the analysis of relapse of T-cell LBL patients treated with BFM protocols, long-term survival was only achieved in a few patients (4 of 28 patients) who were able to undergo allogeneic SCT [39]. Survival improved slightly over the last years in T-LBL patients treated on intensive relapse protocols and currently reaches 27% 8-year OS. However, cure for most patients is unattainable, and more effective treatments for T-cell LBL patients are urgently needed [40]. Intensifying induction chemotherapy and improved molecular characterization [41,42] might lead to more efficient therapies. While the therapeutic effect of mediastinal irradiation has not been confirmed in pediatric patients, some reports presented the efficacy of mediastinal irradiation for selected adult patients who responded insufficiently to induction chemotherapy [43,44]. However, a general recommendation of radiation during early induction is not feasible, since systemic therapy might be postponed, increasing the risk of systemic relapse in that rapidly proliferating disease. The current approach of the NHL BFM group includes a mediastinal boost combined with TBI in case of a detectable mediastinal mass before HSCT. Since 309 T-ALL relapses have been reported from 1983 to 2015 and mediastinal relapse is common in most T-ALL relapses (at first diagnosis up to 60% present with mediastinal mass [45]), mediastinal relapse patient numbers might be underestimated in our OEMR cohort.

It has always been a matter of debate if OEMR requires additional local consolidation including radiation. Since treatment in our cohort was triggered by local poor response or by specific localization such as mediastinal or eye/orbit, only 17 patients, the minority nonresponders, were treated with radiotherapy; thus, the impact of local irradiation on outcome cannot be determined in this retrospective analysis.

In the ALL-REZ BFM 2002 trial, patients with isolated extramedullary relapse did not have an indication for allogeneic HSCT due to acceptable outcome for patients without bone marrow involvement [46]. Nevertheless, patients with isolated OEMR and a T-cell immunophenotype experience such a dismal outcome that chemotherapy alone is no longer an acceptable approach. Current recommendations include HSCT as definitive consolidation in very early and early isolated EM relapsed ALL patients. Evaluation of that approach is ongoing [47,48].

The current analysis includes patients from 1983 to 2015. The vast majority of these patients have not been deeply molecularly characterized. Treatments have been based on established chemotherapeutic schedules, irradiation and HSCT. Current immunologic approaches in relapsed/refractory treatment include daratumumab, blinatumomab, inotuzumab and CAR T-cell approaches [49–52]. Although the efficacy of these agents in the BM compartment has been clearly demonstrated, efficacy in EM localizations is less clear. Further prospective investigations will show if relapse patterns change, if EM relapse is observed more frequently and if additional consolidative elements need to be combined with immunotherapeutic approaches to prevent EM relapse and improve long-term outcome.

5. Conclusions

This retrospective analysis presented the outcome of ALL and LBL relapses in extramedullary compartments other than CNS or testis of which little is known so far. We were able to show that OEMR confers an independent risk for inferior pEFS and pOS and that OEMR subgroups differ significantly in regard to demographic patterns and outcome. Of high importance, we are able to show that established risk stratification can be applied to OEMR patients and these should be treated on established protocols and treatment algorithms. HSCT should be performed in all HR T-ALL relapsed patients and HR OEMR patients. Additional radiation might be of benefit in sanctuary sites, i.e., eye and bone. However, most OEMR patients do not relapse at the initial site, highlighting that the systemic disease requires systemic induction and consolidation chemotherapy. International efforts need to be established to enable robust treatment recommendations on radiation. In that regard, response assessment by positron emission tomography (PET), being of established value in adult lymphoma [47], could exert its diagnostic value even though it is not yet established in pediatric ALL and NHL patients. PET could provide additional information on the viability of the tumor and enable treating physicians to assess local response more exactly.

Due to the scarcity of disease and high heterogeneity, international collaboration is needed to prospectively evaluate treatment, define response criteria and substantially improve outcome of pediatric OEMR ALL patients [53].

Supplementary Materials: The following are available online at https://www.mdpi.com/article/10.3390/jcm10225292/s1, Figure S1: Distribution of OEMR, Figure S2: T-ALL relapses, Table S1: Genetic characteristics, Table S2: Radiation in non-OEMR and OEMR patients.

Author Contributions: Conceptualization, C.v.S., A.L., A.A., C.C.-S. and A.v.S.; methodology, A.v.S., A.L. and I.G.S.; software, I.G.S.; validation, I.G.S., A.v.S., C.E.; formal analysis, I.G.S.; investigation, A.L., C.v.S., I.G.S., A.A., J.-P.B., B.B., G.H., G.M., L.S. and C.E.; resources, A.v.S.; data curation, I.G.S., A.L., C.v.S., A.A. and A.v.S.; writing—original draft preparation, A.L. and C.v.S.; writing—review and editing, A.v.S. and C.E.; visualization, I.G.S.; supervision, C.P., A.v.S., C.C.-S. and C.E.; project administration, A.v.S.; funding acquisition, A.v.S. All authors have read and agreed to the published version of the manuscript.

Funding: This research was funded by Deutsche Kinderkrebsstiftung Deutsche Krebshilfe and José Carreras Leukämie Stiftung.

Institutional Review Board Statement: The study was conducted according to the guidelines of the Declaration of Helsinki and approved by the Institutional Review Board of the Charité-Universitätsmedizin Berlin and Landesamt für Gesundheit und Soziales Berlin.

Informed Consent Statement: Informed consent was obtained from all subjects involved in the study.

Acknowledgments: We thank all funding and collaboration partners within the ALL-REZ consortium and patients and parents providing their informed consent on enrolment into clinical trials and registries.

Conflicts of Interest: The authors have no competing interest. The authors declare no conflict of interest.

References

1. Gaudichon, J.; Jakobczyk, H.; Debaize, L.; Cousin, E.; Galibert, M.D.; Troadec, M.B.; Gandemer, V. Mechanisms of extramedullary relapse in acute lymphoblastic leukemia: Reconciling biological concepts and clinical issues. *Blood Rev.* **2019**, *36*, 40–56. [CrossRef] [PubMed]
2. Pui, C.H. Central nervous system disease in acute lymphoblastic leukemia: Prophylaxis and treatment. *Hematol. Am. Soc. Hematol. Educ. Program* **2006**, *2006*, 142–146. [CrossRef]
3. Wofford, M.M.; Smith, S.D.; Shuster, J.J.; Johnson, W.; Buchanan, G.R.; Wharam, M.D.; Ritchey, A.K.; Rosen, D.; Haggard, M.E.; Golembe, B.L.; et al. Treatment of occult or late overt testicular relapse in children with acute lymphoblastic leukemia: A Pediatric Oncology Group study. *J. Clin. Oncol.* **1992**, *10*, 624–630. [CrossRef]
4. Murray, J.C.; Gmoser, D.J.; Barnes, D.A.; Oshman, D.; Hawkins, H.K.; Gresik, M.V.; Dreyer, Z.E. Isolated bone relapse during hematologic remission in childhood acute lymphoblastic leukemia: Report of a metatarsal relapse and review of the literature. *Med. Pediatr. Oncol.* **1994**, *23*, 153–157. [CrossRef] [PubMed]
5. Padmanjali, K.S.; Bakhshi, S.; Thavaraj, V.; Karak, A.K.; Arya, L.S. Bone relapse in acute lymphoblastic leukemia. *Indian J. Pediatr.* **2004**, *71*, 555–557. [CrossRef]
6. Curto, M.L.; D'Angelo, P.; Jankovic, M.; Fugardi, M.G.; Ziino, O.; Casale, F. Isolated ocular relapse in childhood acute lymphoblastic leukemia during continuing complete remission. *Haematologica* **1996**, *81*, 47–50. [PubMed]
7. Taylor, C.W.; Taylor, R.E.; Kinsey, S.E. Leukemic infiltration of the orbit: Report of three cases and literature review. *Pediatr. Hematol. Oncol.* **2005**, *22*, 415–422. [CrossRef]
8. MacLean, H.; Clarke, M.P.; Strong, N.P.; Kernahan, J.; Ashraf, S. Primary ocular relapse in acute lymphoblastic leukemia. *Eye* **1996**, *10 Pt 6*, 719–722. [CrossRef] [PubMed]
9. Nadel, J.; Meredith, T.; Anthony, C.; Sivasubramaniam, V.; Jabbour, A. Isolated myocardial relapse of Philadelphia-positive acute lymphoblastic leukaemia causing myocarditis: A case report. *Eur. Heart J. Case Rep.* **2018**, *2*, yty104. [CrossRef]
10. Veys, D.; Norton, A.; Ainsworth, J.R.; Amrolia, P.; Lucchini, G. Isolated Intraocular Relapse of Pediatric B-cell Precursor Acute Lymphoblastic Leukaemia Following Chimeric Antigen Receptor T-lymphocyte Therapy. *Cureus* **2020**, *12*, e10937. [CrossRef]
11. Dix, D.B.; Anderson, R.A.; McFadden, D.E.; Wadsworth, L.D. Pleural relapse during hematopoietic remission in childhood acute lymphoblastic leukemia. *J. Pediatr. Hematol. Oncol.* **1997**, *19*, 470–472. [CrossRef] [PubMed]
12. Esmaeli, B.; Medeiros, L.J.; Myers, J.; Champlin, R.; Singh, S.; Ginsberg, L. Orbital mass secondary to precursor T-cell acute lymphoblastic leukemia: A rare presentation. *Arch. Ophthalmol.* **2001**, *119*, 443–446. [CrossRef]
13. Hinkle, A.S.; Dinndorf, P.A.; Bulas, D.I.; Kapur, S. Relapse of acute lymphoblastic leukemia in the inferior rectus muscle of the eye. *Cancer* **1994**, *73*, 1757–1760. [CrossRef]
14. Jankovic, M.; Conter, V.; Pretto, G.; Placa, F.; D'Incalci, M.; Masera, G. Isolated bilateral anterior chamber eye relapse in a child with acute lymphoblastic leukemia. *Med. Pediatr. Oncol.* **1995**, *25*, 109–112. [CrossRef]
15. Kebaili, K.; Manel, A.M.; Chapelon, C.; Taylor, P.; Philippe, N.; Bertrand, Y. Renal enlargement as presentation of isolated renal relapse in childhood leukemia. *J. Pediatr. Hematol. Oncol.* **2000**, *22*, 454–456. [CrossRef] [PubMed]
16. Ly-Sunnaram, B.; Henry, C.; Gandemer, V.; Mee, F.L.; Burtin, F.; Blayau, M.; Cayuela, J.M.; Oster, M.; Clech, P.; Rambeau, M.; et al. Late ovarian relapse of TEL/AML1 positive ALL confirming that TEL deletion is a secondary event in leukemogenesis. *Leuk. Res.* **2005**, *29*, 1089–1094. [CrossRef]
17. Mateo, J.; Abarzuza, R.; Nunez, E.; Cristobal, J.A. Bilateral optic nerve infiltration in acute lymphoblastic leukemia in remission. *Arch. Soc. Esp. Oftalmol.* **2007**, *82*, 167–170. [CrossRef] [PubMed]
18. Millot, F.; Klossek, J.M.; Brizard, F.; Brizard, A.; Vandermarq, P.; Babin, P.; Guilhot, F. Recurrence of childhood acute lymphoblastic leukemia presenting as a tumor of the middle ear: A case report. *J. Pediatr. Hematol. Oncol.* **1997**, *19*, 351–353. [CrossRef]
19. Qamruddin, K.; Hassan, S.; Khurshid, M. Case of pelvic relapse in a child suffering from acute lymphoblastic leukemia. *J. Pak. Med. Assoc.* **1995**, *45*, 193–194.
20. Rush, M.; Toth, B.B.; Pinkel, D. Clinically isolated mandibular relapse in childhood acute leukemia. *Cancer* **1990**, *66*, 369–372. [CrossRef]

21. Todo, K.; Morimoto, A.; Osone, S.; Nukina, S.; Ohtsuka, T.; Ishida, H.; Yoshihara, T.; Todo, S. Isolated relapse of acute lymphoblastic leukemia in the breast of a young female. *Pediatr. Hematol. Oncol.* **2008**, *25*, 607–613. [CrossRef]
22. Tsuruchi, N.; Okamura, J. Childhood acute lymphoblastic leukemia relapse in the uterine cervix. *J. Pediatr. Hematol. Oncol.* **1996**, *18*, 311–313. [CrossRef] [PubMed]
23. Uderzo, C.; Santamaria, M.; Locasciulli, A.; Merati, I.; Di Lelio, A.; Conter, V.; Masera, G. Abdominal mass as manifestation of isolated extramedullary relapse in a child with acute lymphoblastic leukemia (ALL). *Haematologica* **1987**, *72*, 545–547.
24. Gunes, G.; Goker, H.; Demiroglu, H.; Malkan, U.Y.; Buyukasik, Y. Extramedullary relapses of acute leukemias after allogeneic hematopoietic stem cell transplantation: Clinical features, cumulative incidence, and risk factors. *Bone Marrow Transplant.* **2019**, *54*, 595–600. [CrossRef]
25. Bunin, N.J.; Pui, C.H.; Hustu, H.O.; Rivera, G.K. Unusual extramedullary relapses in children with acute lymphoblastic leukemia. *J. Pediatr.* **1986**, *109*, 665–668. [CrossRef]
26. Kim, J.Y.; Im, S.A.; Lee, J.H.; Lee, J.W.; Chung, N.G.; Cho, B. Extramedullary Relapse of Acute Myeloid and Lymphoid Leukemia in Children: A Retrospective Analysis. *Iran. J. Pediatr.* **2016**, *26*, e1711. [CrossRef] [PubMed]
27. Bene, M.C.; Castoldi, G.; Knapp, W.; Ludwig, W.D.; Matutes, E.; Orfao, A.; van't Veer, M.B. Proposals for the immunological classification of acute leukemias. European Group for the Immunological Characterization of Leukemias (EGIL). *Leukemia* **1995**, *9*, 1783–1786. [PubMed]
28. Seeger, K.; Adams, H.P.; Buchwald, D.; Beyermann, B.; Kremens, B.; Niemeyer, C.; Ritter, J.; Schwabe, D.; Harms, D.; Schrappe, M.; et al. TEL-AML1 fusion transcript in relapsed childhood acute lymphoblastic leukemia. The Berlin-Frankfurt-Munster Study Group. *Blood* **1998**, *91*, 1716–1722. [CrossRef]
29. Einsiedel, H.G.; von Stackelberg, A.; Hartmann, R.; Fengler, R.; Schrappe, M.; Janka-Schaub, G.; Mann, G.; Hahlen, K.; Gobel, U.; Klingebiel, T.; et al. Long-term outcome in children with relapsed ALL by risk-stratified salvage therapy: Results of trial acute lymphoblastic leukemia-relapse study of the Berlin-Frankfurt-Munster Group 87. *J. Clin. Oncol.* **2005**, *23*, 7942–7950. [CrossRef]
30. von Stackelberg, A.; Hartmann, R.; Buhrer, C.; Fengler, R.; Janka-Schaub, G.; Reiter, A.; Mann, G.; Schmiegelow, K.; Ratei, R.; Klingebiel, T.; et al. High-dose compared with intermediate-dose methotrexate in children with a first relapse of acute lymphoblastic leukemia. *Blood* **2008**, *111*, 2573–2580. [CrossRef]
31. Eckert, C.; von Stackelberg, A.; Seeger, K.; Groeneveld, T.W.; Peters, C.; Klingebiel, T.; Borkhardt, A.; Schrappe, M.; Escherich, G.; Henze, G. Minimal residual disease after induction is the strongest predictor of prognosis in intermediate risk relapsed acute lymphoblastic leukaemia—Long-Term results of trial ALL-REZ BFM P95/96. *Eur. J. Cancer* **2013**, *49*, 1346–1355. [CrossRef]
32. Eckert, C.; Henze, G.; Seeger, K.; Hagedorn, N.; Mann, G.; Panzer-Grumayer, R.; Peters, C.; Klingebiel, T.; Borkhardt, A.; Schrappe, M.; et al. Use of allogeneic hematopoietic stem-cell transplantation based on minimal residual disease response improves outcomes for children with relapsed acute lymphoblastic leukemia in the intermediate-risk group. *J. Clin. Oncol.* **2013**, *31*, 2736–2742. [CrossRef]
33. Meyr, F.; Escherich, G.; Mann, G.; Klingebiel, T.; Kulozik, A.; Rossig, C.; Schrappe, M.; Henze, G.; von Stackelberg, A.; Hitzler, J. Outcomes of treatment for relapsed acute lymphoblastic leukaemia in children with Down syndrome. *Br. J. Haematol.* **2013**, *162*, 98–106. [CrossRef] [PubMed]
34. Peters, C.; Schrappe, M.; von Stackelberg, A.; Schrauder, A.; Bader, P.; Ebell, W.; Lang, P.; Sykora, K.W.; Schrum, J.; Kremens, B.; et al. Stem-cell transplantation in children with acute lymphoblastic leukemia: A prospective international multicenter trial comparing sibling donors with matched unrelated donors-The ALL-SCT-BFM-2003 trial. *J. Clin. Oncol.* **2015**, *33*, 1265–1274. [CrossRef]
35. van der Wijk, A.E.; Canning, P.; van Heijningen, R.P.; Vogels, I.M.C.; van Noorden, C.J.F.; Klaassen, I.; Schlingemann, R.O. Glucocorticoids exert differential effects on the endothelium in an in vitro model of the blood-retinal barrier. *Acta Ophthalmol.* **2019**, *97*, 214–224. [CrossRef] [PubMed]
36. Gaynon, P.S.; Qu, R.P.; Chappell, R.J.; Willoughby, M.L.; Tubergen, D.G.; Steinherz, P.G.; Trigg, M.E. Survival after relapse in childhood acute lymphoblastic leukemia: Impact of site and time to first relapse–the Children's Cancer Group Experience. *Cancer* **1998**, *82*, 1387–1395. [CrossRef]
37. Tallen, G.; Ratei, R.; Mann, G.; Kaspers, G.; Niggli, F.; Karachunsky, A.; Ebell, W.; Escherich, G.; Schrappe, M.; Klingebiel, T.; et al. Long-term outcome in children with relapsed acute lymphoblastic leukemia after time-point and site-of-relapse stratification and intensified short-course multidrug chemotherapy: Results of trial ALL-REZ BFM 90. *J. Clin. Oncol.* **2010**, *28*, 2339–2347. [CrossRef]
38. Ninane, J.; Taylor, D.; Day, S. The eye as a sanctuary in acute lymphoblastic leukaemia. *Lancet* **1980**, *1*, 452–453. [CrossRef]
39. Burkhardt, B.; Reiter, A.; Landmann, E.; Lang, P.; Lassay, L.; Dickerhoff, R.; Lakomek, M.; Henze, G.; von Stackelberg, A. Poor outcome for children and adolescents with progressive disease or relapse of lymphoblastic lymphoma: A report from the berlin-frankfurt-muenster group. *J. Clin. Oncol.* **2009**, *27*, 3363–3369. [CrossRef]
40. Burkhardt, B.; Taj, M.; Garnier, N.; Minard-Colin, V.; Hazar, V.; Mellgren, K.; Osumi, T.; Fedorova, A.; Myakova, N.; Verdu-Amoros, J.; et al. Treatment and Outcome Analysis of 639 Relapsed Non-Hodgkin Lymphomas in Children and Adolescents and Resulting Treatment Recommendations. *Cancers* **2021**, *13*, 2075. [CrossRef]
41. Khanam, T.; Sandmann, S.; Seggewiss, J.; Ruether, C.; Zimmermann, M.; Norvil, A.B.; Bartenhagen, C.; Randau, G.; Mueller, S.; Herbrueggen, H.; et al. Integrative genomic analysis of pediatric T-cell lymphoblastic lymphoma reveals candidates of clinical significance. *Blood* **2021**, *137*, 2347–2359. [CrossRef]

42. Burkhardt, B.; Hermiston, M.L. Lymphoblastic lymphoma in children and adolescents: Review of current challenges and future opportunities. *Br. J. Haematol.* **2019**, *185*, 1158–1170. [CrossRef]
43. Cortelazzo, S.; Intermesoli, T.; Oldani, E.; Ciceri, F.; Rossi, G.; Pogliani, E.M.; Mattei, D.; Romani, C.; Cortelezzi, A.; Borlenghi, E.; et al. Results of a lymphoblastic leukemia-like chemotherapy program with risk-adapted mediastinal irradiation and stem cell transplantation for adult patients with lymphoblastic lymphoma. *Ann. Hematol.* **2012**, *91*, 73–82. [CrossRef]
44. Dabaja, B.S.; Ha, C.S.; Thomas, D.A.; Wilder, R.B.; Gopal, R.; Cortes, J.; Bueso-Ramos, C.; Hess, M.A.; Cox, J.D.; Kantarjian, H.M. The role of local radiation therapy for mediastinal disease in adults with T-cell lymphoblastic lymphoma. *Cancer* **2002**, *94*, 2738–2744. [CrossRef]
45. Karrman, K.; Johansson, B. Pediatric T-cell acute lymphoblastic leukemia. *Genes Chromosomes Cancer* **2017**, *56*, 89–116. [CrossRef] [PubMed]
46. Bader, P.; Kreyenberg, H.; Henze, G.H.; Eckert, C.; Reising, M.; Willasch, A.; Barth, A.; Borkhardt, A.; Peters, C.; Handgretinger, R.; et al. Prognostic value of minimal residual disease quantification before allogeneic stem-cell transplantation in relapsed childhood acute lymphoblastic leukemia: The ALL-REZ BFM Study Group. *J. Clin. Oncol.* **2009**, *27*, 377–384. [CrossRef]
47. Zhao, J.; Qiao, W.; Wang, C.; Wang, T.; Xing, Y. Therapeutic evaluation and prognostic value of interim hybrid PET/CT with (18)F-FDG after three to four cycles of chemotherapy in non-Hodgkin's lymphoma. *Hematology* **2007**, *12*, 423–430. [CrossRef] [PubMed]
48. Eckert, P.; Johs, A.; Semrau, J.D.; DiSpirito, A.A.; Richardson, J.; Sarangi, R.; Herndon, E.; Gu, B.; Pierce, E.M. Spectroscopic and computational investigations of organometallic complexation of group 12 transition metals by methanobactins from Methylocystis sp. SB2. *J. Inorg. Biochem.* **2021**, *223*, 111496. [CrossRef]
49. Bride, K.L.; Vincent, T.L.; Im, S.Y.; Aplenc, R.; Barrett, D.M.; Carroll, W.L.; Carson, R.; Dai, Y.; Devidas, M.; Dunsmore, K.P.; et al. Preclinical efficacy of daratumumab in T-cell acute lymphoblastic leukemia. *Blood* **2018**, *131*, 995–999. [CrossRef] [PubMed]
50. Locatelli, F.; Zugmaier, G.; Rizzari, C.; Morris, J.D.; Gruhn, B.; Klingebiel, T.; Parasole, R.; Linderkamp, C.; Flotho, C.; Petit, A.; et al. Effect of Blinatumomab vs Chemotherapy on Event-Free Survival Among Children With High-risk First-Relapse B-Cell Acute Lymphoblastic Leukemia: A Randomized Clinical Trial. *JAMA* **2021**, *325*, 843–854. [CrossRef] [PubMed]
51. Bhojwani, D.; Sposto, R.; Shah, N.N.; Rodriguez, V.; Yuan, C.; Stetler-Stevenson, M.; O'Brien, M.M.; McNeer, J.L.; Quereshi, A.; Cabannes, A.; et al. Inotuzumab ozogamicin in pediatric patients with relapsed/refractory acute lymphoblastic leukemia. *Leukemia* **2019**, *33*, 884–892. [CrossRef] [PubMed]
52. Maude, S.L.; Laetsch, T.W.; Buechner, J.; Rives, S.; Boyer, M.; Bittencourt, H.; Bader, P.; Verneris, M.R.; Stefanski, H.E.; Myers, G.D.; et al. Tisagenlecleucel in Children and Young Adults with B-Cell Lymphoblastic Leukemia. *N. Engl. J. Med.* **2018**, *378*, 439–448. [CrossRef] [PubMed]
53. Pui, C.H.; Tang, J.Y.; Yang, J.J.; Chen, S.J.; Chen, Z. International Collaboration to Save Children With Acute Lymphoblastic Leukemia. *J. Glob. Oncol.* **2019**, *5*, 1–2. [CrossRef] [PubMed]

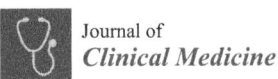

Article

Genetic Variation in *ABCC4* and *CFTR* and Acute Pancreatitis during Treatment of Pediatric Acute Lymphoblastic Leukemia

Thies Bartram [1,2], Peter Schütte [2], Anja Möricke [1], Richard S. Houlston [3], Eva Ellinghaus [4], Martin Zimmermann [2], Anke Bergmann [5], Britt-Sabina Löscher [4], Norman Klein [2], Laura Hinze [2], Stefanie V. Junk [2], Michael Forster [4], Claus R. Bartram [6], Rolf Köhler [6], Andre Franke [4], Martin Schrappe [1], Christian P. Kratz [2], Gunnar Cario [1] and Martin Stanulla [2,*]

[1] Department of Pediatrics, University Hospital Schleswig-Holstein, 24105 Kiel, Germany; thyssen2@gmx.de (T.B.); a.moericke@pediatrics.uni-kiel.de (A.M.); m.schrappe@pediatrics.uni-kiel.de (M.S.); gunnar.cario@uksh.de (G.C.)
[2] Department of Pediatric Hematology and Oncology, Hannover Medical School, 30625 Hannover, Germany; schuette.peter@mh-hannover.de (P.S.); Zimmermann.Martin@mh-hannover.de (M.Z.); klein.norman4@gmail.com (N.K.); hinze.laura@mh-hannover.de (L.H.); junk.stefanie@mh-hannover.de (S.V.J.); Kratz.Christian@mh-hannover.de (C.P.K.)
[3] Division of Genetics and Epidemiology, Institute of Cancer Research, Sutton SM2 5NG, UK; richard.houlston@icr.ac.uk
[4] Institute of Clinical Molecular Biology, Kiel University, 24118 Kiel, Germany; e.ellinghaus@ikmb.uni-kiel.de (E.E.); b.loescher@ikmb.uni-kiel.de (B.-S.L.); m.forster@ikmb.uni-kiel.de (M.F.); a.franke@mucosa.de (A.F.)
[5] Department of Human Genetics, Hannover Medical School, 30625 Hannover, Germany; bergmann.anke@mh-hannover.de
[6] Department of Human Genetics, University Hospital Heidelberg, 69120 Heidelberg, Germany; cr_bartram@med.uni-heidelberg.de (C.R.B.); Rolf.Koehler@med.uni-heidelberg.de (R.K.)
* Correspondence: stanulla.martin@mh-hannover.de; Tel.: +49-511-532-7978

Abstract: Background: Acute pancreatitis (AP) is a serious, mechanistically not entirely resolved side effect of L-asparaginase-containing treatment for acute lymphoblastic leukemia (ALL). To find new candidate variations for AP, we conducted a genome-wide association study (GWAS). Methods: In all, 1,004,623 single-nucleotide variants (SNVs) were analyzed in 51 pediatric ALL patients with AP (cases) and 1388 patients without AP (controls). Replication used independent patients. Results: The top-ranked SNV (rs4148513) was located within the *ABCC4* gene (odds ratio (OR) 84.1; $p = 1.04 \times 10^{-14}$). Independent replication of our 20 top SNVs was not supportive of initial results, partly because rare variants were neither present in cases nor present in controls. However, results of combined analysis (GWAS and replication cohorts) remained significant (e.g., rs4148513; OR = 47.2; $p = 7.31 \times 10^{-9}$). Subsequently, we sequenced the entire *ABCC4* gene and its close relative, the cystic fibrosis associated *CFTR* gene, a strong AP candidate gene, in 48 cases and 47 controls. Six AP-associated variants in *ABCC4* and one variant in *CFTR* were detected. Replication confirmed the six *ABCC4* variants but not the *CFTR* variant. Conclusions: Genetic variation within the *ABCC4* gene was associated with AP during the treatment of ALL. No association of AP with *CFTR* was observed. Larger international studies are necessary to more conclusively assess the risk of rare clinical phenotypes.

Keywords: acute lymphoblastic leukemia; L-asparaginase; acute pancreatitis; polymorphism; SNV; *ABCC4*; *CFTR*

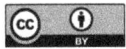

1. Introduction

Acute lymphoblastic leukemia (ALL) is the most common pediatric malignancy and represents approximately 25% of cancers and 80% of all leukemias diagnosed in children and adolescents [1,2]. Contemporary treatment extends over a period of 2 to 3 years and usually consists of combination chemotherapy, which is substituted in small proportions of patients by cranial irradiation or allogeneic hematopoietic stem cell transplantation [3,4]. Timely application of therapy is important to secure optimal treatment effect and outcome but is often compromised by undesired side effects leading to treatment interruptions. Early severe side effects related to the treatment of ALL encompass a variety of specific complications, such as bacterial, viral, and fungal infections; hemostaseological problems; and side effects that can be attributed to specific drugs [5]. Examples of drug-specific toxicities observed during the treatment of ALL are methotrexate-related encephalopathy, steroid-treatment-related avascular bone necrosis, topoisomerase-II-associated secondary acute myeloid leukemia, and acute pancreatitis (AP) developing in the context of L-asparaginase (L-asp) application [6–10].

The mechanism of action of L-asp is the depletion of the extracellular amino acid asparagine by the hydrolysis of asparagine to aspartic acid and ammonia. The depletion results in the inhibition of protein synthesis by malignant cells, such as lymphoblasts, leading to cell death due to the inability to synthesize endogenous asparagine. L-asp used for the treatment of ALL is derived from either *Escherichia coli* (*E. coli*) (native or PEGylated L-asp) or *Erwinia chrysanthemi* [7,8,11], both being associated with AP. The mechanism of AP in association with L-asp is poorly understood. Although L-asp is believed to be the main reason for developing AP, other cytotoxic chemotherapeutics, including 6-mercaptopurine, glucocorticoids, and cytarabine, have been associated with AP, as well [12–15]. Suggested published risk factors for developing AP associated with L-asp treatment include, for example, higher age at diagnosis, acute hypertriglyceridemia, and genetic polymorphisms [11,16–18]. Support for an underlying genetic predisposition comes from the observation that a few applications of L-asp are sufficient to initiate AP and that there is a high probability of recurrence after re-exposure to L-asp [11].

So far, genetic linkage and candidate gene studies have identified several genes (e.g., *PRSS1, PRSS2, SPINK1, CTRC, CASR,* and *CFTR*) that could be associated with chronic, hereditary, and hyperlipidemic pancreatitis. Until recently, no specific loci associated with AP had been identified [11,16,19]. However, meanwhile, genome-wide association studies (GWAS) have identified single-nucleotide variants in the genes *CPA2, ULK2,* and *PRSS1* as being associated with L-asp-associated AP in pediatric ALL [20–22]. Here, we present our results from a GWAS on the etiology of AP in childhood ALL by comparing 51 patients with AP to 1388 control patients without symptoms of AP.

2. Materials and Methods
2.1. Study Individuals

Patients included in this study were 1 to 18 years of age and enrolled in the European AIEOP-BFM ALL 2000 multicenter clinical trial on the treatment of pediatric ALL conducted in Austria, Germany, Italy, and Switzerland [23,24]. Diagnostics and treatment in AIEOP-BFM ALL 2000 have been described previously [23–27]. Briefly, the AIEOP-BFM ALL 2000 patients were stratified into three branches (standard, intermediate, and high risk). Risk group stratification included minimal residual disease (MRD) analysis and required two MRD targets with sensitivities of $\leq 10^{-4}$. Standard-risk patients were MRD-negative on treatment days 33 (TP1) and 78 (TP2) and had no high-risk criteria. High-risk patients had residual disease ($\geq 10^{-3}$) at TP2. MRD-intermediate-risk patients had positive MRD detection at either one or both time points but at a level of $<10^{-3}$ at TP2. Although MRD analysis was the main stratification criterion in AIEOP-BFM ALL 2000, established high-risk parameters were also retained: patients with a poor response to prednisone or $\geq 5\%$ leukemic blasts in the bone marrow on day 33 or positivity for a t(9;22) or t(4;11) or their molecular equivalents (*BCR-ABL1* or *MLL-AF4* gene fusions) were stratified into the high-risk group independent of their MRD results. Treatment details of AIEOP-BFM ALL 2000 are given in Table S1.

Diagnosis of AP was based on the presence of two of the following three clinical symptoms [28]: (1) abdominal pain consistent with acute pancreatitis (acute onset of a persistent, severe, epigastric pain often radiating to the back), (2) serum lipase activity (or amylase activity) at least three times greater than the upper limit of normal, and (3) characteristic findings of AP on abdominal computed tomography, magnetic resonance imaging, or transabdominal ultrasonography or surgical findings consistent with AP.

2.2. DNA Isolation

During the course of treatment, bone marrow and/or blood samples were collected for remission evaluation at defined time points. Morphologically leukemia-cell-free samples with MRD levels of $\leq 10^{-3}$ were selected from these time points and used for DNA isolation using previously described standard techniques [26,27,29]. DNA yielded by this procedure was regarded as a germline DNA surrogate.

2.3. Single-Nucleotide Variant (SNV) Genotyping for Genome-Wide Screening

The GWAS was conducted in 54 childhood ALL patients with AP (cases) and 1435 patients without AP (controls). DNA was genotyped using Human1M-Duo BeadChips (Illumina, San Diego, CA, USA) containing 1,048,711 SNV markers. To avoid false positive data, 44,088 SNVs were excluded due to poor call rate (CR) (<95%) and/or deviation from Hardy–Weinberg equilibrium in the controls ($p > 0.001$). Furthermore, 37 patients (cases/controls) were excluded due to poor genotyping (CR < 95%) and cryptical relationship (IBS-distance > 0.8). Additionally, a multidimensional scaling analysis (MDS) identified 13 patients (cases/controls) with a non-European background. These subjects were also excluded from the study (Figure S1). The quality control finally resulted in a cohort size of 51 cases and 1388 controls.

Two methodological approaches were used to identify candidate SNVs for AP in this GWAS. First, only SNVs with a p-value smaller than 1×10^{-7}, a minimum of one genotyping call in each group of cases and controls, and no restriction of minor allele frequency (MAF) were included. The second approach differed from the first by only including those SNVs with a MAF of more than 0.5%. Minimal evidence of an overall inflation of the test statistics due to population stratification with a moderate genomic inflation factor (approach 1: $\lambda = 1.09$; approach 2: $\lambda = 1.10$) was found (Figure S2).

To confirm the top 20 SNVs from the GWAS, a replication analysis was conducted in an independent patient set of 54 AP cases (selected from both ALL BFM 2000 and AIEOP BFM ALL 2009 study cohorts) and 225 controls (patients with no history of AP from the ALL BFM 2000 cohort). Candidate SNVs were genotyped using the SNVlex multiplex and TaqMan technology (Applied Biosystems, Foster City, CA, USA).

2.4. Gene Sequencing

To fine-map *ATP-binding cassette sub-family C member 4* (*ABCC4*); 281,605 base pairs) and to evaluate the *ABCC4*-related *cystic fibrosis conductance regulator* (*CFTR*); 188,702 base pairs) gene as a candidate for AP predisposition, the two genes were completely sequenced in a cohort of 48 cases and 47 controls selected from the above-described GWAS and replication cohorts depending on the availability of sufficient amounts of non-malignant DNA. Next-generation sequencing (NGS) was conducted on a HiSeq2000 platform (Illumina) using the HaloPlex Illumina 100 kit (Agilent Technologies, Santa Clara, CA, USA) according to the manufacturer's recommendations. The reads were mapped against the human reference genome build hg19 using BWA [30], sorted, converted to bam format, and indexed with SAMtools [31]. Local realignment around InDels and base quality score recalibration were performed with the GATK [32] according to their best practice recommendations, followed by variant calling and variant quality score recalibration. Data were analyzed using the program Integrative Genomic Viewer version 2.3.25 (www.broadinstitute.org/igv/ (accessed on 20 October 2021)) [33,34]. For identification of potential candidate SNVs, regions with a poor sequencing rate (<90%) were excluded. Follow-up SNVs in independent patients from ALL BFM 2000 and AIEOP BFM ALL 2009 with available non-malignant DNA (most of which were part of the initial GWAS and replication cohorts) were analyzed by a

Sanger sequencing using an automated fluorescent sequencer (Applied Biosystems 3730xl DNA Analyzer). All data referring to chromosomal positions were based on GRCh37/hg19 assembly.

2.5. Plotting

Regional association plots were created for the GWAS SNVs using a modified version of deBakker's R script (Figure 1, Figures S3 and S4) by using GWAS SNVs as well as imputed SNVs (if possible). The imputation was done using gPLINK version 2.050 in combination with PLINK v1.07 (www.pngu.mgh.harvard.edu/purcell/plink/ (accessed on 20 October 2021)) [35]. For this purpose, genotypes of autosomal SNVs based on data of 1000 genomes were used. As an input for imputation, only SNVs from the GWAS that passed the above-mentioned quality controls were included.

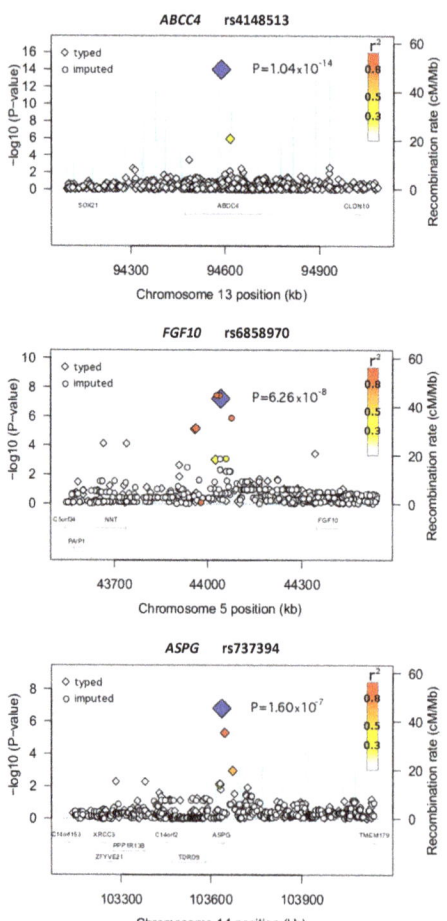

Figure 1. Regional plots of the loci *ABCC4*, *FGF10*, and *ASPG*. Plots of the negative decadic logarithm of the combined *p*-values obtained in the GWAS are shown. The data were imputed with CEU haplotypes generated by the 1000 Genomes Project (August 2010 release) as a reference. A window of ±500 kb around the lead SNVs (blue solid diamonds) is indicated. The magnitude of the linkage disequilibrium with the central SNV measured by r^2 is reflected by the color of each SNV symbol (color coding: see the upper-right corner of the plot). Recombination activity (in centimorgans (cM) per Mb) is depicted by a blue line. Positions are given as NCBI's build coordinates.

2.6. Statistical Analyses

Associations between patient characteristics were evaluated using Fisher's exact or χ^2-tests. The GWAS was assessed using gPLINK. Associations of variations detected by NGS and the replication analyses in the respective cohorts used unconditional logistic regression analysis or Fisher's exact test. Quality control and identity-by-state analysis of the GWAS data was evaluated by gPLINK and R statistics version 2.15.1 (www.r-project.org (accessed on 20 October 2021)). To estimate the European ancestry of the GWAS cohort, the multidimensional scaling analysis was evaluated using R statistics with HapMap CEU, YRI, and JRT/CHB cohorts as reference ancestral populations. Computations were performed using IBM SPSS statistics (IBM Corp., Version 21.0.0, Armonk, NY, USA) and R statistics.

3. Results

3.1. GWAS-Based Identification and Replication of Genomic SNVs Associated with AP

In our GWAS cohort, the incidence of AP was 3.6%, which was in the range of the reported incidence of childhood-ALL-therapy-associated pancreatitis (0.7–18%) [6,7,10]. One previously described clinical risk factor associated with AP development during the treatment of childhood ALL is higher patient age, which was also observed in our analysis (Table 1) [7,11,17,18]. No significant associations of AP with the treatment risk group were detected (Table 1).

Table 1. Clinical characteristics of 1439 patients with ALL from trial AIEOP-BFM ALL 2000 (GWAS cohort) according to the acute pancreatitis (AP) status.

	Patients with AP (n = 51) n (%)	Patients without AP (n = 1388) n (%)	p-Value [d]
Gender			
Male	32 (62.7)	792 (57.1)	
Female	19 (37.3)	596 (42.9)	0.42
Age at diagnosis (years)			
1–6	19 (37.2)	755 (54.4)	
6 to <10	9 (17.6)	248 (17.9)	
≥10	23 (45.1)	385 (27.7)	0.02
Initial WBC [a] (µL)			
<10,000	21 (41.2)	579 (41.7)	
10,000–20,000	11 (21.6)	220 (15.9)	
20,000–50,000	7 (13.7)	242 (17.4)	
≥50,000	12 (23.5)	347 (25.0)	0.70
Immunophenotype			
B	37 (72.5)	1065 (76.7)	
T	14 (27.5)	304 (21.9)	0.56
Other/unknown	0	19 (1.4)	
Treatment risk group			
Standard	13 (25.5)	418 (30.1)	
Intermediate	25 (49.0)	723 (52.1)	
High	13 (25.5)	246 (17.7)	0.37
Unknown	0	1 (0.1)	
ETV6/RUNX1			
Neg	45 (88.2)	1149 (82.8)	
Pos	1 (2.0)	94 (6.8)	0.25
Unknown	5 (9.8)	145 (10.4)	

Table 1. Cont.

	Patients with AP (n = 51) n (%)	Patients without AP (n = 1388) n (%)	p-Value [d]
BCR/ABL			
Neg	50 (98.0)	1304 (93.9)	
Pos	1 (2.0)	24 (1.7)	0.26
Unknown	0	60 (4.3)	
MLL rearrangement			
Neg	46 (90.2)	1213 (87.4)	
Pos	0	4 (0.3)	0.85
Unknown	5 (9.8)	171 (12.3)	
Prednisone response [c]			
Good	43 (84.3)	1201 (86.5)	
Poor	8 (15.7)	174 (12.5)	0.70
Unknown	0	13 (0.9)	
DNA index [b]			
<1.16	24 (47.1)	651 (46.9)	
≥1.16	2 (7.7)	158 (11.4)	0.21
Unknown	25 (49.0)	579 (41.7)	
Timepoint of AP diagnosis [e,f]			
Induction/consolidation (weeks 1–10)	30 (58.8)	–	
CNS-directed therapy (weeks 12–20)	5 (9.8)	–	
Re-induction (weeks 22–28)	16 (31.4)	–	–

[a] WBC, white blood cell count at diagnosis. [b] Ratio of DNA content of leukemic G^0/G^1 cells to normal diploid lymphocytes. [c] Good: <1000 leukemic blood blasts/μL on treatment day 8; poor: ≥1000 μL^{-1}. [d] χ^2—or Fisher's exact test. [e] L-asparaginase application during induction/consolidation and re-induction. [f] Only a few patients (<10%) developed AP after the first dose of L-asp. The majority of cases (>80%) were of severe phenotype [28], and L-asp activity levels were not available for most of them.

As mentioned above, our study used two methodological approaches to detect potential associations for developing AP. In the first approach, six SNVs fulfilled the predefined criteria for significance (Table 1; Figure 1 and Figure S3). An intronic SNV in the *ABCC4* gene (rs4148513) demonstrated the strongest association with AP ($p = 1.04 \times 10^{-14}$; OR = 84.09) (Figure 1; Table 2). Of interest, besides rs4148513, another SNV in *ABCC4* was independently and highly associated with AP in the GWAS (rs4148500; $p = 7.23 \times 10^{-6}$) (Table 2). Other genes with significant associations in the first GWAS approach included *SEMA3D*, *C15orf41*, *COG5*, *ST7*, and *UPF1*.

In the second approach, 13 highly significant SNVs were identified (Table 3; Figure 1 and Figure S4). The SNV with the strongest association (rs6858970) was detected close to the *fibroblast growth factor 10* (*FGF10*) gene ($p = 6.26 \times 10^{-8}$; OR = 8.61) (Figure 1; Table 3). Another highly associated SNV in this approach was rs737394 ($p = 1.59 \times 10^{-7}$; OR = 3.19), an SNV located on an intronic region of the *asparaginase homolog (S. cerevisiae)* (*ASPG*) gene (Figure 1; Table 3)). Other SNVs identified by the second approach were located on or in the vicinity of genes associated with mechanisms and pathways such as cell growth, cell differentiation, and cell death (Table 3).

Table 2. Top SNVs associated with AP identified by genome-wide association analysis and replicated by Sanger sequencing; approach 1.

Chr. Position (bp)	dbSNP ID	Nearby Genes (Relative Position)	A1/A2	Genome-Wide Association Study 1388 Controls 51 Cases			Replication 225 Controls 54 Cases			Combined Analysis GWAS + Replication 1613 Controls 105 Cases		
				AF$_{A1}$ Contr. AF$_{A1}$ Cases	OR (95% CI)	p-Value [a]	AF$_{A1}$ Contr. AF$_{A1}$ Cases	OR (95% CI)	p-Value [a]	AF$_{A1}$ Contr. AF$_{A1}$ Cases	OR (95% CI)	p-Value [a]
13 95790353	rs4148513	ABCC4 (within gene)	A/G	0.0004 0.0294	84.09 (8.67–815.6)	1.04×10^{-14}	0 0	NA	NA	0.0003 0.0144	47.20 (4.89–455.70)	7.31×10^{-9}
7 85465201	rs17160216	SEMA3D (±714 kb)	G/A	0.0007 0.0294	42.03 (6.95–254.4)	8.28×10^{-12}	0.0022 0	NA	NA	0.0009 0.0144	15.72 (3.15–78.38)	6.29×10^{-6}
15 36372995	rs698457	C15orf41 (±499 kb)	G/T	0.0032 0.0490	15.85 (5.21–48.17)	6.75×10^{-11}	0.0022 0.0094	4.26 (0.26–68.62)	0.63	0.0031 0.0289	9.55 (3.44–26.53)	1.27×10^{-7}
7 106850181	rs6963190	COG5 (within gene)	T/C	0.0022 0.0392	18.84 (5.23–67.85)	4.21×10^{-10}	0.0022 0.0094	4.28 (0.26–68.92)	0.27	0.0022 0.0240	11.33 (3.56–36.00)	2.22×10^{-7}
7 116857547	rs7804397	ST7 (within gene)	T/G	0.0011 0.0294	28.01 (5.58–140.50)	7.23×10^{-10}	0 0	NA	NA	0.0009 0.0144	15.72 (3.15–78.38)	6.29×10^{-6}
19 18942559	rs2238652	UPF1 (within gene)	T/C	0.0011 0.0294	28.01 (5.58–140.50)	7.23×10^{-10}	0.0022 0.0093	4.20 (0.26–67.63)	0.26	0.0012 0.0191	15.64 (3.88–62.99)	2.12×10^{-7}
13 95818288	rs4148500	ABCC4 (within gene)	T/C	0.0040 0.0392	10.26 (3.21–32.79)	7.23×10^{-6}	0.0067 0	NA	NA	0.0043 0.0192	4.50 (1.47–13.79)	3.94×10^{-3}

Abbreviations: A1, minor allele; A2, major allele; AF, allele frequency; Chr., chromosome; CI, confidence interval; NA, not analyzed; OR, odds ratio. [a] Allele-based χ^2-test (1 degree of freedom); chromosomal location is based on hg19.

Table 3. Top SNVs associated with AP identified by genome-wide association analysis and replicated by Sanger sequencing; approach 2.

Chr. Position (bp)	dbSNP ID	Nearby Genes (Relative Position)	A1/A2	Genome-Wide Association Study 1388 Controls 51 Cases				Replication 225 Controls 54 Cases				Combined Analysis GWAS + Replication 1613 Controls 105 Cases			
				AF$_{A1}$ Contr. AF$_{A1}$ Cases	OR	(95% CI)	p-Value [a]	AF$_{A1}$ Contr. AF$_{A1}$ Cases	OR	(95% CI)	p-Value [a]	AF$_{A1}$ Contr. AF$_{A1}$ Cases	OR	(95% CI)	p-Value [a]
5 44005497	rs6858970	FGF10 (±300 kb)	T/G	0.0072 0.0588	8.61	(3.38–21.93)	6.26×10^{-8}	0.0111 0.0094	0.85	(0.10–7.33)	0.88	0.0078 0.0337	4.46	(1.90–10.43)	1.64×10^{-4}
1 118847717	rs12402476	SPAG17 (±120 kb)	A/G	0.0072 0.0588	8.61	(3.38–21.92)	6.34×10^{-8}	0.0089 0.0094	1.06	(0.12–9.60)	0.96	0.0074 0.0337	4.64	(1.98–10.91)	1.08×10^{-4}
19 58214147	rs34282745	ZNF154 (within gene)	C/T	0.0382 0.1471	4.34	(2.42–7.77)	7.40×10^{-8}	0.0422 0.0377	0.89	(0.30–2.67)	0.83	0.0388 0.0914	2.49	(1.51–4.13)	2.44×10^{-4}
14 104505922	rs737394	ASPG (within gene)	C/A	0.1013 0.2647	3.19	(2.02–5.04)	1.59×10^{-7}	0.1000 0.0755	0.73	(0.34–1.61)	0.44	0.1011 0.1683	1.80	(1.23–2.63)	2.22×10^{-3}
7 88513041	rs2214632	ZNF804B (within gene)	A/G	0.178 0.3824	2.86	(1.90–4.31)	1.80×10^{-7}	0.1622 0.1226	0.72	(0.38–1.36)	0.31	0.1758 0.2500	1.56	(1.13–2.17)	6.49×10^{-3}
11 130264278	rs7480329	ADAMTS8 (±10.5 kb)	A/G	0.0490 0.1667	3.88	(2.24–6.72)	1.97×10^{-7}	0.0400 0.0189	0.46	(0.11–2.02)	0.29	0.0477 0.0914	2.01	(1.22–3.30)	5.32×10^{-3}
4 170030472	rs17658514	SH3RF1 (within gene)	T/C	0.0328 0.1275	4.31	(2.32–8.00)	4.94×10^{-7}	0.0378 0.0185	0.48	(0.11–2.11)	0.32	0.0335 0.0714	2.22	(1.27–3.88)	4.16×10^{-3}
4 170092033	rs13118066	SH3RF1 (within gene)	C/A	0.0328 0.1275	4.3	(2.32–7.99)	5.02×10^{-7}	0.0378 0.0189	0.49	(0.11–2.15)	0.34	0.0335 0.0721	2.24	(1.28–3.92)	3.72×10^{-3}
9 120052359	rs7026867	ASTN2 (within gene)	C/A	0.0083 0.0588	7.48	(2.98–18.80)	5.19×10^{-7}	0.0044 0	NA		0.49	0.0078 0.0289	3.80	(1.54–9.38)	1.82×10^{-3}
17 46688371	rs16942475	HOXB7 (within gene)	C/T	0.0422 0.1471	3.92	(2.20–6.98)	6.65×10^{-7}	0.0622 0.0463	0.73	(0.28–1.94)	0.53	0.0450 0.0952	2.24	(1.37–3.65)	9.67×10^{-4}

Table 3. Cont.

Chr. Position (bp)	dbSNP ID	Nearby Genes (Relative Position)	A1/A2	Genome-Wide Association Study 1388 Controls 51 Cases			Replication 225 Controls 54 Cases			Combined Analysis GWAS + Replication 1613 Controls 105 Cases		
				AF$_{A1}$ Contr. AF$_{A1}$ Cases	OR (95% CI)	p-Value [a]	AF$_{A1}$ Contr. AF$_{A1}$ Cases	OR (95% CI)	p-Value [a]	AF$_{A1}$ Contr. AF$_{A1}$ Cases	OR (95% CI)	p-Value [a]
4 1720312	rs798752	TMEM129 (within gene)	A/C	0.0177 0.0882	5.36 (2.56–11.24)	6.83×10^{-7}	0.0200 0.0094	0.47 (0.06–3.72)	0.46	0.0181 0.0481	2.75 (1.38–5.46)	2.63×10^{-3}
9 90169981	rs6560001	DAPK1 (within gene)	C/T	0.1445 0.3235	2.83 (1.85–4.35)	6.92×10^{-7}	0.1556 0.1604	1.04 (0.58–1.85)	0.90	0.1460 0.2404	1.85 (1.33–2.58)	2.35×10^{-4}
12 92833965	rs17837141 *	CLLU1 (±9.2 kb)	C/A	0.0144 0.0784	5.82 (2.65–12.77)	7.19×10^{-7}	– –	–	–	– –	–	–

Abbreviations: A1, minor allele; A2, major allele; AF, allele frequency; Chr, chromosome; CI, confidence interval; NA, odds ratio cannot be estimated; OR, odds ratio. [a] Allele-based χ^2-test (1 degree of freedom); * validation analysis of rs17837141 failed; chromosomal location is based on hg19. Replication analysis for the seven SNVs from NGS involved independent patients from ALL-BFM 2000 and AIEOP BFM ALL 2009 ($n = 45$ cases; $n = 45$ controls) with available non-malignant DNA (most of which were part of the initial GWAS and replication cohorts). While for ABCC4, six variants demonstrated a tentative confirmatory behavior in replication analyses, leading to improved significance levels in combined analyses of initial discovery and replication sets, the CFTR SNV did not (Table 4). Five out of six variants localized on ABCC4 had a p-value of 2.4×10^{-2} or less, although one has to acknowledge that four of these variants were highly linked to each other through LD. The most significant variant (rs4773862) had a p-value of 1.3×10^{-2}, with 14 alleles present in the case group and 3 in controls.

Table 4. Top *ABCC4* and *CFTR* SNVs associated with AP identified through next-generation sequencing and replication analysis by Sanger sequencing.

Gene	Variant	A1/A2	Next-Generation Sequencing (Initial)			Sanger (Replication)			Combined Analysis (Initial + Replication)		
			Alleles_controls (A1/A2) Alleles_cases (A1/A2)	OR (95% CI)	p-Value [a]	Alleles_controls (A1/A2) Alleles_cases (A1/A2)	OR (95% CI)	p-Value [a]	Alleles_controls (A1/A2) Alleles_cases (A1/A2)	OR (95% CI)	p-Value [a]
ABCC4	rs34839857	GA/G	(7/81) (21/73)	3.33 (1.34–8.29)	0.01	(8/64) (11/63)	1.40 (0.53–3.70)	0.50	(15/145) (32/136)	2.28 (1.18–4.39)	0.01
ABCC4	rs4773864	T/C	(2/90) (9/87)	4.66 (0.98–22.16)	0.05	(1/78) (4/78)	3.85 (0.42–35.21)	0.23	(3/165) (13/165)	4.33 (1.21–15.49)	0.02
ABCC4	rs4773862	T/C	(2/92) (9/87)	4.76 (1.00–22.64)	0.05	(1/81) (5/75)	5.4 (0.62–47.29)	0.13	(3/173) (14/162)	4.98 (1.41–17.66)	0.01
ABCC4	rs2027444	T/C	(2/92) (9/87)	4.76 (1.00–22.64)	0.05	(1/81) (5/79)	5.13 (0.59–44.87)	0.14	(3/173) (14/166)	4.86 (1.37–17.23)	0.01
ABCC4	rs79230687	G/A	(2/92) (9/87)	4.76 (1.00–22.64)	0.05	(1/81) (5/79)	5.14 (0.59–44.87)	0.14	(3/173) (14/166)	4.86 (1.37–17.23)	0.01
CFTR	rs62469434	A/G	(2/92) (11/85)	5.95 (1.28–27.64)	0.02	(7/75) (4/80)	0.54 (0.15–1.90)	0.34	(9/167) (15/165)	1.69 (0.72–3.96)	0.23
ABCC4	rs2389226	C/A or T	(2/92) (9/87)	4.76 (1.00–22.64)	0.05	(1/79) (5/77)	5.13 (0.59–44.92)	0.14	(3/171) (14/164)	4.87 (1.37–17.2)	0.01
CFTR	rs55831234	G/A	(0/90) (3/91)	NA	0.25 *	(1/87) (2/90)	1.93 (0.17–21.71)	0.59	(1/177) (5/181)	4.89 (0.57–42.27)	0.15

Abbreviations: A1, minor allele; A2, major allele; CI, confidence interval; NA, odds ratio cannot be estimated; OR, odds ratio. [a] Unconditional logistic regression analysis; * Fisher's exact test, as logistic regression analysis cannot be performed.

In total, 20 SNVs were detected by our two GWAS approaches. Six of them were found to be located in intergenic regions, whereas 14 SNVs were discovered directly on a gene (Table 2, Table 3, and Table S2). All of these 20 SNVs were genotyped in additional independent patient samples (54 cases with AP and 225 controls without AP). However, none of the 20 SNVs yielded significant results in replication experiments (Tables 2 and 3). The most significant SNV of the GWAS from the first approach (rs4148513) was neither detected in an additional case nor detected in an additional control individual.

3.2. SNVs from Candidate Gene Studies and GWAS

We investigated all SNVs present on our array platform that were located on or in the vicinity of those genes previously associated with changes in susceptibility to pancreatitis, including *CFTR*, *CTRC*, *PRSS2*, *SPINK1*, *CASR*, and the recently reported variants in AP-associated carboxypeptidase A2-encoding gene *CPA2*, in *unc-51 like autophagy activating kinase 2*-encoding gene *ULK2*, and in *serine protease 1*-encoding gene *PRSS1* [20–22] but could not replicate any of the previously described significant associations (Table S3).

3.3. Fine-Mapping of Potential AP-Associated Variants by Sequencing the ABCC4 and CFTR Genes

Out of the 20 SNVs, the 2 with the highest significance in the GWAS approach were located on the *ABCC4* gene. *ABCC4* is a member of the superfamily of ATP-binding cassette (ABC) transporters, which also includes *CFTR*. Since patients with cystic fibrosis are prone to developing pancreatic problems, including pancreatitis, *CFTR* is a relevant candidate gene for pancreatitis in non-CF patients. The relationship to *ABCC4* as well as the candidate gene status of *CFTR* for AP led us to include both genes, *ABCC4* and *CFTR*, in a targeted NGS-based sequencing approach applied to 48 cases with AP and 47 controls without AP. In total, seven SNVs were significantly associated with AP according to the significance criteria mentioned above (see Section 2; Table 4). All NGS-based SNVs with significant associations were confirmed by Sanger sequencing. Six of the seven variants were located on the *ABCC4* gene and only one on the *CFTR* gene. One of the most significantly associated variants was the insertion rs34839857 ($p = 1.0 \times 10^{-2}$) in *ABCC4*, with 21 alleles present in the case group and 7 in controls. Results by genotype for the seven SNVs are given in Table S4 (Table S5 demonstrates the below-described replication and Table S6 the joint analysis of both cohorts used in fine-mapping analysis). Linkage disequilibrium (LD) analyses are demonstrated in Tables S7 and S8. The top candidate SNV from the GWAS showed no LD with any of the newly NGS identified *ABCC4* SNVs.

4. Discussion

It is assumed that chemotherapeutic drugs (mainly L-asp) are the main trigger for AP in the therapeutic course of childhood ALL [6–11,13,36]. In our analyses, we were able to confirm higher age as a previously published risk factor for developing AP associated with L-asp treatment (Table 1) [7,11,17,18]. In contrast, we did not detect significant associations of AP with the treatment risk group. Several studies have analyzed the effect of risk stratification for ALL treatment as a risk factor for AP with controversial results [36–38]. The observed positive associations are most likely explained by higher doses of L-asp being applied in high-risk patients [36,37]. In comparison to standard- and intermediate-risk patients, our high-risk patients also received higher cumulative doses of L-asp (Table S1). Despite higher frequencies of AP in high-risk patients observed in our study, no significant differences could be detected. This is most likely due to a lack of power in our relatively small sample set.

In addition to demographic or clinical risk factors, there is evidence of genetic factors contributing to the pathophysiology of AP as a severe treatment complication. In our first GWAS approach with no restrictions on MAF, the strongest association was observed for an SNV located on the *ABCC4* gene. *ABCC4* belongs to the ABC transporter superfamily, which mediates the efflux of drugs and plays an important role in the development of drug resistance. *ABCC4* itself is known to mediate the transport of different chemotherapeutic drugs out of the cell (e.g., 6-mercaptopurine and methotrexate) [39–42]. Therefore, variability in *ABCC4* activity may affect pharmacokinetics of *ABCC4* transport substrates and consequently modulate drug effects. Of importance in the context of our findings, *ABCC4* is highly expressed in the pancreas [39,43]. In addition, in a recent study using a rat model to study AP, Ventimiglia and colleagues described a protective role of atrial natriuretic factor (ANF) mediated by cAMP extrusion through *ABCC4* and suggested that the regulation of *ABCC4* by ANF could be relevant to maintaining pancreatic acinar cell homeostasis [44].

The top-ranked SNV in our second GWAS approach, which included SNVs with a MAF of more than 0.5%, was located in the vicinity of *FGF10*, a gene belonging to the fibroblast growth factor family. Members of this group take part in the regulation of cell growth and cell differentiation. In addition, the *FGF*-family is suspected to be involved in pancreatic diseases such as pancreatic cancer, chronic pancreatitis, and acute pancreatitis [45–47]. The *FGF10* gene itself is required for the normal development of the pancreas [47,48]. In a publication of Ishiwata et al., the authors proposed that *FGF10* together with *FGF7* may contribute to the regeneration and differentiation of acinar cells and the angiogenesis of AP [49]. However, despite *FGF10* being a plausible candidate for a role in the pathophysiology of AP, our replication analysis did not support the initial findings.

As mentioned above, one of the most serious adverse events of L-asp treatment is AP. L-asp catalyzes the hydrolysis of asparagine into aspartate and ammonia. The human genome encodes at least three enzymes that can catalyze this reaction, *asparaginase homolog (S. cerevisiae) (ASPG)*, *aspartylglucosaminidase (AGA)*, and *asparaginase like 1 (ASRGL1)* [50]. Of interest, one SNV selected for further follow-up after our initial GWAS screen was located on the gene *ASPG*. This little studied gene has sequence similarity at the N-terminal domain with the *E. coli* types I and II asparaginase [51,52]. It has also been shown that HEK293 cells exhibit asparaginase activity when they are transfected with the cDNA of *ASPG* [53]. Although purely hypothetical, this initial finding, which did not hold in replication analysis, may justify some follow-up investigations of *ASPG* activity in the context of AP development.

We investigated all SNVs present on the GWAS SNV array that were located on or in the vicinity of the genes known to be associated with changes in susceptibility to pancreatitis, including *CFTR*, *CTRC*, *PRSS2*, *SPINK1*, and *CASR*, but did not find any significant association. Therefore, these previously described candidate genes for chronic pancreatitis may not play distinct roles in AP. However, we also failed to detect any association with *CPA2*, *ULK2*, and *PSSR1*, three recently reported AP-associated genes [20–22] (Table S3). Regarding this, our analyses may have been hampered by suboptimal SNV coverage of these candidates on our array (e.g., *CFTR*: 140 SNVs in or ±50 kb up and downstream of the gene) and the fact that hardly any of the few well-known SNVs previously associated with pancreatitis, including the top *CPA2* SNV, were actually present on our platform. LD information on this *CPA2* variant (rs199695765) could not be obtained, probably due to its rareness, so there can be no conclusions drawn from *CPA2* variants present on O1MQR. However, one of the recently published *PRSS1* variants was genotyped, showing no association to the AP phenotype (as shown in Table S3). The other published variant is not present on O1MQR but in perfect LD with the first one. The previously published *ULK2* variant rs281366 was also not genotyped on O1MQR but Table S3 lists several SNVs, for example rs205111, rs9895806, and rs9914674, that are highly linked to the published variant. In summary, our GWAS setting could not replicate the associations of rare or common SNVs to the phenotype of AP that was identified in previously published GWA studies.

Replication of the 20 top candidate SNVs from our GWAS was, unfortunately, not successful. The reasons are manifold, including the fact that our GWAS included rare variants with a low MAF. GWAS analyses often begin by discarding all genotypes for SNVs with a MAF of less than 10%, which results in an enormous loss of data. Low-MAF SNVs are associated with technical and statistical problems, such as lower genotyping rates and inflated false-positive results [53]. The decision to include rare alleles in our analyses was based on the hypothesis that AP is a rare clinical phenotype and may be associated with rare SNVs. From a methodological perspective on GWAS analyses, our practical approach is supported by investigations demonstrating nominally significant results occurring significantly less often than expected for low-MAF SNVs, resulting in a conservative bias [54,55]. However, despite positive arguments to include SNVs of low MAF, our replication cohorts may have been virtually too small to reliably detect enough cases carrying rare variants. For example, the highest-ranked SNV in our GWAS (rs4148513) occurred in three cases and one control only and was not detected in a single individual of the entire validation cohort. Nevertheless, combined data from our GWAS and the validation cohorts still demonstrated strong associations of initially identified candidate variations with AP, supporting the assumption that the initially detected SNVs might truly play a role in the development of AP.

Lending additional support to our findings from initial experiments, we conducted fine-mapping of *ABCC4* by sequencing the entire gene. *ABCC4* was chosen because of our GWAS findings and its simultaneous candidate status based on biological function (see above). As a second candidate gene for pancreatitis, *CFTR* was chosen for sequencing [56–58]. *CFTR* also belongs to the ABC transporter superfamily and plays a role in water and salt transport at the plasma membrane of epithelial cells. Mutations in *CFTR* lead to cystic fibrosis (CF) commonly affecting the lungs, liver, intestine, and pancreas [59]. Moreover, variants within *CFTR* associated with pancreatitis were found in patients without additional symptoms of CF [19,60]. *CFTR* as a genetic risk factor for AP and chronic pancreatitis was linked with trypsin activation and survival in pancreatitis patients [60,61]. Of particular interest, in replication analysis of seven candidate SNVs in *ABCC4* and *CFTR* detected through NGS, all six *ABCC4* variants demonstrated similar effects regarding point estimates while the *CFTR* SNV did not. Its consistent behavior in our different analytical approaches, including genotype analysis, implies that *ABCC4* might truly be associated with AP.

To conclude, for the first time, we were able to associate germline genetic variation in *ABCC4* with the risk of AP during treatment for childhood ALL. Our results demonstrate that *ABCC4* was consistently related to AP in GWAS as well as in fine-mapping analyses by NGS, supporting a true role of *ABCC4* in the development of AP. However, our study on a rare phenotype in a rare disease also clearly demonstrates that international joint efforts are needed to more reliably assess genetic risk factors for AP and other rare toxicities observed in childhood ALL by using larger pooled patient cohorts.

Supplementary Materials: The following are available online at https://www.mdpi.com/article/10.3390/jcm10214815/s1: Table S1. Treatment details of protocol AIEOP-BFM ALL 2000. Table S2. Additional information on top AP-associated SNV from GWAS and fine-mapping (NGS) analyses. Table S3. SNV within the *CPA2, PRSS1 and ULK2* genes previously identified by GWAS analyses and their association with AP in our cohort. Table S4. Genotype frequencies and association with risk of AP for SNV derived from fine-mapping by NGS analyses in the initial cohort. Table S5. Genotype frequencies and association with risk of AP for SNV derived from fine-mapping by NGS analyses in the replication cohort. Table S6: Genotype frequencies and association with risk of AP for SNV derived from fine-mapping by NGS analyses in the combined cohort (initial and replication). Table S7. Linkage disequilibrium of top *ABCC4* SNV from GWAS and fine-mapping analyses. Table S8. Linkage disequilibrium of *CFTR* SNV. Figure S1. Identification of individuals in the GWA scan of non-European ancestry. Figure S2. Quantile-quantile (Q-Q) plots showing observed vs. expected distribution of *p*-values for association of the GWAS-SNVs with Acute Pancreatitis (AP). Figure S3. Regional plots of the loci of the SNVs identified within the first approach of the GWAS of AP patients and controls (with the exception of the SNV located on the gene *ABCC4*, which is represented in Figure 1 in the article). Figure S4. Regional plots of the loci of the SNVs identified within the second approach of the GWAS of AP patients and controls (with the exception of the SNVs located on the genes *FGF10* and *ASPG*, which are represented in Figure 1 in the article).

Author Contributions: C.R.B.: Data provision and the final approval of the manuscript. T.B.: Collection and assembly of data, data analysis and interpretation, laboratory analyses, manuscript writing, and the final approval of the manuscript. A.B.: Collection and assembly of data and the final approval of the manuscript. G.C.: Collection and assembly of data and the final approval of the manuscript. E.E.: Data analysis and interpretation and the final approval of the manuscript. M.F.: Data analysis and interpretation and the final approval of the manuscript. A.F.: Data interpretation and the final approval of the manuscript. L.H.: Data analysis and the final approval of the manuscript. R.S.H.: Data analysis and interpretation and the final approval of the manuscript. S.V.J.: Data analysis and the final approval of the manuscript. N.K.: Collection and assembly of data and the final approval of the manuscript. R.K.: Collection and assembly of data and the final approval of the manuscript. C.P.K.: Data interpretation and the final approval of the manuscript. A.M.: Collection and assembly of data and the final approval of the manuscript. B.-S.L.: Laboratory analysis, data interpretation, and the final approval of the manuscript. M.S.(Martin Schrappe): Collection and assembly of data and the final approval of the manuscript. P.S.: Data analysis, manuscript writing, and the final approval of the manuscript. M.S.(Martin Stanulla): Conception and design of study, collection, assembly and interpretation of data, supervision of research, manuscript writing, and the final approval of the manuscript. M.Z.: Data analysis, data interpretation, and the final approval of the manuscript. All authors have read and agreed to the published version of the manuscript.

Funding: The project was funded by Madeleine Schickedanz-Kinderkrebsstiftung, Deutsche José Carreras Leukämie-Stiftung (DJCLS R 15/04), TRANSCALL2, ERA-NET TRANSCAN/European Commission under the 7th Framework Programme (FP7), and Verein für krebskranke Kinder Hannover e.V.

Institutional Review Board Statement: The study was approved by the Institutional Review Boards of Hannover Medical School, Hannover (Nr. 2522), and the Medical Faculty of the Christian Albrechts University, Kiel, Germany (A 177/09), and conducted according to the guidelines of the Declaration of Helsinki.

Informed Consent Statement: Informed consent was obtained from the legal representatives of all subjects involved in the study.

Data Availability Statement: Datasets of the current study are not publicly available but are available from the corresponding author on reasonable request.

Acknowledgments: We thank all participating patients, their families, and all personnel involved in AIEOP-BFM ALL-BFM 2000.

Conflicts of Interest: The authors declare no conflict of interest.

References

1. Pui, C.H.; Evans, W.E. Treatment of acute lymphoblastic leukemia. *N. Engl. J. Med.* **2006**, *354*, 166–178. [CrossRef]
2. Redaelli, A.; Laskin, B.L.; Stephens, J.M.; Botteman, M.F.; Pashos, C.L. A systematic literature review of the clinical and epidemiological burden of acute lymphoblastic leukaemia (ALL). *Eur. J. Cancer Care* **2005**, *14*, 53–62. [CrossRef]
3. Pui, C.H.; Robison, L.L.; Look, A.T. Acute lymphoblastic leukaemia. *Lancet* **2008**, *371*, 1030–1043. [CrossRef]
4. Stanulla, M.; Schrappe, M. Treatment of childhood acute lymphoblastic leukemia. *Semin. Hematol.* **2009**, *46*, 52–63. [CrossRef]
5. Vagace, J.M.; Gervasini, G. Chemotherapy toxicity in patients with acute leukemia. In *Acute Leukemia—The Scientists Perspective and Challenge*; Antica, M., Ed.; InTechOpen: Rijeka, Croatia, 2011; pp. 391–414.
6. Alvarez, O.A.; Zimmerman, G. Pegaspargase-induced pancreatitis. *Med. Pediatr. Oncol.* **2000**, *34*, 200–205. [CrossRef]
7. Knoderer, H.M.; Robarge, J.; Flockhart, D.A. Predicting asparaginase-associated pancreatitis. *Pediatr. Blood Cancer* **2007**, *49*, 634–639. [CrossRef] [PubMed]
8. Laugel, V.; Escande, B.; Entz-Werle, N.; Mazingue, F.; Ferster, A.; Bertrand, Y.; Missud, F.; Lutz, P. [Severe acute pancreatitis in children receiving asparaginase: Multicenter retrospective study]. *Arch. Pediatr.* **2005**, *12*, 34–41. [CrossRef] [PubMed]
9. Sadoff, J.; Hwang, S.; Rosenfeld, D.; Ettinger, L.; Spigland, N. Surgical pancreatic complications induced by L-asparaginase. *J. Pediatr. Surg.* **1997**, *32*, 860–863. [CrossRef]
10. Sahu, S.; Saika, S.; Pai, S.K.; Advani, S.H. L-asparaginase (Leunase) induced pancreatitis in childhood acute lymphoblastic leukemia. *Pediatr. Hematol. Oncol.* **1998**, *15*, 533–538. [CrossRef]
11. Raja, R.A.; Schmiegelow, K.; Frandsen, T.L. Asparaginase-associated pancreatitis in children. *Br. J. Haematol.* **2012**, *159*, 18–27. [CrossRef]
12. Altman, A.J.; Dinndorf, P.; Quinn, J.J. Acute pancreatitis in association with cytosine arabinoside therapy. *Cancer* **1982**, *49*, 1384–1386. [CrossRef]
13. Halalsheh, H.; Bazzeh, F.; Alkayed, K.; Salami, K.; Madanat, F. 6-Mercaptopurine-induced recurrent acute pancreatitis in children with acute lymphoblastic leukemia/lymphoma. *J. Pediatr. Hematol. Oncol.* **2013**, *35*, 470–472. [CrossRef]

14. Riemenschneider, T.A.; Wilson, J.F.; Vernier, R.L. Glucocorticoid-induced pancreatitis in children. *Pediatrics* **1968**, *41*, 428–437.
15. Varma, M.R.; Mathew, S.; Krishnadas, D.; Vinayakumar, K.R. Imatinib-induced pancreatitis. *Indian J. Pharmacol.* **2010**, *42*, 50–52. [CrossRef]
16. Whitcomb, D.C. Genetic aspects of pancreatitis. *Annu. Rev. Med.* **2010**, *61*, 413–424. [CrossRef]
17. Kearney, S.L.; Dahlberg, S.E.; Levy, D.E.; Voss, S.D.; Sallan, S.E.; Silverman, L.B. Clinical course and outcome in children with acute lymphoblastic leukemia and asparaginase-associated pancreatitis. *Pediatr. Blood Cancer* **2009**, *53*, 162–167. [CrossRef] [PubMed]
18. Rank, C.U.; Wolthers, B.O.; Grell, K.; Albertsen, B.K.; Frandsen, T.L.; Overgaard, U.M.; Toft, N.; Nielsen, O.J.; Wehner, P.S.; Harila-Saari, A.; et al. Asparaginase-Associated Pancreatitis in Acute Lymphoblastic Leukemia: Results From the NOPHO ALL2008 Treatment of Patients 1–45 Years of Age. *J. Clin. Oncol.* **2020**, *38*, 145–154. [CrossRef]
19. Ooi, C.Y.; Gonska, T.; Durie, P.R.; Freedman, S.D. Genetic testing in pancreatitis. *Gastroenterology* **2010**, *138*, 2202–2206. [CrossRef] [PubMed]
20. Liu, C.; Yang, W.; Devidas, M.; Cheng, C.; Pei, D.; Smith, C.; Carroll, W.L.; Raetz, E.A.; Bowman, W.P.; Larsen, E.C.; et al. Clinical and Genetic Risk Factors for Acute Pancreatitis in Patients With Acute Lymphoblastic Leukemia. *J. Clin. Oncol.* **2016**, *34*, 2133–2140. [CrossRef] [PubMed]
21. Wolthers, B.O.; Frandsen, T.L.; Abrahamsson, J.; Albertsen, B.K.; Helt, L.R.; Heyman, M.; Jónsson, Ó.G.; Kõrgvee, L.T.; Lund, B.; Raja, R.A.; et al. Asparaginase-associated pancreatitis: A study on phenotype and genotype in the NOPHO ALL2008 protocol. *Leukemia* **2017**, *31*, 325–332. [CrossRef]
22. Wolthers, B.O.; Frandsen, T.L.; Patel, C.J.; Abaji, R.; Attarbaschi, A.; Barzilai, S.; Colombini, A.; Escherich, G.; Grosjean, M.; Krajinovic, M.; et al. Trypsin-encoding *PRSS1-PRSS2* variations influence the risk of asparaginase-associated pancreatitis in children with acute lymphoblastic leukemia: A Ponte di Legno toxicity working group report. *Haematologica* **2019**, *104*, 556–563. [CrossRef] [PubMed]
23. Conter, V.; Bartram, C.R.; Valsecchi, M.G.; Schrauder, A.; Panzer-Grümayer, R.; Möricke, A.; Aricò, M.; Zimmermann, M.; Mann, G.; De Rossi, G.; et al. Molecular response to treatment redefines all prognostic factors in children and adolescents with B-cell precursor acute lymphoblastic leukemia: Results in 3184 patients of the AIEOP-BFM ALL 2000 study. *Blood* **2010**, *115*, 3206–3214. [CrossRef] [PubMed]
24. Schrappe, M.; Valsecchi, M.G.; Bartram, C.R.; Schrauder, A.; Panzer-Grümayer, R.; Möricke, A.; Parasole, R.; Zimmermann, M.; Dworzak, M.; Buldini, B.; et al. Late MRD response determines relapse risk overall and in subsets of childhood T-cell ALL: Results of the AIEOP-BFM-ALL 2000 study. *Blood* **2011**, *118*, 2077–2084. [CrossRef] [PubMed]
25. Stanulla, M.; Dagdan, E.; Zaliova, M.; Möricke, A.; Palmi, C.; Cazzaniga, G.; Eckert, C.; Te Kronnie, G.; Bourquin, J.P.; Bornhauser, B.; et al. IKZF1(plus) Defines a New Minimal Residual Disease-Dependent Very-Poor Prognostic Profile in Pediatric B-Cell Precursor Acute Lymphoblastic Leukemia. *J. Clin. Oncol.* **2018**, *36*, 1240–1249. [CrossRef]
26. Stanulla, M.; Schaeffeler, E.; Möricke, A.; Buchmann, S.; Zimmermann, M.; Igel, S.; Schmiegelow, K.; Flotho, C.; Hartmann, H.; Illsinger, S.; et al. Hepatic sinusoidal obstruction syndrome and short-term application of 6-thioguanine in pediatric acute lymphoblastic leukemia. *Leukemia* **2021**, *35*, 2650–2657. [CrossRef]
27. Meissner, B.; Bartram, T.; Eckert, C.; Trka, J.; Panzer-Grümayer, R.; Hermanova, I.; Ellinghaus, E.; Franke, A.; Möricke, A.; Schrauder, A.; et al. Frequent and sex-biased deletion of SLX4IP by illegitimate V(D)J-mediated recombination in childhood acute lymphoblastic leukemia. *Hum. Mol. Genet.* **2014**, *23*, 590–601. [CrossRef]
28. Banks, P.A.; Bollen, T.L.; Dervenis, C.; Gooszen, H.G.; Johnson, C.D.; Sarr, M.G.; Tsiotos, G.G.; Vege, S.S. Acute Pancreatitis Classification Working Group. Classification of acute pancreatitis—2012: Revision of the Atlanta classification and definitions by international consensus. *Gut* **2013**, *62*, 102–111. [CrossRef]
29. Ellinghaus, E.; Stanulla, M.; Richter, G.; Ellinghaus, D.; te Kronnie, G.; Cario, G.; Cazzaniga, G.; Horstmann, M.; Panzer Grümayer, R.; Cavé, H.; et al. Identification of germline susceptibility loci in ETV6-RUNX1-rearranged childhood acute lymphoblastic leukemia. *Leukemia* **2012**, *26*, 902–909. [CrossRef]
30. Li, H.; Durbin, R. Fast and accurate short read alignment with Burrows-Wheeler transform. *Bioinformatics* **2009**, *25*, 1754–1760. [CrossRef]
31. Li, H.; Handsaker, B.; Wysoker, A.; Fennell, T.; Ruan, J.; Homer, N.; Marth, G.; Abecasis, G.; Durbin, R. 1000 Genome Project Data Processing Subgroup. The Sequence Alignment/Map format and SAMtools. *Bioinformatics* **2009**, *25*, 2078–2079. [CrossRef]
32. McKenna, A.; Hanna, M.; Banks, E.; Sivachenko, A.; Cibulskis, K.; Kernytsky, A.; Garimella, K.; Altshuler, D.; Gabriel, S.; Daly, M. The Genome Analysis Toolkit: A MapReduce framework for analyzing next-generation DNA sequencing data. *Genome Res.* **2010**, *20*, 1297–1303. [CrossRef] [PubMed]
33. Robinson, J.T.; Thorvaldsdóttir, H.; Winckler, W.; Guttman, M.; Lander, E.S.; Getz, G.; Mesirov, J.P. Integrative genomics viewer. *Nat. Biotechnol.* **2011**, *29*, 24–26. [CrossRef] [PubMed]
34. Thorvaldsdóttir, H.; Robinson, J.T.; Mesirov, J.P. Integrative Genomics Viewer (IGV): High-performance genomics data visualization and exploration. *Brief Bioinform.* **2013**, *14*, 178–192. [CrossRef] [PubMed]
35. Purcell, S.; Neale, B.; Todd-Brown, K.; Thomas, L.; Ferreira, M.A.; Bender, D.; Maller, J.; Sklar, P.; de Bakker, P.I.; Daly, M.J. PLINK: A tool set for whole-genome association and population-based linkage analyses. *Am. J. Hum. Genet.* **2007**, *81*, 559–575. [CrossRef] [PubMed]

36. Treepongkaruna, S.; Thongpak, N.; Pakakasama, S.; Pienvichit, P.; Sirachainan, N.; Hongeng, S. Acute pancreatitis in children with acute lymphoblastic leukemia after chemotherapy. *J. Pediatr. Hematol. Oncol.* **2009**, *31*, 812–815. [CrossRef] [PubMed]
37. Samarasinghe, S.; Dhir, S.; Slack, J.; Iyer, P.; Wade, R.; Clack, R.; Vora, A.; Goulden, N. Incidence and outcome of pancreatitis in children and young adults with acute lymphoblastic leukaemia treated on a contemporary protocol, UKALL 2003. *Br. J. Haematol.* **2013**, *162*, 710–713. [CrossRef]
38. Raja, R.A.; Schmiegelow, K.; Albertsen, B.K.; Prunsild, K.; Zeller, B.; Vaitkeviciene, G.; Abrahamsson, J.; Heyman, M.; Taskinen, M.; Harila-Saari, A. Asparaginase-associated pancreatitis in children with acute lymphoblastic leukaemia in the NOPHO ALL2008 protocol. *Br. J. Haematol.* **2014**, *165*, 126–133. [CrossRef]
39. Borst, P.; de Wolf, C.; van de Wetering, K. Multidrug resistance-associated proteins 3, 4, and 5. *Pflugers Arch.* **2007**, *453*, 661–673. [CrossRef] [PubMed]
40. Chen, Z.S.; Lee, K.; Walther, S.; Raftogianis, R.B.; Kuwano, M.; Zeng, H.; Kruh, G.D. Analysis of methotrexate and folate transport by multidrug resistance protein 4 (ABCC4): MRP4 is a component of the methotrexate efflux system. *Cancer Res.* **2002**, *62*, 3144–3150. [PubMed]
41. Janke, D.; Mehralivand, S.; Strand, D.; Gödtel-Armbrust, U.; Habermeier, A.; Gradhand, U.; Fischer, C.; Toliat, M.R.; Fritz, P.; Zanger, U.M. 6-mercaptopurine and 9-(2-phosphonyl-methoxyethyl) adenine (PMEA) transport altered by two missense mutations in the drug transporter gene ABCC4. *Hum. Mutat.* **2008**, *29*, 659–669. [CrossRef]
42. Russel, F.G.; Koenderink, J.B.; Masereeuw, R. Multidrug resistance protein 4 (MRP4/ABCC4): A versatile efflux transporter for drugs and signalling molecules. *Trends Pharmacol. Sci.* **2008**, *29*, 200–207. [CrossRef]
43. König, J.; Hartel, M.; Nies, A.T.; Martignoni, M.E.; Guo, J.; Büchler, M.W.; Friess, H.; Keppler, D. Expression and localization of human multidrug resistance protein (ABCC) family members in pancreatic carcinoma. *Int. J. Cancer* **2005**, *115*, 359–367. [CrossRef] [PubMed]
44. Ventimiglia, M.S.; Najenson, A.C.; Perazzo, J.C.; Carozzo, A.; Vatta, M.S.; Davio, C.A.; Bianciotti, L.G. Blockade of Multidrug Resistance-Associated Proteins Aggravates Acute Pancreatitis and Blunts Atrial Natriuretic Factor's Beneficial Effect in Rats: Role of MRP4 (ABCC4). *Mol. Med.* **2015**, *21*, 58–67. [CrossRef] [PubMed]
45. Ebert, M.; Yokoyama, M.; Ishiwata, T.; Friess, H.; Büchler, M.W.; Malfertheiner, P.; Korc, M. Alteration of fibroblast growth factor and receptor expression after acute pancreatitis in humans. *Pancreas* **1999**, *18*, 240–246. [CrossRef] [PubMed]
46. Kornmann, M.; Beger, H.G.; Korc, M. Role of fibroblast growth factors and their receptors in pancreatic cancer and chronic pancreatitis. *Pancreas* **1998**, *17*, 169–175. [CrossRef]
47. Nandy, D.; Mukhopadhyay, D. Growth factor mediated signaling in pancreatic pathogenesis. *Cancers* **2011**, *3*, 841–871. [CrossRef]
48. Bhushan, A.; Itoh, N.; Kato, S.; Thiery, J.P.; Czernichow, P.; Bellusci, S.; Scharfmann, R. Fgf10 is essential for maintaining the proliferative capacity of epithelial progenitor cells during early pancreatic organogenesis. *Development* **2001**, *128*, 5109–5117. [CrossRef] [PubMed]
49. Ishiwata, T.; Naito, Z.; Lu, Y.P.; Kawahara, K.; Fujii, T.; Kawamoto, Y.; Teduka, K.; Sugisaki, Y. Differential distribution of fibroblast growth factor (FGF)-7 and FGF-10 in L-arginine-induced acute pancreatitis. *Exp. Mol. Pathol.* **2002**, *73*, 181–190. [CrossRef] [PubMed]
50. Nomme, J.; Su, Y.; Konrad, M.; Lavie, A. Structures of apo and product-bound human L-asparaginase: Insights into the mechanism of autoproteolysis and substrate hydrolysis. *Biochemistry* **2012**, *51*, 6816–6826. [CrossRef]
51. Menniti, M.; Iuliano, R.; Föller, M.; Sopjani, M.; Alesutan, I.; Mariggiò, S.; Nofziger, C.; Perri, A.M.; Amato, R.; Blazer-Yost, B. 60kDa lysophospholipase, a new Sgk1 molecular partner involved in the regulation of ENaC. *Cell Physiol. Biochem.* **2010**, *26*, 587–596. [CrossRef]
52. Sugimoto, H.; Odani, S.; Yamashita, S. Cloning and expression of cDNA encoding rat liver 60-kDa lysophospholipase containing an asparaginase-like region and ankyrin repeat. *J. Biol. Chem.* **1998**, *273*, 12536–12542. [CrossRef] [PubMed]
53. Lam, A.C.; Schouten, M.; Aulchenko, Y.S.; Haley, C.S.; de Koning, D.J. Rapid and robust association mapping of expression quantitative trait loci. *BMC Proc.* **2007**, *1* (Suppl. 1), S144. [CrossRef] [PubMed]
54. Gorlov, I.P.; Gorlova, O.Y.; Sunyaev, S.R.; Spitz, M.R.; Amos, C.I. Shifting paradigm of association studies: Value of rare single-nucleotide polymorphisms. *Am. J. Hum. Genet.* **2008**, *82*, 100–112. [CrossRef]
55. Tabangin, M.E.; Woo, J.G.; Martin, L.J. The effect of minor allele frequency on the likelihood of obtaining false positives. *BMC Proc.* **2009**, *3* (Suppl. 7), S41. [CrossRef]
56. Cohn, J.A.; Friedman, K.J.; Noone, P.G.; Knowles, M.R.; Silverman, L.M.; Jowell, P.S. Relation between mutations of the cystic fibrosis gene and idiopathic pancreatitis. *N. Engl. J. Med.* **1998**, *339*, 653–658. [CrossRef] [PubMed]
57. Whitcomb, D.C.; Ermentrout, G.B. A mathematical model of the pancreatic duct cell generating high bicarbonate concentrations in pancreatic juice. *Pancreas* **2004**, *29*, e30–e40. [CrossRef]
58. Hegyi, P.; Maléth, J.; Venglovecz, V.; Rakonczay, Z., Jr. Pancreatic ductal bicarbonate secretion: Challenge of the acinar Acid load. *Front. Physiol.* **2011**, *2*, 36. [CrossRef]
59. Riordan, J.R.; Rommens, J.M.; Kerem, B.; Alon, N.; Rozmahel, R.; Grzelczak, Z.; Zielenski, J.; Lok, S.; Plavsic, N.; Chou, J.L.; et al. Identification of the cystic fibrosis gene: Cloning and characterization of complementary DNA. *Science* **1989**, *245*, 1066–1073. [CrossRef] [PubMed]

60. Schneider, A.; Larusch, J.; Sun, X.; Aloe, A.; Lamb, J.; Hawes, R.; Cotton, P.; Brand, R.E.; Anderson, M.A.; Money, M.E. Combined bicarbonate conductance-impairing variants in CFTR and SPINK1 variants are associated with chronic pancreatitis in patients without cystic fibrosis. *Gastroenterology* **2011**, *140*, 162–171. [CrossRef]
61. Mounzer, R.; Whitcomb, D.C. Genetics of acute and chronic pancreatitis. *Curr. Opin. Gastroenterol.* **2013**, *29*, 544–551. [CrossRef] [PubMed]

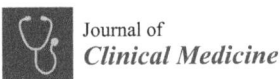

Journal of Clinical Medicine

Review

Blinatumomab in Pediatric Acute Lymphoblastic Leukemia—From Salvage to First Line Therapy (A Systematic Review)

Manon Queudeville * and Martin Ebinger

Department I–General Pediatrics, Hematology/Oncology, Children's Hospital, University Hospital Tübingen, 72076 Tübingen, Germany; martin.ebinger@med.uni-tuebingen.de
* Correspondence: manon.queudeville@med.uni-tuebingen.de

Abstract: Acute lymphoblastic leukemia is by far the most common malignancy in children, and new immunotherapeutic approaches will clearly change the way we treat our patients in future years. Blinatumomab is a bispecific T-cell-engaging antibody indicated for the treatment of relapsed/refractory acute lymphoblastic leukemia (R/R-ALL). The use of blinatumomab in R/R ALL has shown promising effects, especially as a bridging tool to hematopoietic stem cell transplantation. For heavily pretreated patients, the response to one or two cycles of blinatumomab ranges from 34% to 66%. Two randomized controlled trials have very recently demonstrated an improved reduction in minimal residual disease as well as an increased survival for patients treated with blinatumomab compared to standard consolidation treatment in first relapse. Current trials using blinatumomab frontline for high-risk patients or as a consolidation treatment post-transplant will show whether efficacy is even higher in less heavily pretreated patients. Due to the distinct pattern of adverse events compared to high-dose conventional chemotherapy, blinatumomab could play an important role for patients with a risk for severe chemotherapy-associated toxicities. This systematic review discusses all published results for blinatumomab in children as well as all ongoing clinical trials.

Keywords: acute lymphoblastic leukemia; immunotherapy; bispecific T-cell engager (BiTE)

1. Introduction

Blinatumomab is a bispecific T-cell engaging (BiTE) antibody linking the targeting regions of two antibodies directed against CD19 and CD3. CD19 is expressed by the precursor-B-ALL cells, and CD3 is the constant part of the T-cell receptor (TCR) complex that mediates T-cell receptor signaling. Blinatumomab, therefore, leads to a very close linkage between malignant B cells and T cells, a cytolytic synapse forming in the close contact zone [1]. Multiple, bivalent binding leads to a strong stimulus of the engaged T cell which is independent of the TCR specificity and of MHC class I antigen presentation or other costimulatory factors [2,3]. The strong activation of engaged T cells leads to direct and serial lysis. Furthermore, blinatumomab induces the polyclonal proliferation of activated T cells, which leads to an increased activity of blinatumomab 1 to 2 days after the onset of application [3].

The US Food and Drug Administration (FDA) approved blinatumomab for the treatment of adults and children with B-cell precursor acute lymphoblastic leukemia in first or second complete remission with minimal residual disease (MRD) greater than or equal to 0.1% as well as for relapsed or refractory ALL. The indication according to the European Medicines Agency (EMA) limits the use of blinatumomab to pediatric patients aged one year or older with Philadelphia chromosome negative CD19 positive B-precursor ALL, which is refractory or in relapse after receiving at least two prior therapies or in relapse after receiving prior allogeneic hematopoietic stem cell transplantation (HSCT).

There is still considerable paucity of pediatric data for the use of blinatumomab, and the results of a preponderance of adult trials as well as numerous adult reviews cannot simply be transferred to the pediatric setting. It is widely accepted that pediatric and adult ALL are biologically different with distinct underlying genetic alterations [4,5]. The relapse rate and prognosis are markedly worse in adults [6–8] and co-morbidities in adult patients might lead to a different profile of adverse events. Moreover, due to the maturation and expansion of the immune system during the first years of life, lymphocyte subpopulations vary during childhood and differ from adult numbers in relative and absolute size [9], which could affect the activity of blinatumomab.

Rationale for the review: Only four reviews have been published on the use of blinatumomab in the pediatric population [10–13]. The first three reviews were published several years ago; the very recent review by Shukla and Sulis focuses on high-risk relapsed B-ALL with an excellent summary on the evolvement of treatment in high-risk relapsed ALL. The authors particularly discuss both randomized controlled trials published in the same issue of the *Journal of the American Medical Association* (*JAMA*).

Other pediatric reviews focus on immunotherapy in general [14–16], only one of which is less than a year old [17] and a great number of reviews combine adult and pediatric data.

Objective: To provide a comprehensive overview of all published data concerning the use of blinatumomab in children and to summarize all current clinical trials open to pediatric patients.

2. Materials and Methods

A PubMed literature search using the terms "blinatumomab and pediatric or children" was performed. The search yielded 127 results by mid-March 2021. In addition, the database ClinicalTrials.gov and EU Clinical Trials Register were searched using blinatumomab and leukemia with "child" as eligibility criteria. The search revealed 25 clinical trials. Four of the clinical trials have been completed and have been published and were, therefore, present in both lists. Of the records screened, 87 were immediately excluded, mostly because they were obviously only focused on adults or on non-Hodgkin lymphoma; we also excluded all manuscripts on nursing and drug preparation as well as all review articles. Of the 61 full-text articles and studies assessed for eligibility, several case reports were excluded because they described single adult patients with adverse events or because the original articles did not contain any clinical information (basic research). Please see the PRISMA flow diagram in Figure 1.

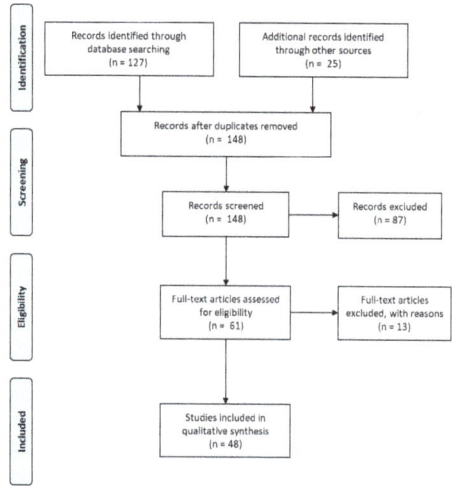

Figure 1. PRISMA flow chart [18].

3. Results

3.1. Efficacy

The first descriptions of the use of blinatumomab in the pediatric population were two small case series of patients with a relapse of ALL after allogeneic HSCT. Handgretinger and colleagues showed that complete remission (CR) after blinatumomab-induced donor T-cell activation in three pediatric patients with post-transplant relapsed ALL was possible [19]. In an extended investigation three years later, nine patients treated with blinatumomab for relapse post-HSCT were analyzed of which six achieved a CR and three did not respond [20].

Until two years ago, there was only one phase I/II study published for the treatment of R/R ALL in pediatric patients (open-label, single-arm phase I/II study at 26 European and US centers NCT01471782). Patients included had refractory or relapsed ALL with >25% bone marrow blasts. The authors showed that blinatumomab clearly demonstrated anti-leukemic activity as a single agent in children with R/R-ALL: among the 70 patients who received the recommended dosage, 27 (39%; 95% CI, 27% to 51%) achieved complete remission within the first two cycles, 14 (52%) of whom achieved complete minimal residual disease response [21]. Furthermore, the follow-up study showed that allogeneic HSCT before or after blinatumomab was associated with a positive effect on survival [22]. In a post hoc analysis day 15 bone marrow minimal residual disease (MRD) predicted complete MRD response to blinatumomab within the first two treatment cycles so that patients with BM MRD $\geq 10^{-4}$ at day 15, being predictive of survival, could potentially pursue alternative therapies, such as dose escalation or combination therapies, to achieve deeper remission [23].

Locatelli and colleagues compared the efficacy of blinatumomab from the single-arm, phase I/II study with that of historical standard of care (SOC) therapy in comparison with three historical comparator groups from North America, Australia and Europe. Single-agent blinatumomab treatment was associated with longer overall survival (OS) and a trend for higher CR in comparison with SOC chemotherapy [24].

Simultaneously, results on the safety and efficacy of blinatumomab in an open-label, single-arm, expanded access international study of pediatric patients with CD19-positive R/R BCPALL were published (RIALTO trial, NCT02187354) [25]. In contrast to the first open label study, patients with a lower tumor burden (≥ 5% blasts or <5% blasts but with MRD level $\geq 10^{-3}$) were eligible. Of the 110 patients in the study, 69 patients had CR as the best response in the first two cycles; of these, 45 (65%) proceeded to allogeneic HSCT. There was a trend toward improved OS and relapse-free survival (RFS) for patients who received allogeneic HSCT after blinatumomab compared with those who did not. Median OS for all patients (n = 110) was 13.1 months (95% CI 10.2–21.3), with a median follow up of 17.4 months. For all patients reaching or maintaining CR in the first two cycles of blinatumomab (n = 69), median RFS was 8.5 months (95% CI 4.4—not evaluable), with a median follow up of 11.2 months.

Over the last two to three years, there have been several case series, single-center experiences or single-country evaluations on the use of blinatumomab in children with R/R ALL. Mouttet and colleagues encouragingly described durable remissions in nine patients with TCF3-HLF-positive ALL, most of whom were treated early in the first consolidation with blinatumomab as a bridge to HSCT [26]. This rare subtype of childhood ALL is usually characterized by a high rate of treatment failure, despite treatment intensification and HSCT. Similarly, Keating and colleagues describe 15 patients in which blinatumomab given prior to transplant reduces MRD and results in favorable leukemia-free survival, toxicity and overall survival [27].

Blinatumomab has also successfully been used to treat patients with a high risk for chemotherapy-related adverse events, such as a patient with Down syndrome [28] or patients who experienced overwhelming chemotherapy-associated toxicity during induction therapy. In these patients, blinatumomab served as a bridge to further cytostatic therapy [29]. Infants with ALL are another vulnerable group; the leukemias often harbor

KMT2A rearrangements and have a high risk for treatment failure and relapse. The last international Interfant trials unfortunately could not improve the outcome of patients below one year of age [30,31]. Clesham and colleagues report on 11 patients with KMT2A-rearranged infant ALL [32]. Nine patients became MRD negative, and two patients had a >1-log reduction in MRD prior to HSCT. Three-year EFS and OS post-transplant were 47% and 81%, respectively, comparing favorably with historical outcomes in this subgroup of patients. Four patients relapsed, one of which was MRD-positive pretransplant. One patient relapsed with lineage-switch to monoblastic acute myeloid leukemia and died shortly after.

Colleagues from Spain describe 27 patients treated with blinatumomab and/or inotuzumab, demonstrating that both immunotherapies can induce deep remissions, and blinatumomab can serve as an effective bridging therapy during severe infections [33]. Colleagues from Greece published their experience with nine patients with R/R ALL [34]. They observed a response with morphological CR in 6/9 patients (66.7%) after one cycle of blinatumomab. A successful bridging to HSCT was feasible in 5/9 patients (55.6%), but the median RFS and OS remained low (3.0 and 8.7 months, respectively). Correspondingly, colleagues in Japan conducted an open-label phase 1b study in nine patients [35]. No dose-limiting toxicities were reported; morphological remission within the first two treatment cycles was 56%; one patient had a minimal residual disease response. We described our own single-center experience in 38 patients with R/R-ALL in Tübingen and observed a response to blinatumomab in 13/38 patients (34%) [36]. To date, nine patients (24%) are alive and in complete molecular remission with a median follow-up time of 54 months (8.9–113 months). All survivors underwent haploidentical hematopoietic stem cell transplantation after treatment with blinatumomab. Sutton and colleagues very recently published the Australian experience with blinatumomab in children with R/R-ALL and high-risk genetics [37]. Overall, MRD response was 58%, median follow up was 26 months (14–42 months), 83% proceeded to HSCT and inferior progression-free survival (PFS) was associated with MRD positivity and KMT2A-rearranged leukemia.

In March 2021, the first results of two randomized controlled trials investigating blinatumomab in pediatric patients with ALL were published back to back in JAMA. Brown and colleagues describe the effect of postreinduction therapy consolidation with blinatumomab versus chemotherapy in patients with first relapse of ALL [38]. All patients received a 4-week reinduction chemotherapy course, followed by randomized assignment to receive two cycles of blinatumomab or two cycles of multiagent chemotherapy, each followed by HSCT. The Children's Oncology Group conducted this randomized phase 3 clinical trial at hospitals in the US, Canada, Australia and New Zealand (NCT02101853). Eligible patients included those aged 1 to 30 years with B-ALL first relapse. Among 208 randomized patients (median age, 9 years; 97 [47%] females), 118 (57%) completed the randomized therapy. Randomization was terminated at the recommendation of the data and safety monitoring committee without meeting stopping rules for efficacy or futility due to a concern of loss of clinical equipoise. The blinatumomab group presented obvious advantages, such as improved disease-free and overall survival, higher rate of negative MRD and lower rates of serious adverse events. With 2.9 years of median follow up, 2-year disease-free survival was 54.4% for the blinatumomab group vs. 39.0% for the chemotherapy group (hazard ratio for disease progression or mortality, 0.70 [95% CI, 0.47–1.03]; 1-sided p = 0.03). Two-year overall survival was 71.3% for the blinatumomab group vs. 58.4% for the chemotherapy group (hazard ratio for mortality, 0.62 [95% CI, 0.39–0.98]; 1-sided p = 0.02). In conclusion, postreinduction treatment with blinatumomab did not result in a statistically significant difference in disease-free survival, but the differences between the blinatumomab group and the chemotherapy group in overall survival (71.3% vs. 58.4%) and MRD negativity (75% vs. 32%) were both statistically significant.

The second trial is reported by Locatelli and colleagues [39]. Centers in Europe, Australia and Israel enrolled 108 children older than 28 days and younger than 18 years with high-risk first-relapse B-ALL in morphologic complete remission (M1 marrow, <5%

blasts) or with M2 marrow (blasts ≥ 5% and <25%) at randomization: (NCT02393859). Patients were randomized to receive one cycle of blinatumomab or chemotherapy for the third consolidation. A total of 108 patients were randomized, and all patients were included in the analysis. Enrollment was terminated early because it met a prespecified stopping criterion for superiority of the blinatumomab group. After a median of 22.4 months of follow up (IQR, 8.1–34.2), the incidence of events in the blinatumomab vs. consolidation chemotherapy group was 31% vs. 57% (log-rank $p < 0.001$; hazard ratio [HR], 0.33 [95% CI, 0.18–0.61]). Deaths occurred in eight patients (14.8%) in the blinatumomab group and 16 (29.6%) in the consolidation chemotherapy group. The overall survival HR was 0.43 (95% CI, 0.18–1.01). Minimal residual disease remission was observed in more patients in the blinatumomab vs. consolidation chemotherapy group (90% [44/49] vs. 54% [26/48]), and more patients in the blinatumomab group were able to proceed to HSCT. Among children with high-risk first-relapse B-ALL, treatment with one cycle of blinatumomab compared with standard intensive multidrug chemotherapy before allogeneic HSCT resulted in an improved EFS at a median of 22.4 months of follow up. The benefit of blinatumomab was observed in all analyzed subgroups and was especially noticeable for patients with an early relapse.

Please see Table 1 for a list of publications concerning blinatumomab in ALL.

Table 1. Table with all articles published on use of blinatumomab in pediatric ALL.

Author	Year	Ref.[1]	Patients	Title
Handgretinger	2011	[19]	3 R/R-ALL patients post-HSCT	CR after blinatumomab-induced donor T-cell activation in three pediatric patients with post-transplant relapsed ALL
Schlegel	2014	[20]	9 R/R-ALL patients post-HSCT	Pediatric post-transplant R/R BCP ALL leukemia shows durable remission by therapy with the T-cell engaging bispecific antibody blinatumomab
Von Stackelberg	2016	[21]	93 R/R patients (70 with recommended dosage)	Phase I/phase II study of blinatumomab in pediatric patients with R/R ALL
Mejstříková	2017	[40]	18 patients (4 with CD19-negative relapse)	CD19-negative relapse of pediatric BCP-ALL following blinatumomab treatment
Zoghbi	2017	[41]	case report	Lineage switch under blinatumomab treatment of relapsed common ALL without MLL rearrangement
Wadhwa	2018	[28]	case report	Blinatumomab activity in a patient with Down syndrome BCP-ALL
Gore	2018	[22]	70 R/R-ALL patients	Survival after blinatumomab treatment in pediatric patients with R/R BCP-ALL
Wölfl	2018	[42]	case report	Spontaneous reversion of a lineage switch following an initial blinatumomab-induced ALL-to-AML switch in MLL-rearranged infant ALL
Mouttet	2019	[26]	9 TCF3/HLF	Durable remissions in TCF3-HLF positive acute lymphoblastic leukemia with blinatumomab and SCT
Keating	2019	[27]	15 children MRD-positive before HSCT	Reducing minimal residual disease with blinatumomab prior to HSCT for pediatric patients with ALL
Elitzur	2019	[29]	11 pediatric patients with overwhelming chemotherapy-associated toxicity	Blinatumomab as a bridge to further therapy in case of overwhelming toxicity in pediatric BCP-ALL
Brown	2019	[23]	59 patients of the MT103-205 study (NCT01471782)	Day 15 bone marrow MRD predicts response to blinatumomab
Locatelli	2020	[24]	70 patients of the MT103-205 study (NCT01471782)	Blinatumomab versus historical standard therapy in pediatric patients with R/R Ph-negative BCP-ALL
Locatelli	2020	[25]	110 R/R-ALL patients	Blinatumomab in pediatric patients with R/R ALL: results of the RIALTO trial, an expanded access study

Table 1. Cont.

Author	Year	Ref.[1]	Patients	Title
Mikhailova	2020	[43]	90 patients	Immunophenotypic changes of leukemic blasts in children with R/R- ALL who have been treated with blinatumomb
Contreras	2020	[33]	27 children/young adults treated with blinatumomab and/or inotuzumab	Clinical utilization of blinatumomab and inotuzumab immunotherapy in children with relapsed or refractory B-ALL
Clesham	2020	[32]	11 infants	Blinatumomab for infant ALL
Horibe	2020	[35]	9 children	A phase 1 study of blinatumomab in Japanese children
Ampatzidou	2020	[34]	9 children	Insights from the Greek experience of the use of Blinatumomab in pediatric R/R ALL
Queudeville	2021	[36]	38 R/R-ALL patients	Blinatumomab in pediatric patients with relapsed/refractory B-cell precursor acute lymphoblastic leukemia
Sutton	2021	[37]	24 R/R-ALL patients outside of clinical trials	Outcomes for Australian children with relapsed/refractory acute lymphoblastic leukaemia treated with blinatumomab
Brethon	2021	[44]	case report	Targeting 2 antigens as a promising strategy in mixed phenotype acute leukemia: combination with blinatumomab with gemtuzumab ozogamicin in an infant with KMT2A-rearraged leukemia
Brown	2021	[38]	208 pts, 1 to 30 years	Effect of Postreinduction Therapy Consolidation with Blinatumomab vs. Chemotherapy on Disease-Free Survival in Children, Adolescents, and Young Adults with First relapse of B-Cell Acute Lymphoblastic Leukemia NCT02101853
Locatelli	2021	[39]	108 pts, 28 days to 18 years	Effect of Blinatumomab vs. Chemotherapy on Event-Free Survival Among Children with High-risk First-Relapse B-Cell Acute Lymphoblastic Leukemia: A Randomized Clinical Trial NCT02393859

[1] References according to mention in this article.

3.2. Adverse Events

Cytokine release syndrome (CRS) and neurotoxicity are the most feared adverse events under therapy with blinatumomab. The first pediatric study by von Stackelberg and colleagues described cytopenias as being by far the most common adverse events, obviously mostly preexisting in patients with R/R-ALL. Cytokine release syndrome (CRS) of higher grades was only seen in 4/70 (6%) patients, and 17 patients had neurologic/neuropsychiatric events, mostly tremor, dizziness and somnolence. In nine patients (13%), neurologic events were considered to be treatment related. All events were of grade 2 and resolved; two patients interrupted treatment due to grade 2 seizures, but there were no permanent discontinuations caused by neurologic events [21].

Our own single-center retrospective evaluation showed that cytopenias and febrile reactions were the most common adverse events. Half of the patients experienced CRS, but only 7/38 (18%) of grade ≥3 [36]. High grades of CRS were especially seen in patients who did not receive steroid premedication before blinatumomab, and we demonstrated a clear association between high tumor load and the development of CRS. Neurotoxicity was seen in seven patients (18%); only two patients discontinued blinatumomab therapy due to generalized seizures.

A case series in 11 infants described three patients with grade 1-2 CRS and one patient with neurotoxicity (confusion and somnolence); symptoms were resolved by interrupting the blinatumomab infusion [32].

In newly published RCTs, Brown and colleagues describe blinatumomab-related adverse events with overall 22% CRS, 11% encephalopathy and 4% seizures but only one case of grade ≥3 CRS or seizure each and two cases of higher-grade encephalopathy. Other rates of notable serious adverse events were much less common in the blinatumomab group compared to the chemotherapy group: infection (15% vs. 65%), febrile neutropenia (5% vs. 58%), sepsis (2% vs. 27%) and mucositis (1% vs. 28%) [38].

Locatelli and colleagues reported an incidence of serious adverse events of 24.1% vs. 43.1% in a blinatumomab vs. consolidation chemotherapy group. The incidence of adverse events grade ≥3 was also lower in the blinatumomab group (57.4% vs. 82.4%). The most frequently reported adverse events were neurologic symptoms and seizure (each 3.7%) in the blinatumomab group and febrile neutropenia (17.6%) in the consolidation chemotherapy group. Only two patients in the blinatumomab group and one in the consolidation chemotherapy group experienced CRS at less than grade 3.

3.3. CD19 Expression

CD19-negative relapses of pediatric BCP-ALL following blinatumomab treatment were first described in 2017 from a phase I/II study: four patients experienced CD19-negative relapse after prior blinatumomab-induced hematologic remission, and one patient showed CD19-negative progression during treatment after 10 days in cycle 1 with blasts showing a monocytic phenotype [40].

In the retrospective evaluation of our own 38 patients in Tübingen, none of the patients displayed a CD19-negative subclone detectable by flow cytometry before receiving a first cycle of blinatumomab. Sixteen patients had CD19-positive relapse. One patient experienced a CD19-negative relapse after the second cycle was completed. Another patient's leukemia did not express CD19 by flow cytometric analysis during the second cycle. Interestingly, the leukemic cells quickly regained normal CD19 expression after cessation of blinatumomab [36]. One patient with *KMT2A* translocation showed myeloid differentiation in addition to the disappearance of CD19 under treatment with blinatumomab and spontaneous conversion back to a CD19-positive immunophenotype after the discontinuation of blinatumomab.

A study analyzing immunophenotypic changes in leukemic cells at relapse in 90 pediatric R/R ALL patients treated with blinatumomab showed that in 21 cases, leukemia cells at relapse were CD19 positive, whereas in six cases, they were CD19 negative [43]. Three children (two with *KMT2A* gene rearrangement and one with germline *KMT2A*) developed relapse through lineage switch to CD19-negative acute myeloid leukemia, mixed phenotypic acute leukemia and unclassifiable leukemia. This switch in immunophenotype has previously been described in case reports by others [42,45]. One case report also describes such a lineage switch following blinatumomab in a young girl post-HSCT whose leukemia did not harbor *KMT2A* rearrangement [41].

The Australian group described two patients with CD19-negative relapses, one of which also harbored a *KMT2A* rearrangement and showed myeloid differentiation; however, the leukemias of most patients who relapsed remained CD19 positive [37].

3.4. Clinical Trials

Of 78 trials listed on Clinical trills.gov, only 24 include pediatric patients. One trial was only listed in the European registry. All are interventional open-label trials.

In addition to the phase I/II studies in R/R ALL and both recently published phase III randomized controlled trials (RCTs) mentioned above, there are further trials ongoing for patients with a refractory or relapsed leukemia. One study in Japan is still recruiting, with adult data already published [46], but pediatric results still pending (NCT02412306). An observational retrospective study sponsored by Amgen for children and adults with Ph-chromosome-negative R/R ALL was completed, but there are no published results yet (NCT02783651). Checkpoint inhibitors might increase T-cell proliferation and enhance the mechanism of action of blinatumomab. Adolescents and adults with poor-risk R/R ALL are eligible for a trial of the National Cancer Institute where blinatumomab and nivolumab are administered with or without ipilimumab (NCT02879695). Similarly, the Children's

Hospital Medical Center in Cincinnati planned a pilot study to assess the safety, tolerability and preliminary anti-tumor activity of combining pembrolizumab and blinatumomab in children and young adults with R/R ALL (NCT03605589). This study is currently suspended due to slow recruitment, an amendment is pending. Moreover, the National Cancer Institute is conducting a phase II trial in children and young adults with first relapse of ALL comparing blinatumomab alone to blinatumomab with nivolumab.

Many studies are investigating blinatumomab in relation to HSCT, either as a bridging element or as a consolidation treatment afterwards. The Medical College of Wisconsin has two ongoing trials: Blina Part 1 explores blinatumomab as a bridging therapy for patients in first or greater relapse (NCT04556084), and Part 2 is focused on blinatumomab after T-cell receptor (TCR) alpha/beta-depleted HSCT (NCT04746209). The University of British Columbia is planning a trial on blinatumomab for MRD in pre-B-ALL patients following HSCT but is not yet recruiting (NCT04044560). Similarly, Seoul national University is planning a single-arm study for patients with persistent or recurrent MRD before HSCT (NCT04604691) but is currently not recruiting. M.D. Anderson Cancer Center are evaluating blinatumomab maintenance following allogeneic HSCT in children and adults (NCT02807883). Equivalently, European colleagues included an add-on study for blinatumomab post-HSCT into the ALL SCTped 2012 study (NCT04785547). St. Jude Children's Research Hospital is currently conducting two trials for several hematological malignancies receiving naïve T-cell-depleted haploidentical HSCT. The first study combines TCRgamma/delta T cells and memory T cells with the selected use of blinatumomab in relapsed/refractory malignancies (NCT02790515). The second couples a TCRalpha/beta-depleted progenitor cell graft with an additional memory T-cell donor lymphocyte infusion (DLI), plus the selected use of blinatumomab a week after DLI (NCT03849651).

Blinatumomab has also found its way into the frontline treatment of ALL in children. In the United States, the M.D. Anderson Cancer Center is recruiting adolescents aged 14 years and older for a phase II trial with blinatumomab and combination chemotherapy as frontline therapy (NCT02877303) and patients in the same age group for a phase II trial combining blinatumomab with inotuzumab ozogamicin (NCT02877303). The TOTAL Therapy XVII of St. Jude Children's Research Hospital is open for children aged 1 to 18 years (NCT03117751). The National Cancer Institute phase III trial includes patients aged 1 to 31 years (NCT03914625). Both studies include patients with Philadelphia-chromosome-positive (Ph+) leukemias. The federal research institute of pediatric hematology, oncology and immunology in Russia are also conducting an interventional trial with one course of blinatumomab in consolidation therapy as the experimental arm (NCT04723342). Simultaneously, several large randomized multicenter phase III trials in Europe are investigating blinatumomab as a frontline treatment. ALLTogether1 is a treatment study protocol for children and young adults (1–45 years of age) using a sequential assignment to therapy (NCT04307576), and AIEOP-BFM ALL 2017 is open for children aged below 18 years using a factorial assignment (NCT03643276). Colleagues from the Netherlands are conducting a pilot study to test the feasibility, safety and efficacy of adding blinatumomab to the Interfant-06 backbone in infants with *KMT2A(MLL)*-rearranged ALL (EudraCT 2016-004674-17, no NCT identifier). Together with the AIEOP-BFM ALL 2017 study, these are currently the only frontline randomized clinical trials including infants with ALL.

Please see Table 2 for a list of all clinical trials of blinatumomab in pediatric patients.

Table 2. Table containing all ongoing clinical trials with blinatumomab for pediatric patients.

Clinical Trials Identifier	Other Study ID Numbers	Ref. [1]	Title	Age	Status
NCT01471782	MT103-205 2010-024264-18 (Eudra-CT)	[21]	Clinical Study With Blinatumomab in Pediatric and Adolescent Patients With Relapsed/Refractory B-precursor Acute Lymphoblastic Leukemia	Up to 17 years (child)	completed
NCT02187354	RIALTO 2014-001700-21 (EudraCT)	[25]	Expanded Access Protocol-Blinatumomab in Pediatric & Adolescent Subjects with Relapsed/Refractory B-precursor ALL (RIALTO)	Up to 17 years (child)	completed
NCT02783651	20150253		A Study of Patients with Ph-Chromosome-negative Relapsed or Refractory Acute Lymphoblastic Leukemia in the US	Child, adult	completed
NCT02879695	NCI-2016-01300 (CTRP)		Blinatumomab and Nivolumab With or Without Ipilimumab in Treating Patients With Poor-Risk Relapsed or Refractory CD19+ Precursor B-Lymphoblastic Leukemia	16 years and older	recruiting
NCT02393859	2014-002476-92 (EudraCT)	[39]	Phase 3 Trial of Blinatumomab vs. Standard Chemotherapy in Pediatric Subjects With High-Risk (HR) First Relapse B-precursor Acute Lymphoblastic Leukemia (ALL)	Up to 17 years (child)	active, not recruiting
NCT04546399	NCI-2020-06813 (CTRP)		A Study to Compare Blinatumomab Alone to Blinatumomab With Nivolumab in Patients Diagnosed With First Relapse B-Cell Acute Lymphoblastic Leukemia (B-ALL)	1 to 31 years (child, adult) Including Down syndrome patients	recruiting
NCT03914625	NCI-2019-02187 (CTRP)		A Study to Investigate Blinatumomab in Combination With Chemotherapy in Patients With Newly Diagnosed B-Lymphoblastic Leukemia	1 to 31 years (child, adult) Including Down syndrome patients	recruiting
NCT02101853	NCI-2014-00631 (CTRP) COG-AALL1331	[38]	Blinatumomab in Treating Younger Patients With Relapsed B-cell Acute Lymphoblastic Leukemia	1 to 31 years (child, adult)	Active, not recruiting
NCT02877303	NCI-2017-00596 (CTRP)		Blinatumomab and Combination Chemotherapy as Frontline Therapy in Treating Patients With B Acute Lymphoblastic Leukemia	14 years and older	recruiting
NCT02790515	REF2HCT NCI-2016-00812 (CTRP)		Provision of TCRγδ T Cells and Memory T Cells Plus Selected Use of Blinatumomab in Naïve T-cell Depleted Haploidentical Donor Hematopoietic Cell Transplantation for Hematologic Malignancies Relapsed or Refractory Despite Prior Transplantation	Up to 21 years	recruiting
NCT03849651	HAP2HCT		TCRαβ-depleted Progenitor Cell Graft With Additional Memory T-cell DLI, Plus Selected Use of Blinatumomab, in Naive T-cell Depleted Haploidentical Donor Hematopoietc Cell Transplantation for Hematologic Malignancies	Up to 21 years	recruiting

Table 2. Cont.

Clinical Trials Identifier	Other Study ID Numbers	Ref. [1]	Title	Age	Status
NCT04307576	ALLTogether1 2018-001795-38 (EudraCT)		ALLTogether1—A Treatment Study Protocol of the ALLTogether Consortium for Children and Young Adults (1–45 Years of Age) With Newly Diagnosed Acute Lymphoblastic Leukaemia (ALL)	1 to 45 years	recruiting
NCT03643276	AIEOP-BFM ALL 2017 2016-001935-12 (EudraCT)		Treatment Protocol for Children and Adolescents With Acute Lymphoblastic Leukemia-AIEOP-BFM ALL 2017	Up to 17 years	recruiting
NCT03117751	TOT17 NCI-2017-00582 (CTRP)		Total Therapy XVII for Newly Diagnosed Patients With Acute Lymphoblastic Leukemia and Lymphoma	1 to 18 years	recruiting
	2016-004674-17 (EudraCT) ML59901.078.17		A pilot study to test the feasibility, safety and efficacy of the addition of the BiTE antibody Blinatumomab to the Interfant-06 backbone in infants with MLL-rearranged acute lymphoblastic leukemia. A collaborative study of the Interfant network	Up to 17 years	recruiting
NCT04604691			Blinatumomab in Pediatric B-cell Acute Lymphoblastic Leukemia (ALL) with Minimal Residual Disease (MRD)		Not yet recruiting
NCT03605589			Pembro and Blina combination in Pediatric and Young Adult Patients With Relapsed/Refractory Acute Leukemia or Lymphoma	1 to 40 years	Suspended, slow recruitment, amendment pending
NCT04723342	ALL-MB 2019 Pilot		Treatment of Children and Adolescents With Primary B-precursor Acute Lymphoblastic Leukemia With Combination Chemotherapy and Immunotherapy	1–18 years	recruiting
NCT04556084	Blina Part 1		Blinatumomab Bridging Therapy	Up to 25 years	recruiting
NCT04746209	Blina Part 2		Blinatumomab After TCR Alpha Beta/CD19 Depleted HCT	Up to 25 years	not yet recruiting
NCT02807883	NCI-2016-01182		Blinatumomab Maintenance Following Allogeneic Hematopoietic Cell Transplantation for Patients With Acute Lymphoblastic Leukemia	1 to 70 years	active, not recruiting
NCT02412306	20130265		Study of Blinatumomab in Japanese Patients With Relapsed/Refractory B-precursor Acute Lymphoblastic Leukemia	<18 years for pediatric subjects	recruiting
NCT02877303	2014-0845 NCI-2017-00596		Blinatumomab, Inotuzumab Ozogamicin, and Combination Chemotherapy as Frontline Therapy in Treating Patients With B Acute Lymphoblastic Leukemia	14 years and older	recruiting
NCT04044560	H19-00893 CTTC 1902		Blinatumomab for MRD in Pre-B-ALL Patients Following Stem Cell Transplant (OZM-097)	1 year and older (children and adults)	not yet recruiting
NCT04785547	FORUM Add-on Blina post TX		ALL SCTped 2012 FORUM Add-on Study Blina Post HSCT	6 months to 21 years	recruiting

[1] References according to mention in this article.

4. Discussion

The results of the phase I/II study and several single-institution or national retrospective evaluations show that children with R/R-ALL show a response to blinatumomab ranging from 34–38% [21,36] to around 60% [25,37]. In almost all studies published to date, there is evidence or at least a trend of improved survival if blinatumomab is administered prior to or after allogeneic HSCT [22,25,26,32,36].

The results of both phase III RCTs in children with first relapse of ALL confirm the superiority of blinatumomab in achieving MRD-negativity before HSCT and even show evidence for an advantage in overall survival [38,39], while inducing less severe adverse events compared to conventional chemotherapy. These results definitely warrant the inclusion of blinatumomab into relapse protocols before HSCT.

The prognostic importance of achieving MRD negativity prior to HSCT has been well established [47]. Response rates for blinatumomab in R/R-ALL are encouraging, but they are still insufficient. Survival outcomes for the non-responding patients remain extremely poor [48,49]. Combination therapies with other antibodies, such as inotuzumab ozogamicin, will hopefully overcome problems of CD19-escape (current trial NCT02877303). Administering donor lymphocyte infusions in a haploidentical setting (NCT02790515 and NCT03849651) or adding a checkpoint inhibitor, such as PD-1- or CTLA-4-inhibitors, could enhance the efficacy of blinatumomab (NCT02879695, NCT04546399 and NCT03605589).

Overall, adverse events are much less common under blinatumomab compared to conventional chemotherapy [38,39]. Additionally, even specific blinatumomab-related toxicities, such as CRS and neurotoxicity, only rarely necessitate the interruption of therapy [20,31,35]. This observation makes blinatumomab an ideal drug for selected use in vulnerable patients, such as children with Down syndrome, with a high risk for chemotherapy-related mortality [50] or other patients experiencing overwhelming toxicities [29]. To date, only two case reports have described the benefit of using blinatumomab in Down syndrome children [28,29]. No Down syndrome patients were included in the pediatric RCT for R/R-ALL, but several frontline trials are enabling Down syndrome patients with high-risk features access to upfront treatment with blinatumomab (NCT03643276, NCT04307576 and NCT03117751). This approach might also prove to be a worthwhile strategy in the group of patients with underlying genetic defects, such as chromosomal instability or defects in DNA-damage repair.

On the other hand, patients with ALL harboring almost incurable translocations, such as TCF3/HLF-fusion, are also directly eligible for receiving blinatumomab upfront, as these patients are known to display a high rate of treatment failure with conventional chemotherapy [51]. The promising results of durable remissions in nine patients with TCF3/HLF-positive leukemia confer great hopes [26].

Philadelphia-chromosome-positive (Ph+) patients comprise another important subgroup. Patients with Ph+ leukemia have a poor outcome and are, therefore, treated with high-risk regimens, including a tyrosine kinase inhibitor targeting the BCR/ABL-fusion [52]. Continuous concomitant medication with imatinib or dasatinib leads to an important increase in adverse events, necessitating alternative therapeutic options. Sutton and colleagues observed relatively good outcomes for patients with Philadelphia-positive or Philadelphia-like ALL treated with blinatumomab [37]. Unfortunately, most upfront trials with blinatumomab for children open today do not include patients with Ph+ ALL, with the exception of Total Therapy XVII (NCT03117751).

Infants with ALL are a unique subgroup of patients; infant leukemias often harbor *KMT2A* rearrangement and also display high relapse rates and unsatisfying outcomes [30,31]. Clesham and colleagues described 11 infants treated with blinatumomab; treatment was well tolerated, and complete MRD responses were seen in the majority of cases. All children received HSCT, and the 12-month EFS compares favorably with historical outcomes [32]. In contrast, in an Australian study, infants with *KMT2A*-rearranged leukemia had poor outcomes with an MRD response rate of only 44% [37]. This disparity might be explained by pretreatment or tumor burden differences prior to treatment. One

European study is currently adding blinatumomab treatment to the Inferfant-06 backbone (EudraCT 2016-004674-17), and the frontline AIEOP-ALL BFM trial also includes infants (NCT03643276). The results will hopefully clarify the utility of blinatumomab in these patients, and also regarding the lineage switch with the outgrowth of myeloid leukemia that several groups have described for *KMT2A*-rearranged leukemias under the selective pressure of blinatumomab [36,42,45]. The combination of targeting two antigens might be a strategy in such cases. A recent case report describes the successful combination of blinatumomab with gemtuzumab ozogamicin in an infant with *KMT2A*-rearraged mixed phenotypic leukemia [44].

The first mention of blinatumomab in three pediatric patients was published ten years ago in 2011 [19], followed by the description of nine children receiving blinatumomab after relapse post-HSCT [20]. It took a further two years until the publication of the phase I/II trial [21]. The first results of RCTs for the use of blinatumomab in children with first relapse of ALL were published this year [38,39]. Current front-line trials are investigating blinatumomab in children with standard-risk ALL (NCT03914625, NCT02877303); others only apply blinatumomab to standard-risk patients with residual disease at the end of induction therapy (NCT03117751) or intermediate and high-risk ALL (NCT0363276). Results from these trials will show whether replacing part of the classic chemotherapy with blinatumomab is feasible without impairing EFS. The prognosis of standard-risk leukemia patients is excellent; risk-stratified therapy has reduced late morbidity and mortality [53]. Direct treatment-related morbidity and mortality, especially due to infections, cardio-metabolic dysfunction, hepatotoxicity, osteonecrosis and asparaginase-associated problems, such as coagulation disorders and pancreatitis, remain an important issue. Replacing steroids and cytostatic drugs with immunotherapeutics, such as blinatumomab, might help reduce these problems.

Compared to treatment with chimeric antigen receptor (CAR) T cells, blinatumomab has a few advantages: it is an off-the-shelf product; it is less expensive; the short half-life enables the precise control of serum levels; and a quick reduction is possible in the case of an adverse event, such as neurotoxicity or CRS. Outpatient delivery by a portable minipump enables a good health-related quality of life. The direct comparison of blinatumomab with CAR T cells or other immunotherapies, such as inotuzumab ozogamicin, are lacking, and further studies are necessary to help determine at which point each therapeutic option might yield the best results. However, it has been shown that sequential treatment is often feasible, in both directions [54,55].

5. Conclusions

Patients in currently published studies and case series have all been heavily pretreated, and today, blinatumomab has evolved to being a first-line salvage therapy in many centers, but there are still only two RCTs published with results in the pediatric setting for the use of blinatumomab in first relapse or even in a situation with rising MRD levels. All available data in R/R-ALL suggest a necessity for HSCT after a bridging therapy with blinatumomab. Ongoing trials will show whether blinatumomab is capable of inducing lasting remissions without a following allogeneic HSCT or constitutes a suitable maintenance therapy post-HSCT. Adult data suggest that not all MRD responders necessarily require a transplant [56].

Many questions remain unanswered. Some have recently been pointed out by Shukla and Sulis [13], such as the following: when is the optimal time to introduce blinatumomab, and how many cycles are needed? Current frontline protocols have different approaches (blinatumomab after or instead of consolidation therapy; one versus two cycles). Does blinatumomab have a value as a consolidation treatment in non-high-risk patients with negative MRD in terms of reducing the relapse rate? Why do some patients respond and others do not? This is definitely not merely due to the loss of the target antigen CD19.

Ongoing trials will hopefully clarify these questions in the near future.

Funding: This research received no external funding.

Conflicts of Interest: M.E. received honoraria from Amgen.

References

1. Brischwein, K.; Schlereth, B.; Guller, B.; Steiger, C.; Wolf, A.; Lutterbuese, R.; Offner, S.; Locher, M.; Urbig, T.; Raum, T.; et al. MT110: A novel bispecific single-chain antibody construct with high efficacy in eradicating established tumors. *Mol. Immunol.* **2006**, *43*, 1129–1143. [CrossRef] [PubMed]
2. Offner, S.; Hofmeister, R.; Romaniuk, A.; Kufer, P.; Baeuerle, P.A. Induction of regular cytolytic T cell synapses by bispecific single-chain antibody constructs on MHC class I-negative tumor cells. *Mol. Immunol.* **2006**, *43*, 763–771. [CrossRef] [PubMed]
3. Hoffmann, P.; Hofmeister, R.; Brischwein, K.; Brandl, C.; Crommer, S.; Bargou, R.; Itin, C.; Prang, N.; Baeuerle, P.A. Serial killing of tumor cells by cytotoxic T cells redirected with a CD19-/CD3-bispecific single-chain antibody construct. *Int. J. Cancer* **2005**, *115*, 98–104. [CrossRef]
4. Pui, C.H.; Evans, W.E. Acute lymphoblastic leukemia. *N. Engl. J. Med.* **1998**, *339*, 605–615. [CrossRef]
5. Greaves, M. Molecular genetics, natural history and the demise of childhood leukaemia. *Eur. J. Cancer* **1999**, *35*, 1941–1953. [CrossRef]
6. Gokbuget, N.; Hoelzer, D. Recent approaches in acute lymphoblastic leukemia in adults. *Rev. Clin. Exp. Hematol.* **2002**, *6*, 114–141. [CrossRef] [PubMed]
7. Schrappe, M.; Camitta, B.; Pui, C.H.; Eden, T.; Gaynon, P.; Gustafsson, G.; Janka-Schaub, G.E.; Kamps, W.; Masera, G.; Sallan, S.; et al. Long-term results of large prospective trials in childhood acute lymphoblastic leukemia. *Leukemia* **2000**, *14*, 2193–2194. [CrossRef]
8. Gokbuget, N.; Dombret, H.; Ribera, J.M.; Fielding, A.K.; Advani, A.; Bassan, R.; Chia, V.; Doubek, M.; Giebel, S.; Hoelzer, D.; et al. International reference analysis of outcomes in adults with B-precursor Ph-negative relapsed/refractory acute lymphoblastic leukemia. *Haematologica* **2016**, *101*, 1524–1533. [CrossRef]
9. Comans-Bitter, W.M.; de Groot, R.; van den Beemd, R.; Neijens, H.J.; Hop, W.C.; Groeneveld, K.; Hooijkaas, H.; van Dongen, J.J. Immunophenotyping of blood lymphocytes in childhood. Reference values for lymphocyte subpopulations. *J. Pediatr.* **1997**, *130*, 388–393. [CrossRef]
10. Hoffman, L.M.; Gore, L. Blinatumomab, a Bi-Specific Anti-CD19/CD3 BiTE((R)) Antibody for the Treatment of Acute Lymphoblastic Leukemia: Perspectives and Current Pediatric Applications. *Front. Oncol.* **2014**, *4*, 63. [CrossRef]
11. Franca, R.; Favretto, D.; Granzotto, M.; Decorti, G.; Rabusin, M.; Stocco, G. Epratuzumab and Blinatumomab as Therapeutic Antibodies for Treatment of Pediatric Acute Lymphoblastic Leukemia: Current Status and Future Perspectives. *Curr. Med. Chem.* **2017**, *24*, 1050–1065. [CrossRef] [PubMed]
12. Algeri, M.; Del Bufalo, F.; Galaverna, F.; Locatelli, F. Current and future role of bispecific T-cell engagers in pediatric acute lymphoblastic leukemia. *Expert Rev. Hematol.* **2018**, *11*, 945–956. [CrossRef]
13. Shukla, N.; Sulis, M.L. Blinatumomab for Treatment of Children With High-risk Relapsed B-Cell Acute Lymphoblastic Leukemia. *JAMA* **2021**, *325*, 830–832. [CrossRef] [PubMed]
14. Inaba, H.; Pui, C.H. Immunotherapy in pediatric acute lymphoblastic leukemia. *Cancer Metastasis Rev.* **2019**, *38*, 595–610. [CrossRef] [PubMed]
15. Foster, J.B.; Maude, S.L. New developments in immunotherapy for pediatric leukemia. *Curr. Opin. Pediatr.* **2018**, *30*, 25–29. [CrossRef] [PubMed]
16. Bautista, F.; Van der Lugt, J.; Kearns, P.R.; Mussai, F.J.; Zwaan, C.M.; Moreno, L. The development of targeted new agents to improve the outcome for children with leukemia. *Expert Opin. Drug Discov.* **2016**, *11*, 1111–1122. [CrossRef] [PubMed]
17. Jasinski, S.; De Los Reyes, F.A.; Yametti, G.C.; Pierro, J.; Raetz, E.; Carroll, W.L. Immunotherapy in Pediatric B-Cell Acute Lymphoblastic Leukemia: Advances and Ongoing Challenges. *Paediatr. Drugs* **2020**, *22*, 485–499. [CrossRef] [PubMed]
18. Moher, D.; Liberati, A.; Tetzlaff, J.; Altman, D.G.; Group, P. Preferred reporting items for systematic reviews and meta-analyses: The PRISMA statement. *PLoS Med.* **2009**, *6*, e1000097. [CrossRef]
19. Handgretinger, R.; Zugmaier, G.; Henze, G.; Kreyenberg, H.; Lang, P.; von Stackelberg, A. Complete remission after blinatumomab-induced donor T-cell activation in three pediatric patients with post-transplant relapsed acute lymphoblastic leukemia. *Leukemia* **2011**, *25*, 181–184. [CrossRef]
20. Schlegel, P.; Lang, P.; Zugmaier, G.; Ebinger, M.; Kreyenberg, H.; Witte, K.E.; Feucht, J.; Pfeiffer, M.; Teltschik, H.M.; Kyzirakos, C.; et al. Pediatric posttransplant relapsed/refractory B-precursor acute lymphoblastic leukemia shows durable remission by therapy with the T-cell engaging bispecific antibody blinatumomab. *Haematologica* **2014**, *99*, 1212–1219. [CrossRef]
21. von Stackelberg, A.; Locatelli, F.; Zugmaier, G.; Handgretinger, R.; Trippett, T.M.; Rizzari, C.; Bader, P.; O'Brien, M.M.; Brethon, B.; Bhojwani, D.; et al. Phase I/Phase II Study of Blinatumomab in Pediatric Patients With Relapsed/Refractory Acute Lymphoblastic Leukemia. *J. Clin. Oncol.* **2016**, *34*, 4381–4389. [CrossRef]
22. Gore, L.; Locatelli, F.; Zugmaier, G.; Handgretinger, R.; O'Brien, M.M.; Bader, P.; Bhojwani, D.; Schlegel, P.G.; Tuglus, C.A.; von Stackelberg, A. Survival after blinatumomab treatment in pediatric patients with relapsed/refractory B-cell precursor acute lymphoblastic leukemia. *Blood Cancer J.* **2018**, *8*, 80. [CrossRef] [PubMed]

23. Brown, P.A.; Ji, L.; Xu, X.; Devidas, M.; Hogan, L.; Borowitz, M.J.; Raetz, E.A.; Zugmaier, G.; Sharon, E.; Gore, L.; et al. A Randomized Phase 3 Trial of Blinatumomab Vs. Chemotherapy As Post-Reinduction Therapy in High and Intermediate Risk (HR/IR) First Relapse of B-Acute Lymphoblastic Leukemia (B-ALL) in Children and Adolescents/Young Adults (AYAs) Demonstrates Superior Efficacy and Tolerability of Blinatumomab: A Report from Children's Oncology Group Study AALL1331. *Blood* **2019**, *134*, LBA-1. [CrossRef]
24. Locatelli, F.; Whitlock, J.A.; Peters, C.; Chen-Santel, C.; Chia, V.; Dennis, R.M.; Heym, K.M.; Katz, A.J.; Kelsh, M.A.; Sposto, R.; et al. Blinatumomab versus historical standard therapy in pediatric patients with relapsed/refractory Ph-negative B-cell precursor acute lymphoblastic leukemia. *Leukemia* **2020**, *34*, 2473–2478. [CrossRef]
25. Locatelli, F.; Zugmaier, G.; Mergen, N.; Bader, P.; Jeha, S.; Schlegel, P.G.; Bourquin, J.P.; Handgretinger, R.; Brethon, B.; Rossig, C.; et al. Blinatumomab in pediatric patients with relapsed/refractory acute lymphoblastic leukemia: Results of the RIALTO trial, an expanded access study. *Blood Cancer J.* **2020**, *10*, 77. [CrossRef] [PubMed]
26. Mouttet, B.; Vinti, L.; Ancliff, P.; Bodmer, N.; Brethon, B.; Cario, G.; Chen-Santel, C.; Elitzur, S.; Hazar, V.; Kunz, J.; et al. Durable remissions in TCF3-HLF positive acute lymphoblastic leukemia with blinatumomab and stem cell transplantation. *Haematologica* **2019**, *104*, e244–e247. [CrossRef] [PubMed]
27. Keating, A.K.; Gossai, N.; Phillips, C.L.; Maloney, K.; Campbell, K.; Doan, A.; Bhojwani, D.; Burke, M.J.; Verneris, M.R. Reducing minimal residual disease with blinatumomab prior to HCT for pediatric patients with acute lymphoblastic leukemia. *Blood Adv.* **2019**, *3*, 1926–1929. [CrossRef] [PubMed]
28. Wadhwa, A.; Kutny, M.A.; Xavier, A.C. Blinatumomab activity in a patient with Down syndrome B-precursor acute lymphoblastic leukemia. *Pediatr. Blood Cancer* **2018**, *65*. [CrossRef] [PubMed]
29. Elitzur, S.; Arad-Cohen, N.; Barzilai-Birenboim, S.; Ben-Harush, M.; Bielorai, B.; Elhasid, R.; Feuerstein, T.; Gilad, G.; Gural, A.; Kharit, M.; et al. Blinatumomab as a bridge to further therapy in cases of overwhelming toxicity in pediatric B-cell precursor acute lymphoblastic leukemia: Report from the Israeli Study Group of Childhood Leukemia. *Pediatr. Blood Cancer* **2019**, *66*, e27898. [CrossRef] [PubMed]
30. Pieters, R.; Schrappe, M.; De Lorenzo, P.; Hann, I.; De Rossi, G.; Felice, M.; Hovi, L.; LeBlanc, T.; Szczepanski, T.; Ferster, A.; et al. A treatment protocol for infants younger than 1 year with acute lymphoblastic leukaemia (Interfant-99): An observational study and a multicentre randomised trial. *Lancet* **2007**, *370*, 240–250. [CrossRef]
31. Pieters, R.; De Lorenzo, P.; Ancliffe, P.; Aversa, L.A.; Brethon, B.; Biondi, A.; Campbell, M.; Escherich, G.; Ferster, A.; Gardner, R.A.; et al. Outcome of Infants Younger Than 1 Year With Acute Lymphoblastic Leukemia Treated With the Interfant-06 Protocol: Results From an International Phase III Randomized Study. *J. Clin. Oncol.* **2019**, *37*, 2246–2256. [CrossRef]
32. Clesham, K.; Rao, V.; Bartram, J.; Ancliff, P.; Ghorashian, S.; O'Connor, D.; Pavasovic, V.; Rao, A.; Samarasinghe, S.; Cummins, M.; et al. Blinatumomab for infant acute lymphoblastic leukemia. *Blood* **2020**, *135*, 1501–1504. [CrossRef]
33. Contreras, C.F.; Higham, C.S.; Behnert, A.; Kim, K.; Stieglitz, E.; Tasian, S.K. Clinical utilization of blinatumomab and inotuzumab immunotherapy in children with relapsed or refractory B-acute lymphoblastic leukemia. *Pediatr. Blood Cancer* **2021**, *68*, e28718. [CrossRef]
34. Ampatzidou, M.; Kattamis, A.; Baka, M.; Paterakis, G.; Anastasiou, T.; Tzanoudaki, M.; Kaisari, A.; Avgerinou, G.; Doganis, D.; Papadakis, V.; et al. Insights from the Greek experience of the use of Blinatumomab in pediatric relapsed and refractory acute lymphoblastic leukemia patients. *Neoplasma* **2020**, *67*, 1424–1430. [CrossRef]
35. Horibe, K.; Morris, J.D.; Tuglus, C.A.; Dos Santos, C.; Kalabus, J.; Anderson, A.; Goto, H.; Ogawa, C. A phase 1b study of blinatumomab in Japanese children with relapsed/refractory B-cell precursor acute lymphoblastic leukemia. *Int. J. Hematol.* **2020**, *112*, 223–233. [CrossRef]
36. Queudeville, M.; Schlegel, P.; Heinz, A.T.; Lenz, T.; Doring, M.; Holzer, U.; Hartmann, U.; Kreyenberg, H.; von Stackelberg, A.; Schrappe, M.; et al. Blinatumomab in pediatric patients with relapsed/refractory B-cell precursor acute lymphoblastic leukemia. *Eur. J. Haematol.* **2021**, *106*, 473–483. [CrossRef] [PubMed]
37. Sutton, R.; Pozza, L.D.; Khaw, S.L.; Fraser, C.; Revesz, T.; Chamberlain, J.; Mitchell, R.; Trahair, T.N.; Bateman, C.M.; Venn, N.C.; et al. Outcomes for Australian children with relapsed/refractory acute lymphoblastic leukaemia treated with blinatumomab. *Pediatr. Blood Cancer* **2021**, *68*, e28922. [CrossRef] [PubMed]
38. Brown, P.A.; Ji, L.; Xu, X.; Devidas, M.; Hogan, L.E.; Borowitz, M.J.; Raetz, E.A.; Zugmaier, G.; Sharon, E.; Bernhardt, M.B.; et al. Effect of Postreinduction Therapy Consolidation With Blinatumomab vs Chemotherapy on Disease-Free Survival in Children, Adolescents, and Young Adults With First Relapse of B-Cell Acute Lymphoblastic Leukemia: A Randomized Clinical Trial. *JAMA* **2021**, *325*, 833–842. [CrossRef]
39. Locatelli, F.; Zugmaier, G.; Rizzari, C.; Morris, J.D.; Gruhn, B.; Klingebiel, T.; Parasole, R.; Linderkamp, C.; Flotho, C.; Petit, A.; et al. Effect of Blinatumomab vs Chemotherapy on Event-Free Survival Among Children With High-risk First-Relapse B-Cell Acute Lymphoblastic Leukemia: A Randomized Clinical Trial. *JAMA* **2021**, *325*, 843–854. [CrossRef] [PubMed]
40. Mejstrikova, E.; Hrusak, O.; Borowitz, M.J.; Whitlock, J.A.; Brethon, B.; Trippett, T.M.; Zugmaier, G.; Gore, L.; von Stackelberg, A.; Locatelli, F. CD19-negative relapse of pediatric B-cell precursor acute lymphoblastic leukemia following blinatumomab treatment. *Blood Cancer J.* **2017**, *7*, 659. [CrossRef] [PubMed]
41. Zoghbi, A.; Zur Stadt, U.; Winkler, B.; Muller, I.; Escherich, G. Lineage switch under blinatumomab treatment of relapsed common acute lymphoblastic leukemia without MLL rearrangement. *Pediatr. Blood Cancer* **2017**, *64*. [CrossRef]

42. Wolfl, M.; Rasche, M.; Eyrich, M.; Schmid, R.; Reinhardt, D.; Schlegel, P.G. Spontaneous reversion of a lineage switch following an initial blinatumomab-induced ALL-to-AML switch in MLL-rearranged infant ALL. *Blood Adv.* **2018**, *2*, 1382–1385. [CrossRef]
43. Mikhailova, E.; Gluhanyuk, E.; Illarionova, O.; Zerkalenkova, E.; Kashpor, S.; Miakova, N.; Diakonova, Y.; Olshanskaya, Y.; Shelikhova, L.; Novichkova, G.; et al. Immunophenotypic changes of leukemic blasts in children with relapsed/refractory B-cell precursor acute lymphoblastic leukemia, who have been treated with Blinatumomab. *Haematologica* **2020**. [CrossRef] [PubMed]
44. Brethon, B.; Lainey, E.; Caye-Eude, A.; Grain, A.; Fenneteau, O.; Yakouben, K.; Roupret-Serzec, J.; Le Mouel, L.; Cave, H.; Baruchel, A. Case Report: Targeting 2 Antigens as a Promising Strategy in Mixed Phenotype Acute Leukemia: Combination of Blinatumomab With Gemtuzumab Ozogamicin in an Infant With a KMT2A-Rearranged Leukemia. *Front. Oncol.* **2021**, *11*, 637951. [CrossRef]
45. Aldoss, I.; Song, J.Y. Extramedullary relapse of KMT2A(MLL)-rearranged acute lymphoblastic leukemia with lineage switch following blinatumomab. *Blood* **2018**, *131*, 2507. [CrossRef]
46. Kiyoi, H.; Morris, J.D.; Oh, I.; Maeda, Y.; Minami, H.; Miyamoto, T.; Sakura, T.; Iida, H.; Tuglus, C.A.; Chen, Y.; et al. Phase 1b/2 study of blinatumomab in Japanese adults with relapsed/refractory acute lymphoblastic leukemia. *Cancer Sci.* **2020**, *111*, 1314–1323. [CrossRef]
47. Bader, P.; Kreyenberg, H.; Henze, G.H.; Eckert, C.; Reising, M.; Willasch, A.; Barth, A.; Borkhardt, A.; Peters, C.; Handgretinger, R.; et al. Prognostic value of minimal residual disease quantification before allogeneic stem-cell transplantation in relapsed childhood acute lymphoblastic leukemia: The ALL-REZ BFM Study Group. *J. Clin. Oncol.* **2009**, *27*, 377–384. [CrossRef]
48. Tallen, G.; Ratei, R.; Mann, G.; Kaspers, G.; Niggli, F.; Karachunsky, A.; Ebell, W.; Escherich, G.; Schrappe, M.; Klingebiel, T.; et al. Long-term outcome in children with relapsed acute lymphoblastic leukemia after time-point and site-of-relapse stratification and intensified short-course multidrug chemotherapy: Results of trial ALL-REZ BFM 90. *J. Clin. Oncol.* **2010**, *28*, 2339–2347. [CrossRef] [PubMed]
49. von Stackelberg, A.; Volzke, E.; Kuhl, J.S.; Seeger, K.; Schrauder, A.; Escherich, G.; Henze, G.; Tallen, G.; Group, A.-R.B.S. Outcome of children and adolescents with relapsed acute lymphoblastic leukaemia and non-response to salvage protocol therapy: A retrospective analysis of the ALL-REZ BFM Study Group. *Eur. J. Cancer* **2011**, *47*, 90–97. [CrossRef] [PubMed]
50. Buitenkamp, T.D.; Izraeli, S.; Zimmermann, M.; Forestier, E.; Heerema, N.A.; van den Heuvel-Eibrink, M.M.; Pieters, R.; Korbijn, C.M.; Silverman, L.B.; Schmiegelow, K.; et al. Acute lymphoblastic leukemia in children with Down syndrome: A retrospective analysis from the Ponte di Legno study group. *Blood* **2014**, *123*, 70–77. [CrossRef]
51. Minson, K.A.; Prasad, P.; Vear, S.; Borinstein, S.; Ho, R.; Domm, J.; Frangoul, H. t(17;19) in Children with Acute Lymphocytic Leukemia: A Report of 3 Cases and a Review of the Literature. *Case Rep. Hematol.* **2013**, *2013*, 563291. [CrossRef] [PubMed]
52. Biondi, A.; Schrappe, M.; De Lorenzo, P.; Castor, A.; Lucchini, G.; Gandemer, V.; Pieters, R.; Stary, J.; Escherich, G.; Campbell, M.; et al. Imatinib after induction for treatment of children and adolescents with Philadelphia-chromosome-positive acute lymphoblastic leukaemia (EsPhALL): A randomised, open-label, intergroup study. *Lancet Oncol.* **2012**, *13*, 936–945. [CrossRef]
53. Dixon, S.B.; Chen, Y.; Yasui, Y.; Pui, C.H.; Hunger, S.P.; Silverman, L.B.; Ness, K.K.; Green, D.M.; Howell, R.M.; Leisenring, W.M.; et al. Reduced Morbidity and Mortality in Survivors of Childhood Acute Lymphoblastic Leukemia: A Report From the Childhood Cancer Survivor Study. *J. Clin. Oncol.* **2020**, *38*, 3418–3429. [CrossRef] [PubMed]
54. Tambaro, F.P.; Khazal, S.; Nunez, C.; Ragoonanan, D.; Tewari, P.; Petropoulos, D.; Kebriaei, P.; Wierda, W.G.; Mahadeo, K.M. Complete remission in refractory acute lymphoblastic leukemia using blinatumomab after failure of response to CD-19 chimeric antigen receptor T-cell therapy. *Clin. Case Rep.* **2020**, *8*, 1678–1681. [CrossRef] [PubMed]
55. Danylesko, I.; Chowers, G.; Shouval, R.; Besser, M.J.; Jacoby, E.; Shimoni, A.; Nagler, A.; Avigdor, A. Treatment with anti CD19 chimeric antigen receptor T cells after antibody-based immunotherapy in adults with acute lymphoblastic leukemia. *Curr. Res. Transl. Med.* **2020**, *68*, 17–22. [CrossRef] [PubMed]
56. Sigmund, A.M.; Sahasrabudhe, K.D.; Bhatnagar, B. Evaluating Blinatumomab for the Treatment of Relapsed/Refractory ALL: Design, Development, and Place in Therapy. *Blood Lymphat. Cancer* **2020**, *10*, 7–20. [CrossRef] [PubMed]

Review

Development of CAR T Cell Therapy in Children—A Comprehensive Overview

Michael Boettcher [1], Alexander Joechner [2,3], Ziduo Li [3], Sile Fiona Yang [3] and Patrick Schlegel [2,3,4,*]

1. Department of Pediatric Surgery, University Medical Centre Mannheim, University of Heidelberg, 69117 Heidelberg, Germany; michael.boettcher@umm.de
2. School of Medical Sciences, Faculty of Medicine and Health, University of Sydney, Sydney 2006, Australia; ajoechner@cmri.org.au
3. Cellular Cancer Therapeutics Unit, Children's Medical Research Institute, Sydney 2145, Australia; cli@cmri.org.au (Z.L.); syang@cmri.org.au (S.F.Y.)
4. Department of Pediatric Hematology and Oncology, Westmead Children's Hospital, Sydney 2145, Australia
* Correspondence: patrick.schlegel@sydney.edu.au

Abstract: CAR T cell therapy has revolutionized immunotherapy in the last decade with the successful establishment of chimeric antigen receptor (CAR)-expressing cellular therapies as an alternative treatment in relapsed and refractory CD19-positive leukemias and lymphomas. There are fundamental reasons why CAR T cell therapy has been approved by the Food and Drug administration and the European Medicines Agency for pediatric and young adult patients first. Commonly, novel therapies are developed for adult patients and then adapted for pediatric use, due to regulatory and commercial reasons. Both strategic and biological factors have supported the success of CAR T cell therapy in children. Since there is an urgent need for more potent and specific therapies in childhood malignancies, efforts should also include the development of CAR therapeutics and expand applicability by introducing new technologies. Basic aspects, the evolution and the drawbacks of childhood CAR T cell therapy are discussed as along with the latest clinically relevant information.

Keywords: evolution of CAR T cells; FDA-approved CAR products; TcR versus CAR; limitations and complications of CAR T cell therapy; future directions of CAR T cell therapy

1. Introduction

CAR T cell therapy has revolutionized immunotherapy in the last decade with the successful establishment of chimeric antigen receptor (CAR)-expressing cellular therapies as an alternative treatment in relapsed and refractory (r/r) homogeneously CD19-positive leukemias and lymphomas [1–3]. There are fundamental reasons why CAR T cell therapy has been approved by the Food and Drug administration (FDA) in the USA and the European Medicines Agency (EMA) for pediatric and young adult patients, as well as adult patients whose clinical data usually pave the way for translation of novel therapies into the clinic for children. Commonly, novel therapies are developed for the larger adult patient cohort, and then adapted for pediatric use, due to regulatory and commercial reasons [4,5]. Both strategic and biological factors have supported the development of CAR T cell therapy in children. The higher clinical relevance of CD19-positive malignancies in children compared to adults is one of the pivotal factors. B-cell acute lymphoblastic leukemia (B-ALL) is the most common pediatric malignancy, with a prevalence of up to 25% of cancers in all childhood cancers [6]. In contrast, the prevalence of all cancers in adults is below 0.5%, and B-cell non-Hodgkin's lymphoma (NHL) represents approximately 3.6% of adult cancers [7,8]. Despite the unprecedented success story of ALL treatment in childhood, with 5 year overall survival rates exceeding 90% in contemporary treatment optimization studies [9], prognosis for r/r patients and patients with high-risk predispositions is still dismal [10]. Therefore, there is an urgent need for improved and more specific therapies in r/r ALL to reduce the adverse event profile and prolong survival. Furthermore, the susceptibility of B-ALL to CAR T cell therapy is significantly higher [2] than that of chronic lymphoblastic leukemia (CLL) [11] and a broad variety of B-lineage-derived lymphomas [12].

In general, pediatric ALL is an unmatched success story in cancer treatment, with high overall survival (OS) rates throughout the Western world, drastically increasing from no chance of survival in the 1950s, ~10% OS in the 1960s, ~40% OS in the 1970s, ~65% in the 1980s, to survival rates above 90% today [9]. The main reason for the excellent survival rates is the sophisticated chemotherapy protocols that have been initiated and optimized over the last seven decades [13]. Moreover, major advances have been achieved with the development and improvement of allogeneic hematopoietic stem cell transplantation (allo-HSCT) [14] and immunotherapy with the bispecific T cell engager therapy (BiTE) blinatumomab (CD3XCD19) [15,16], which is currently trialed in patients with precursor B-ALL as an alternative to conventional intensive and toxic chemotherapies, and in patients who are at high risk of relapse post chemotherapy in the clinical trial AIEOP-BFM ALL 2017 (NCT03643276).

CD19-CAR T cell therapy has been a medical breakthrough in the treatment of pediatric ALL, demonstrated by its outstanding clinical success, which exceeds previous therapies including allo-HSCT and blinatumomab treatment in r/r patients considered to be incurable with a shortened life expectancy [2,17]. CD19-targeted CAR-expressing T cells (CD19-CAR-T) were able to cure pediatric patients with a single-agent infusion trialed as the last resort after blinatumomab therapy [2]. Subsequent exploration of CD19-CAR-T cell treatment also demonstrated success in r/r ALL patients post allo-HSCT after infusion of true-allogeneic CD19-CAR T cells (donor-derived) [18] and pseudo-allogeneic (posttransplant recipient-derived) CD19-CAR T cells [19]. In the landmark clinical trials NCT01626495 and NCT01029366, autologous CD19-CAR-T treatment resulted in a high response rate (90% complete remission induction) and a 50% long-term event-free survival, despite recruitment of a limited number (N = 25) of patients [2]. These unprecedented clinical data in CAR T cell trials have led to the FDA approval of the first CD19-CAR-T cell therapy in children and young adults with B-ALL in 2017.

To date, the clinical development of CAR T cell therapy has only been successful (beyond case reports) in B-lineage-derived acute and chronic hematologic malignancies [2,3,20]. The overwhelming and convincing clinical benefits over other existing treatments in r/r B-lineage malignancies have led to FDA and/or EMA approvals of more CD19-, as well as BCMA-targeted CAR therapeutics (Table 1). To date, r/r B-ALL [21], r/r diffuse large B-cell lymphoma (DLBCL) [22,23], r/r follicular lymphoma (FL) [22,23], mantle cell lymphoma (MCL) [24] and r/r multiple myeloma (MM) [25] can be treated successfully with the FDA-approved CAR products. Amongst the four approved CD19-CAR-T cell products, data to support the choice of the optimal therapy for different B-lineage-derived cancers are lacking, and further evaluation in clinical trials will be required to identify a treatment algorithm that enables timely and optimal use of these CAR T cell treatments [26]. The clinical success of CD19-CAR-T cell therapy has led to great expectations of translating CAR T cell strategies beyond B-lineage malignancies.

The future directions of CAR T cell therapy are to develop advanced CAR technologies to overcome the current limitations in CAR-mediated immunotherapy, which are toxicities and limited or lack of efficacy. Toxicities that arise from CAR T cell therapy include acute life-threatening complications, such as cytokine release syndrome (CRS) [27,28], immune effector cell-associated neurotoxicity syndrome (ICANS) [28] and mid-term and long-term side effects caused by profound B-cell aplasia that requires human IgG substitution to prevent severe infectious complications [29].

The long-term efficacy of CAR T cell therapy may be improved by addressing treatment failure due to antigen escape in pediatric patients. Relapses in approximately 25% of patients can be accounted for by antigen loss or downregulation, lineage switch or primary target antigen heterogeneity [30], lack of persistence and fitness of cells and resistance to CAR T cell therapy due to immunosuppressive factors such as immune checkpoint inhibition (PD-1), poor trafficking and tumor infiltration [31]. Chen et al. were able to identify gene signatures of TCF7 and IFN response genes in CD19-CAR-T cell products for pediatric patients to predict CAR T cell persistence, which is associated with long-term survival. Constant IFN signaling negatively impacts on CAR T cell performance. Thus, elucidating the underlying molecular determinants of clinical CAR T cell function may facilitate improving the clinical efficacy of CAR T cell therapy by adapting CAR T cell manufacturing to induce a favorable gene expression profile or by introducing novel genetic modifications [32]. Moreover, T cell exhaustion and senescence impact on the performance of T cells and CAR T cells. T cell senescence and restoration of T cell function are determinants of longevity and anticancer function but seem to be more evident in elderly patients than in children [33]. In solid cancers, immunosuppressive ligands and soluble factors, low oxygen and glucose levels in the tumor microenvironment (TME) have been identified to be the most important factors that limit the anticancer activity of CAR T therapeutics [34].

This review will provide insights into the molecular architecture and function of CAR T cells and touch on new advanced CAR technologies, as well as elucidating the importance of target antigens, the historic development of CAR technology and T cell receptor immunology. Further, the FDA/EMA-approved products will be reviewed to introduce the state-of-the-art CAR T cell therapy in children hitherto, covering major complications, relapse patterns and challenges of current CAR T cell concepts.

Table 1. FDA-approved CAR T cell products.

Name	Target Antigen	Brand	FDA Approval	Indications
Tisagenlecleucel	CD19	Kymriah	August 2017 May 2018	r/r B-cell precursor ALL, r/r large B-cell lymphoma
Axicabtagene ciloleucel	CD19	Yescarta	October 2017 March 2021	r/r large B-cell lymphoma r/r follicular lymphoma
Brexucabtagene autoleucel	CD19	Tecartus	July 2020 October 2021	r/r MCL (July 2020) r/r B-cell precursor ALL (Oct 2021)
Lisocabtagene maraleucel	CD19	Breyanzi	February 2021	r/r large B-cell lymphoma
Idecabtagene vicleucel	BCMA	Abecma	March 2021	r/r MM
Ciltacabtagene autoleucel	BCMA	Carvykti	February 2022	r/r MM

2. Methods

We used open-source medical and clinical trial databases including PubMed and Clinicaltrials.gov (accessed on 25 March 2022) to extract the information presented and discussed in this review article.

3. Molecular Architecture of CAR Receptors

CAR T cells are artificially generated transgenic cells that express a hybrid in silico designed de novo dimeric immune receptor. The basic architecture of CAR receptors is an extracellular antigen recognition domain, a spacer domain, a transmembrane domain, and an intracellular signaling domain [35]. Each domain of a CAR receptor has been intensively studied and variations have been designed and established successfully. It is noteworthy that critical steps in the development of CAR receptors were necessary to make CAR T cells potent therapeutics being capable of curing patients [36,37].

The main function and idea of CAR receptors are obviously to enable immune effector cells such as T cells and NK cells to be specifically redirected to cancer cells overexpressing the target antigen in a major histocompatibility complex (MHC)-independent manner [38,39]. scFv-based CAR receptors may also be constructed to target peptides presented by the MHC, for instance HLA-A2/NY-ESO-1 [40]. In Figure 1, the CAR architecture is illustrated and indicates established domain-variations.

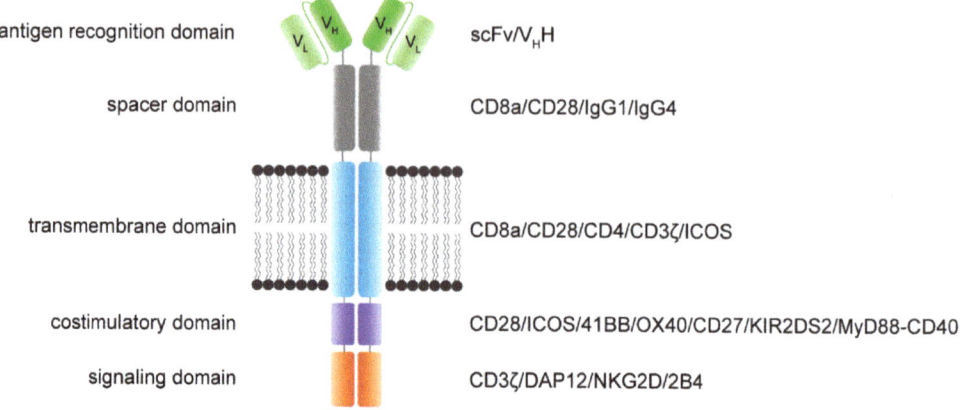

Figure 1. Functional modules of CAR receptors.

A schematic illustration of a second-generation CAR receptor. CAR receptors are comprised of several modules indicated in different colors—the antigen recognition domain, which usually consists of an antibody-derived scFv or V_HH, the spacer domain of variable length, configuration, and flexibility, connecting the antigen recognition domain to the transmembrane domain. The transmembrane domain robustly anchors the CAR in the phospholipid bilayer cell membrane and is linked to the intracellular parts of the artificial immune receptor. Thus, another important role of the transmembrane domain is to facilitate the mechanic signal transduction into the cell. The intracellular costimulatory domains and signaling domain transform the activation signal via a signaling cascade into the cell to activate downstream signaling that results in various effector functions such as cytolysis, cytokine secretion and proliferation. scFv: single-chain variable fragment; V_HH: heavy chain variable fragment of a single-domain antibody; V_L: variable fragment of the light chain; V_H: variable fragment of the heavy chain.

A CAR is a modular structure typically consisting of an extracellular antigen-binding domain linked by a spacer region to a transmembrane domain, attached to one or more intracellular activation domains. In general, every subunit of a CAR can significantly change the properties and function of the CAR receptor. CAR design has evolved over the last three decades, with the goal to improve CAR T cell efficacy, persistence, and safety.

The extracellular recognition domain in most CAR receptors is derived from the variable segments of the antibody light and heavy chains. They are constructed in line with peptide linkers [35,38] to assemble in a single-chain variable fragment (scFv) format. In general, scFvs are less stable in their configuration compared to the Fab region of antibodies [41]. Most antibodies in the past were generated by immunization of mice [42]. Today, fully human antibodies can be generated [43]. Single-domain VH binders (sdFv) based on human libraries or camelid binders or alternative formats can also be used as recognition domains [44]. The advantage of camelid sdFv is the reduced genetic load (half the size), reduced immunogenicity and the reduced tendency for aggregation while retaining the same specificity and affinity [45]. For hidden epitopes, the sdFv may be advantageous for the initial interaction of the targeted epitope compared to scFv based targeting due to less steric hinderance, higher solubility and the stability. Further, ligand-based CAR recognition domains have been introduced to target BCMA via trimeric APRIL [46], and the small chlorotoxin, a naturally derived 36-amino-acid-long peptide found in the venom of the death stalker scorpion leiurus quinquestriatus, which selectively binds to primary brain cancers is used for the treatment of glioblastoma (GBM) [47]. The basic requirement of recognition domains is the specific and rapid binding to the targeted antigen with the recognition domain to facilitate the CAR engagement.

The structural domains including the spacer (also called hinge) and transmembrane domains stabilize the receptor and allow the functional presentation of the recognition domain. They shape the extracellular configuration of the receptor and connect the extracellular domains to the intracellular modules of the receptor to facilitate an efficient mechanistic signal transduction to the intracellular signaling domains. Various protein subunits derived from CD8a, CD28, and IgG hinge regions also in combination with IgG CH_2 and CH_3 domains and others have been utilized as spacer domains, which have shown distinct properties. The most frequently used transmembrane domains are derived from the CD8a and CD28 [48].

The intracellular signaling domains usually contain one or more costimulatory domains and a signaling domain. Costimulatory domains are mainly derived from two families, namely the immunoglobulin superfamily, which is represented by CD28 and ICOS, and the tumor necrosis factor receptor superfamily (TNFR) represented by 4-1BB, OX40 and CD27. Signaling domains are mainly derived from the CD3ζ chain, while alternative signaling domains such as DAP12 have been used [49–51].

4. Exponential Evolution in CAR T Cell Development

The early development of CAR receptors was hampered by the limited speed in molecular and synthetic biology in the late 1980s to perform high-throughput screenings [35]. The basic technologies required for CAR generation have evolved rapidly and made CAR manufacturing a standard GMP procedure [52] that can be partially automated today [53]. In the past decade, CAR patenting activity has exponentially increased by 100-fold from academic institutions and pharmaceutical companies [54], demonstrating the clinical and commercial impact of CAR T cell therapy today. Advancements in synthetic biology and gene synthesis technology has come to speed and allows screening of large gene libraries with thousands of different CAR constructs in a very short time nowadays, making the work much more time-efficient and studying detailed variations of CAR receptors possible. For instance, CAR receptor signaling can be systematically evaluated in response to combinations and mutations in costimulatory domains, transcriptional regulation enhancement and perturbation, gene knockdowns, knockouts, and knockins, which could not be addressed in the past in a timely manner [55,56]. Moreover, the refinement of phage display [57] and deimmunization strategies [58,59] have dawned a new era of generating binding sequences such as scFvs according to biological requirements at a high pace, compared to conventional laborious methods including mouse immunization followed by hybridoma screening, single-B-cell screening, and the use of transgenic mice with fully human variable regions to discover fully human mAbs through mouse immunization and screening [42,60].

5. The Evolution of CAR Receptors

The evolution of CAR T cells is illustrated in Figure 2. The original concept of a T body, considered as the prototype of a CAR, was invented by Eshhar et al. in the 1980s [35]; following that, the first scFv-based CARs, which were also created by Eshhar et al. in the early 1990s [38]. The critical step in the evolution of CAR T cells was the introduction of a costimulatory domain in the late 1990s by various CAR labs all around the world to mature from a first- to second-generation CAR [37]. From today's perspective, first-generation CARs remain historic anecdotes.

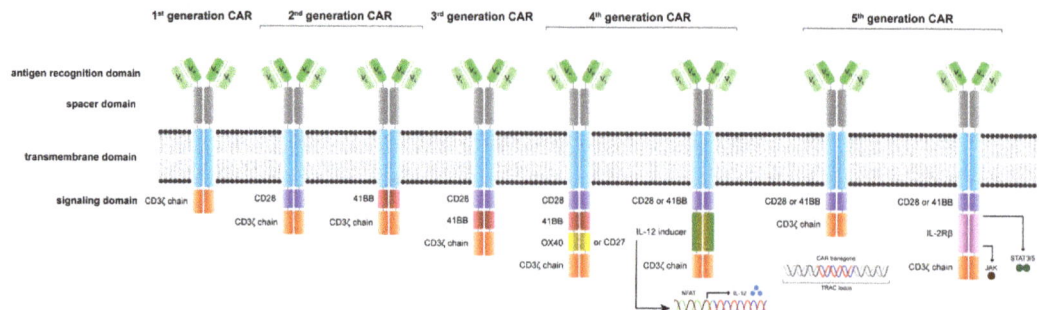

Figure 2. Evolution of CAR receptors.

In the evolution of CAR design, the number of intracellular signaling domains were increased in later generations to enhance the potency and persistence of the CAR T cells. The extracellular domain is comprised of an antigen recognition domain, followed by the spacer, the transmembrane domain and the intracellular signaling domains. First-generation CAR T cells relied on the signaling of the CD3ζ chain only, whereas second-generation CARs incorporate two signaling domains, and third-generation CARs three signaling domains. The nomenclature of higher CAR T cell generations or next-generation CAR T cell technologies is not clearly defined. Fourth-generation CAR constructs may incorporate four signaling domains, may incorporate an inducible suicide switch (iCasp9) [61] or may conditionally secrete cytokines such as IL-12 in a CAR activation-dependent manner under an inducible promotor containing NFAT, NF$_K$B or AP-1 responsive elements [62]. Site-specific CAR transgene integration at the TRAC locus leads to a functional collapse of the CD3 complex (TcR knockout, abrogation of GvHD) and may facilitate a more physiological CAR expression [63] and can be considered a fifth-generation CAR T technology. Additionally, the integration of IL-2Rß signaling that allows JAK/STAT pathway activation has been used under the term fifth-generation CAR technology [64]. Most used and validated costimulatory signaling domains include CD28, 4-1BB, OX40 and CD27 or a combination thereof. CD3ζ chain signaling is the most common signaling component of CAR receptors to date. CAR: chimeric antigen receptor. V_H/V_L: variable heavy chain and variable light chain of a single-chain variable fragment (scFv).

Although CAR technology has gone through a fast human-made scientific evolution, awareness of the rather slow progress in CAR technology shall change our language around CAR T cells being a novel kind of treatment. In recent years, high-throughput synthetic biology has come to speed and has led to a significant acceleration in the development of applied molecular genetics [55,56].

The early first-generation CARs demonstrated limited activity due to various factors, largely attributable to failure in generating high-quality CAR products and the design of the molecular structure of CARs [38]. First-generation CARs comprised only a CD3ζ chain signaling domain, which lead to poor signal transduction, resulting in antigen-specific in vitro activation of CAR T cells that have cancer cell killing activity, but lack the ability for sufficient proliferation and engraftment in vivo [65]. Costimulatory domains derived from activating immune co-receptors such as the CD28 family and the TNF-receptor family are introduced in second-generation CARs [36,37], resulting in a sufficient signal transduction that leads to a stronger activation, cytokine production, proliferation, persistence and increased fitness of CAR-expressing effector T cells [36,37,65,66]. All currently FDA/EMA-approved CAR products are second-generation CAR-T cell products. They are illustrated in Figure 3 and will be discussed in a later section. Additional attempts to improve the potency of CAR constructs are illustrated in Figure 2. Yet, there are numerous other technologies that are not included in this review.

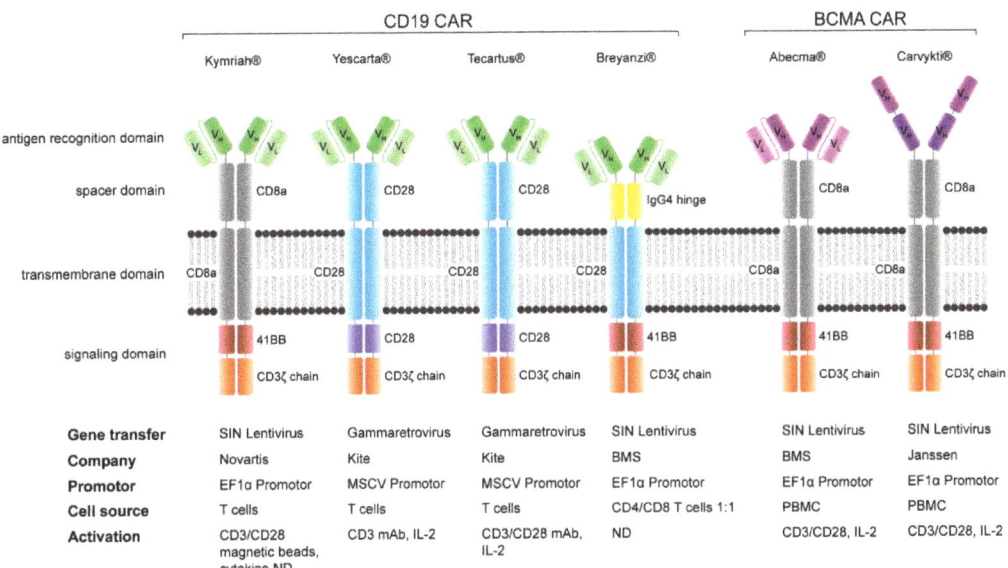

Figure 3. FDA-approved CAR T cell products.

6. Link of CAR Architecture and Function

The CAR architecture and its modules define the function of CAR receptors. The overall performance of CAR-expressing cells is defined by the cell type and cell origin (NK cells [67] versus T cells [68]), and the immunophenotype representing the multiplicity of interacting immune receptors [69]. The subunits of a CAR are clearly correlated with their primary as well as secondary functions. Shaping CAR function is possible; however, complete control of CAR function by architecture design is impossible because artificial proteins have their own properties and always lack evolutionary-based optimization.

The primary function and performance of a CAR are antigen recognition and engagement of the CAR-expressing cell with the target cell, the activation of the effector cell, polarization, formation of the cytolytic synapse, the initiation of cytotoxic action and induction of apoptosis in the target cell-mediated by the CAR, as well as the alteration of the gene expression and the persistent genetic imprint. The secondary function of CAR-expressing cells is more complex and more difficult to assess, simply for the factor of time. Long-term persistence, cellular metabolism, and its impact on cell fate are defined by non-immediate interactions and mechanisms. Most of the clinically relevant knowledge that we acquired about CAR-expressing cells is from applications in humans [70]. The translation from mice to human is the most challenging step. Curing mice is "easy" compared to curing humans. Mice are fantastic models to understand the biology of CARs, but real understanding is gained through human applications. As a result, despite accelerated development in preclinical sciences including gene synthesis, large high-throughput data acquisition and analysis technologies supported by artificial intelligence, only time-consuming clinical trials that take years to complete will reveal the truth of CARs in the context of human patients. Hence, clinical trials present the bottleneck in CAR development, especially in rare cancers with low patient numbers such as in pediatrics [70,71]. Nonetheless, all the excellent preclinical work provide the objectives and the rationale to run the most promising clinical trials and consequently save time in the development of next-generation CAR therapeutics.

The basic and simplified principle of a CAR receptor is to make an effector cell, e.g., a T cell, specifically engage with a target cell that expresses the targeted antigen, for instance CD19. By recognizing and binding to the target antigen, the CAR-expressing cell is strongly attached in close proximity at approximately 10–40 nm distance to the target cell, a distance comparable to TcR–pMHC interactions [72,73]. The CAR receptor is constructed in a way that it transduces an activation signal into the CAR T cells, which in most cases mimics the response of a T cell receptor (TcR) via CD3ζ chain signaling. Basically, the mechanic lever of the CAR receptor leads to a signal transduction into the T cell, mimicking TcR signaling, which triggers a complex downstream signaling machinery with a multitude of effector functions within minutes [74]. Thus, a CAR is hijacking the function of the TcR to efficiently target surface expressed antigens in a MHC-independent non-restricted manner. However, CARs are not as good as canonical TcRs. Given the fact that TcRs are perfected by evolution over several hundred millions of years [75] and CAR technology has only a short history of development of 30 years [35,38], the results we have achieved using CARs are quite remarkable. On the other hand, failures in CAR development have taught us to appreciate the importance of the biology of effector cells, especially of T cells, and cancer biology in order to advance CAR therapeutics to the next level. This topic is discussed further in the review article by Waldman et al. "A guide to cancer immunotherapy: from T cell basic science to clinical practice" [76].

7. CD19—A Curse and Blessing

CAR T cell functions have been widely studied in CD19-CARs. So, why is that the case? The answer is shockingly simple—because CD19-CAR-Tcells work remarkably well. Several factors have facilitated successful treatment with CD19-CAR-T cells.

7.1. CD19 Antigen

One crucial factor is the suitability of CD19 to serve as a CAR-targeted antigen [2,3]. The optimal cancer antigen is differentially overexpressed in cancer tissues and is not co-expressed on vitally essential tissues, and it is homogeneously expressed at high levels in all cancer cells [77]. Furthermore, it shows stable antigen expression irrespective of the cell cycle or treatment with no escape mechanism such as downregulation or loss of the antigen, and the antigen must be accessible for a CAR expressed by an effector cell [78,79] and not only by a soluble protein such as an antibody. On these premises, CD19 is not the perfect CAR antigen as patients treated with CD19-CAR-T cells develop immune escape variants. Nonetheless, CD19 is the best CAR target antigen available to date in terms of clinical efficacy [80].

CD19 is almost a perfect antigen with high expression levels in a large fraction of acute and chronic B-lineage-derived malignancies [81] with high and stable expression from early progenitor cells to late maturated B cells [77]. Besides, the generally high antigen density of CD19 in the range of several thousand molecules per cell (4000–25,000/cell) in BCP-ALL [82]. CD19 is a high-quality antigen because of the small size of its extracellular domain (271 amino acids), the configuration of the extracellular domain and the easy accessibility of its targeted epitope [83,84]. In multiply relapsed disease, patients may experience CD19$_{low}$ (several hundred molecules per cell) or negative leukemia, yet the expression level in most cases still exceeds the expression of CD22, an alternative CAR-targeted antigen [83,84]. To recruit CAR-T cells to lyse target cells under optimized in vitro conditions, as low as 200 molecules per cell can be sufficient. However, to induce cytokine secretion, 10× more molecules are required [85] and the activation threshold clearly depends on the CAR architecture, especially the costimulatory domain and of course also on the targeted antigen [86].

High-affinity anti-CD19 antibodies have been generated by immunization of mice. CD19 carries several immunogenic epitopes, with one prominent epitope (around loop [87–95]), against which numerous high-affinity antibody clones (FMC63, AB1, B4, 4G7, HD37, BU12, F974A2, and SJ25) have been generated [96]. The most commonly used scFv in CD19-CAR-T cells is based on the murine FMC63 clone [26] which binds CD19 at a picomolar affinity (0.32 nM) [97]. Fortunately, the FMC63-based scFvs do not show any tendency for tonic signaling in the context of CAR-expressing cells [98]. All

FDA/EMA-approved CD19-CAR-T products are based on the murine FMC63 recognition domain (scFv) [26].

7.2. CD19 in Comparison to Other Leukemia-Associated Antigens

The distance of the T cell to the target cell is critical for optimal effector function. In native T cells, the TcR–pMHC interaction occurs at a distance of approximately 15 nm [99,100]. For optimal CAR T cell engagement, the distance between the CAR T cell and the target cell is also a determining factor of CAR function [101]. CD19 appears to be an optimal CAR target antigen compared to other interesting alternatives such as CD22 [102].

The spatial distance of T cells engaging with virus-infected or cancerous cells via T cell receptor (TcR) engagement is approximately 15 nm. Most CAR receptors mimic the function of the TcR via CD3ζ chain signaling. FDA/EMA-approved CAR products are optimized to operate at the distance of TcR–MHC synapses. If the distance between the effector cell and the target cell is too long, the formation of the cytolytic synapse is impaired and CAR targeting is non-efficient which results in poor CAR function. Thus, choosing the best suitable targeted epitope is critical for the function of CAR T cells targeted to proteins with a large extracellular domain. However, target antigens cannot be modified and therefore the CAR receptor must be adapted perfectly to engage with the target antigen and initiate the formation of the cytolytic synapse. CAR function in CD19 and BCMA-targeting CARs is supported by the small extracellular domain. CD22 CARs require targeting of a proximal epitope, since targeting a distal epitope of the large extracellular domain hinders the formation of a cytolytic synapse [103,104]. The proximal epitope is recognized by the mouse antibody clone m971. More distal epitopes are targeted by the mouse antibody clones HA22 and BL2 which do not translate in any relevant effector function used in CAR-expressing cells [104]. In the FDA/EMA-approved CAR-T cell products, the recognition domain for CD19-CAR-T cells is based on a scFv, derived from the mouse anti-CD19 antibody clone FMC63 [21], and in idecabtagene vicleucel Abecma®, the only BCMA-CAR-T cell product on the market to date, was constructed from the mouse anti-BCMA antibody clone C11D5.3.

Alternative target antigens in the treatment of BCP-ALL are CD20, CD22, CD38 and CD79B. The expression level varies significantly between CD10$^+$ and CD10$^-$ BCP ALL, with unfavorable prognosis of CD10$^-$ leukemia [105]. CD38 is homogenously expressed across BCP-ALL, whereas CD22 has a higher expression in CD10$^+$ BCP-ALL, and CD20 is expressed only in CD10$^+$ in 42% of patients [106].

In patients who experienced CD19-negative relapse after CD19-CAR-T cell treatment, CD22-targeted CAR T cells are able to induce complete remissions [107]. However, the expression of CD22 in general is lower than CD19 and leukemia-free survival is significantly lower than in CD19-CAR-T cell therapy [104]. Due to the high risk of relapse post CD22-CAR-T cell therapy, subsequent allogeneic stem cell transplantation in molecular remission is highly recommended as patients are unlikely to survive without consolidation therapy by allo-HSCT [84]. Relapsed patients showed a significantly reduced CD22 expression at diagnosis compared to the pre-treatment condition, which is indicative of the selective evolutionary pressure. Thus, combinatorial CD19-CD22 bivalent CAR T cells may reduce the risk for leukemia recurrence and are studied in clinical trials in children and adults [80]. In preclinical models, trispecific CD19-CD20-CD22 CAR T cells can control heterogenous cancers [108,109]; however, antigen loss remains the major cause of CAR T cell resistance also in dual-targeted CAR therapies [80]. Strategies to specifically increase the target antigen expression by co-administration of medications, such as Bryostatin1 to increase CD22 levels, can improve CAR T cell performance, but curing patients will depend on a robust target antigen expression [110]. In preclinical models, CD20 [111], CD22 [84], CD38 [112] and CD79B [87] CAR T cells have been proven efficacious and are used in clinical trials to treat B-lineage malignancies. CD38 CAR T cells can also be used for the treatment of T ALL and AML [113], but they are associated with a broader spectrum of toxicities in the lymphoid and myeloid compartment and leads to fratricide of early T cell progenitor cells [112]. In Figure 4, the structural properties of the CAR target antigens CD19, BCMA and CD22 are illustrated.

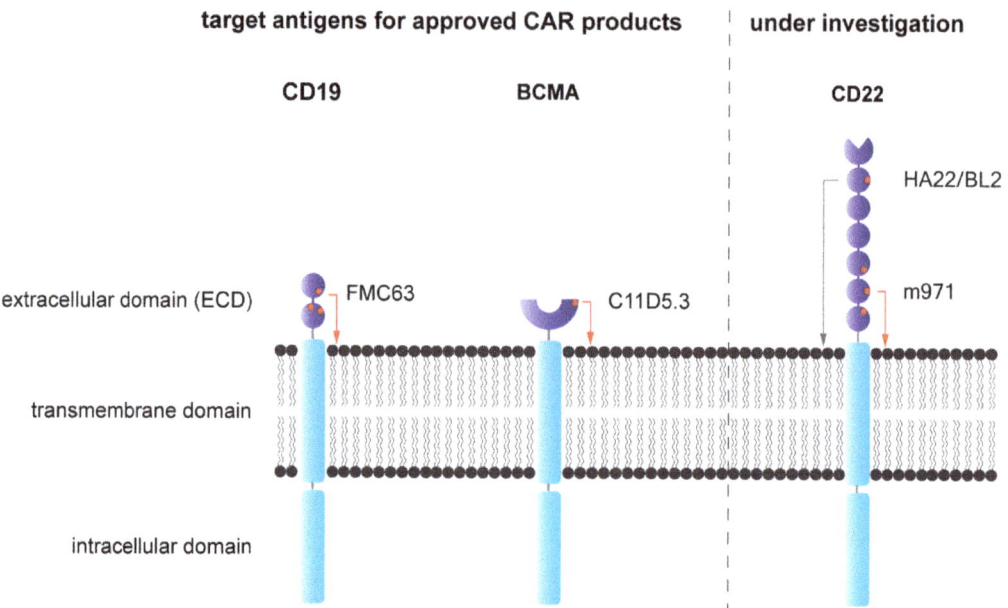

Figure 4. Mechanistic challenges of CAR-targeted antigens.

The use of CAR T cells for the treatment of acute myeloid leukemia (AML) is challenging due to dramatic on-target off-tumor toxicities. The most effective AML-associated CAR-targeted antigens such as CD33 and CD123 are co-expressed in hematopoietic progenitor cells [114]. Strong activity of CD33- [115] or CD123-CAR-T cells can lead to profound depletion of the myeloid compartment [116,117] that is acceptable only for a limited time frame within the range of several weeks because lethal infectious complications including systemic and invasive bacterial and fungal infections result from mid-term agranulocytosis, which is a major cause for transplant-related mortality in allogeneic stem cell transplantation with delayed myeloid immune reconstitution [118]. Many cancer-associated overexpressed antigens cannot be targeted continuously on a tissue-depletion level, because lethal inflammatory complications can lead to organ failure. Thus, transient targeting may provide a solution for targeting non-exclusive overexpressed antigens as CAR targets.

8. A Paradigm without a Shift—Affinity and CAR Performance

In the context of CAR-mediated cancer targeting, predominantly the affinity of the recognition domain, but also the signaling as well as the structural domains determine the CAR activation threshold to the corresponding target antigen density, which allows the CAR to successfully recognize and engage with low antigen-expressing cancer cells [86,119,120]. As immune escape mediated by downregulation or any functional antigen loss is the major cause of relapse in CD19-CAR-T cell-treated patients, it appears favorable for CD19-CAR-T cells to also engage with $CD19_{low}$-expressing cancer cells [2,78,121] at the price of on-target off-tumor toxicity on healthy cells, e.g., neurons with low CD19 expression. High-affinity CD19-CAR-T cells (FMC63, K_D 0.32 nM) may have a lower risk of antigen escape variants as a result of reduced CD19 antigen expression required to be recognized and eliminated by high-affinity CD19-CAR-T cells, compared to moderately reduced-affinity CD19-CAR-T cells (CAT19) [2,97]. Conversely, the severe neurotoxicity (ICANS) can be ameliorated by using reduced-affinity CD19-CAR-T cells (CAT19, K_D 14 nM), which may however not engage with $CD19_{low}$-expressing cancer cells on the other end. Despite that CAT19 CD19-CAR-T cells have been reported to show a greater tendency for rapid expansion and persistence compared to high-affinity CD19-CAR-T cells based on (FMC63), the commonly observed life-threatening toxicities CRS and ICANS occurred significantly less [97]. However, comparing the outcome of high-affinity versus reduced-affinity CD19-CAR-T cell-treated patients, event-free survival revealed substantial differences. Under the current circumstances with limited clinical data available, the most relevant and alarming discriminator of high- versus reduced-affinity CD19-CAR-T cell-treated patients seems to be the significantly increased risk of CD19-negative and $CD19_{low}$ relapse in the reduced-affinity CAT19 CD19-CAR-T-treated cohort (35%, 5/14 pts) [97] compared to 10–20% in high-affinity FMC63-based CD19-CAR-T-treated patients [2]. With regard to mediating tumor lysis via secondary mechanisms, cytokine secretion plays an important role to facilitate the elimination of $antigen_{low}$ and antigen-negative tumor cell populations [122], and thus activation thresholds based on the variables antigen density, scFv affinity and signaling also determine the performance of CAR T cells in antigen-negative cancer cells [30,86].

8.1. Comparison of the T Cell Receptor and a Chimeric Antigen Receptor

The recognition domain is one of the subunits responsible for determining the antigen-density activation threshold in CAR-expressing immune cells [101]. The signaling domains also have an impact on the antigen-density threshold [86]. As discussed above, in comparison to TcRs, the activation threshold of CAR receptors is at least a 100-fold higher [123]. This means 100-fold more antigens on the cell surface are necessary to engage a CAR T cell compared to native unmodified T cells via TcR engagement [124]. Even though TcRs have an affinity in the micromolar range (1 to 50 uM), the signaling, especially the ZAP70 recruitment of the CD3ζ chain, is much more efficient in native TcRs compared to artificial CAR receptors [125]. In general, TcR-mediated and CAR-mediated targeting involve two separate mechanisms with the same goal to eliminate aberrant cells. While TcRs are highly specific to changes in the genome, e.g., mutations or foreign non-human proteins, CARs recognize cancer-associated antigens. The level of aberrant peptides presented by MHC (pMHC) in cancer is very low [126], inconsistent and heterogenous compared to pMHC in virus-infected cells [127]. In virus-infected cells, the interaction of TcR and MHC is more potent and still the total number of available pMHC complexes often is lower than the minimum target antigen expression required for substantial CAR engagement [84,86,127]. These comparisons are important and drives major implications on how to reconstruct new artificial receptors with higher sensitivity [123,128]. Despite TcRs having the superior capability for lower target antigen density, CAR-expressing cells are extraordinary in their performance, as CAR receptors facilitate antigen-specific immune responses in a novel mode of action that native T cells with their TcRs cannot achieve. CAR signaling must be adapted to the expressed antigen density in wise consideration of the targeted antigen to balance efficacy and toxicity [129,130]. Therefore, the super high sensitivity of TcR-mediated targeting for the target antigen CD19 would potentially lead to self-destruction of vitally essential tissues including CD19+ cells in the CNS. High-sensitivity CAR designs may also drive exhaustion due to the abundance and consecutive overactivation during the targeting process [129]. T cells, unlike CAR-T cells, are designed to detect and function on a low or very low-antigen pMHC frequency level [123]. In general, depending on the targeted antigen, CAR function requires adaptation to the expression level of the targeted antigen. As there are no exclusive surface expressed cancer antigens (MHC independent), the sensitivity of the CAR has to be fine-tuned and adapted to react robustly with cancer cells and shall not engage with healthy tissue at best, if the target antigen is co-expressed on vitally essential tissues [97,119]. In some respects, the almost exclusive target antigens CD19, CD20 and CD22 for B-lineage-derived cells are exceptions, as the B-lineage compartment can be regarded as non-vitally essential tissue [131]. CAR receptors by nature cover a different range of target antigen density than TcRs and to date the activation threshold has not been successfully tuned to the same sensitivity level as TcRs [123]. The clou of

CAR-mediated targeting is not to find a way to make a CAR another variant of a TcR, which it is not, but rather to appreciate the limitations of CAR targeting and identify smart combinations of CAR targeting to increase the potency of CAR technologies [80,132].

8.2. Requirement for CAR Optimization per Antigen

For every target antigen, the challenge is to identify the best CAR architecture with an optimized sensitivity for that particular target antigen to balance anticancer activity and on-target off-tumor toxicity in order to prevent fatal complications [130]. The threshold is thought to be above the low threshold target antigen density of CD19 [129]. To date, no CAR T has been identified to target at a lower antigen threshold density (molecules per cell surface) than CD19-CARs and most likely the target antigen threshold for most antigens will be in the range of several 1000 molecules per cell and above [30,84,86]. Understanding the complexity of CAR targeting requires rethinking and thinking beyond CD19. Even though CD20, CD22 and BCMA are almost exclusive B-lineage-derived antigens, the targeting is less potent and reveal the molecular challenge in CAR T cell therapy, which are the identification and fine-tuning of the most efficient CAR T cells in an approach tailored to the target antigen expression. It is noteworthy that high-affinity CARs compared to low-affinity CARs show an improved recognition capability of low-expressed target antigens. On the other hand, they are more likely to exhaust, and long-term persistence may be impaired. Further, CRS and ICANS are more common in high-affinity CD19-CAR-Tcells [97]. As a result, patients who receive low-affinity CD19-CAR-T cell treatment appear to be at a higher risk to experience $CD19_{low}$ and CD19-negative leukemia recurrence which is less common in high-affinity CD19-CAR-T cell therapy [2,97].

Generally speaking, the sweet spot of CAR targeting is reached at the point where cancer is specifically targeted, while the CARs are not overactivated, lose their fitness through exhaustion and lack persistence. There is a need to achieve a target antigen-specific balance to facilitate robust anticancer immunity with acceptable on-target off-tumor toxicity [119]. Current CAR concepts are limited in their ability to meet these complex and dynamic criteria, but next-generation CAR designs with the ability of combinatorial targeting may solve some of these problems [132].

9. Immunogenicity of CAR Products

Originally, CAR receptors used to be artificial immune receptors composed of murine and human protein sequences making them a chimeric receptor. Today, fully human CAR receptors can be generated [133], which should be appreciated in the nomenclature of artificial immune receptors. This may seem to be a minor difference in the molecular anatomy and evolution of CAR receptors, considering the few changes of the amino acid residues only in the recognition domain, the single-chain variable fragment (scFv) [134].

However, these minor differences in immunogenicity may as well be one of the key changes, making CAR-expressing cells applicable to a broader range of antigens with reduced risk of antibody-mediated CAR rejection [135]. Another way of potentially decreasing the immunogenicity of a recognition domain is to reduce the size and simplify the structure to single-domain heavy-chain-only binding domains [136]. By CAR-specific depletion of the antibody producing cells including the B cells and the plasma cells, CAR effector cells targeting B-lineage malignancies inherently suppress the generation of anti-CAR antibodies. However, antitransgene rejection of CAR T cells has been observed in CD19- and CD20-CAR-T cells [137] as well as in CAR-T cells targeted to non-B-lineage-associated antigens[131]. Thus, the function of the B-lineage compartment is dramatically impaired by CAR T cell therapy targeted to B-lineage-associated antigens such as CD19, CD20, CD22 and BCMA [138,139].

Anti-CAR humoral response is capable of rejecting non-human proteins, especially those highly expressed and accessible on the cell surface such as CAR receptors on CAR-expressing cells distributed in the whole body [103]. Besides the production of immunoglobulins, B-lineage-derived cells are regarded as professional antigen-presenting cells (APCs) to ensure effective production of high-affinity antigen-specific antibodies while minimizing the production of non-specific antibodies and auto-antibodies [140]. As CAR receptors are expressed at very high levels > 50,000 molecules per cell [141], presentation of non-human immunogenic peptide sequences by MHC bears the risk of T cell-mediated immune rejection. Thus, the risk of T-cell-mediated CAR elimination is also reduced by depleting B-lineage-derived cells which act as antigen-presenting cells.

Targeting non-B-lineage-associated antigens does not impact on the B-cell compartment and thus does not inhibit its function. Logically, both the risk of immune rejection of CAR-expressing cells via antibodies targeted to the murine extracellular component of the CAR as well as T cell-mediated CAR rejection are higher in CAR T cells targeting antigens that do not suppress the humoral immune response.

Potent strategies to reduce the risk of immune-mediated rejection of CAR-expressing cells include deimmunization, humanization and the generation of fully human CAR sequences [58,133,142]. In theory, fully human CAR constructs should not be recognized as foreign proteins and trigger an immune response. The truth, however, is that immune rejection may occur in response to any synthetic protein as it is of non-human origin and in the light of autoimmune phenomena, we know that naturally present physiological human proteins may be attacked by the immune system as a result of cross-reactivity with immune responses against pathogens (virus, bacteria, fungus) [143]. Errors in the maturation of immune cells may cause transient or chronic autoinflammation, partially leading to devastating autoimmune diseases such as Crohn's disease [144,145]. The development of antidrug antibodies against the fully human anti-TNFα antibody adalimumab is associated with treatment failure [146]. Nonetheless, all mentioned strategies to reduce the immunogenicity of foreign proteins have been proven efficacious.

10. Comparison of FDA/EMA-Approved CAR-T Cell Products

The CD19-targeting FDA/EMA-approved CAR-T cell products are constructed in distinct architectures, even though they share the same recognition domain derived from the murine FMC63 IgG2a antibody clone with the same orientation (VL-VH) of the single-chain variable fragment (scFv) [21]. Despite these differences, all CD19-CAR-T cell constructs—tisagenlecleucel (marketing name Kymriah®), axicabtagene ciloleucel (marketing name Yescarta®), brexucabtagene autoleucel (marketing name Tecartus®), and lisocabtagene maraleucel (marketing name Breyanzi®)—have demonstrated outstanding clinical performance in various B-lineage malignancies [2,3,22–24,147,148]. Tisagenlecleucel was FDA approved and later approved by the EMA based on the findings in the clinical trial "Study of Efficacy and Safety of CTL019 in Pediatric ALL Patients (ELIANA)" with the ClinicalTrials.gov identifier: NCT02435849, funded by Novartis [2,21,149]. Recently, the BCMA-targeted CAR T cell product idecabtagene vicleucel (marketing name Abecma®) was US-FDA approved for the treatment of multiple myeloma with identical molecular architecture to the CD19-CAR T cell product tisagenlecleucel [21,25,150].

Currently, six different CAR T cell products are approved by the US-FDA and/or the EMA for the treatment of refractory patients with B-lineage-derived cancers including ALL, lymphomas, and multiple myeloma. All products are based on a second-generation CAR architecture with one costimulatory domain and CD3ζ as the signaling domain. Interestingly, the CD19-CAR-T cell products use different spacer, transmembrane and costimulatory domains. Kymriah® is approved for use in pediatric patients and young adults (<25 years). The integrated table provides details on the gene transfer, the marketing company, the constitutive promotor, the cell source and information about the activation and culturing conditions if accessible. VH/L: heavy/Light chain of single-chain variable fragment (scFv). SIN Lentivirus: Self-inactivating Lentivirus. PBMC: peripheral blood mononuclear cell. ND: not disclosed.

Evidently, CD19 is a perfectly well-suited CAR target antigen with different CAR constructs being efficacious for patient treatments [26,78,151]. This is not the case for most CAR-targeted antigens, which prove to be more challenging for various biological reasons, including the expression level [83] and expression in cancerous tissue as well as vitally essential tissues, the size of the extracellular domain [102], configuration and accessibility (hidden epitopes) of the targeted antigen [84,104,152]. The most obvious difference of the CD19 CAR constructs lies in the costimulatory domains 4-1BB or CD28 which lead to a differential gene expression signature of >200 genes [153], despite the shared bidirectional activation of the NF-kB and mTOR pathway with the induction of proinflammatory cytokine production such as IL-2 and IL-6 as well as the expression and activation of antiapoptotic proteins such as BCL-xL [154–156]. The biological consequences of CD28 and/or 4-1BB costimulation are diverse, with distinct differences in response kinetics, cell cycling, clonal expansion, survival, metabolism, and long-term persistence in vitro and in vivo.

Depending on the requirements of the CAR, the features of CD28 or 4-1BB costimulation may be advantageous [157]. Costimulation by a receptor of the TNFR family such as 4-1BB leads to increased oxidative metabolism, mitochondrial biogenesis and mitochondrial fitness and capacity associated with the pronounced maturation in central memory T cells with enhanced persistence, whereas costimulation by the CD28 family leads to increased glycolytic metabolism, reduced mitochondrial biogenesis, fitness and capacity associated with the maturation to effector memory T cells with shortened persistence [158]. The strongest activating costimulatory domain is CD28. Clinically, CD28 costimulation leads to a more rapid expansion of the CAR T cells accompanied by life-threatening adverse events such as cytokine release syndrome (CRS) and immune effector cell-associated neurotoxicity syndrome (ICANS) [159]. Preclinical studies have revealed that CD28-costimulated CAR T cells express higher levels of exhaustion markers such as PD-1, TIM3 and LAG3 compared to 4-1BB-costimulated CAR T cells [120,160]. To date, there are no sufficient biological data available in a clinical setting to allow a conclusive comparative analysis of CD28 versus 4-1BB costimulation in CAR T cells. Despite the unclear data landscape in preclinical models with regard to enhanced persistence of CAR T cells, most likely due to the short observation time of less than 3 months in most mouse studies [157,161], greater persistence in 4-1BB-costimulated CD19-CAR T compared to CD28-costimulated cells were observed in various clinical trials and are in general accepted, even though the value of CD19-CAR persistence remains elusive and seems to be cancer-specific [2,3,162]. In adult patients with B-NHL lymphomas and B-ALL, CD19-CAR T long-term persistence does not correlate with response to treatment and long-term cancer-free survival [163], whereas in pediatric ALL patients, persistence for over 6 months appears to be the determining factor for long-term leukemia clearance or leukemia recurrence in case of shorter CAR persistence [2]. Thus, in pediatric and adolescent patients, 4-1BB costimulation in CD19-CAR-T cell therapy may be superior compared to CD28 costimulation for the treatment of B-cell precursor ALL.

11. State-of-the-Art CAR T Cell Therapy in Children

Outcome of relapsed and refractory BCP-ALL remains poor at approximately 40% with a median survival of 14 months despite the use of allogeneic hematopoietic stem cell transplantation and the emergence of novel therapies in recent years [164–166]. CD19-targeted therapies including the bispecific T cell engager (BiTE) therapy blinatumomab and the even more potent CD19-CAR-T cell therapy have been proven efficacious in heavily pre-treated patients, albeit with severe but widely accepted toxicities due to the lack of alternative treatment options [2,167]. As outlined above, the main reason why CD19 qualifies for highly potent and long-term immunotherapy is the differential overexpression of CD19 on malignant blasts compared to the low expression levels on vitally essential tissues, such as low-level expression on neural tissues [168,169]. Tisagenlecleucel therapy provides cures to patients who were considered incurable until CD19-CAR-T cells were used in a substantial number of patients and continuously showed high complete remission induction rates and durable leukemia-free survival [2,17,78,149].

11.1. Clinical Indication for CD19-CAR-T Cell Product Tisagenlecleucel (CTL019, Kymriah®)

The indication for treatment with tisagenlecleucel in children and young adults (3 to 25 years) is relapsed or refractory pediatric B-cell ALL. Tisagenlecleucel treatment is approved for autologous CAR T cell therapy only. The major eligibility criteria include the presence of >5% blasts at screening, second or subsequent bone marrow relapse, or bone marrow relapse after allogeneic hematopoietic stem cell transplantation and must be ≥6 months from HSCT. The definition of refractory is not achieving an initial complete remission after two cycles of standard chemotherapy regimen (primary refractory) [21,149].

11.2. Tisagenlecleucel Therapy

According to inclusion and exclusion criteria, eligible patients are identified and required to undergo unstimulated mononuclear cell apheresis. Subsequently, the apheresis products are evaluated first for manufacturability, before the patient is approved eligible for tisagenlecleucel treatment. In the meantime, patients receive an individual bridging therapy according to the treating physician [21]. An overview of treatment with CAR T cells including the lymphodepletion, the most common adverse events and the pathophysiology of CRS and ICANS is illustrated in Figure 5.

After clearance of the patient-individual CD19-CAR-T cell product tisagenlecleucel, the patient undergoes a preparative lymphodepleting chemotherapy. Lymphodepletion includes 4 doses of fludarabine (Flu) at 30 mg/m^2 and 2 doses of cyclophosphamide (Cy) at 500 mg/m^2. Lymphodepletion paves the way for CAR T cell engraftment by eradication of immunosuppressive cells such as regulatory T cells (T$_{REG}$) and myeloid-derived suppressor cells (MDSCs), which leads to enhanced expression of costimulatory ligands on cancer cells, reduced elimination of relevant T cell homeostatic cytokine levels such as (IL-2, IL-7 and IL-15) thus promoting the initial anticancer immune response, exponential proliferation, robust engraftment and persistence of CAR T cells [170]. This may also induce immune tolerance and prevent rejection of chimeric transgene cells. Tisagenlecleucel may be infused into the patient from 2 to 14 days after completion of the (Flu/Cy) non-myeloablative lymphodepletion. CAR T cells are infused at 0.2 to 5.0 × 10^6 tisagenlecleucel transduced viable T cells per kg body weight for patients ≤ 50 kg, or 0.1 to 2.5 × 10^8 tisagenlecleucel transduced viable T cells for patients > 50 kg) [21,149].

It is noteworthy that a significant proportion of pediatric BCP-ALL patients do not survive while waiting for the production and preparation of CAR T cell products. In the ELIANA trial NCT02435849, a total of 107 patients were screened, 92 were enrolled, but only 75 (70%) underwent infusion [149] which meant 32 (30%) patients did not receive the CAR T cell treatment. Multiple factors contributed to the significantly reduced number of patients who finally received the tisagenlecleucel (CTL019) product including biological reasons, but also infrastructural reasons and time, which has a determining role in some patients' lives. Centralized versus decentralized manufacturing is an ongoing discussion in the field. Decentralized on-time manufacturing may shorten the waiting time for the CAR T cell product and may reduce costs [171]. On the other hand, implementing tisagenlecleucel CAR T cell therapy earlier in the treatment algorithm will improve the outcome of CAR T cell therapy [172]. Hence, the success of CD19-CAR-T cell therapy using tisagenlecleucel was significantly lower when all enrolled patients (intent-to-treat) were taken into account, compared to exclusively analyzing patients who received the CAR T cell product. In the clinical trial NCT02028455, the decentralized CAR manufacturing improved the intent-to-treat to >90% [173] compared to 70% in the ELIANA trial [149]. Notably, the real-world outcomes for tisagenlecleucel showed the same efficacy and even a higher safety profile than in the pivotal study [174]. First presented data of brexucabtagene autoleucel by Wayne et al. in pediatric patients also demonstrated a reliable remission induction rate and an impressive leukapheresis to product release time of 14 days. Not unexpectedly, higher grades of CRS were observed (≥3 adverse events in 100% of patients); and among responders, CAR T cells were undetectable by 3 months post infusion [175]. Even though there is still a need for major improvements, it is beyond question that CD19-CAR-T cells and tisagenlecleucel especially are novel therapeutics that have contributed significantly to better outcome and prolonged survival in r/r pediatric BCP-ALL patients.

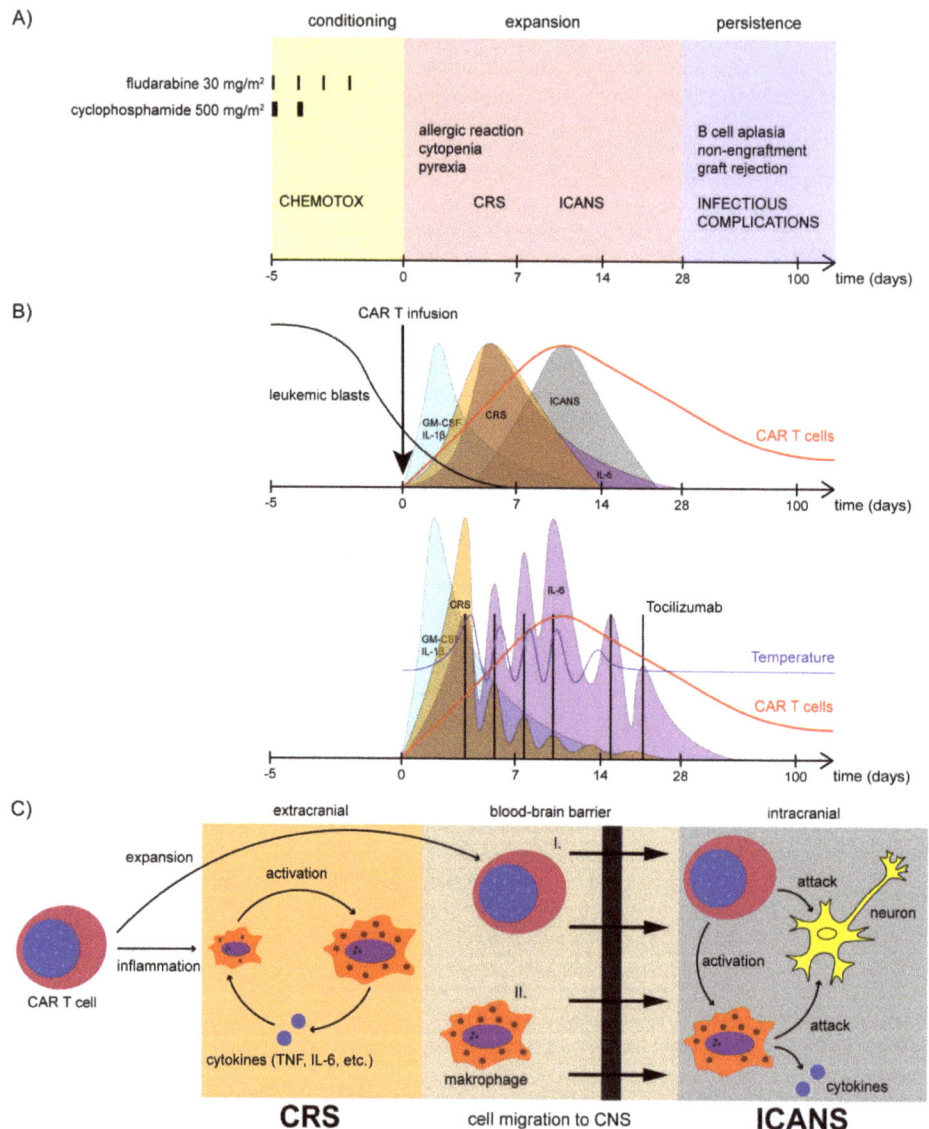

Figure 5. CAR T cell treatment and complications.

11.3. Follow-Up Patient Care Post Tisagenlecleucel Infusion

Usually, patients are closely monitored after tisagenlecleucel infusion for the first 28 days [21]. The follow-up intervals are extended in due course comparable to follow-up intervals common in autologous HSCT. However, patients are required to receive regular immunoglobulin replacement in case of sustained tisagenlecleucel persistence and consecutive B-cell aplasia that can cause chronic hypogammaglobulinemia-dependent humoral immune deficiency [131].

11.4. Allogeneic HSCT versus CD19-CAR-T Cell Therapy

It is difficult to make a direct comparison of clinical efficacy between allogeneic HSCT and CD19-CAR-T cell therapy, as HSCT improves outcomes in specific ALL populations, while CD19-CAR-T cell therapy has demonstrated efficacy in patients who failed allogeneic HSCT and/or are not eligible for HSCT [176]. Tisagenlecleucel CAR T cells exhibit impressive antitumor efficacy with superior complete remission induction of 81–90% and overall survival rates of 67–76% at 12 months, superior to conventional chemotherapy or HSCT [2,149,177]. In patients with high CD19 expression and no escape variants, CD19-CAR-T cell therapy is associated with less toxicity and superior leukemia-free survival than after HSCT. It is noteworthy that the combination of blinatumomab and HSCT also results in excellent survival rates in patients with complete MRD response [178]. Patients who show a tendency to develop CD19-negative tumor cell populations, e.g., during blinatumomab treatment, are likely to fail CD19-CAR-T cell therapy as well [2]. CD19-CAR-T cells cannot provide durable remissions for patients with CD19-negative cancer. In this case or if CD19-CAR-T cells do not persist > 6 months after infusion in BCP-ALL (but not for DLBCL), consolidative allogeneic HSCT may be a valid strategy to improve the outcome at the price of chemotoxicity from the conditioning regimen [2,179] and posttransplant complications such as acute and chronic GvHD as well as infectious complications [180]. Further, CD19-negative relapse post tisagenlecleucel occurs in 10–20% of patients [2]. Despite limited data available to date, CD22-CAR-T cell therapy is an option for patients who failed CD19-CAR-T cell therapy, with a high complete remission (MRD$^-$) induction rate (61%). Yet, patients who do not undergo a consolidative allogeneic HSCT seem to be at very high risk of relapse [84,181]. Thus, CAR T cell therapy may be used for remission induction therapy in these patients and allow patients to proceed for an allogeneic HSCT in complete MRD-negative remission that cannot be achieved by any other treatment in chemorefractory patients for consolidation therapy [176,179]. Bivalent CAR T cell technologies address antigen escape but have not proven to solve the antigen question rigorously [80].

11.5. Cytokine Release Syndrome

In early-phase post CAR T cell administration, most patients develop an immune reaction with unspecific clinical symptoms such as fever, rigors, malaise, and anorexia [182]. Fever can reach high grades for a week or longer and may be accompanied by multiorgan dysfunction including dyspnea, lung edema, hepatic, and renal dysfunction as well as heart dysfunction, which can consequently lead to a life-threatening clinical state with multiorgan failure and death [183,184]. Today, cytokine release syndrome (CRS) can be treated successfully if CRS is detected at an early stage and the specific anti-inflammatory treatment is initiated without delay utilizing tocilizumab to block the IL-6 signaling and corticosteroids to dampen the overall immune response and dampen the CAR T cell function [182,185].

The conditioning regimen fosters the increased production and secretion of the TH1-associated cytokines IL-2, IL-7 and IL-15 after CAR T cell engagement with targeted antigen-positive cells. In stage one (1), the highly activated CAR T cells lyse target cells, secrete cytokines, and undergo polyclonal exponential proliferation. The cytokines promote survival and ongoing proliferation of the CAR T cells, and in parallel co-activate monocytes and macrophages which are capable of producing massive amounts of cytokines in any tissue. The systemic activation and secretion of cytokines by CAR T cells as well as monocytes and macrophages drive local CRS to become a systemic CRS. Thus, the second stage (2) of CRS is introduced by a second wave of cytokines which is predominantly characterized by high serum levels of GM-CSF and the pleiotropic cytokine IL-6, an early detection marker of CRS. In the third stage (3), CRS can evolve dynamically into a life-threatening cytokine storm based on the autocrine, paracrine and systemically paracrine pyramid activation system [186]. CRS may develop over a couple of days but may be initiated immediately after CAR T cell administration. Secondary, life-threatening neurotoxic complications usually develop during the course of CRS, but may also develop in patients with mild CRS or in patients with absent CRS [187]. The clinically predominant features of CRS may depend on the systemic involvement of different body compartments and organs [184]. The higher the grade of inflammation, the more severe the specific immune response. The secondary recruitment of accessory cells including monocytes, macrophages and endothelial cells further exacerbates CRS, leading to the increased risk of direct organ toxicity [186]. In the beginning of CRS, the brain is protected from primary and secondary involvement of CRS by the blood–brain barrier. The migration of CAR T cells to the brain is slower compared to other compartments of the body. In due course, the endothelial cells of the omnipresent vascular system contribute to CRS complications by expressing Ang-2 and *von Willebrand factor* triggered by IL-1 and IL-6 [188]. This makes the blood–brain barrier porous, allowing cytokines to intrude the central nervous system and affect the brain with increasing concentrations [186]. There is evidence that higher CAR T cell numbers and higher cytokine levels in the CNS promote ICANS. Yet, the complex pathophysiology of ICANS make it difficult to discern the severity of ICANS with simple measures such as cell numbers or with cytokine levels. Nonetheless, there is a clear correlation between the incidence of neurotoxicity and CRS [189]. In general, ICANS may be regarded as a local CRS of the brain. The main reason why the treatment and pre-emptive treatment utilizing the IL-6 receptor blocking antibody tocilizumab significantly reduces the risk for extracranial CRS, but not intracranial CRS (ICANS) is the lack of ability to reach sufficient blocking concentrations in the brain (approximately 1% of peripheral extracranial concentration) [190]. The clinical grading and management of CRS are well described in the article "Current approaches in the grading and management of cytokine release syndrome after chimeric antigen receptor T-cell therapy" [191].

11.6. Neurotoxicity

A range of neurologic symptoms after CAR T cell administration including headache, tremor, speech impairment, confusion, delirium, and reduced consciousness (lethargy, stupor, obtundation) are in the scope of the clinical presentation of ICANS [28]. B-ALL patients are at higher risk than lymphoma patients to develop ICANS even though the exact mechanisms for the development of severe ICANS are not well understood and severe CRS is one of the main risk factors for ICANS [28,192].

CD19 is a B-cell receptor (BCR) co-receptor almost exclusively expressed in the B-lineage compartment. Even though there is low expression of CD19 on neural tissues [168], the actual clinically relevant on-target off-tumor toxicity in neural tissue is limited to the very early phase of the treatment after infusion of the cells. ICANS usually develops on day 4–6 post CAR infusion and lasts for up to 14 days [193] during the exponential proliferation phase of highly activated CD19-CAR-T cells. It is the main cause of life-threatening events and fatalities especially in CD19-CAR-T cell treatments with CD28 as costimulatory domain [188,194]. There is an association between serum concentrations of IL-15, a key cytokine for T cell expansion and survival, and the development of ICANS [28]. Neurotoxicity due to cerebral edema lead to the termination of the phase II ROCKET JCAR015 CD19-CAR-T cell trial treating adult patients with r/r ALL [195]. The mechanism of neurotoxicity caused by CD19-CAR-T cell therapy is not fully understood and various factors appear to impact on the susceptibility and severity such as bone marrow disease burden, the use of cyclophosphamide and fludarabine for lymphodepletion, and the presence of any pre-existing neurologic comorbidity [187,188,194].

11.7. Macrophage-Associated Hyperinflammation

There are several distinct life-threatening inflammatory syndromes associated with macrophage-derived pathological hyperinflammation characterized by high persistent fever, cytopenia, liver dysfunction with coagulopathy accompanied by high cytokine levels (IL-1β, IL-6, IL-18, TNF, and IFNγ), hypertriglyceridaemia and hyperferritinaemia [196]. These are hemophagocytic lymphohistiocytosis (HLH) and macrophage activation syndrome (MAS) mostly triggered by viral infections, rheumatological diseases and inherited lymphoid immune cell dysregulation [197–199] or a gain-of-function mutation in the inflammasome component gene NLRC4 [200]; and in the era of T cell immunotherapies, HLH and MAS are also initiated via BiTE [201] and CAR T cell therapy [181].

A biphasic inflammatory response was observed after CD22-CAR-T cell therapy, with a self-resolving initial CRS and signs of HLH features. In a second wave, driven by a secondary CAR T cell expansion, patients developed HLH/MAS-like symptoms dissociated from the first CRS phase [181]. Morris et al. suggested a unique pathophysiology [202] but the clinical pattern may as well be a recurrence of the initial CRS with a triggered HLH/MAS component induced by the very same mechanism.

Major complications following CAR T cell therapy over the course of 180 days after infusion. (Figure 5A) Different phases of treatment with CAR T cells: conditioning (yellow) with lymphodepleting chemotherapy starts with 4 doses of fludarabine 30 mg/m^2 and two doses of cyclophosphamide 500 mg/m^2. CAR T cells are administered on day 0 and go through an expansion phase (red). After clearing the tumor cells, the CAR T cells enter the persistence phase (blue). Major complications are CRS and ICANS, both manifesting in the first days after treatment with CAR T cells. (Figure 5B) Kinetics of leukemic blasts (black) and CAR T cells (red) after conditioning and infusion of CAR T cells. Blast count starts to drop slightly after lymphodepleting chemotherapy and decreases rapidly after infusion of CAR T cells. CAR T cell count starts to rise exponentially shortly after infusion and reaches peak values at approximately day +10. After clearing tumor cells from patients' blood, CAR T cell count drops again but remains detectable on a low level for several months. Depicted on the upper half are the kinetics of cytokine secretion and development of CRS/ICANS without intervention. Secretion of GM-CSF and IL-1β (light blue) rises almost immediately after infusion of CAR T cells and peaks rapidly followed by an equally rapid decrease, IL-6 secretion (purple) starts to increase shortly after and peaks at the same time as CRS (orange) is most likely to occur; after which, IL-6 drops but remains on an elevated level for some time. Peak level of IL-6 correlates to the severity of CRS. ICANS (grey) typically occurs a bit later than CRS and is connected to migration of CAR T cells to the neural compartment. Treatment of severe CRS consists of inhibition of IL-6 signaling with tocilizumab (indicated by black bars), a blocking monoclonal antibody targeting the membrane bound and soluble IL-6 receptor. After injection of tocilizumab, IL-6 decreases shortly but accumulates over time as elimination by receptor internalization is inhibited as well. Normalization of body temperature and amelioration of CRS symptoms can be observed immediately or within a few hours after administration of tocilizumab. In the case of severe CRS, the effect of anti-IL-6 therapy can wear off and multiple injections are required for treatment. Indication for subsequent application of tocilizumab is re-occurrence of fever which is followed by an increase in IL-6 and exacerbation of CRS symptoms. (Figure 5C) Pathophysiology of CRS/ICANS. Expansion of CAR T cells results in inflammation in the extracerebral compartment (orange), which activates resting macrophages into cytokine-producing macrophages (TNF, IL-6, etc.). These cytokines stimulate other macrophages to produce more cytokines in series, resulting in a vicious cycle of stimulation and cytokine secretion. This so-called macrophage activation syndrome (MAS) is the major trigger for CRS in CAR T cell therapy. During expansion, CAR T cells migrate through the blood–brain barrier (light brown) into the intracerebral compartment (grey) followed by activated macrophages evoking intracerebral MAS. Consecutively, these effector cells start to attack neurological tissue, leading to neurological damage, which is observed clinically as ICANS. CAR: chimeric antigen receptor. CAR T: chimeric antigen receptor T cells. CRS: cytokine release syndrome. ICANS: immune effector cell-associated neurotoxicity syndrome. TNF: tumor-necrosis factor. IL-1ß: Interleukin 1-beta. GM-CSF: granulocyte-macrophage-colony-stimulating factor.

11.8. B-Cell Aplasia

CD19-CAR-T cell-mediated B-cell aplasia results in reduced immunoglobulin levels, which requires treatment by IgG replacement. Due to the fundamental understanding of the immune system and the well-established technologies to purify antibodies from healthy donors, the immune protective function of the B-lineage compartment can be substituted by regular immunoglobulin infusions [149] to prevent infections and are associated with improved quality of life in antibody deficiency [203]. Hypogammaglobulinemia post CD19-CAR-T cell therapy seems to be more pronounced and cause more complications in children than in adults. Continued B-cell aplasia and subsequent hypogammaglobulinemia are linked to CD19-CAR performance and persistence, which is dependent on the product that was used for the treatment of the underlying disease [131,139]. Tisagenlecleucel incorporating a 4-1BB costimulatory domain tends to persist longer than axicabtagene ciloleucel with a CD28 costimulatory domain [2,3]. Only tisagenlecleucel is approved for the treatment in children and young adults (<25 years) [21]. Infectious complications post CD19-CAR-T cell therapy are of multifactorial origin. Strategic combinatorial medications including antiviral, antifungal and antibacterial therapy in a time- and risk-adapted approach can prevent infectious complications. IgG replacement on a regular basis can reduce the risk for high grade infections [131,204].

11.9. Relapse Patterns in Pediatric CD19-CAR-T Cell Therapy

The main cause of death after tisagenlecleucel treatment according to the ELIANA trial NCT02435849 is relapse at a rate of 68% (13/19 patients). Only one patient in the ELIANA trial (1/19 patients, 5%) died from a directly linked tisagenlecleucel toxicity that caused cerebral hemorrhage during coagulopathy in the context of CRS (15 days after infusion). The other patients died from infectious complications including HHV-6-caused encephalitis and systemic mycosis in association with prolonged neutropenia as well as from complications that occur subsequent to therapies of the primary disease [149]. Undoubtedly, many complications are rather caused by the poor clinical state of patients when they qualify for CD19-CAR-T cell therapy according to the current treatment criteria.

There are various strategies to reduce the probability of adverse events during CAR T cell therapy, but the most straight forward approach to improve safety is to implement CAR T cell therapy earlier in the treatment algorithm of r/r B-lineage ALL in children and young adults [172]. Consequently, patients will be in better condition than after intensive chemotherapy and allogeneic HSCT [2,176,177]. Reducing the risk of relapse would bring the highest impact on improving outcomes of CD19-CAR-T cell therapy, since most patients die from the leukemia recurrence, but not of CAR T cell induced complications. Therefore, addressing the question of "How to prevent relapse?" will bring most benefits to our patients, and understanding the current relapse pattern (illustrated in Figure 6) will direct the strategies that are most promising for improving patient outcome.

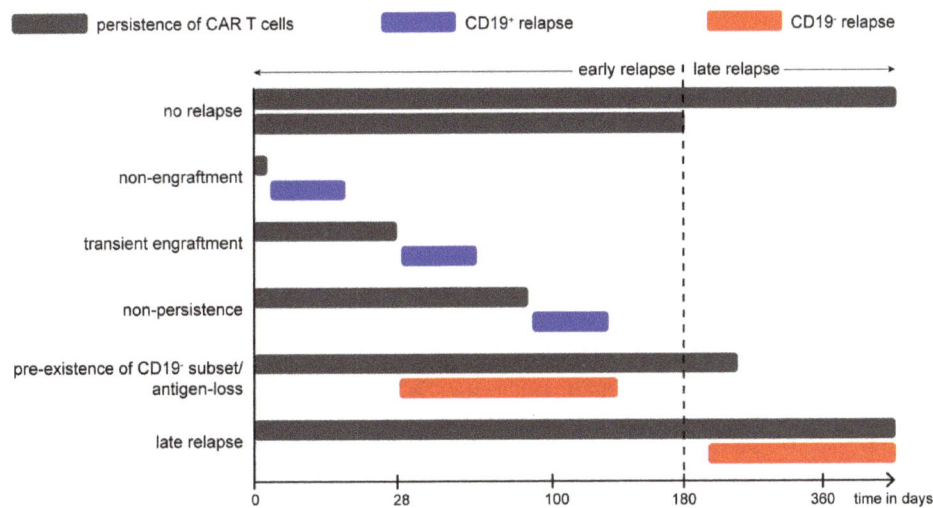

Figure 6. Relapse pattern after CD19-CAR-T cell therapy in BCP-ALL.

The interplay of CD19+ B-lineage ALL blasts in childhood ALL and CD19-CAR-T cells define the relapse pattern after this highly potent targeted therapy. Early and late relapse may be distinguished at day +180 after CAR T cell infusion; however, the mechanism of relapse is strongly dependent **firstly** on the antileukemic performance [2] of the CAR T cells, and **secondly** on the pre-existence or development of CD19− leukemic subsets as a result of the selection pressure [121]. In children with acute B-lineage ALL, the optimal scenario is the induction of complete molecular remission and maintenance beyond 6 months after CAR T cell infusion. These patients have a high chance of achieving long-term remission and leukemia-free survival. Patients whose CAR T cells have poor antileukemic performance of their CAR T cells, indicated in the figure by non-engraftment, transient engraftment, non-persistence and/or lack of exponential expansion, tend to develop CD19+ relapses. Without the selection pressure exerted by CD19-CAR-T cells, BCP-ALL blasts maintain CD19 expression. Patients whose CAR T cells have high antileukemic activity, as per the definition above, do not experience CD19+ relapse. Nonetheless, 10–20% of patients develop CD19− relapses. There are two major independent mechanisms on how CD19− relapse may occur. Pre-existence of CD19− blasts prior to CD19-CAR-T cells at a very low frequency has been identified as a primary resistance mechanism [205], while the other mechanism is the development of CD19− subsets over time via lineage switch or antigen escape (loss of the targeted epitope, alternative splicing of CD19 or downregulation of CD19) [30,84,206]. Grey: persistence of CAR T cells. Blue: CD19-positive relapse. Red: CD19-negative relapse.

Relapse patterns post CD19-CAR-T cell therapy can be classified by the expression status of CD19, but remain elusive and difficult to predict. Nonetheless, there are known determinants of CD19+ and CD19− relapses. The key discriminators are leukemic burden at the initiation of treatment with CD19-CAR-T cells (MRD > 10^{-2} versus MRD < 10^{-3}), previous exposure to blinatumomab and duration of B-cell aplasia [207].

As known from alternative CD19-targeted therapies including CD19 antibody therapy and BiTE therapy using blinatumomab, insufficient leukemia control leads to an increased risk of CD19− relapse and extramedullary leukemia formation, driven by the evolutionary pressure put on leukemia [16,82]. Incomplete clearance of BCP-ALL by blinatumomab may also predict resistance to CD19-CAR-T cell therapy [2,207]. In the beginning of CD19-CAR-T cell therapy, it was observed that patients with a higher leukemia burden would facilitate a better engraftment of CD19-CAR-T cells and thus CAR T cell therapy would be more successful. This early observation has been disproved in B-ALL. It has been demonstrated that patients with a lower leukemia burden show a favorable outcome [163].

Patients with a higher leukemia burden show a different relapse pattern to patients with a lower leukemia burden. Patients with a higher leukemia burden carry more leukemic blasts, leading to faster and more robust engraftment of CD19-CAR-T cells at the cost of more severe adverse events, such as CRS and ICANS [163]. Since the number of leukemic blasts is significantly higher, there is a greater chance of both the pre-existence and emergence of CD19 antigen immune escape variants. Thus, patients with a higher leukemic load tend to relapse with CD19$^-$ leukemia. Conversely, patients with a lower leukemic burden show less rapid and robust engraftment of CD19-CAR-T cells and suffer from less severe adverse events. Due to the less robust or transient engraftment of CD19-CAR-T cells in these patients, CAR T cell performance may be reduced, and patients tend to experience CD19$^+$ relapse (Figure 6) [207].

CD19-CAR-T cell performance and persistence can be monitored efficiently by standard flow cytometric evaluation of B-cell reconstitution. While continuous B-cell aplasia indicates persistence and functionality of CD19-CAR-T cells, patients with B-cell reconstitution at early time after CAR T cell treatment (prior to 6 months post infusion) tend to have a significantly increased risk for CD19$^+$ leukemia recurrence [2,149,163]. However, some patients with co-existence of low B-cell counts and circulating CD19-CAR-T cells remain in remission, which may be partially attributed to the stronger resistance of physiologic B cells to CD19-CAR-T cells than leukemic blasts [2,149,163,207].

11.10. CAR T Cell Trials on Alternative Targets in B-Lineage Malignancies

Relapses can occur in over 60% of patients treated with CD19-CAR-T cells within the first 12 months, despite remarkable initial response rates [149,163]. The majority of these relapses are attributable to immune escape due to CD19 antigen loss or decreased expression [109,208,209]. This has lead to numerous investigations of alternative B-lineage markers including CD20 and CD22 as targets for CAR T cell therapy against B-cell lymphomas. Both CD20 and CD22 are highly expressed in B-cell lymphoblasts, with 50% and 80–90% expression, respectively [210]. CD20 has been extensively studied as a therapeutic target for the treatment of r/r B-cell non-Hodgkin's lymphoma (NHL) and r/r B-ALL, with demonstrated preclinical and clinical efficacy [211]. The clinical success of CD20-CAR-T cells in adult B-cell lymphoma patients is moderate with high relapse rates (>80%), albeit showing favorable initial complete response rates (>50–70%) [212–214]. More promising is the preliminary data from a phase I CD22-CAR-T cell trial in children and young adults, with a 70% complete response rate and a median 6 month relapse-free survival, despite including multiply relapsed patients who had previously relapsed CD19$_{low}$ or CD19$^-$ after CD19-CAR-T cell therapy [84,181]. Unlike in CD19-CAR-T cells, relapses post CD22-CAR-T cell treatment occur mainly due to decreased CD22 expression (antigen downregulation) rather than antigen loss. However, this accentuates the common problem of immune escape as a mechanism of resistance to monovalent CAR T cell therapy and raises the question as to the long-term efficacy of CAR therapy beyond CD19. To counteract the risk of immune escape in B-lineage cancers, bivalent CAR T cells simultaneously targeting CD19-CD22, and CD19-CD20 have been developed and tested in phase I trials [80,111,215–217]. Antileukemic activities and complete remission rates were comparable to monovalent CAR T cells; however, long-term efficacy was not attained due to relapse. Interestingly, the relapses were due to loss or decreased expression of CD19, and not CD22, indicative of a biased selective pressure on CD19 [80]. In another trial utilizing CD19-CD20 tandem-CAR-T cells, CD19 expression was retained in all relapsed patients [217]. These results highlight the presence of multiple resistance mechanisms to CAR T cell therapy.

Driven by the need for additional target antigens to reduce the risk of antigen escape, CD37 and CD79B have emerged as promising novel CAR T cell targets for B-cell malignancies. Both CD37 and CD79B are highly expressed across multiple types of B-cell malignancies. Both CD37- and CD79B-CAR T cells have shown specific and effective antitumor activities in vitro as well as in vivo, which supports further clinical development [87,218,219]. At the time of this review, there is one phase I trial for both anti-CD37- and CD79B-CAR-T cell products in the early phase of recruitment (Table 2).

Table 2. CAR T cell trials for B-lymphoid leukemias (non-CD19 targeting) and AML.

CAR Target	Condition Treated	Eligible Age	Status	ClinicalTrials.gov ID
CD20	B-cell Non-Hodgkin's lymphomas	≥18	Recruiting	NCT03277729
CD20	B-cell lymphoma r/r to anti-CD19-CAR-Ttherapy	14 to 70	Unknown	NCT04036019
CD20	Lymphomas r/r to chemotherapy	≥18, <90	Unknown	NCT01735604
CD22	r/r B-cell lymphoma/leukemia	3 to 39	Recruiting	NCT02315612
CD22	B-ALL	1–30	Recruiting	NCT04088864
CD22	B-ALL	1–24	Recruiting	NCT02650414
CD22	r/r B-ALL	15–70	Recruiting	NCT04150497
CD19, CD20	r/r B-cell lymphoma/leukemia	16–70	Completed	NCT03097770
CD19, CD20	r/r B-cell lymphoma/leukemia	18–70	Active, not recruiting	NCT03019055
CD19, CD20	r/r B-cell lymphoma/leukemia	18–70	Recruiting	NCT04007029
CD19, CD20	r/r B-ALL	1–39	Recruiting	NCT04049383
CD19, CD22	r/r B-cell lymphoma/leukemia	≥18	Recruiting	NCT03233854
CD19, CD22	r/r B-cell lymphoma/leukemia	3–39	Recruiting	NCT03448393
CD19, CD22	r/r B-cell lymphoma/leukemia	6 months to 70	Recruiting	NCT04029038
CD19, CD22	B-cell lymphoma/leukemia	≤30	Recruiting	NCT03330691
CD19, CD22	r/r B-ALL	1–30	Recruiting	NCT03241940
CD37	B and T cell lymphoma/leukemia	≥18	Recruiting	NCT04136275
CD79B	r/r B-ALL, B-cell NHL	No age limit	Not yet recruiting	NCT04609241
CD33	AML	1–35	Recruiting	NCT03971799
CD123	AML	≥12	Recruiting	NCT02159495
CD123	AML	18–65	Recruiting	NCT03190278
CD123	AML	18–70	Recruiting	NCT04014881
CD123	AML	≥18	Active, not recruiting	NCT03766126
CD33, CLL-1, CD123	AML	6 months to 75	Recruiting	NCT04010877
CLL-1	AML	≤75	Recruiting	NCT04219163
CD38	AML	6–65	Recruiting	NCT04351022
CD33, CLL-1	AML/MDS/MPN/CML	No age limit	Recruiting	NCT03795779

11.11. CAR T Cell Therapy for T Cell Malignancies

Among of the most challenging cancers to treat with CAR T cells are T-lineage-derived malignancies. The main reason for this challenge is the co-expression of the target antigens on physiological T cells and progenitors thereof. Targeting of T-lineage-associated antigens leads to fratricide of CAR T cells and physiological T cells, the key immune cell subset of the adaptive immune compartment. Further, separating physiological T cells from malignant T cells during CAR T cell manufacturing has not been solved satisfactorily. There are no T cell-exclusive target antigens that can be targeted with CAR T cells without severely compromising the T cell compartment. However, targeting of CD2, CD5, CD7 and CD38 as well as the constant chains of the T cell receptor TRCB1 or TRCB2 have been used successfully in preclinical models [89,90]. Impressive CD7-CAR-T cell responses (90% remission induction rate) in patients with acute T cell leukemias were reported from the Chinese trial NCT04689659, with 15 out of 20 patients being in remission after a median follow-up of 6 months. CAR T cell persistence was confirmed in month 6 after CAR T cell infusion of $0.5\text{--}1 \times 10^6$/kgBW. Interestingly, physiological CD7-negative T cells expanded and compensated for treatment-related T cell immunodeficiency [91]. Larger cohorts need to be treated to understand the current value of CAR T cell therapy in T-lineage malignancies.

11.12. CAR T Cell Therapy for AML

The lack of cancer-specific antigens is the fundamental biological obstacle limiting the application of CAR T cell therapy in AML. Although AML blasts express various cell surface antigens such as CD33, CD123, CD38 and CLL-1, against which CAR T cells have been developed, these antigens are also expressed by hematopoietic stem or progenitor cells (HSPCs) [92]. Therefore, on-target off-tumor toxicity on HSPCs of these CAR T cells is of great concern, although they have shown potent antitumor activity in preclinical models [93,94]. Prolonged myeloablation resulting from on-target off-tumor toxicity on HSPCs can induce fatal infections in neutropenic fever and bleeding disorders. Strategies to facilitate CAR T cell therapy in AML include using CAR T cells as a remission induction therapy and rescuing the hematopoiesis by allogeneic HSCT. Further, myelotoxicity by CAR T cells can be terminated by CAR T cell ablation via suicide switches, and can be circumvented by generation of gene knockout of the targeted antigen (e.g., CD33) in rescue hematopoietic stem cell grafts [116].

Currently, CAR T cell products for AML that are in clinical trials mostly target CD33, CD38, CD123 and CLL-1 (Table 2). There are limited clinical data published at this stage to allow a thorough appreciation of the safety and efficacy profile of these CAR T cell products, although promising clinical responses have been reported, with myeloablation managed by HSCT [116].

11.13. CAR T Cell Therapy in Solid Tumors

In comparison to hematological cancers, solid tumors pose several unique challenges to CAR T cell therapy. Solid tumors encompassing the majority of cancers exhibit high levels of intrinsic tumor heterogeneity. CAR T cells that target only one antigen therefore are unable to recognize all the cancer cells in the tumor. Target antigens under investigation in solid tumors are always co-expressed at lower levels in vitally essential tissues. Consequently, it is inevitable to cause on-target off-tumor toxicities on healthy tissues [95]. Another major challenge is the highly immunosuppressive tumor microenvironment (TME) inducing T cell inactivation and dysfunction. Thus far, CAR T cell therapies in solid tumors lack clinical efficacy and have caused severe toxicities [31].

Pediatric brain tumors remain the leading cause of cancer-related death in children. CAR T cells have been developed to target the antigens B7-H3 (CD276), GD2, EGFR, IL13Ra2 and HER2 in a range of brain cancers such as medulloblastoma, glioma and ependymoma [220]. GD2-CAR-T cells have shown promising antitumor activity in neuroblastomas and sarcomas [221]. B7-H3 has been characterized as a pan-cancer antigen overexpressed in a variety of solid tumors including neuroblastoma and pediatric sarcomas, for which CD276-CAR-T cells are being investigated [222]. Supported by encouraging preclinical results, these CAR T cells have progressed to phase I clinical trials to assess their safety (Table 3).

Table 3. CAR T cell trials for pediatric solid tumors.

CAR Target	Condition Treated	Eligible Age	Status	ClinicalTrials.gov ID
B7-H3	Pediatric CNS tumors	1–26	Recruiting	NCT04185038
B7-H3	Pediatric solid tumors	≤ 26	Recruiting	NCT04483778
B7-H3	Solid tumors	1–75	Recruiting	NCT04432649
GD2	DIPG/high grade glioma	12 months to 18	Recruiting	NCT04099797
GD2	DIPG/DMG	2–30	Recruiting	NCT04196413
GD2	Osteosarcoma, neuroblastoma	≤ 35	Recruiting	NCT04539366
GD2	Neuroblastoma	12 months to 25	Recruiting	NCT03373097
GD2	Neuroblastoma, sarcoma	1–74	Recruiting	NCT03635632
GD2	Osteosarcoma, neuroblastoma	18 months to 18	Recruiting	NCT03721068
EGFR	Pediatric CNS tumors	≥ 15 and ≤ 26	Recruiting	NCT03638167
EGFR	Pediatric solid tumors	1–30	Recruiting	NCT03618381
EGFRvIII	Hematological and solid tumors	4–70	Recruiting	NCT03638206
HER2	Pediatric CNS tumors	1–26	Recruiting	NCT03500991
HER2	CNS tumors	≥ 3	Recruiting	NCT02442297
IL13Ra2	Pediatric CNS tumors	4–35	Recruiting	NCT04510051
IL13Ra2	Glioma	12–75	Recruiting	NCT02208362

12. Novel CAR T Technologies—The Antigen Question

The remarkable clinical success of CD19- and BCMA-CAR-T cell therapy [2,3,223] is the result of three decades of continuous research effort [35]. Today, the focus has shifted to removing the roadblocks in CAR T cell therapy to facilitate its application in acute myeloid leukemia (AML) and solid cancers. The main goals are to increase the clinical efficacy of CAR T cells while improving safety profiles and reducing the treatment costs [172].

Current limitations in CAR T cell therapy are mainly defined by how conventional CAR T cells operate. Most of the key obstacles are defined by the targeted antigens. The ideal target antigens are homogeneously expressed on all cancer cells, at sufficient levels above the CAR T activation threshold, and are significantly overexpressed in cancerous tissue with low expression in healthy tissues, and no expression in vitally essential tissues to spare toxicities [132]. The pursuit of the perfect antigen is rather far-fetched. The main effort to improve CAR T cell therapy in B-lineage malignancies is to efficiently target beyond CD19 [111,150,181].

As discussed above, the major cause of treatment failure and subsequent death of patients who received CAR T cell therapy in B-lineage cancers is relapse. To address antigen-negative relapse, which occurs in approximately 20% of CD19-CAR-T cell-treated patients (in BCP-ALL) [2], multitargeted CAR T cell products have been developed and are used in various formats as tandem CAR constructs or bicistronic or even tri-valent CAR constructs [80,84,108]. Clinical success of combinatorial CAR constructs is to be demonstrated and first data indicate that the clinical benefit is far less than anticipated. Dual CAR constructs did not show the same efficacy as two single-CAR T cell constructs for the same targeted antigens. The reduced potency seems to increase the chance of antigen low-positive relapse and immune escape variants which may not develop with more potent monotargeted CAR T cell therapies [181]. Further, sequential CD22 targeting in patients who experienced CD19-negative relapse after CD19-CAR-T cell therapy was associated with the emergence of $CD22_{low}$ relapse [84] and did not solve the antigen problem either.

Altogether, the fundamental challenge in CAR T cell therapy is to generate highly potent and safe CAR T cell products targeting non-B-lineage-derived cancers in a clinical setting. There are numerous preclinical studies that have demonstrated efficacy in various cancer models including AML [224], melanoma, lung cancer, brain cancer, osteosarcoma, Ewing sarcoma, prostate cancer [225], pancreatic cancer [226], and liver cancer [227]; however, clinical translation has not been successful [222]. Major advancements in CAR T cell therapy are expected, once multitargeted approaches facilitate the treatment of antigen heterogenous cancers.

12.1. Indirect CAR Technologies

One elegant way to overcome immune escape in CAR T cell therapy is a multi-targeted approach utilizing indirect CAR technologies. Adapter CAR technologies are two-component CAR technologies. The first component is comprised of a universal CAR T cell and the second component consists of adapter molecules that link the CAR receptors to the overexpressed tumor-associated antigen, leading to the recruitment and engagement of the CAR-expressing cells (Figure 7). The effector functions are the same as in conventional CAR T cells.

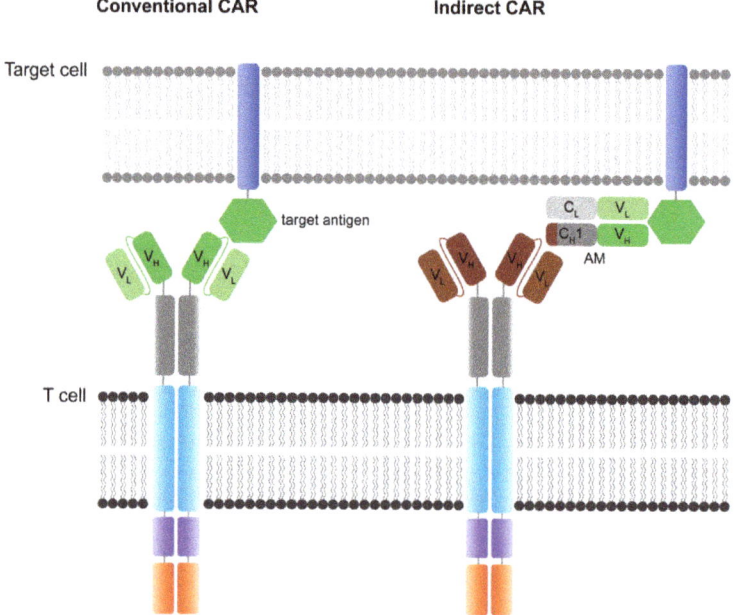

Figure 7. The designs of conventional and indirect CAR T cell technologies.

Conventional CAR T cells directly recognize the targeted antigen with their antigen recognition domain, which in most CAR constructs is a scFv. Indirect CAR technologies aim to highly specifically target exclusive *neo-antigens* incorporated on the adapter molecules as tags, such as peptides or LLE or chemical agents, on the adapter molecule to facilitate a clean off-state during the absence of the activating adapter molecules and a clean on-state during the presence of the adapter molecules and the target antigens. In the case of using non-exclusive antigens, such as alpha-fetoprotein cross reactivity and blocking phenomena can be induced. For the adapter CAR T cell system to function properly, the adapter CAR effector cell, the adapter molecule, and the target need to assemble correctly. This mechanism is more complex and dependent on more variables compared to the direct targeting of a conventional CAR. On the other hand, adapter CAR technologies are versatile and can facilitate features which are not achievable with conventional CAR targeting. These features include the safety and efficacy aspects determined by the nature of the on and off switches, the universal targeting (one CAR for all antigens), combinatorial targeting and more physiologic recruitment of the CAR-expressing cells. To date, conventional and indirect CAR technologies shall be regarded as complementary to each other. If adapter CAR technologies reach the same level of efficacy as conventional CAR technologies, they are likely to substitute conventional CARs for the clear advantages arising from the flexible technology.

There are numerous sophisticated adapter CAR technologies that have been developed over the last decade with distinct functional properties. They may be grouped into different CAR systems: (**I**) CARs that make use of the high-affinity CD16 (FCGR3A) V158 variant [228] in combination with antibodies or Fc-engineered antibodies [229], (**II**) scFv-based CARs targeting a tag on the adapter molecules, such as a the chemical compound FITC [230,231], peptides [232,233], alpha-fetoprotein (AFP) [234] or naturally occurring vitamins such as biotin [132,235], and (**III**) non-scFv-based binding domains such as streptavidin-derived avidin [236] or leucine zippers [237], and (**IV**) ligand-based CARs that are recruited via bivalent adapter molecules [238]. Putting aside the details in the distinct mode of actions, adapter CAR technologies may be considered to be advanced versions of antibody-dependent cellular cytotoxicity.

All listed strategies aim to overcome the obstacles of conventional CAR T cell therapy and can facilitate universal targeting (one CAR for all target antigens), combinatorial targeting and transient targeting. The switch-on and switch-off mechanism provides both enhanced safety and efficacy.

In the CAR T cell community, the main criticism arises from the added physiological complexity of adapter CAR systems. Conventional CAR T cells are always equipped with the recognition domain, whereas adapter CAR T cells are *"blind"* without the adapter molecules. Thus, adapter CAR T cells need to assemble correctly with the adapter molecule and the targeted antigen before they become functional. There is clear evidence that the adapter molecule format and size will impact on the distribution and elimination kinetics, the pharmacokinetics and pharmacodynamics [239]. Human IgG antibodies are mainly eliminated via intracellular catabolism by lysosomal degradation after pinocytosis, unspecific endocytosis, or by receptor-mediated endocytosis [240], whereas low-molecular-weight antibody fragments or fusion proteins below 70 kDa [241] are filtered and usually reabsorbed and metabolized in the proximal tubule of the nephron [239].

Certain body compartments are less accessible than others and it remains uncertain how adapter molecules may penetrate into the CNS [242], the testicles, and cancer tissues [243–245]. In many cancers, such as leukemias, primary brain cancers and brain metastasis, intracranial anticancer activity will be crucial for long-term tumor control [2]. On the other hand, antibodies have been shown to be functional beyond the blood–brain barrier such as immune checkpoint inhibitors (antibodies) and blinatumomab; however, their ability to penetrate the CNS is discussed controversially [245–247].

The advantages of adapter CAR technologies though are apparent. They provide solutions to overcome the major limitations in CAR T cell therapy. With regard to tissue penetration of adapter molecules, the reduced size of adapter molecules in the Fab or scFv formats have been used successfully in various adapter CAR technologies [232,248]. There are various strategies to overcome the blood–brain barrier in order to reach effective concentrations in cancer tissues, the testicular tissue and the CNS. Firstly, there is an obvious pharmacodynamic advantage of adapter molecules (for adapter CAR T cells) over blinatumomab. Adapter molecules can be administered at significantly higher doses than BiTEs, because no relevant unspecific activation of adapter CAR T cells is induced by adapter molecules in absence of the target [132,232]. In contrast, the maximum tolerated dose of blinatumomab defined by the study "Clinical Study With Blinatumomab in Patients With Relapsed/Refractory Diffuse Large B-cell Lymphoma (DLBCL)" (NCT01741792) in adults is 60 ug/m^2/day, reaching serum concentrations of 3 ng/mL, up to a maximum applied dose of 90 ug/m^2/day, reaching 3.5 ng/mL [249]. The recommended blinatumomab dose for the treatment of BCP-ALL in children is 5–15 ug/m^2/day, reaching serum concentrations of 0.6 ng/mL [167]. By increasing the dose significantly for instance by

1000-fold to more than 100 ng/mL, the adapter molecule penetration into the CNS and cancer tissues would be increased [243]. Secondly, intrathecal, intraventricular or intratumoral applications [250] of adapter molecules and CAR T cells have been shown for mesothelioma [251] and glioblastoma [252] and appear to be feasible and would help to overcome the blood–brain barrier or blood-cancer barrier through changing the application route [190,253]. Intrathecal application of chemotherapy in the treatment of leukemias is a standard procedure for both treatment of leukemic CNS involvement as well as CNS prophylaxis [254].

The low clinical tolerability of BiTEs clearly limits the potency of these fantastic new drugs, and if higher concentrations could be tolerated, the advantages of complex adapter CAR technologies compared to bispecific immune cell recruiting fusion proteins would be significantly reduced. In this scenario, BiTEs would most likely make the race for many applications as they are off-the-shelf products, need fewer complex infrastructures, making them cheaper to produce, handle and apply, and still have shown great clinical efficacy, despite being underdosed for toxicity reasons. The real-life clinical experience, however, will not support using BiTEs at their optimal concentrations in human patients [249]. Despite that adapter CAR T cell technologies will have to prove their superiority over blinatumomab in resistant CD19$^+$ leukemias and lymphomas, they have a very promising prospect as adapter CAR technologies have the chance to overcome the unspecific BiTE toxicities beyond CD19 targeting. Bispecific antibodies including BiTEs have not been convincingly successful in other leukemias such as AML [255], even though they demonstrated promising in vitro efficacy in primary AMLs at 5 ng/mL [256].

12.2. Technologies to Improve the Safety of CAR T Cells

Major CAR T cell infusion-related side effects comprise systemic inflammatory responses derived from rapid T cell expansion and on-target off-tumor effects. By expressing a targetable truncated antigen on CAR T cells (e.g., EGFR) and infusion of the corresponding antibodies (e.g., cetuximab), the elimination of the engineered CAR T cells can be achieved [257]. Another safety switch makes use of the inducible Caspase 9 (iCasp9) suicide gene, which offers a fast onset and more specific elimination of highly activated CAR T cells with high levels of transgene expression [258,259]. Sterner et al. studied granulocyte-macrophage colony-stimulating factor (GM-CSF) disruption by CRISPR/Cas9 in preclinical murine models and showed that neutralizing GM-CSF by lenzilumab is a potential strategy to abrogate CD19-CAR-T-related CRS without inhibition of CAR T cell function [260].

Discriminating normal tissues from cancer cells by the usage of logic gating of CARs can eliminate the on-target off-tumor effects. One example is the synNotch gating [261]. A synNotch receptor recognizes the first antigen which triggers the expression of a CAR toward a second tumor antigen. The recognition of both antigens enables the activation of T cells. The slow activation and degradation kinetics are the major limitations for further clinical application. Another strategy for combined sensing of two or more tumor antigens is to split the primary CD3ζ and the costimulatory domain into two separate chimeric receptors that are introduced into the same T cell [258,262].

Recent studies have substantiated the feasibility of controlling CAR functions via small-molecule interactions. Modulation of CAR functions can be achieved by using dimerizing agents as on switches and off switches [263], as well as on switches leading to a conformational change in the variable recognition domains induced by methotrexate that functions as an off switch [264]. In preclinical models, CAR T cell functions were shown to be tightly controlled via a pharmacological on/off switch using the tyrosine kinase inhibitor dasatinib. Dasatinib can abrogate CAR-mediated effector functions such as cytokine secretion, proliferation, and cytolysis rapidly with regular dosing. After termination of dasatinib exposure, CAR functions were fully restored, and even synergistic effects potentiating CAR function have been observed. In contrast to corticosteroid therapy in CRS, application of dasatinib would be distinguished from the other strategies to ablate CAR T cells [265,266].

With respect to the current developments in CAR T cell therapy, translational and practical approaches will help to improve patient safety. Optimizing the CD4/CD8 composition in CAR T cell products and reducing the number of accessory cells can reduce life-threatening CRS and ICANS while retaining the potency of CAR T cell products [181,267]. The development of ICANS in patients treated with the CD19-CAR-T cell product axicabtagene ciloleucel is associated with the number of accessory cells in the product and not with the number of CAR T cells. These cells may be referred to as ICANS-associated cells and carry a distinct monocyte-like transcriptional signature [267].

12.3. Armored Modules to Increase CAR T Cell Performance in TME

The production of inhibitory cytokines is employed by the tumor cells to create an immunosuppressive tumor microenvironment (TME) and evade the anticancer immune response. To protect CAR T cells from the immunosuppressive TME, engineered cytokine factor blockades have been developed in the format of cytokine switch receptors or dominant-negative receptors (DNR). For example, interleukin-4 (IL-4) is a key cytokine that controls the differentiation of T cells to the TH2 effector cells, which promotes and maintains an immunosuppressive environment and abrogates the anticancer immune response [268]. IL-4-IL-7 switch receptors transform the inhibitory IL-4 signal into a proinflammatory IL-7 signal with proliferative potential, promoting fitness, youth, and survival of T cells [269]. Another important immunosuppressive cytokine is TGFβ, which has been associated with in tumor progression and metastasis formation in several types of cancers. Upon expression of the DNR TGF-βRII in CAR T cells, enhanced cytokine secretion, resistance to exhaustion and improved long-term in vivo persistence have been observed in human prostate cancer mouse models of PSMA-CAR-TGF-ßRII-DNR-T cells [270].

Immune checkpoint inhibition by therapeutic antibodies unleashes the T cell antitumor immunity of T cells. Multiple strategies to achieve engineered PD-1 checkpoint blockade have been developed. Engineered PD1-CD28 switch receptors [271], secretion of blocking PD-1-targeted scFv [272] or antibodies by CAR T cells [273], shRNA knockdown of PD-1 and DNR of PD-1 have been shown to overcome immune checkpoint inhibition [274]. These potentiating CAR technologies and strategies have demonstrated the ability to increase the CAR effector functions in preclinical models [275,276]. Multiple genetic receptor modifications in CAR T cells have already reached the clinic, as exemplified by the "Study of CRISPR-Cas9 Mediated PD-1 and TCR Gene-knocked Out Mesothelin-directed CAR-T Cells in Patients With Mesothelin Positive Multiple Solid Tumors" (NCT03545815) that demonstrates feasibility with proof-of-concept experiments in preclinical models and with early preliminary clinical response data in a limited number of patients demonstrating feasibility [276]. Furthermore, advanced gene editing technology fuels the endeavors of donor-independent CAR T cell therapy by enabling gene knockouts of the TRAC and ß-microglobulin gene, which consequently eliminate the T cell receptors and the MHCs, leading to abrogation of GvHD and prevention of T cell-mediated rejections, respectively [277,278]. These genetic modifications may promote donor-independent allogeneic application of CAR therapeutics in the future. However, the T cell receptors and immune checkpoint receptors are important homeostatic receptors involved in the physiological functions of T cells, for which further investigation to fully understand the impact of these modifications on co-signaling pathways is imperative in order to ensure patient safety, and to create the most efficacious transgenic T cell therapy [279,280]. Site-specific integration of CAR transgenes into the TRAC locus using engineered endonucleases or CRISPR/Cas9 in combination with AAV templates or single-stranded DNA and electroporation for gene delivery has been established [63,281]. Integration of the CAR in the TRAC locus under the expression modulation of the TcR has demonstrated an activation-dependent transgene expression, which has shown to be advantageous compared to constitutive CAR expression in preclinical models and a step forward towards universal allogeneic CAR T cell therapy by disruption of the endogenous TcR [63,282]. However, to date, there is no proof that this new approach will improve CAR T cell therapy in humans. Despite the amazingly sophisticated technology, CARs will not be able to substitute the constitutive signaling function of the TcR [280]. Other strategies attempt to integrate the CARs in various ways to achieve the assembly within the native CD3 T cell receptor complex and make use of the TcR machinery [283,284], but these approaches are accompanied by other obstacles, such as TcR mispairing, overstimulation, and lack of space for antigen-specific receptor optimization.

CAR T cells engineered to secrete cytokines such as IL-12 [285] and IL-18 [286] or express tethered IL15-IL15RA [287] have proven to augment CAR T cell functions and are regarded as the fourth generation of CAR T cells. CARs that induce cytokine secretion upon recognition of the antigens are referred to as TRUCKs [62] and may overcome the toxic limitations of highly and constitutively expressed potent cytokines.

13. Conclusions

CAR T cell therapy has become a highly valued treatment in pediatric patients with r/r B-lineage malignancies. Thus far, CD19 is the best target antigen for CAR T cell therapy which has lead to cures for patients who were considered incurable. This unprecedented clinical success has ignited worldwide efforts to broaden the application of CAR T cell therapy beyond targeting CD19. On the other hand, we have learned our lessons from CD19-CAR-T cell therapy [288] and recognized the drawback that every new CAR, targeting a different antigen other than CD19, will need to go through a rigorous and lengthy development and optimization program. Identifying the best suitable target antigens for each cancer and solving the antigen challenges for CAR T cell therapy are the most important strategies in the development of novel CAR T cell therapies [132,289].

Furthermore, economic aspects constantly change the competitive landscape of adoptive cell therapy. Despite the remarkable complete response rates in CD19-CAR-T cell therapy in children and young adults [2], it has been argued that the initial treatment costs and secondary costs are too high, and strategies to reduce manufacturing costs [290], treatment costs and secondary costs such as immunoglobulin replacements have to be carefully addressed [291,292]. We need to succeed in increasing the potency and safety of CAR T cell products and expand CAR T cell-based immunotherapy to other cancers. Next-generation CAR T cell technologies, including adapter CAR technologies, have the chance to overcome some of the current clinical and economic limitations and transform CAR T cell therapy into a treatment platform with versatile functions and applications in cancer and beyond.

Author Contributions: Conceptualization, P.S.; P.S., M.B., Z.L., S.F.Y., A.J. writing—original draft preparation, P.S., M.B., Z.L., S.F.Y., A.J. writing—review and editing, P.S., M.B., Z.L., S.F.Y., A.J.; visualization, A.J., P.S.; supervision, P.S.; project administration, P.S.; funding acquisition, P.S. All authors have read and agreed to the published version of the manuscript.

Funding: This research received no external funding.

Institutional Review Board Statement: Not applicable.

Informed Consent Statement: Not applicable.

Data Availability Statement: Not applicable.

Conflicts of Interest: M.B., A.J., Z.L. and S.F.Y. declare no conflict of interest. P.S. is coinventor of a patent application focusing on adapter CAR technology.

References

1. Singh, A.K.; McGuirk, J.P. CAR T cells: Continuation in a revolution of immunotherapy. *Lancet Oncol.* **2020**, *21*, e168–e178. [CrossRef]
2. Maude, S.L.; Frey, N.; Shaw, P.A.; Aplenc, R.; Barrett, D.M.; Bunin, N.J.; Chew, A.; Gonzalez, V.E.; Zheng, Z.; Lacey, S.F.; et al. Chimeric Antigen Receptor T Cells for Sustained Remissions in Leukemia. *N. Engl. J. Med.* **2014**, *371*, 1507–1517. [CrossRef] [PubMed]

3. Neelapu, S.S.; Locke, F.L.; Bartlett, N.L.; Lekakis, L.J.; Miklos, D.B.; Jacobson, C.A.; Braunschweig, I.; Oluwole, O.O.; Siddiqi, T.; Lin, Y.; et al. Axicabtagene Ciloleucel CAR T-Cell Therapy in Refractory Large B-Cell Lymphoma. *N. Engl. J. Med.* **2017**, *377*, 2531–2544. [CrossRef] [PubMed]
4. Spadoni, C. Pediatric Drug Development: Challenges and Opportunities. *Curr. Res. Clin. Exp.* **2018**, *90*, 119–122. [CrossRef] [PubMed]
5. Joseph, P.D.; Craig, J.C.; Caldwell, P.H.Y. Clinical trials in children. *Br. J. Clin. Pharmacol.* **2015**, *79*, 357–369. [CrossRef] [PubMed]
6. Kakaje, A.; Alhalabi, M.; Ghareeb, A.; Karam, B.; Mansour, B.; Zahra, B.; Hamdan, O. Rates and trends of childhood acute lymphoblastic leukaemia: An epidemiology study. *Sci. Rep.* **2020**, *10*, 6756. [CrossRef]
7. Siegel, R.L.; Miller, K.D.; Fuchs, H.E.; Jemal, A. Cancer Statistics, 2021. *CA Cancer J. Clin.* **2021**, *71*, 7–33. [CrossRef]
8. Terwilliger, T.; Abdul-Hay, M. Acute lymphoblastic leukemia: A comprehensive review and 2017 update. *Blood Cancer J.* **2017**, *7*, e577. [CrossRef]
9. Inaba, H.; Mullighan, C.G. Pediatric acute lymphoblastic leukemia. *Haematologica* **2020**, *105*, 2524–2539. [CrossRef]
10. Reismüller, B.; Peters, C.; Dworzak, M.N.; Pötschger, U.; Urban, C.; Meister, B.; Schmitt, K.; Dieckmann, K.; Gadner, H.; Attarbaschi, A.; et al. Outcome of children and adolescents with a second or third relapse of acute lymphoblastic leukemia (ALL): A population-based analysis of the Austrian ALL-BFM (Berlin-Frankfurt-Münster) study group. *J. Pediatr. Hematol. Oncol.* **2013**, *35*, e200–e204. [CrossRef]
11. Lemal, R.; Tournilhac, O. State-of-the-art for CAR T-cell therapy for chronic lymphocytic leukemia in 2019. *J. ImmunoTher. Cancer* **2019**, *7*, 202. [CrossRef] [PubMed]
12. Schuster, S.J.; Bishop, M.R.; Tam, C.S.; Waller, E.K.; Borchmann, P.; McGuirk, J.P.; Jäger, U.; Jaglowski, S.; Andreadis, C.; Westin, J.R.; et al. Tisagenlecleucel in Adult Relapsed or Refractory Diffuse Large B-Cell Lymphoma. *N. Engl. J. Med.* **2018**, *380*, 45–56. [CrossRef] [PubMed]
13. Pui, C.-H.; Evans, W.E. A 50-year journey to cure childhood acute lymphoblastic leukemia. *Semin. Hematol.* **2013**, *50*, 185–196. [CrossRef] [PubMed]
14. Brissot, E.; Rialland, F.; Cahu, X.; Strullu, M.; Corradini, N.; Thomas, C.; Blin, N.; Thebaud, E.; Chevallier, P.; Moreau, P.; et al. Improvement of overall survival after allogeneic hematopoietic stem cell transplantation for children and adolescents: A three-decade experience of a single institution. *Bone Marrow Transplant.* **2016**, *51*, 267–272. [CrossRef]
15. Handgretinger, R.; Zugmaier, G.; Henze, G.; Kreyenberg, H.; Lang, P.; Von Stackelberg, A. Complete remission after blinatumomab-induced donor T-cell activation in three pediatric patients with post-transplant relapsed acute lymphoblastic leukemia. *Leukemia* **2011**, *25*, 181–184. [CrossRef]
16. Patrick, S.; Peter, L.; Gerhard, Z.; Martin, E.; Hermann, K.; Kai-Erik, W.; Judith, F.; Matthias, P.; Heiko-Manuel, T.; Christina, K.; et al. Pediatric posttransplant relapsed/refractory B-precursor acute lymphoblastic leukemia shows durable remission by therapy with the T-cell engaging bispecific antibody blinatumomab. *Haematologica* **2014**, *99*, 1212–1219.
17. Lee, D.W.; Kochenderfer, J.N.; Stetler-Stevenson, M.; Cui, Y.K.; Delbrook, C.; Feldman, S.A.; Fry, T.J.; Orentas, R.; Sabatino, M.; Shah, N.N.; et al. T cells expressing CD19 chimeric antigen receptors for acute lymphoblastic leukaemia in children and young adults: A phase 1 dose-escalation trial. *Lancet* **2015**, *385*, 517–528. [CrossRef]
18. Kebriaei, P.; Singh, H.; Huls, M.H.; Figliola, M.J.; Bassett, R.; Olivares, S.; Jena, B.; Dawson, M.J.; Kumaresan, P.R.; Su, S.; et al. Phase I trials using Sleeping Beauty to generate CD19-specific CAR T cells. *J. Clin. Investig.* **2016**, *126*, 3363–3376. [CrossRef]
19. Turtle, C.J.; Hanafi, L.-A.; Berger, C.; Gooley, T.A.; Cherian, S.; Hudecek, M.; Sommermeyer, D.; Melville, K.; Pender, B.; Budiarto, T.M.; et al. CD19 CAR–T cells of defined CD4+:CD8+ composition in adult B cell ALL patients. *J. Clin. Investig.* **2016**, *126*, 2123–2138. [CrossRef]
20. Turtle, C.J.; Hay, K.; Hanafi, L.-A.; Li, D.; Cherian, S.; Chen, X.; Wood, B.; Lozanski, A.; Byrd, J.C.; Heimfeld, S.; et al. Durable Molecular Remissions in Chronic Lymphocytic Leukemia Treated With CD19-Specific Chimeric Antigen Receptor–Modified T Cells After Failure of Ibrutinib. *J. Clin. Oncol.* **2017**, *35*, 3010–3020. [CrossRef]
21. KYMRIAH® (Tisagenlecleucel) [Package Insert]; Novartis: Basel, Switzerland, 2017.
22. YESCARTA® (Axicabtagene Ciloleucel) [Package Insert]; Kite: Los Angeles, CA, USA, 2017.
23. BREYANZI® (Lisocabtagene Maraleucel) [Package Insert]; Bristol Myers Squibb: New York, NY, USA, 2021.
24. TECARTUS® (Brexucabtagene Autoleucel) [Package Insert]; Kite: Los Angeles, CA, USA, 2021.
25. ABECMA® (Idecabtagene Vicleucel) [Package Insert]; Myers Squibb: New York, NY, USA, 2021.
26. Quintás-Cardama, A. What CAR Will Win the CD19 Race? *Mol. Cancer Ther.* **2019**, *18*, 498–506. [CrossRef]
27. Schuster, S.J.; Maziarz, R.T.; Rusch, E.S.; Li, J.; Signorovitch, J.E.; Romanov, V.V.; Locke, F.L.; Maloney, D.G. Grading and management of cytokine release syndrome in patients treated with tisagenlecleucel in the JULIET trial. *Blood Adv.* **2020**, *4*, 1432–1439. [CrossRef]
28. Sheth, V.S.; Gauthier, J. Taming the beast: CRS and ICANS after CAR T-cell therapy for ALL. *Bone Marrow Transplant.* **2021**, *56*, 552–566. [CrossRef]
29. Wudhikarn, K.; Palomba, M.L.; Pennisi, M.; Garcia-Recio, M.; Flynn, J.R.; Devlin, S.M.; Afuye, A.; Silverberg, M.L.; Maloy, M.A.; Shah, G.L.; et al. Infection during the first year in patients treated with CD19 CAR T cells for diffuse large B cell lymphoma. *Blood Cancer J.* **2020**, *10*, 79. [CrossRef]

30. Majzner, R.G.; Mackall, C.L. Tumor Antigen Escape from CAR T-cell Therapy. *Cancer Discov.* **2018**, *8*, 1219–1226. [CrossRef]
31. Wagner, J.; Wickman, E.; DeRenzo, C.; Gottschalk, S. CAR T Cell Therapy for Solid Tumors: Bright Future or Dark Reality? *Mol. Ther.* **2020**, *28*, 2320–2339. [CrossRef]
32. Chen, G.M.; Chen, C.; Das, R.K.; Gao, P.; Chen, C.-H.; Bandyopadhyay, S.; Ding, Y.-Y.; Uzun, Y.; Yu, W.; Zhu, Q.; et al. Integrative Bulk and Single-Cell Profiling of Premanufacture T-cell Populations Reveals Factors Mediating Long-Term Persistence of CAR T-cell Therapy. *Cancer Discov.* **2021**, *11*, 2186–2199. [CrossRef]
33. Kasakovski, D.; Xu, L.; Li, Y. T cell senescence and CAR-T cell exhaustion in hematological malignancies. *J. Hematol. Oncol.* **2018**, *11*, 91. [CrossRef]
34. Martinez, M.; Moon, E.K. CAR T Cells for Solid Tumors: New Strategies for Finding, Infiltrating, and Surviving in the Tumor Microenvironment. *Front. Immunol.* **2019**, *10*, 128. [CrossRef]
35. Gross, G.; Waks, T.; Eshhar, Z. Expression of immunoglobulin-T-cell receptor chimeric molecules as functional receptors with antibody-type specificity. *Proc. Natl. Acad. Sci. USA* **1989**, *86*, 10024–10028. [CrossRef]
36. Milone, M.C.; Fish, J.D.; Carpenito, C.; Carroll, R.G.; Binder, G.K.; Teachey, D.; Samanta, M.; Lakhal, M.; Gloss, B.; Danet-Desnoyers, G.; et al. Chimeric Receptors Containing CD137 Signal Transduction Domains Mediate Enhanced Survival of T Cells and Increased Antileukemic Efficacy In Vivo. *Mol. Ther.* **2009**, *17*, 1453–1464. [CrossRef]
37. Gong, M.C.; Latouche, J.-B.; Krause, A.; Heston, W.D.; Bander, N.H.; Sadelain, M. Cancer Patient T Cells Genetically Targeted to Prostate-Specific Membrane Antigen Specifically Lyse Prostate Cancer Cells and Release Cytokines in Response to Prostate-Specific Membrane Antigen. *Neoplasia* **1999**, *1*, 123–127. [CrossRef]
38. Eshhar, Z.; Waks, T.; Gross, G.; Schindler, D.G. Specific activation and targeting of cytotoxic lymphocytes through chimeric single chains consisting of antibody-binding domains and the gamma or zeta subunits of the immunoglobulin and T-cell receptors. *Proc. Natl. Acad. Sci. USA* **1993**, *90*, 720–724. [CrossRef]
39. Goverman, J.; Gomez, S.M.; Segesman, K.D.; Hunkapiller, T.; Laug, W.E.; Hood, L. Chimeric immunoglobulin-T cell receptor proteins form functional receptors: Implications for T cell receptor complex formation and activation. *Cell* **1990**, *60*, 929–939. [CrossRef]
40. Ochi, T.; Maruta, M.; Tanimoto, K.; Kondo, F.; Yamamoto, T.; Kurata, M.; Fujiwara, H.; Masumoto, J.; Takenaka, K.; Yasukawa, M. A single-chain antibody generation system yielding CAR-T cells with superior antitumor function. *Commun. Biol.* **2021**, *4*, 273. [CrossRef]
41. Kang, T.H.; Seong, B.L. Solubility, Stability, and Avidity of Recombinant Antibody Fragments Expressed in Microorganisms. *Front. Microbiol.* **2020**, *11*, 1927. [CrossRef]
42. Asensio, M.A.; Lim, Y.W.; Wayham, N.; Stadtmiller, K.; Edgar, R.C.; Leong, J.; Leong, R.; Mizrahi, R.A.; Adams, M.S.; Simons, J.F.; et al. Antibody repertoire analysis of mouse immunization protocols using microfluidics and molecular genomics. *mAbs* **2019**, *11*, 870–883. [CrossRef]
43. Lonberg, N. Fully human antibodies from transgenic mouse and phage display platforms. *Curr. Opin. Immunol.* **2008**, *20*, 450–459. [CrossRef]
44. Zajc, C.U.; Salzer, B.; Taft, J.M.; Reddy, S.T.; Lehner, M.; Traxlmayr, M.W. Driving CARs with alternative navigation tools—The potential of engineered binding scaffolds. *FEBS J.* **2021**, *288*, 2103–2118. [CrossRef]
45. Asaadi, Y.; Jouneghani, F.F.; Janani, S.; Rahbarizadeh, F. A comprehensive comparison between camelid nanobodies and single chain variable fragments. *Biomark. Res.* **2021**, *9*, 87. [CrossRef]
46. Schmidts, A.; Ormhøj, M.; Choi, B.D.; Taylor, A.O.; Bouffard, A.A.; Scarfò, I.; Larson, R.C.; Frigault, M.J.; Gallagher, K.; Castano, A.P.; et al. Rational design of a trimeric APRIL-based CAR-binding domain enables efficient targeting of multiple myeloma. *Blood Adv.* **2019**, *3*, 3248–3260. [CrossRef]
47. Wang, D.; Starr, R.; Chang, W.-C.; Aguilar, B.; Alizadeh, D.; Wright, S.L.; Yang, X.; Brito, A.; Sarkissian, A.; Ostberg, J.R.; et al. Chlorotoxin-directed CAR T cells for specific and effective targeting of glioblastoma. *Sci. Transl. Med.* **2020**, *12*, eaaw2672. [CrossRef]
48. Jayaraman, J.; Mellody, M.P.; Hou, A.J.; Desai, R.P.; Fung, A.W.; Pham, A.H.T.; Chen, Y.Y.; Zhao, W. CAR-T design: Elements and their synergistic function. *EBioMedicine* **2020**, *58*, 102931. [CrossRef]
49. Zhang, H.; Zhao, P.; Huang, H. Engineering better chimeric antigen receptor T cells. *Exp. Hematol. Oncol.* **2020**, *9*, 34. [CrossRef]
50. Ng, Y.-Y.; Tay, J.C.; Li, Z.; Wang, J.; Zhu, J.; Wang, S. T Cells Expressing NKG2D CAR with a DAP12 Signaling Domain Stimulate Lower Cytokine Production While Effective in Tumor Eradication. *Mol. Ther.* **2020**, *29*, 75–85. [CrossRef]
51. Guedan, S.; Calderon, H.; Posey, A.D., Jr.; Maus, M.V. Engineering and Design of Chimeric Antigen Receptors. *Mol. Ther. Methods Clin. Dev.* **2019**, *12*, 145–156. [CrossRef]
52. Tyagarajan, S.; Spencer, T.; Smith, J. Optimizing CAR-T Cell Manufacturing Processes during Pivotal Clinical Trials. *Mol. Ther. Methods Clin. Dev.* **2020**, *16*, 136–144. [CrossRef]
53. Jackson, Z.; Roe, A.; Sharma, A.A.; Lopes, F.B.T.P.; Talla, A.; Kleinsorge-Block, S.; Zamborsky, K.; Schiavone, J.; Manjappa, S.; Schauner, R.; et al. Automated Manufacture of Autologous CD19 CAR-T Cells for Treatment of Non-hodgkin Lymphoma. *Front. Immunol.* **2020**, *11*, 1941. [CrossRef]
54. Jürgens, B.; Clarke, N.S. Evolution of CAR T-cell immunotherapy in terms of patenting activity. *Nat. Biotechnol.* **2019**, *37*, 370–375. [CrossRef]

55. Yang, J.; Kim, B.; Kim, G.Y.; Jung, G.Y.; Seo, S.W. Synthetic biology for evolutionary engineering: From perturbation of genotype to acquisition of desired phenotype. *Biotechnol. Biofuels* **2019**, *12*, 113. [CrossRef]
56. Kunjapur, A.M.; Pfingstag, P.; Thompson, N.C. Gene synthesis allows biologists to source genes from farther away in the tree of life. *Nat. Commun.* **2018**, *9*, 4425. [CrossRef]
57. Petrenko, V.A. Landscape Phage: Evolution from Phage Display to Nanobiotechnology. *Viruses* **2018**, *10*, 311. [CrossRef]
58. Winter, G.; Harris, W.J. Humanized antibodies. *Trends Pharmacol. Sci.* **1993**, *14*, 139–143. [CrossRef]
59. Zinsli, L.V.; Stierlin, N.; Loessner, M.J.; Schmelcher, M. Deimmunization of protein therapeutics—Recent advances in experimental and computational epitope prediction and deletion. *Comput. Struct. Biotechnol. J.* **2021**, *19*, 315–329. [CrossRef]
60. Laffleur, B.; Pascal, V.; Sirac, C.; Cogné, M. Production of Human or Humanized Antibodies in Mice. *Mol. Radio-Oncol.* **2012**, *901*, 149–159.
61. Zhou, X.; Tu, S.; Wang, C.; Huang, R.; Deng, L.; Song, C.; Yue, C.; He, Y.; Yang, J.; Liang, Z.; et al. Phase I Trial of Fourth-Generation Anti-CD19 Chimeric Antigen Receptor T Cells Against Relapsed or Refractory B Cell Non-Hodgkin Lymphomas. *Front. Immunol.* **2020**, *11*, 564099. [CrossRef]
62. Chmielewski, M.; Kopecky, C.; Hombach, A.A.; Abken, H. IL-12 Release by Engineered T Cells Expressing Chimeric Antigen Receptors Can Effectively Muster an Antigen-Independent Macrophage Response on Tumor Cells That Have Shut Down Tumor Antigen Expression. *Cancer Res.* **2011**, *71*, 5697–5706. [CrossRef]
63. Eyquem, J.; Mansilla-Soto, J.; Giavridis, T.; van der Stegen, S.J.C.; Hamieh, M.; Cunanan, K.M.; Odak, A.; Gönen, M.; Sadelain, M. Targeting a CAR to the TRAC locus with CRISPR/Cas9 enhances tumour rejection. *Nature* **2017**, *543*, 113–117. [CrossRef]
64. Kim, D.W.; Cho, J.-Y. Recent Advances in Allogeneic CAR-T Cells. *Biomolecules* **2020**, *10*, 263. [CrossRef]
65. Savoldo, B.; Ramos, C.A.; Liu, E.; Mims, M.P.; Keating, M.J.; Carrum, G.; Kamble, R.T.; Bollard, C.M.; Gee, A.P.; Mei, Z.; et al. CD28 costimulation improves expansion and persistence of chimeric antigen receptor–modified T cells in lymphoma patients. *J. Clin. Investig.* **2011**, *121*, 1822–1826. [CrossRef]
66. Maher, J.; Brentjens, R.J.; Gunset, G.; Rivière, I.; Sadelain, M. Human T-lymphocyte cytotoxicity and proliferation directed by a single chimeric TCRζ/CD28 receptor. *Nat. Biotechnol.* **2002**, *20*, 70–75. [CrossRef]
67. Xie, G.; Dong, H.; Liang, Y.; Ham, J.D.; Rizwan, R.; Chen, J. CAR-NK cells: A promising cellular immunotherapy for cancer. *EBioMedicine* **2020**, *59*, 102975. [CrossRef]
68. Davila, M.L.; Brentjens, R.J. CD19-Targeted CAR T cells as novel cancer immunotherapy for relapsed or refractory B-cell acute lymphoblastic leukemia. *Clin. Adv. Hematol. Oncol. HO* **2016**, *14*, 802–808.
69. Sommermeyer, D.; Hudecek, M.; Kosasih, P.L.; Gogishvili, T.; Maloney, D.G.; Turtle, C.J.; Riddell, S.R. Chimeric antigen receptor-modified T cells derived from defined CD8+ and CD4+ subsets confer superior antitumor reactivity in vivo. *Leukemia* **2016**, *30*, 492–500. [CrossRef]
70. Xu, X.; Huang, S.; Xiao, X.; Sun, Q.; Liang, X.; Chen, S.; Zhao, Z.; Huo, Z.; Tu, S.; Li, Y. Challenges and Clinical Strategies of CAR T-Cell Therapy for Acute Lymphoblastic Leukemia: Overview and Developments. *Front. Immunol.* **2021**, *11*, 569117. [CrossRef]
71. Hartmann, J.; Schüßler-Lenz, M.; Bondanza, A.; Buchholz, C.J. Clinical development of CAR T cells—challenges and opportunities in translating innovative treatment concepts. *EMBO Mol. Med.* **2017**, *9*, 1183–1197. [CrossRef]
72. Mariuzza, R.A.; Agnihotri, P.; and Orban, J. The structural basis of T-cell receptor (TCR) activation: An enduring enigma. *J. Biol. Chem.* **2020**, *295*, 914–925. [CrossRef]
73. Li, R.; Ma, C.; Cai, H.; Chen, W. The CAR T-Cell Mechanoimmunology at a Glance. *Adv. Sci.* **2020**, *7*, 2002628. [CrossRef]
74. Davenport, A.J.; Cross, R.S.; Watson, K.A.; Liao, Y.; Shi, W.; Prince, H.M.; Beavis, P.A.; Trapani, J.A.; Kershaw, M.H.; Ritchie, D.S.; et al. Chimeric antigen receptor T cells form nonclassical and potent immune synapses driving rapid cytotoxicity. *Proc. Natl. Acad. Sci. USA* **2018**, *115*, E2068–E2076. [CrossRef]
75. Papadopoulou, M.; Tieppo, P.; McGovern, N.; Gosselin, F.; Chan, J.K.Y.; Goetgeluk, G.; Dauby, N.; Cogan, A.; Donner, C.; Ginhoux, F.; et al. TCR Sequencing Reveals the Distinct Development of Fetal and Adult Human Vγ9Vδ2 T Cells. *J. Immunol.* **2019**, *203*, 1468–1479. [CrossRef]
76. Waldman, A.D.; Fritz, J.M.; Lenardo, M.J. A guide to cancer immunotherapy: From T cell basic science to clinical practice. *Nat. Rev. Immunol.* **2020**, *20*, 651–668. [CrossRef]
77. Scheuermann, R.; Racila, E. CD19 Antigen in Leukemia and Lymphoma Diagnosis and Immunotherapy. *Leuk. Lymphoma* **1995**, *18*, 385–397. [CrossRef]
78. Maude, S.L.; Teachey, D.; Porter, D.L.; Grupp, S.A. CD19-targeted chimeric antigen receptor T-cell therapy for acute lymphoblastic leukemia. *Blood* **2015**, *125*, 4017–4023. [CrossRef]
79. Hammer, O. CD19 as an attractive target for antibody-based therapy. *mAbs* **2012**, *4*, 571–577. [CrossRef]
80. Spiegel, J.Y.; Patel, S.; Muffly, L.; Hossain, N.M.; Oak, J.; Baird, J.H.; Frank, M.J.; Shiraz, P.; Sahaf, B.; Craig, J.; et al. CAR T cells with dual targeting of CD19 and CD22 in adult patients with recurrent or refractory B cell malignancies: A phase 1 trial. *Nat. Med.* **2021**, *27*, 1419–1431. [CrossRef]
81. Ginaldi, L.; De Martinis, M.; Matutes, E.; Farahat, N.; Morilla, R.; Catovsky, D. Levels of expression of CD19 and CD20 in chronic B cell leukaemias. *J. Clin. Pathol.* **1998**, *51*, 364–369. [CrossRef]
82. Seidel, U.J.E.; Schlegel, P.; Grosse-Hovest, L.; Hofmann, M.; Aulwurm, S.; Pyz, E.; Schuster, F.R.; Meisel, R.; Ebinger, M.; Feuchtinger, T.; et al. Reduction of Minimal Residual Disease in Pediatric B-lineage Acute Lymphoblastic Leukemia by an Fc-optimized CD19 Antibody. *Mol. Ther.* **2016**, *24*, 1634–1643. [CrossRef]

83. Qin, H.; Ramakrishna, S.; Nguyen, S.; Fountaine, T.J.; Ponduri, A.; Stetler-Stevenson, M.; Yuan, C.M.; Haso, W.; Shern, J.F.; Shah, N.N.; et al. Preclinical Development of Bivalent Chimeric Antigen Receptors Targeting Both CD19 and CD22. *Mol. Ther. Oncolytics* **2018**, *11*, 127–137. [CrossRef]
84. Fry, T.J.; Shah, N.N.; Orentas, R.J.; Stetler-Stevenson, M.; Yuan, C.M.; Ramakrishna, S.; Wolters, P.; Martin, S.; Delbrook, C.; Yates, B.; et al. CD22-targeted CAR T cells induce remission in B-ALL that is naive or resistant to CD19-targeted CAR immunotherapy. *Nat. Med.* **2018**, *24*, 20–28. [CrossRef]
85. Watanabe, K.; Terakura, S.; Martens, A.C.; van Meerten, T.; Uchiyama, S.; Imai, M.; Sakemura, R.; Goto, T.; Hanajiri, R.; Imahashi, N.; et al. Target Antigen Density Governs the Efficacy of Anti–CD20-CD28-CD3 ζ Chimeric Antigen Receptor–Modified Effector CD8$^+$ T Cells. *J. Immunol.* **2015**, *194*, 911–920. [CrossRef]
86. Majzner, R.G.; Rietberg, S.P.; Sotillo, E.; Dong, R.; Vachharajani, V.T.; Labanieh, L.; Myklebust, J.H.; Kadapakkam, M.; Weber, E.W.; Tousley, A.M.; et al. Tuning the Antigen Density Requirement for CAR T-cell Activity. *Cancer Discov.* **2020**, *10*, 702–723. [CrossRef] [PubMed]
87. Ormhøj, M.; Scarfò, I.; Cabral, M.L.; Bailey, S.; Lorrey, S.J.; Bouffard, A.A.; Castano, A.P.; Larson, R.C.; Riley, L.S.; Schmidts, A.; et al. Chimeric Antigen Receptor T Cells Targeting CD79b Show Efficacy in Lymphoma with or without Cotargeting CD19. *Clin. Cancer Res.* **2019**, *25*, 7046–7057. [CrossRef]
88. Ding, S.; Mao, X.; Cao, Y.; Wang, N.; Xu, H.; Zhou, J. Targeting CD79b for Chimeric Antigen Receptor T-Cell Therapy of B-Cell Lymphomas. *Target. Oncol.* **2020**, *15*, 365–375. [CrossRef] [PubMed]
89. Teachey, D.T.; Hunger, S.P. Anti-CD7 CAR T cells for T-ALL: Impressive early-stage efficacy. *Nat. Rev. Clin. Oncol.* **2021**, *18*, 677–678. [CrossRef] [PubMed]
90. Maciocia, P.; A Wawrzyniecka, P.; Philip, B.; Ricciardelli, I.; Akarca, A.U.; Onuoha, S.C.; Legut, M.; Cole, D.; Sewell, A.K.; Gritti, G.; et al. Targeting the T cell receptor β-chain constant region for immunotherapy of T cell malignancies. *Nat. Med.* **2017**, *23*, 1416–1423. [CrossRef] [PubMed]
91. Pan, J.; Tan, Y.; Wang, G.; Deng, B.; Ling, Z.; Song, W.; Seery, S.; Zhang, Y.; Peng, S.; Xu, J.; et al. Donor-Derived CD7 Chimeric Antigen Receptor T Cells for T-Cell Acute Lymphoblastic Leukemia: First-in-Human, Phase I Trial. *J. Clin. Oncol.* **2021**, *39*, 3340–3351. [CrossRef] [PubMed]
92. Cummins, K.; Gill, S. Will CAR T cell therapy have a role in AML? Promises and pitfalls. *Semin. Hematol.* **2019**, *56*, 155–163. [CrossRef] [PubMed]
93. Gill, S.; Tasian, S.; Ruella, M.; Shestova, O.; Li, Y.; Porter, D.L.; Carroll, M.; Danet-Desnoyers, G.; Scholler, J.; Grupp, S.A.; et al. Preclinical targeting of human acute myeloid leukemia and myeloablation using chimeric antigen receptor–modified T cells. *Blood* **2014**, *123*, 2343–2354. [CrossRef]
94. Kim, M.Y.; Yu, K.-R.; Kenderian, S.S.; Ruella, M.; Chen, S.; Shin, T.-H.; Aljanahi, A.A.; Schreeder, D.; Klichinsky, M.; Shestova, O.; et al. Genetic Inactivation of CD33 in Hematopoietic Stem Cells to Enable CAR T Cell Immunotherapy for Acute Myeloid Leukemia. *Cell* **2018**, *173*, 1439–1453.e19. [CrossRef]
95. Hou, A.J.; Chen, L.C.; Chen, Y.Y. Navigating CAR-T cells through the solid-tumour microenvironment. *Nat. Rev. Drug Discov.* **2021**, *20*, 531–550. [CrossRef]
96. Teplyakov, A.; Obmolova, G.; Luo, J.; Gilliland, G.L. Crystal structure of B-cell co-receptor CD19 in complex with antibody B43 reveals an unexpected fold. *Proteins Struct. Funct. Bioinform.* **2018**, *86*, 495–500. [CrossRef] [PubMed]
97. Ghorashian, S.; Kramer, A.M.; Onuoha, S.; Wright, G.; Bartram, J.; Richardson, R.; Albon, S.J.; Casanovas-Company, J.; Castro, F.; Popova, B.; et al. Enhanced CAR T cell expansion and prolonged persistence in pediatric patients with ALL treated with a low-affinity CD19 CAR. *Nat. Med.* **2019**, *25*, 1408–1414. [CrossRef] [PubMed]
98. Long, A.H.; Haso, W.M.; Shern, J.F.; Wanhainen, K.M.; Murgai, M.; Ingaramo, M.; Smith, J.P.; Walker, A.J.; Kohler, M.E.; Venkateswara, V.R.; et al. 4-1BB costimulation ameliorates T cell exhaustion induced by tonic signaling of chimeric antigen receptors. *Nat. Med.* **2015**, *21*, 581–590. [CrossRef] [PubMed]
99. Garcia, K.C.; Degano, M.; Stanfield, R.L.; Brunmark, A.; Jackson, M.R.; Peterson, P.A.; Teyton, L.; Wilson, I.A. An αβ T Cell Receptor Structure at 2.5 υ and Its Orientation in the TCR-MHC Complex. *Science* **1996**, *274*, 209–219. [CrossRef]
100. Garboczi, D.N.; Ghosh, P.; Utz, U.; Fan, Q.R.; Biddison, W.E.; Wiley, D.C. Structure of the complex between human T-cell receptor, viral peptide and HLA-A2. *Nature* **1996**, *384*, 134–141. [CrossRef]
101. Watanabe, N.; Bajgain, P.; Sukumaran, S.; Ansari, S.; Heslop, H.E.; Rooney, C.M.; Brenner, M.K.; Leen, A.M.; Vera, J.F. Fine-tuning the CAR spacer improves T-cell potency. *OncoImmunology* **2016**, *5*, e1253656. [CrossRef]
102. Long, A.H.; Haso, W.M.; Orentas, R.J. Lessons learned from a highly-active CD22-specific chimeric antigen receptor. *OncoImmunology* **2013**, *2*, e23621. [CrossRef]
103. James, S.E.; Greenberg, P.D.; Jensen, M.C.; Lin, Y.; Wang, J.; Till, B.G.; Raubitschek, A.A.; Forman, S.J.; Press, O.W. Antigen Sensitivity of CD22-Specific Chimeric TCR Is Modulated by Target Epitope Distance from the Cell Membrane. *J. Immunol.* **2008**, *180*, 7028–7038. [CrossRef]
104. Haso, W.; Lee, D.W.; Shah, N.N.; Stetler-Stevenson, M.; Yuan, C.M.; Pastan, I.H.; Dimitrov, D.S.; Morgan, R.A.; Fitzgerald, D.J.; Barrett, D.M.; et al. Anti-CD22–chimeric antigen receptors targeting B-cell precursor acute lymphoblastic leukemia. *Blood* **2013**, *121*, 1165–1174. [CrossRef]

105. Möricke, A.; Ratei, R.; Ludwig, W.-D.; Harbott, J.; Borkhardt, A.; Viehmann, S.; Zimmermann, M.; Gadner, H.; Riehm, H.; Schrappe, M. Prognostic Factors in CD10 Negative Precursor B-Cell Acute Lymphoblastic Leukemia in Children: Data from Three Consecutive Trials ALL-BFM 86, 90, and 95. *Blood* **2004**, *104*, 1957. [CrossRef]
106. Sędek, Ł.; Bulsa, J.; Sonsala, A.; Twardoch, M.; Wieczorek, M.; Malinowska, I.; Derwich, K.; Niedźwiecki, M.; Sobol-Milejska, G.; Kowalczyk, J.R.; et al. The immunophenotypes of blast cells in B-cell precursor acute lymphoblastic leukemia: How different are they from their normal counterparts? *Cytom. Part B Clin. Cytom.* **2014**, *86*, 329–339. [CrossRef] [PubMed]
107. Baird, J.H.; Frank, M.J.; Craig, J.; Patel, S.; Spiegel, J.Y.; Sahaf, B.; Oak, J.S.; Younes, S.F.; Ozawa, M.G.; Yang, E.; et al. CD22-directed CAR T-cell therapy induces complete remissions in CD19-directed CAR–refractory large B-cell lymphoma. *Blood* **2021**, *137*, 2321–2325. [CrossRef] [PubMed]
108. Schneider, D.; Xiong, Y.; Wu, D.; Hu, P.; Alabanza, L.; Steimle, B.; Dropulić, B. Trispecific CD19-CD20-CD22-targeting duoCAR-T cells eliminate antigen-heterogeneous B cell tumors in preclinical models. *Sci. Transl. Med.* **2021**, *13*, eabc6401. [CrossRef] [PubMed]
109. Fousek, K.; Watanabe, J.; Joseph, S.K.; George, A.; An, X.; Byrd, T.T.; Morris, J.; Luong, A.; Martínez-Paniagua, M.A.; Sanber, K.; et al. CAR T-cells that target acute B-lineage leukemia irrespective of CD19 expression. *Leukemia* **2021**, *35*, 75–89. [CrossRef] [PubMed]
110. Ramakrishna, S.; Highfill, S.L.; Walsh, Z.; Nguyen, S.M.; Lei, H.; Shern, J.F.; Qin, H.; Kraft, I.L.; Stetler-Stevenson, M.; Yuan, C.M.; et al. Modulation of Target Antigen Density Improves CAR T-cell Functionality and Persistence. *Clin. Cancer Res.* **2019**, *25*, 5329–5341. [CrossRef] [PubMed]
111. Tong, C.; Zhang, Y.; Liu, Y.; Ji, X.; Zhang, W.; Guo, Y.; Han, X.; Ti, D.; Dai, H.; Wang, C. Optimized tandem CD19/CD20 CAR-engineered T cells in refractory/relapsed B-cell lymphoma. *Blood* **2020**, *136*, 1632–1644. [CrossRef] [PubMed]
112. Guo, Y.; Feng, K.; Tong, C.; Jia, H.; Liu, Y.; Wang, Y.; Ti, D.; Yang, Q.; Wu, Z.; Han, W. Efficiency and side effects of anti-CD38 CAR T cells in an adult patient with relapsed B-ALL after failure of bi-specific CD19/CD22 CAR T cell treatment. *Cell. Mol. Immunol.* **2020**, *17*, 430–432. [CrossRef]
113. Jyoti, N.; Maria, T.; de Regina, J.-K.; Ruud, W.J.R.; Pino, J.P.; Huipin, Y.; de Bruijn, J.D.; Ossenkoppele, G.J.; Zweegman, S.; Smit, L.; et al. CD38 as a therapeutic target for adult acute myeloid leukemia and T-cell acute lymphoblastic leukemia. *Haematologica* **2019**, *104*, e100–e103.
114. Haubner, S.; Perna, F.; Köhnke, T.; Schmidt, C.; Berman, S.; Augsberger, C.; Schnorfeil, F.M.; Krupka, C.; Lichtenegger, F.S.; Liu, X.; et al. Coexpression profile of leukemic stem cell markers for combinatorial targeted therapy in AML. *Leukemia* **2019**, *33*, 64–74. [CrossRef]
115. Tambaro, F.P.; Singh, H.; Jones, E.; Rytting, M.; Mahadeo, K.M.; Thompson, P.; Daver, N.; DiNardo, C.; Kadia, T.; Garcia-Manero, G.; et al. Autologous CD33-CAR-T cells for treatment of relapsed/refractory acute myelogenous leukemia. *Leukemia* **2021**, *35*, 3282–3286. [CrossRef]
116. Mardiana, S.; Gill, S. CAR T Cells for Acute Myeloid Leukemia: State of the Art and Future Directions. *Front. Oncol.* **2020**, *10*, 697. [CrossRef] [PubMed]
117. Baroni, M.L.; Martinez, D.S.; Aguera, F.G.; Ho, H.R.; Castella, M.; Zanetti, S.; Hernandez, T.V.; De La Guardia, R.D.; Castaño, J.; Anguita, E.; et al. 41BB-based and CD28-based CD123-redirected T-cells ablate human normal hematopoiesis in vivo. *J. Immunother. Cancer* **2020**, *8*, e000845. [CrossRef] [PubMed]
118. Styczyński, J.; Ebmt, F.T.I.D.W.P.; Tridello, G.; Koster, L.; Iacobelli, S.; Van Biezen, A.; Van Der Werf, S.; Mikulska, M.; Gil, L.; Cordonnier, C.; et al. Death after hematopoietic stem cell transplantation: Changes over calendar year time, infections and associated factors. *Bone Marrow Transplant.* **2020**, *55*, 126–136. [CrossRef] [PubMed]
119. Liu, X.; Jiang, S.; Fang, C.; Yang, S.; Olalere, D.; Pequignot, E.C.; Cogdill, A.; Li, N.; Ramones, M.; Granda, B.; et al. Affinity-Tuned ErbB2 or EGFR Chimeric Antigen Receptor T Cells Exhibit an Increased Therapeutic Index against Tumors in Mice. *Cancer Res.* **2015**, *75*, 3596–3607. [CrossRef]
120. Du, H.; Hirabayashi, K.; Ahn, S.; Kren, N.P.; Montgomery, S.A.; Wang, X.; Tiruthani, K.; Mirlekar, B.; Michaud, D.; Greene, K.; et al. Antitumor Responses in the Absence of Toxicity in Solid Tumors by Targeting B7-H3 via Chimeric Antigen Receptor T Cells. *Cancer Cell* **2019**, *35*, 221–237.e8. [CrossRef]
121. Xu, X.; Sun, Q.; Liang, X.; Chen, Z.; Zhang, X.; Zhou, X.; Li, M.; Tu, H.; Liu, Y.; Tu, S.; et al. Mechanisms of Relapse After CD19 CAR T-Cell Therapy for Acute Lymphoblastic Leukemia and Its Prevention and Treatment Strategies. *Front. Immunol.* **2019**, *10*, 2664. [CrossRef]
122. Kagoya, Y.; Tanaka, S.; Guo, T.; Anczurowski, M.; Wang, C.-H.; Saso, K.; Butler, M.O.; Minden, M.D.; Hirano, N. A novel chimeric antigen receptor containing a JAK–STAT signaling domain mediates superior antitumor effects. *Nat. Med.* **2018**, *24*, 352–359. [CrossRef]
123. Salter, A.I.; Rajan, A.; Kennedy, J.J.; Ivey, R.G.; Shelby, S.A.; Leung, I.; Templeton, M.L.; Muhunthan, V.; Voillet, V.; Sommermeyer, D.; et al. Comparative analysis of TCR and CAR signaling informs CAR designs with superior antigen sensitivity and in vivo function. *Sci. Signal.* **2021**, *14*, eabe2606. [CrossRef]
124. Watanabe, K.; Kuramitsu, S.; Posey, A.D., Jr.; June, C.H. Expanding the Therapeutic Window for CAR T Cell Therapy in Solid Tumors: The Knowns and Unknowns of CAR T Cell Biology. *Front. Immunol.* **2018**, *9*, 2486. [CrossRef]
125. Dong, R.; A Libby, K.; Blaeschke, F.; Fuchs, W.; Marson, A.; Vale, R.D.; Su, X. Rewired signaling network in T cells expressing the chimeric antigen receptor (CAR). *EMBO J.* **2020**, *39*, e104730. [CrossRef]

126. Stopfer, L.E.; Gajadhar, A.S.; Patel, B.; Gallien, S.; Frederick, D.T.; Boland, G.M.; Sullivan, R.J.; White, F.M. Absolute quantification of tumor antigens using embedded MHC-I isotopologue calibrants. *Proc. Natl. Acad. Sci. USA* **2021**, *118*, 2111173118. [CrossRef] [PubMed]
127. Croft, N.; Smith, S.A.; Wong, Y.C.; Tan, C.T.; Dudek, N.L.; Flesch, I.E.A.; Lin, L.C.W.; Tscharke, D.C.; Purcell, A.W. Kinetics of Antigen Expression and Epitope Presentation during Virus Infection. *PLOS Pathog.* **2013**, *9*, e1003129. [CrossRef] [PubMed]
128. Walker, A.J.; Majzner, R.G.; Zhang, L.; Wanhainen, K.; Long, A.H.; Nguyen, S.M.; Lopomo, P.; Vigny, M.; Fry, T.J.; Orentas, R.J.; et al. Tumor Antigen and Receptor Densities Regulate Efficacy of a Chimeric Antigen Receptor Targeting Anaplastic Lymphoma Kinase. *Mol. Ther.* **2017**, *25*, 2189–2201. [CrossRef] [PubMed]
129. Heitzeneder, S.; Bosse, K.R.; Zhu, Z.; Zhelev, D.; Majzner, R.G.; Radosevich, M.T.; Dhingra, S.; Sotillo, E.; Buongervino, S.; Pascual-Pasto, G.; et al. GPC2-CAR T cells tuned for low antigen density mediate potent activity against neuroblastoma without toxicity. *Cancer Cell* **2022**, *40*, 53–69.e9. [CrossRef] [PubMed]
130. A Morgan, R.; Yang, J.C.; Kitano, M.; E Dudley, M.; Laurencot, C.M.; A Rosenberg, S. Case Report of a Serious Adverse Event Following the Administration of T Cells Transduced With a Chimeric Antigen Receptor Recognizing ERBB2. *Mol. Ther.* **2010**, *18*, 843–851. [CrossRef]
131. Hill, J.A.; Giralt, S.; Torgerson, T.R.; Lazarus, H.M. CAR-T—And a side order of IgG, to go?—Immunoglobulin replacement in patients receiving CAR-T cell therapy. *Blood Rev.* **2019**, *38*, 100596. [CrossRef]
132. Seitz, C.M.; Mittelstaet, J.; Atar, D.; Hau, J.; Reiter, S.; Illi, C.; Kieble, V.; Engert, F.; Drees, B.; Bender, G.; et al. Novel adapter CAR-T cell technology for precisely controllable multiplex cancer targeting. *OncoImmunology* **2021**, *10*, 2003532. [CrossRef]
133. Sommermeyer, D.; Hill, T.; Shamah, S.M.; Salter, A.; Chen, Y.; Mohler, K.M.; Riddell, S.R. Fully human CD19-specific chimeric antigen receptors for T-cell therapy. *Leukemia* **2017**, *31*, 2191–2199. [CrossRef]
134. Muzard, J.; Bouabdelli, M.; Zahid, M.; Ollivier, V.; Lacapère, J.J.; Jandrot-Perrus, M.; Billiald, P. Design and humanization of a murine scFv that blocks human platelet glycoprotein VI in vitro. *FEBS J.* **2009**, *276*, 4207–4222. [CrossRef]
135. Lam, N.; Trinklein, N.D.; Buelow, B.; Patterson, G.H.; Ojha, N.; Kochenderfer, J.N. Anti-BCMA chimeric antigen receptors with fully human heavy-chain-only antigen recognition domains. *Nat. Commun.* **2020**, *11*, 283. [CrossRef]
136. Holliger, P.; Hudson, P.J. Engineered antibody fragments and the rise of single domains. *Nat. Biotechnol.* **2005**, *23*, 1126–1136. [CrossRef] [PubMed]
137. Jensen, M.C.; Popplewell, L.; Cooper, L.J.; DiGiusto, D.; Kalos, M.; Ostberg, J.R.; Forman, S.J. Antitransgene Rejection Responses Contribute to Attenuated Persistence of Adoptively Transferred CD20/CD19-Specific Chimeric Antigen Receptor Redirected T Cells in Humans. *Biol. Blood Marrow Transplant.* **2010**, *16*, 1245–1256. [CrossRef] [PubMed]
138. Wang, Y.; Li, C.; Xia, J.; Li, P.; Cao, J.; Pan, B.; Tan, X.; Li, H.; Qi, K.; Wang, X.; et al. Humoral immune reconstitution after anti-BCMA CAR T-cell therapy in relapsed/refractory multiple myeloma. *Blood Adv.* **2021**, *5*, 5290–5299. [CrossRef]
139. Doan, A.; Pulsipher, M.A. Hypogammaglobulinemia due to CAR T-cell therapy. *Pediatr. Blood Cancer* **2018**, *65*, e26914. [CrossRef]
140. Chen, X.; Jensen, P.E. The role of B lymphocytes as antigen-presenting cells. *Arch. Immunol. Ther. Exp.* **2008**, *56*, 77–83. [CrossRef] [PubMed]
141. Harris, D.T.; Kranz, D.M. Adoptive T Cell Therapies: A Comparison of T Cell Receptors and Chimeric Antigen Receptors. *Trends Pharmacol. Sci.* **2016**, *37*, 220–230. [CrossRef]
142. De Groot, A.S.; Terry, F.; Cousens, L.; Martin, W. Beyond humanization and de-immunization: Tolerization as a method for reducing the immunogenicity of biologics. *Expert Rev. Clin. Pharmacol.* **2013**, *6*, 651–662. [CrossRef]
143. Augustyniak, D.; Majkowska-Skrobek, G.; Roszkowiak, J.; Dorotkiewicz-Jach, A. Defensive and Offensive Cross-Reactive Antibodies Elicited by Pathogens: The Good, the Bad and the Ugly. *Curr. Med. Chem.* **2017**, *24*, 4002–4037. [CrossRef]
144. Polymeros, D.; Bogdanos, D.P.; Day, R.; Arioli, D.; Vergani, D.; Forbes, A. Does Cross-Reactivity between Mycobacterium avium paratuberculosis and Human Intestinal Antigens Characterize Crohn's Disease? *Gastroenterology* **2006**, *131*, 85–96. [CrossRef]
145. Larmonier, C.B.; Shehab, K.W.; Ghishan, F.K.; Kiela, P. T Lymphocyte Dynamics in Inflammatory Bowel Diseases: Role of the Microbiome. *BioMed Res. Int.* **2015**, *2015*, 504638. [CrossRef]
146. Bartelds, G.M.; Krieckaert, C.L.M.; Nurmohamed, M.T.; van Schouwenburg, P.A.; Lems, W.F.; Twisk, J.W.R.; Dijkmans, B.A.C.; Aarden, L.; jan Wolbink, G. Development of Antidrug Antibodies Against Adalimumab and Association With Disease Activity and Treatment Failure During Long-term Follow-up. *JAMA* **2011**, *305*, 1460–1468. [CrossRef] [PubMed]
147. Abramson, J.S.; Palomba, M.L.; Gordon, L.I.; Lunning, M.A.; Wang, M.; Arnason, J.; Mehta, A.; Purev, E.; Maloney, D.G.; Andreadis, C.; et al. Lisocabtagene maraleucel for patients with relapsed or refractory large B-cell lymphomas (TRANSCEND NHL 001): A multicentre seamless design study. *Lancet* **2020**, *396*, 839–852. [CrossRef]
148. Wang, M.; Munoz, J.; Goy, A.; Locke, F.L.; Jacobson, C.A.; Hill, B.T.; Timmerman, J.M.; Holmes, H.; Jaglowski, S.; Flinn, I.W.; et al. KTE-X19 CAR T-Cell Therapy in Relapsed or Refractory Mantle-Cell Lymphoma. *N. Engl. J. Med.* **2020**, *382*, 1331–1342. [CrossRef] [PubMed]
149. Maude, S.L.; Laetsch, T.W.; Buechner, J.; Rives, S.; Boyer, M.; Bittencourt, H.; Bader, P.; Verneris, M.R.; Stefanski, H.E.; Myers, G.D.; et al. Tisagenlecleucel in Children and Young Adults with B-Cell Lymphoblastic Leukemia. *N. Engl. J. Med.* **2018**, *378*, 439–448. [CrossRef] [PubMed]

150. Munshi, N.C.; Anderson, L.D., Jr.; Shah, N.; Madduri, D.; Berdeja, J.; Lonial, S.; Raje, N.; Lin, Y.; Siegel, D.; Oriol, A.; et al. Idecabtagene Vicleucel in Relapsed and Refractory Multiple Myeloma. *N. Engl. J. Med.* **2021**, *384*, 705–716. [CrossRef] [PubMed]
151. Park, J.H.; Geyer, M.B.; Brentjens, R.J. CD19-targeted CAR T-cell therapeutics for hematologic malignancies: Interpreting clinical outcomes to date. *Blood* **2016**, *127*, 3312–3320. [CrossRef] [PubMed]
152. Kenderian, S.; Ruella, M.; Shestova, O.; Klichinsky, M.; Aikawa, V.; Morrissette, J.J.D.; Scholler, J.; Song, D.; Porter, D.L.; Carroll, M.C.; et al. CD33-specific chimeric antigen receptor T cells exhibit potent preclinical activity against human acute myeloid leukemia. *Leukemia* **2015**, *29*, 1637–1647. [CrossRef]
153. Zhong, Q.; Zhu, Y.-M.; Zheng, L.-L.; Shen, H.-J.; Ou, R.-M.; Liu, Z.; She, Y.-L.; Chen, R.; Li, C.; Huang, J.; et al. Chimeric Antigen Receptor-T Cells with 4-1BB Co-Stimulatory Domain Present a Superior Treatment Outcome than Those with CD28 Domain Based on Bioinformatics. *Acta Haematol.* **2018**, *140*, 131–140. [CrossRef] [PubMed]
154. Shao, Z.; Schwarz, H. CD137 ligand, a member of the tumor necrosis factor family, regulates immune responses via reverse signal transduction. *J. Leukoc. Biol.* **2011**, *89*, 21–29. [CrossRef]
155. Esensten, J.H.; Helou, Y.A.; Chopra, G.; Weiss, A.; Bluestone, J.A. CD28 Costimulation: From Mechanism to Therapy. *Immunity* **2016**, *44*, 973–988. [CrossRef]
156. Colombetti, S.; Basso, V.; Mueller, D.; Mondino, A. Prolonged TCR/CD28 Engagement Drives IL-2-Independent T Cell Clonal Expansion through Signaling Mediated by the Mammalian Target of Rapamycin. *J. Immunol.* **2006**, *176*, 2730–2738. [CrossRef]
157. Zhao, Z.; Condomines, M.; Van Der Stegen, S.J.C.; Perna, F.; Kloss, C.C.; Gunset, G.; Plotkin, J.; Sadelain, M. Structural Design of Engineered Costimulation Determines Tumor Rejection Kinetics and Persistence of CAR T Cells. *Cancer Cell* **2015**, *28*, 415–428. [CrossRef]
158. Kawalekar, O.U.; O'Connor, R.S.; Fraietta, J.A.; Guo, L.; Mcgettigan, S.E.; Posey, A.D.; Patel, P.R.; Guedan, S.; Scholler, J.; Keith, B.; et al. Distinct Signaling of Coreceptors Regulates Specific Metabolism Pathways and Impacts Memory Development in CAR T Cells. *Immunity* **2016**, *44*, 380–390. [CrossRef]
159. Ying, Z.; He, T.; Wang, X.; Zheng, W.; Lin, N.; Tu, M.; Xie, Y.; Ping, L.; Zhang, C.; Liu, W.; et al. Parallel Comparison of 4-1BB or CD28 Co-stimulated CD19-Targeted CAR-T Cells for B Cell Non-Hodgkin's Lymphoma. *Mol. Ther. Oncolytics* **2019**, *15*, 60–68. [CrossRef]
160. Drent, E.; Poels, R.; Ruiter, R.; Van De Donk, N.W.C.J.; Zweegman, S.; Yuan, H.; de Bruijn, J.; Sadelain, M.; Lokhorst, H.M.; Groen, R.W.J.; et al. Combined CD28 and 4-1BB Costimulation Potentiates Affinity-tuned Chimeric Antigen Receptor–engineered T Cells. *Clin. Cancer Res.* **2019**, *25*, 4014–4025. [CrossRef]
161. Li, G.; Boucher, J.C.; Kotani, H.; Park, K.; Zhang, Y.; Shrestha, B.; Wang, X.; Guan, L.; Beatty, N.; Abate-Daga, D.; et al. 4-1BB enhancement of CAR T function requires NF-κB and TRAFs. *JCI Insight* **2018**, *3*, e121322. [CrossRef]
162. Porter, D.L.; Hwang, W.-T.; Frey, N.V.; Lacey, S.F.; Shaw, P.A.; Loren, A.W.; Bagg, A.; Marcucci, K.T.; Shen, A.; Gonzalez, V.; et al. Chimeric antigen receptor T cells persist and induce sustained remissions in relapsed refractory chronic lymphocytic leukemia. *Sci. Transl. Med.* **2015**, *7*, 303ra139. [CrossRef]
163. Park, J.H.; Rivière, I.; Gonen, M.; Wang, X.; Sénéchal, B.; Curran, K.J.; Sauter, C.; Wang, Y.; Santomasso, B.; Mead, E.; et al. Long-Term Follow-up of CD19 CAR Therapy in Acute Lymphoblastic Leukemia. *N. Engl. J. Med.* **2018**, *378*, 449–459. [CrossRef]
164. Gökbuget, N.; Stanze, D.; Beck, J.; Diedrich, H.; Horst, H.-A.; Hüttmann, A.; Kobbe, G.; Kreuzer, K.-A.; Leimer, L.; Reichle, A.; et al. Outcome of relapsed adult lymphoblastic leukemia depends on response to salvage chemotherapy, prognostic factors, and performance of stem cell transplantation. *Blood* **2012**, *120*, 2032–2041. [CrossRef]
165. Martin, A.; Morgan, E.; Hijiya, N. Relapsed or refractory pediatric acute lymphoblastic leukemia: Current and emerging treatments. *Paediatr. Drugs* **2012**, *14*, 377–387. [CrossRef]
166. Sun, W.; Malvar, J.; Sposto, R.; Verma, A.; Wilkes, J.J.; Dennis, R.; Heym, K.; Laetsch, T.W.; Widener, M.; Rheingold, S.R.; et al. Outcome of children with multiply relapsed B-cell acute lymphoblastic leukemia: A therapeutic advances in childhood leukemia & lymphoma study. *Leukemia* **2018**, *32*, 2316–2325. [PubMed]
167. Locatelli, F.; Whitlock, J.A.; Peters, C.; Chen-Santel, C.; Chia, V.; Dennis, R.M.; Heym, K.M.; Katz, A.J.; Kelsh, M.A.; Sposto, R.; et al. Blinatumomab versus historical standard therapy in pediatric patients with relapsed/refractory Ph-negative B-cell precursor acute lymphoblastic leukemia. *Leukemia* **2020**, *34*, 2473–2478. [CrossRef] [PubMed]
168. Parker, K.R.; Migliorini, D.; Perkey, E.; Yost, K.E.; Bhaduri, A.; Bagga, P.; Haris, M.; Wilson, N.E.; Liu, F.; Gabunia, K.; et al. Single-Cell Analyses Identify Brain Mural Cells Expressing CD19 as Potential Off-Tumor Targets for CAR-T Immunotherapies. *Cell* **2020**, *183*, 126–142.e17. [CrossRef] [PubMed]
169. Mejstrikova, E.; Klinger, M.; Markovic, A.; Zugmaier, G.; Locatelli, F. CD19 expression in pediatric patients with relapsed/refractory B-cell precursor acute lymphoblastic leukemia pre- and post-treatment with blinatumomab. *Pediatr. Blood Cancer* **2021**, *68*, e29323. [CrossRef] [PubMed]
170. Neelapu, S.S. CAR-T efficacy: Is conditioning the key? *Blood* **2019**, *133*, 1799–1800. [CrossRef]
171. Harrison, R.P.; Rafiq, Q.A.; Medcalf, N. Centralised versus decentralised manufacturing and the delivery of healthcare products: A United Kingdom exemplar. *Cytotherapy* **2018**, *20*, 873–890. [CrossRef]
172. Maude, S.L. Future directions in chimeric antigen receptor T cell therapy. *Curr. Opin. Pediatr.* **2017**, *29*, 27–33. [CrossRef]
173. Gardner, R.A.; Finney, O.; Annesley, C.; Brakke, H.; Summers, C.; Leger, K.; Bleakley, M.; Brown, C.; Mgebroff, S.; Kelly-Spratt, K.S.; et al. Intent-to-treat leukemia remission by CD19 CAR T cells of defined formulation and dose in children and young adults. *Blood* **2017**, *129*, 3322–3331. [CrossRef]

174. Pasquini, M.C.; Hu, Z.-H.; Curran, K.; Laetsch, T.; Locke, F.; Rouce, R.; Pulsipher, M.A.; Phillips, C.L.; Keating, A.; Frigault, M.J.; et al. Real-world evidence of tisagenlecleucel for pediatric acute lymphoblastic leukemia and non-Hodgkin lymphoma. *Blood Adv.* 2020, *4*, 5414–5424. [CrossRef]
175. EHA2021 Virtual Congress Abstract Book. *HemaSphere* 2021, *5*, e566. [CrossRef]
176. Diorio, C.; Maude, S.L. CAR T cells vs allogeneic HSCT for poor-risk ALL. *Hematology* 2020, *2020*, 501–507. [CrossRef] [PubMed]
177. Gaynon, P.S.; Harris, R.E.; Altman, A.J.; Bostrom, B.C.; Breneman, J.C.; Hawks, R.; Steele, D.; Zipf, T.; Stram, D.O.; Villaluna, D.; et al. Bone Marrow Transplantation Versus Prolonged Intensive Chemotherapy for Children With Acute Lymphoblastic Leukemia and an Initial Bone Marrow Relapse Within 12 Months of the Completion of Primary Therapy: Children's Oncology Group Study CCG-1941. *J. Clin. Oncol.* 2006, *24*, 3150–3156. [CrossRef] [PubMed]
178. Locatelli, F.; Zugmaier, G.; Mergen, N.; Bader, P.; Jeha, S.; Schlegel, P.-G.; Bourquin, J.-P.; Handgretinger, R.; Brethon, B.; Rössig, C.; et al. Blinatumomab In pediatric relapsed/refractory B-cell acute lymphoblastic leukemia: RIALTO expanded access study final analysis. *Blood Adv.* 2022, *6*, 1004–1014. [CrossRef] [PubMed]
179. Jiang, H.; Hu, Y.; Mei, H. Consolidative allogeneic hematopoietic stem cell transplantation after chimeric antigen receptor T-cell therapy for relapsed/refractory B-cell acute lymphoblastic leukemia: Who? When? Why? *Biomark. Res.* 2020, *8*, 66. [CrossRef]
180. Hierlmeier, S.; Eyrich, M.; Wölfl, M.; Schlegel, P.-G.; Wiegering, V. Early and late complications following hematopoietic stem cell transplantation in pediatric patients—A retrospective analysis over 11 years. *PLoS ONE* 2018, *13*, e0204914. [CrossRef]
181. Shah, N.N.; Highfill, S.L.; Shalabi, H.; Yates, B.; Jin, J.; Wolters, P.L.; Ombrello, A.; Steinberg, S.M.; Martin, S.; Delbrook, C.; et al. CD4/CD8 T-Cell Selection Affects Chimeric Antigen Receptor (CAR) T-Cell Potency and Toxicity: Updated Results From a Phase I Anti-CD22 CAR T-Cell Trial. *J. Clin. Oncol.* 2020, *38*, 1938–1950. [CrossRef]
182. Lee, D.W.; A Gardner, R.; Porter, D.L.; Louis, C.U.; Ahmed, N.; Jensen, M.C.; Grupp, S.A.; Mackall, C.L. Current concepts in the diagnosis and management of cytokine release syndrome. *Blood* 2014, *124*, 188–195. [CrossRef]
183. Hay, K.A.; Hanafi, L.-A.; Li, D.; Gust, J.; Liles, W.C.; Wurfel, M.M.; López, J.A.; Chen, J.; Chung, D.; Harju-Baker, S.; et al. Kinetics and biomarkers of severe cytokine release syndrome after CD19 chimeric antigen receptor–modified T-cell therapy. *Blood* 2017, *130*, 2295–2306. [CrossRef]
184. Fitzgerald, J.C.; Weiss, S.; Maude, S.L.; Barrett, D.M.; Lacey, S.F.; Melenhorst, J.J.; Shaw, P.; Berg, R.A.; June, C.H.; Porter, D.L.; et al. Cytokine Release Syndrome After Chimeric Antigen Receptor T Cell Therapy for Acute Lymphoblastic Leukemia. *Crit. Care Med.* 2017, *45*, e124–e131. [CrossRef]
185. Neelapu, S.S.; Tummala, S.; Kebriaei, P.; Wierda, W.; Gutierrez, C.; Locke, F.L.; Komanduri, K.V.; Lin, Y.; Jain, N.; Daver, N.; et al. Chimeric antigen receptor T-cell therapy—Assessment and management of toxicities. *Nat. Rev. Clin. Oncol.* 2018, *15*, 47–62. [CrossRef]
186. Wei, J.; Liu, Y.; Wang, C.; Zhang, Y.; Tong, C.; Dai, G.; Wang, W.; Rasko, J.; Melenhorst, J.J.; Qian, W.; et al. The model of cytokine release syndrome in CAR T-cell treatment for B-cell non-Hodgkin lymphoma. *Signal Transduct. Target. Ther.* 2020, *5*, 134. [CrossRef] [PubMed]
187. Gust, J.; Hay, K.A.; Hanafi, L.-A.; Li, D.; Myerson, D.; Gonzalez-Cuyar, L.F.; Yeung, C.; Liles, W.C.; Wurfel, M.; Lopez, J.A.; et al. Endothelial Activation and Blood–Brain Barrier Disruption in Neurotoxicity after Adoptive Immunotherapy with CD19 CAR-T Cells. *Cancer Discov.* 2017, *7*, 1404–1419. [CrossRef] [PubMed]
188. Siegler, E.L.; Kenderian, S.S. Neurotoxicity and Cytokine Release Syndrome after Chimeric Antigen Receptor T Cell Therapy: Insights Into Mechanisms and Novel Therapies. *Front. Immunol.* 2020, *11*, 1973. [CrossRef] [PubMed]
189. Gust, J.; Ponce, R.; Liles, W.C.; Garden, G.A.; Turtle, C.J. Cytokines in CAR T Cell–Associated Neurotoxicity. *Front. Immunol.* 2020, *11*, 577027. [CrossRef] [PubMed]
190. Nellan, A.; McCully, C.M.L.; Garcia, R.C.; Jayaprakash, N.; Widemann, B.C.; Lee, D.W.; Warren, K.E. Improved CNS exposure to tocilizumab after cerebrospinal fluid compared to intravenous administration in rhesus macaques. *Blood* 2018, *132*, 662–666. [CrossRef]
191. Riegler, L.L.; Jones, G.P.; Lee, D.W. Current approaches in the grading and management of cytokine release syndrome after chimeric antigen receptor T-cell therapy. *Ther. Clin. Risk Manag.* 2019, *15*, 323–335. [CrossRef]
192. Wudhikarn, K.; Bansal, R.; Khurana, A.; Hathcock, M.; Ruff, M.; Carabenciov, I.D.; Braksick, S.A.; Bennani, N.N.; Paludo, J.; Villasboas, J.C.; et al. Characteristics, outcomes, and risk factors of ICANS after axicabtagene ciloleucel: Does age matter? *J. Clin. Oncol.* 2021, *39*, e19556. [CrossRef]
193. Sievers, S.; Watson, G.; Johncy, S.; Adkins, S. Recognizing and Grading CAR T-Cell Toxicities: An Advanced Practitioner Perspective. *Front. Oncol.* 2020, *10*, 885. [CrossRef]
194. Zhao, X.; Yang, J.; Zhang, X.; Lu, X.-A.; Xiong, M.; Zhang, J.; Zhou, X.; Qi, F.; He, T.; Ding, Y.; et al. Efficacy and Safety of CD28- or 4-1BB-Based CD19 CAR-T Cells in B Cell Acute Lymphoblastic Leukemia. *Mol. Ther. Oncolytics* 2020, *18*, 272–281. [CrossRef]
195. JCAR015 in ALL: A Root-Cause Investigation. *Cancer Discov.* 2018, *8*, 4–5.
196. Henderson, L.A.; Cron, R.Q. Macrophage Activation Syndrome and Secondary Hemophagocytic Lymphohistiocytosis in Childhood Inflammatory Disorders: Diagnosis and Management. *Pediatr. Drugs* 2020, *22*, 29–44. [CrossRef] [PubMed]
197. Voskoboinik, I.; Whisstock, J.C.; Trapani, J.A. Perforin and granzymes: Function, dysfunction and human pathology. *Nat. Rev. Immunol.* 2015, *15*, 388–400. [CrossRef] [PubMed]

198. Gadoury-Levesque, V.; Dong, L.; Su, R.; Chen, J.; Zhang, K.; Risma, K.A.; Marsh, R.A.; Sun, M. Frequency and spectrum of disease-causing variants in 1892 patients with suspected genetic HLH disorders. *Blood Adv.* **2020**, *4*, 2578–2594. [CrossRef] [PubMed]
199. Grom, A.A.; Horne, A.; De Benedetti, F. Macrophage activation syndrome in the era of biologic therapy. *Nat. Rev. Rheumatol.* **2016**, *12*, 259–268. [CrossRef]
200. Canna, S.W.; de Jesus, A.A.; Gouni, S.; Brooks, S.R.; Marrero, B.; Liu, Y.; DiMattia, M.A.; Zaal, K.J.M.; Sanchez, G.A.M.; Kim, H.; et al. An activating NLRC4 inflammasome mutation causes autoinflammation with recurrent macrophage activation syndrome. *Nat. Genet.* **2014**, *46*, 1140–1146. [CrossRef]
201. Teachey, D.T.; Rheingold, S.R.; Maude, S.L.; Zugmaier, G.; Barrett, D.M.; Seif, A.E.; Nichols, K.E.; Suppa, E.K.; Kalos, M.; Berg, R.A.; et al. Cytokine release syndrome after blinatumomab treatment related to abnormal macrophage activation and ameliorated with cytokine-directed therapy. *Blood* **2013**, *121*, 5154–5157. [CrossRef]
202. Morris, E.C.; Neelapu, S.S.; Giavridis, T.; Sadelain, M. Cytokine release syndrome and associated neurotoxicity in cancer immunotherapy. *Nat. Rev. Immunol.* **2021**, *22*, 85–96. [CrossRef]
203. A Misbah, S.; Weeratunga, P. Immunoglobulin replacement and quality of life after CAR T-cell therapy. *Lancet Oncol.* **2020**, *21*, e6. [CrossRef]
204. Hill, J.A.; Seo, S.K. How I prevent infections in patients receiving CD19-targeted chimeric antigen receptor T cells for B-cell malignancies. *Blood* **2020**, *136*, 925–935. [CrossRef]
205. Rabilloud, T.; Potier, D.; Pankaew, S.; Nozais, M.; Loosveld, M.; Payet-Bornet, D. Single-cell profiling identifies pre-existing CD19-negative subclones in a B-ALL patient with CD19-negative relapse after CAR-T therapy. *Nat. Commun.* **2021**, *12*, 865. [CrossRef]
206. Weiland, J.; Pal, D.; Case, M.; Irving, J.; Ponthan, F.; Koschmieder, S.; Heidenreich, O.; Von Stackelberg, A.; Eckert, C.; Vormoor, J.; et al. BCP-ALL blasts are not dependent on CD19 expression for leukaemic maintenance. *Leukemia* **2016**, *30*, 1920–1923. [CrossRef] [PubMed]
207. Dourthe, M.-E.; Rabian, F.; Yakouben, K.; Chevillon, F.; Cabannes-Hamy, A.; Méchinaud, F.; Grain, A.; Chaillou, D.; Rahal, I.; Caillat-Zucman, S.; et al. Determinants of CD19-positive vs CD19-negative relapse after tisagenlecleucel for B-cell acute lymphoblastic leukemia. *Leukemia* **2021**, *35*, 3383–3393. [CrossRef] [PubMed]
208. Sotillo, E.; Barrett, D.M.; Black, K.L.; Bagashev, A.; Oldridge, D.; Wu, G.; Sussman, R.; LaNauze, C.; Ruella, M.; Gazzara, M.R.; et al. Convergence of Acquired Mutations and Alternative Splicing of CD19 Enables Resistance to CART-19 Immunotherapy. *Cancer Discov.* **2015**, *5*, 1282–1295. [CrossRef]
209. Gardner, R.; Wu, D.; Cherian, S.; Fang, M.; Hanafi, L.-A.; Finney, O.; Smithers, H.; Jensen, M.C.; Riddell, S.R.; Maloney, D.G.; et al. Acquisition of a CD19-negative myeloid phenotype allows immune escape of MLL-rearranged B-ALL from CD19 CAR-T-cell therapy. *Blood* **2016**, *127*, 2406–2410. [CrossRef] [PubMed]
210. Zhou, Y.; You, M.J.; Young, K.H.; Lin, P.; Lu, G.; Medeiros, L.J.; Bueso-Ramos, C.E. Advances in the molecular pathobiology of B-lymphoblastic leukemia. *Hum. Pathol.* **2012**, *43*, 1347–1362. [CrossRef]
211. Salvaris, R.; Fedele, P. Targeted Therapy in Acute Lymphoblastic Leukaemia. *J. Pers. Med.* **2021**, *11*, 715. [CrossRef]
212. Zhang, W.-Y.; Liu, Y.; Wang, Y.; Wang, C.-M.; Yang, Q.-M.; Zhu, H.-L.; Han, W.-D. Long-term safety and efficacy of CART-20 cells in patients with refractory or relapsed B-cell non-Hodgkin lymphoma: 5-years follow-up results of the phase I and IIa trials. *Signal Transduct. Target. Ther.* **2017**, *2*, 17054. [CrossRef]
213. Liang, A.; Ye, S.; Li, P.; Huang, J.; Zhu, S.; Yao, X.; Zhou, L.; Xu, Y.; Zhu, J.; Zheng, C.; et al. Safety and efficacy of a novel anti-CD20 chimeric antigen receptor (CAR)-T cell therapy in relapsed/refractory (r/r) B-cell non-Hodgkin lymphoma (B-NHL) patients after failing CD19 CAR-T therapy. *J. Clin. Oncol.* **2021**, *39*, 2508. [CrossRef]
214. Shadman, M.; Yeung, C.; Redman, M.; Lee, S.Y.; Lee, D.H.; Ra, S.; Ujjani, C.S.; Dezube, B.J.; Poh, C.; Warren, E.H.; et al. Safety and Efficacy of Third Generation CD20 Targeted CAR-T (MB-106) for Treatment of Relapsed/Refractory B-NHL and CLL. *Blood* **2021**, *138*, 3872. [CrossRef]
215. Schultz, L.M.; Muffly, L.S.; Spiegel, J.Y.; Ramakrishna, S.; Hossain, N.; Baggott, C.; Sahaf, B.; Patel, S.; Craig, J.; Yoon, J.; et al. Phase I Trial Using CD19/CD22 Bispecific CAR T Cells in Pediatric and Adult Acute Lymphoblastic Leukemia (ALL). *Blood* **2019**, *134*, 744. [CrossRef]
216. Shalabi, H.; Yates, B.; Shahani, S.; Qin, H.; HIghfill, S.L.; Panch, S.; Tran, M.; Stroncek, D.; Hoffman, L.; Little, L.; et al. Abstract CT051: Safety and efficacy of CD19/CD22 CAR T cells in children and young adults with relapsed/refractory ALL. *Cancer Res.* **2020**, *80*, CT051.
217. Shah, N.N.; Johnson, B.D.; Schneider, D.; Zhu, F.; Szabo, A.; Keever-Taylor, C.A.; Krueger, W.; Worden, A.A.; Kadan, M.J.; Yim, S.; et al. Bispecific anti-CD20, anti-CD19 CAR T cells for relapsed B cell malignancies: A phase 1 dose escalation and expansion trial. *Nat. Med.* **2020**, *26*, 1569–1575. [CrossRef] [PubMed]
218. Köksal, H.; Dillard, P.; Josefsson, S.E.; Maggadottir, S.M.; Pollmann, S.; Fåne, A.; Blaker, Y.N.; Beiske, K.; Huse, K.; Kolstad, A.; et al. Preclinical development of CD37CAR T-cell therapy for treatment of B-cell lymphoma. *Blood Adv.* **2019**, *3*, 1230–1243. [CrossRef] [PubMed]
219. Scarfò, I.; Ormhøj, M.; Frigault, M.J.; Castano, A.P.; Lorrey, S.; Bouffard, A.A.; Van Scoyk, A.; Rodig, S.J.; Shay, A.J.; Aster, J.C.; et al. Anti-CD37 chimeric antigen receptor T cells are active against B- and T-cell lymphomas. *Blood* **2018**, *132*, 1495–1506. [CrossRef] [PubMed]

220. Patterson, J.D.; Henson, J.C.; Breese, R.O.; Bielamowicz, K.J.; Rodriguez, A. CAR T Cell Therapy for Pediatric Brain Tumors. *Front. Oncol.* **2020**, *10*, 1582. [CrossRef] [PubMed]
221. Richards, R.M.; Sotillo, E.; Majzner, R.G. CAR T Cell Therapy for Neuroblastoma. *Front. Immunol.* **2018**, *9*, 2380. [CrossRef]
222. Majzner, R.G.; Theruvath, J.L.; Nellan, A.; Heitzeneder, S.; Cui, Y.; Mount, C.W.; Rietberg, S.P.; Linde, M.H.; Xu, P.; Rota, C.; et al. CAR T Cells Targeting B7-H3, a Pan-Cancer Antigen, Demonstrate Potent Preclinical Activity Against Pediatric Solid Tumors and Brain Tumors. *Clin. Cancer Res.* **2019**, *25*, 2560–2574. [CrossRef]
223. Raje, N.; Berdeja, J.; Lin, Y.; Siegel, D.; Jagannath, S.; Madduri, D.; Liedtke, M.; Rosenblatt, J.; Maus, M.V.; Turka, A.; et al. Anti-BCMA CAR T-Cell Therapy bb2121 in Relapsed or Refractory Multiple Myeloma. *N. Engl. J. Med.* **2019**, *380*, 1726–1737. [CrossRef]
224. Qin, H.; Yang, L.; Chukinas, J.A.; Shah, N.N.; Tarun, S.; Pouzolles, M.; Chien, C.D.; Niswander, L.M.; Welch, A.R.; Taylor, N.A.; et al. Systematic preclinical evaluation of CD33-directed chimeric antigen receptor T cell immunotherapy for acute myeloid leukemia defines optimized construct design. *J. Immunother. Cancer* **2021**, *9*, e003149. [CrossRef]
225. Wolf, P.; Alzubi, J.; Gratzke, C.; Cathomen, T. The potential of CAR T cell therapy for prostate cancer. *Nat. Rev. Urol.* **2021**, *18*, 556–571. [CrossRef]
226. Akce, M.; Zaidi, M.Y.; Waller, E.K.; El-Rayes, B.F.; Lesinski, G.B. The Potential of CAR T Cell Therapy in Pancreatic Cancer. *Front. Immunol.* **2018**, *9*, 2166. [CrossRef] [PubMed]
227. Bo, M.D.; De Mattia, E.; Baboci, L.; Mezzalira, S.; Cecchin, E.; Assaraf, Y.G.; Toffoli, G. New insights into the pharmacological, immunological, and CAR-T-cell approaches in the treatment of hepatocellular carcinoma. *Drug Resist. Updat.* **2020**, *51*, 100702.
228. Kudo, K.; Imai, C.; Lorenzini, P.; Kamiya, T.; Kono, K.; Davidoff, A.M.; Chng, W.J.; Campana, D. T Lymphocytes Expressing a CD16 Signaling Receptor Exert Antibody-Dependent Cancer Cell Killing. *Cancer Res.* **2014**, *74*, 93–103. [CrossRef] [PubMed]
229. Rataj, F.; Jacobi, S.J.; Stoiber, S.; Asang, F.; Ogonek, J.; Tokarew, N.; Cadilha, B.; Van Puijenbroek, E.; Heise, C.; Duewell, P.; et al. High-affinity CD16-polymorphism and Fc-engineered antibodies enable activity of CD16-chimeric antigen receptor-modified T cells for cancer therapy. *Br. J. Cancer* **2019**, *120*, 79–87. [CrossRef]
230. Tamada, K.; Geng, D.; Sakoda, Y.; Bansal, N.; Srivastava, R.; Li, Z.; Davila, E. Redirecting Gene-Modified T Cells toward Various Cancer Types Using Tagged Antibodies. *Clin. Cancer Res.* **2012**, *18*, 6436–6445. [CrossRef]
231. Ma, J.S.Y.; Kim, J.Y.; Kazane, S.A.; Choi, S.-H.; Yun, H.Y.; Kim, M.S.; Rodgers, D.T.; Pugh, H.M.; Singer, O.; Sun, S.B.; et al. Versatile strategy for controlling the specificity and activity of engineered T cells. *Proc. Natl. Acad. Sci. USA* **2016**, *113*, E450–E458. [CrossRef]
232. Rodgers, D.T.; Mazagova, M.; Hampton, E.N.; Cao, Y.; Ramadoss, N.S.; Hardy, I.R.; Schulman, A.; Du, J.; Wang, F.; Singer, O.; et al. Switch-mediated activation and retargeting of CAR-T cells for B-cell malignancies. *Proc. Natl. Acad. Sci. USA* **2016**, *113*, E459–E468. [CrossRef]
233. Bachmann, M. The UniCAR system: A modular CAR T cell approach to improve the safety of CAR T cells. *Immunol. Lett.* **2019**, *211*, 13–22. [CrossRef]
234. Mu, J.; Edwards, J.; Zaritskaya, L.; Swers, J.; Gupta, A.; LaFleur, D.; Hilbert, D.; Richman, L. Selective targeting of HER2-overexpressing solid tumors with a next-generation CAR-T cell therapy. *J. Clin. Oncol.* **2020**, *38*, 3041. [CrossRef]
235. Grote, S.; Mittelstaet, J.; Baden, C.; Chan, K.C.; Seitz, C.; Schlegel, P.; Kaiser, A.; Handgretinger, R.; Schleicher, S. Adapter chimeric antigen receptor (AdCAR)-engineered NK-92 cells: An off-the-shelf cellular therapeutic for universal tumor targeting. *Oncoimmunology* **2020**, *9*, 1825177. [CrossRef]
236. Urbanska, K.; Lanitis, E.; Poussin, M.; Lynn, R.C.; Gavin, B.P.; Kelderman, S.; Yu, J.; Scholler, N.; Powell, D.J., Jr. A Universal Strategy for Adoptive Immunotherapy of Cancer through Use of a Novel T-cell Antigen Receptor. *Cancer Res.* **2012**, *72*, 1844–1852. [CrossRef] [PubMed]
237. Cho, J.H.; Collins, J.J.; Wong, W.W. Universal Chimeric Antigen Receptors for Multiplexed and Logical Control of T Cell Responses. *Cell* **2018**, *173*, 1426–1438.e11. [CrossRef] [PubMed]
238. Kim, M.S.; Ma, J.S.Y.; Yun, H.; Cao, Y.; Kim, J.Y.; Chi, V.; Wang, D.; Woods, A.; Sherwood, L.; Caballero, D.; et al. Redirection of Genetically Engineered CAR-T Cells Using Bifunctional Small Molecules. *J. Am. Chem. Soc.* **2015**, *137*, 2832–2835. [CrossRef] [PubMed]
239. Ryman, J.T.; Meibohm, B. Pharmacokinetics of Monoclonal Antibodies. *CPT Pharmacomet. Syst. Pharmacol.* **2017**, *6*, 576–588. [CrossRef]
240. Waldmann, T.A.; Strober, W. Metabolism of Immunoglobulins. *Prog. Allergy* **1969**, *13*, 891–903.
241. Knauf, M.J.; Bell, D.P.; Hirtzer, P.; Luo, Z.P.; Young, J.D.; Katre, N.V. Relationship of effective molecular size to systemic clearance in rats of recombinant interleukin-2 chemically modified with water-soluble polymers. *J. Biol. Chem.* **1988**, *263*, 15064–15070. [CrossRef]
242. Lampson, L.A. Monoclonal antibodies in neuro-oncology: Getting past the blood-brain barrier. *mAbs* **2011**, *3*, 153–160. [CrossRef]
243. Cavaco, M.; Gaspar, D.; Castanho, M.A.; Neves, V. Antibodies for the Treatment of Brain Metastases, a Dream or a Reality? *Pharmaceutics* **2020**, *12*, 62. [CrossRef]
244. Cruz, E.; Kayser, V. Monoclonal antibody therapy of solid tumors: Clinical limitations and novel strategies to enhance treatment efficacy. *Biol. Targets Ther.* **2019**, *13*, 33–51. [CrossRef]

245. Davis, K.L.; Mackall, C.L. Immunotherapy for acute lymphoblastic leukemia: From famine to feast. *Blood Adv.* **2016**, *1*, 265–269. [CrossRef]
246. Lenk, L.; Alsadeq, A.; Schewe, D.M. Involvement of the central nervous system in acute lymphoblastic leukemia: Opinions on molecular mechanisms and clinical implications based on recent data. *Cancer Metastasis Rev.* **2020**, *39*, 173–187. [CrossRef] [PubMed]
247. Abid, H.; Watthanasuntorn, K.; Shah, O.; Gnanajothy, R. Efficacy of Pembrolizumab and Nivolumab in Crossing the Blood Brain Barrier. *Cureus* **2019**, *11*, e4446. [CrossRef] [PubMed]
248. Cartellieri, M.; Feldmann, A.; Koristka, S.; Arndt, C.; Loff, S.; Ehninger, A.V.; Von Bonin, M.; Bejestani, E.P.; Ehninger, G.; Bachmann, M.P. Switching CAR T cells on and off: A novel modular platform for retargeting of T cells to AML blasts. *Blood Cancer J.* **2016**, *6*, e458. [CrossRef] [PubMed]
249. Goebeler, M.-E.; Knop, S.; Viardot, A.; Kufer, P.; Topp, M.S.; Einsele, H.; Noppeney, R.; Hess, G.; Kallert, S.; Mackensen, A.; et al. Bispecific T-Cell Engager (BiTE) Antibody Construct Blinatumomab for the Treatment of Patients With Relapsed/Refractory Non-Hodgkin Lymphoma: Final Results From a Phase I Study. *J. Clin. Oncol.* **2016**, *34*, 1104–1111. [CrossRef]
250. . Hong, W.X.; Haebe, S.; Lee, A.S.; Westphalen, C.B.; Norton, J.A.; Jiang, W.; Levy, R. Intratumoral Immunotherapy for Early-stage Solid Tumors. *Clin. Cancer Res.* **2020**, *26*, 3091–3099. [CrossRef]
251. Adusumilli, P.S.; Zauderer, M.G.; Rivière, I.; Solomon, S.B.; Rusch, V.W.; O'Cearbhaill, R.E.; Zhu, A.; Cheema, W.; Chintala, N.K.; Halton, E.; et al. A Phase I Trial of Regional Mesothelin-Targeted CAR T-cell Therapy in Patients with Malignant Pleural Disease, in Combination with the Anti–PD-1 Agent Pembrolizumab. *Cancer Discov.* **2021**, *11*, 2748–2763. [CrossRef]
252. Choi, B.D.; O'Rourke, D.M.; Maus, M.V. Engineering Chimeric Antigen Receptor T cells to Treat Glioblastoma. *Int. J. Target. Ther. Cancer* **2017**, *6*, 22–25.
253. Schulz, H.; Pels, H.; Schmidt-Wolf, I.; Zeelen, U.; Germing, U.; Engert, A. Intraventricular treatment of relapsed central nervous system lymphoma with the anti-CD20 antibody rituximab. *Haematology* **2004**, *89*, 753–754.
254. Sison, E.A.R.; Silverman, L.B. CNS prophylaxis in pediatric acute lymphoblastic leukemia. *Hematology* **2014**, *2014*, 198–201. [CrossRef]
255. Ravandi, F.; Walter, R.B.; Subklewe, M.; Buecklein, V.; Jongen-Lavrencic, M.; Paschka, P.; Ossenkoppele, G.J.; Kantarjian, H.M.; Hindoyan, A.; Agarwal, S.K.; et al. Updated results from phase I dose-escalation study of AMG 330, a bispecific T-cell engager molecule, in patients with relapsed/refractory acute myeloid leukemia (R/R AML). *J. Clin. Oncol.* **2020**, *38*, 7508. [CrossRef]
256. Krupka, C.; Kufer, P.; Kischel, R.; Zugmaier, G.; Bögeholz, J.; Köhnke, T.; Lichtenegger, F.S.; Schneider, S.; Metzeler, K.; Fiegl, M.; et al. CD33 target validation and sustained depletion of AML blasts in long-term cultures by the bispecific T-cell–engaging antibody AMG 330. *Blood* **2014**, *123*, 356–365. [CrossRef] [PubMed]
257. Wang, X.; Chang, W.-C.; Wong, C.W.; Colcher, D.; Sherman, M.; Ostberg, J.R.; Forman, S.J.; Riddell, S.R.; Jensen, M.C. A transgene-encoded cell surface polypeptide for selection, in vivo tracking, and ablation of engineered cells. *Blood* **2011**, *118*, 1255–1263. [CrossRef] [PubMed]
258. Di Stasi, A.; Tey, S.-K.; Dotti, G.; Fujita, Y.; Kennedy-Nasser, A.; Martinez, C.; Straathof, K.; Liu, E.; Durett, A.G.; Grilley, B.; et al. Inducible Apoptosis as a Safety Switch for Adoptive Cell Therapy. *N. Engl. J. Med.* **2011**, *365*, 1673–1683. [CrossRef] [PubMed]
259. Budde, L.E.; Berger, C.; Lin, Y.; Wang, J.; Lin, X.; Frayo, S.E.; Brouns, S.A.; Spencer, D.M.; Till, B.G.; Jensen, M.C.; et al. Combining a CD20 Chimeric Antigen Receptor and an Inducible Caspase 9 Suicide Switch to Improve the Efficacy and Safety of T Cell Adoptive Immunotherapy for Lymphoma. *PLoS ONE* **2013**, *8*, e82742. [CrossRef] [PubMed]
260. Sterner, R.M.; Sakemura, R.; Cox, M.J.; Yang, N.; Khadka, R.H.; Forsman, C.L.; Hansen, M.J.; Jin, F.; Ayasoufi, K.; Hefazi, M.; et al. GM-CSF inhibition reduces cytokine release syndrome and neuroinflammation but enhances CAR-T cell function in xenografts. *Blood* **2019**, *133*, 697–709. [CrossRef]
261. Roybal, K.T.; Rupp, L.J.; Morsut, L.; Walker, W.J.; McNally, K.A.; Park, J.S.; Lim, W.A. Precision Tumor Recognition by T Cells With Combinatorial Antigen-Sensing Circuits. *Cell* **2016**, *164*, 770–779. [CrossRef]
262. Kloss, C.C.; Condomines, M.; Cartellieri, M.; Bachmann, M.; Sadelain, M. Combinatorial antigen recognition with balanced signaling promotes selective tumor eradication by engineered T cells. *Nat. Biotechnol.* **2013**, *31*, 71–75. [CrossRef]
263. Zajc, C.U.; Dobersberger, M.; Schaffner, I.; Mlynek, G.; Pühringer, D.; Salzer, B.; Djinović-Carugo, K.; Steinberger, P.; Linhares, A.D.S.; Yang, N.J.; et al. A conformation-specific ON-switch for controlling CAR T cells with an orally available drug. *Proc. Natl. Acad. Sci. USA* **2020**, *117*, 14926–14935. [CrossRef]
264. Park, S.; Pascua, E.; Lindquist, K.C.; Kimberlin, C.; Deng, X.; Mak, Y.S.L.; Melton, Z.; Johnson, T.O.; Lin, R.; Boldajipour, B.; et al. Direct control of CAR T cells through small molecule-regulated antibodies. *Nat. Commun.* **2021**, *12*, 710. [CrossRef]
265. Weber, E.W.; Lynn, R.C.; Sotillo, E.; Lattin, J.; Xu, P.; Mackall, C.L. Pharmacologic control of CAR-T cell function using dasatinib. *Blood Adv.* **2019**, *3*, 711–717. [CrossRef]
266. Mestermann, K.; Giavridis, T.; Weber, J.; Rydzek, J.; Frenz, S.; Nerreter, T.; Mades, A.; Sadelain, M.; Einsele, H.; Hudecek, M. The tyrosine kinase inhibitor dasatinib acts as a pharmacologic on/off switch for CAR T cells. *Sci. Transl. Med.* **2019**, *11*, eaau5907. [CrossRef] [PubMed]
267. Deng, Q.; Han, G.; Puebla-Osorio, N.; Ma, M.C.J.; Strati, P.; Chasen, B.; Dai, E.; Dang, M.; Jain, N.; Yang, H.; et al. Characteristics of anti-CD19 CAR T cell infusion products associated with efficacy and toxicity in patients with large B cell lymphomas. *Nat. Med.* **2020**, *26*, 1878–1887. [CrossRef] [PubMed]

268. Li-Weber, M.; Krammer, P.H. Regulation of IL4 gene expression by T cells and therapeutic perspectives. *Nat. Rev. Immunol.* **2003**, *3*, 534–543. [CrossRef] [PubMed]
269. Mohammed, S.; Sukumaran, S.; Bajgain, P.; Watanabe, N.; Heslop, H.E.; Rooney, C.M.; Brenner, M.K.; Fisher, W.E.; Leen, A.M.; Vera, J.F. Improving Chimeric Antigen Receptor-Modified T Cell Function by Reversing the Immunosuppressive Tumor Microenvironment of Pancreatic Cancer. *Mol. Ther.* **2017**, *25*, 249–258. [CrossRef]
270. Kloss, C.C.; Lee, J.; Zhang, A.; Chen, F.; Melenhorst, J.J.; Lacey, S.F.; Maus, M.V.; Fraietta, J.A.; Zhao, Y.; June, C.H. Dominant-Negative TGF-beta Receptor Enhances PSMA-Targeted Human CAR T Cell Proliferation And Augments Prostate Cancer Eradication. *Mol. Ther.* **2018**, *26*, 1855–1866. [CrossRef]
271. Liu, X.; Ranganathan, R.; Jiang, S.; Fang, C.; Sun, J.; Kim, S.; Newick, K.; Lo, A.; June, C.H.; Zhao, Y.; et al. A Chimeric Switch-Receptor Targeting PD1 Augments the Efficacy of Second-Generation CAR T Cells in Advanced Solid Tumors. *Cancer Res.* **2016**, *76*, 1578–1590. [CrossRef]
272. Rafiq, S.; Yeku, O.O.; Jackson, H.J.; Purdon, T.J.; Van Leeuwen, D.G.; Drakes, D.J.; Song, M.; Miele, M.M.; Li, Z.; Wang, P.; et al. Targeted delivery of a PD-1-blocking scFv by CAR-T cells enhances anti-tumor efficacy in vivo. *Nat. Biotechnol.* **2018**, *36*, 847–856. [CrossRef]
273. Suarez, E.R.; de Chang, K.; Sun, J.; Sui, J.; Freeman, G.J.; Signoretti, S.; Zhu, Q.; Marasco, W.A. Chimeric antigen receptor T cells secreting anti-PD-L1 antibodies more effectively regress renal cell carcinoma in a humanized mouse model. *Oncotarget* **2016**, *7*, 34341–34355. [CrossRef]
274. Cherkassky, L.; Morello, A.; Villena-Vargas, J.; Feng, Y.; Dimitrov, D.S.; Jones, D.R.; Sadelain, M.; Adusumilli, P.S. Human CAR T cells with cell-intrinsic PD-1 checkpoint blockade resist tumor-mediated inhibition. *J. Clin. Investig.* **2016**, *126*, 3130–3144. [CrossRef]
275. Rupp, L.J.; Schumann, K.; Roybal, K.T.; Gate, R.E.; Ye, C.J.; Lim, W.A.; Marson, A. CRISPR/Cas9-mediated PD-1 disruption enhances anti-tumor efficacy of human chimeric antigen receptor T cells. *Sci. Rep.* **2017**, *7*, 737. [CrossRef]
276. Wang, Z.; Li, N.; Feng, K.; Chen, M.; Zhang, Y.; Liu, Y.; Yang, Q.; Nie, J.; Tang, N.; Zhang, X.; et al. Phase I study of CAR-T cells with PD-1 and TCR disruption in mesothelin-positive solid tumors. *Cell. Mol. Immunol.* **2021**, *18*, 2188–2198. [CrossRef] [PubMed]
277. Choi, B.D.; Yu, X.; Castano, A.P.; Darr, H.; Henderson, D.B.; Bouffard, A.A.; Larson, R.C.; Scarfò, I.; Bailey, S.R.; Gerhard, G.M.; et al. CRISPR-Cas9 disruption of PD-1 enhances activity of universal EGFRvIII CAR T cells in a preclinical model of human glioblastoma. *J. Immunother. Cancer* **2019**, *7*, 304. [CrossRef] [PubMed]
278. Poirot, L.; Philip, B.; Schiffer-Mannioui, C.; Le Clerre, D.; Chion-Sotinel, I.; Derniame, S.; Potrel, P.; Bas, C.; Lemaire, L.; Galetto, R.; et al. Multiplex Genome-Edited T-cell Manufacturing Platform for "Off-the-Shelf" Adoptive T-cell Immunotherapies. *Cancer Res.* **2015**, *75*, 3853–3864. [CrossRef] [PubMed]
279. Riley, J.L. PD-1 signaling in primary T cells. *Immunol. Rev.* **2009**, *229*, 114–125. [CrossRef]
280. Stenger, D.; Stief, T.A.; Kaeuferle, T.; Willier, S.; Rataj, F.; Schober, K.; Vick, B.; Lotfi, R.; Wagner, B.; Grünewald, T.G.P.; et al. Endogenous TCR promotes in vivo persistence of CD19-CAR-T cells compared to a CRISPR/Cas9-mediated TCR knockout CAR. *Blood* **2020**, *136*, 1407–1418. [CrossRef]
281. Roth, T.L.; Puig-Saus, C.; Yu, R.; Shifrut, E.; Carnevale, J.; Li, P.J.; Hiatt, J.; Saco, J.; Krystofinski, P.; Li, H.; et al. Reprogramming human T cell function and specificity with non-viral genome targeting. *Nature* **2018**, *559*, 405–409. [CrossRef]
282. MacLeod, D.T.; Antony, J.; Martin, A.J.; Moser, R.J.; Hekele, A.; Wetzel, K.J.; Brown, A.E.; Triggiano, M.A.; Hux, J.A.; Pham, C.D.; et al. Integration of a CD19 CAR into the TCR Alpha Chain Locus Streamlines Production of Allogeneic Gene-Edited CAR T Cells. *Mol. Ther.* **2017**, *25*, 949–961. [CrossRef]
283. Liu, Y.; Liu, G.; Wang, J.; Zheng, Z.-Y.; Jia, L.; Rui, W.; Huang, D.; Zhou, Z.-X.; Zhou, L.; Wu, X.; et al. Chimeric STAR receptors using TCR machinery mediate robust responses against solid tumors. *Sci. Transl. Med.* **2021**, *13*, abb5191. [CrossRef]
284. Baeuerle, P.A.; Ding, J.; Patel, E.; Thorausch, N.; Horton, J.; Gierut, J.; Scarfo, I.; Choudhary, R.; Kiner, O.; Krishnamurthy, J.; et al. Synthetic TRuC receptors engaging the complete T cell receptor for potent anti-tumor response. *Nat. Commun.* **2019**, *10*, 2087. [CrossRef]
285. Koneru, M.; Purdon, T.J.; Spriggs, D.; Koneru, S.; Brentjens, R.J. IL-12 secreting tumor-targeted chimeric antigen receptor T cells eradicate ovarian tumors in vivo. *OncoImmunology* **2015**, *4*, e994446. [CrossRef]
286. Hu, B.; Ren, J.; Luo, Y.; Keith, B.; Young, R.M.; Scholler, J.; Zhao, Y.; June, C.H. Augmentation of Antitumor Immunity by Human and Mouse CAR T Cells Secreting IL-18. *Cell Rep.* **2017**, *20*, 3025–3033. [CrossRef] [PubMed]
287. Hurton, L.V.; Singh, H.; Najjar, A.M.; Switzer, K.C.; Mi, T.; Maiti, S.; Olivares, S.; Rabinovich, B.; Huls, H.; Forget, M.-A.; et al. Tethered IL-15 augments antitumor activity and promotes a stem-cell memory subset in tumor-specific T cells. *Proc. Natl. Acad. Sci. USA* **2016**, *113*, E7788–E7797. [CrossRef] [PubMed]
288. Majzner, R.G.; Mackall, C.L. Clinical lessons learned from the first leg of the CAR T cell journey. *Nat. Med.* **2019**, *25*, 1341–1355. [CrossRef] [PubMed]
289. Sterner, R.C.; Sterner, R.M. CAR-T cell therapy: Current limitations and potential strategies. *Blood Cancer J.* **2021**, *11*, 69. [CrossRef]
290. Yang, J.; He, J.; Zhang, X.; Wang, Z.; Zhang, Y.; Cai, S.; Sun, Z.; Ye, X.; He, Y.; Shen, L.; et al. A Feasibility and Safety Study of a New CD19-Directed Fast CAR-T Therapy for Refractory and Relapsed B Cell Acute Lymphoblastic Leukemia. *Blood* **2019**, *134*, 825. [CrossRef]

291. Whittington, M.D.; McQueen, R.B.; Ollendorf, D.A.; Kumar, V.M.; Chapman, R.H.; Tice, J.; Pearson, S.D.; Campbell, J.D. Long-term Survival and Value of Chimeric Antigen Receptor T-Cell Therapy for Pediatric Patients With Relapsed or Refractory Leukemia. *JAMA Pediatr.* **2018**, *172*, 1161–1168. [CrossRef]
292. Sarkar, R.R.; Gloude, N.J.; Schiff, D.; Murphy, J.D. Cost-Effectiveness of Chimeric Antigen Receptor T-Cell Therapy in Pediatric Relapsed/Refractory B-Cell Acute Lymphoblastic Leukemia. *JNCI J. Natl. Cancer Inst.* **2019**, *111*, 719–726. [CrossRef]

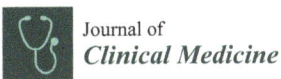

Article

Engineering of CD19 Antibodies: A CD19-TRAIL Fusion Construct Specifically Induces Apoptosis in B-Cell Precursor Acute Lymphoblastic Leukemia (BCP-ALL) Cells In Vivo

Dorothee Winterberg [1,2,†], Lennart Lenk [1,†], Maren Oßwald [2], Fotini Vogiatzi [1], Carina Lynn Gehlert [2], Fabian-Simon Frielitz [3], Katja Klausz [2], Thies Rösner [2], Thomas Valerius [2], Anna Trauzold [4], Matthias Peipp [2], Christian Kellner [5,‡] and Denis Martin Schewe [1,*,‡]

1. ALL-BFM Study Group, Department of Pediatrics I, Christian-Albrechts University Kiel and University Medical Center Schleswig-Holstein, Arnold-Heller Str. 3, Haus C, 24105 Kiel, Germany; dorothee.winterberg@uksh.de (D.W.); Lennart.lenk@uksh.de (L.L.); Fotini.Vogiatzi@uksh.de (F.V.)
2. Department of Medicine II Christian-Albrechts, Division of Stem Cell Transplantation and Immunotherapy, Campus Kiel, University Kiel and University Hospital Schleswig-Holstein, 24105 Kiel, Germany; osswaldmaren@gmail.com (M.O.); CarinaLynn.Gehlert@uksh.de (C.L.G.); Katja.Klausz@uksh.de (K.K.); Thies.Roesner@uksh.de (T.R.); t.valerius@med2.uni-kiel.de (T.V.); m.peipp@med2.uni-kiel.de (M.P.)
3. Institute for Social Medicine and Epidemiology, University of Lübeck, 23538 Lübeck, Germany; fabian@frielitz.net
4. Institute for Experimental Cancer Research, Christian-Albrechts-University Kiel, 24104 Kiel, Germany; atrauzold@email.uni-kiel.de
5. Department of Transfusion Medicine, Cell Therapeutics and Hemostaseology, LMU University Hospital Munich, 81377 Munich, Germany; Christian.Kellner@med.uni-muenchen.de
* Correspondence: Denis.Schewe@uksh.de; Tel.: +49-431-500-20140
† Contributed equally.
‡ Shared senior authorship.

Abstract: B-cell precursor acute lymphoblastic leukemia (BCP-ALL) is the most frequent malignancy in children and also occurs in adulthood. Despite high cure rates, BCP-ALL chemotherapy can be highly toxic. This type of toxicity can most likely be reduced by antibody-based immunotherapy targeting the CD19 antigen which is commonly expressed on BCP-ALL cells. In this study, we generated a novel Fc-engineered CD19-targeting IgG1 antibody fused to a single chain tumor necrosis factor (TNF)-related apoptosis-inducing ligand (TRAIL) domain (CD19-TRAIL). As TRAIL induces apoptosis in tumor cells but not in healthy cells, we hypothesized that CD19-TRAIL would show efficient killing of BCP-ALL cells. CD19-TRAIL showed selective binding capacity and pronounced apoptosis induction in CD19-positive (CD19$^+$) BCP-ALL cell lines in vitro and in vivo. Additionally, CD19-TRAIL significantly prolonged survival of mice transplanted with BCP-ALL patient-derived xenograft (PDX) cells of different cytogenetic backgrounds. Moreover, simultaneous treatment with CD19-TRAIL and Venetoclax (VTX), an inhibitor of the anti-apoptotic protein BCL-2, promoted synergistic apoptosis induction in CD19$^+$ BCP-ALL cells in vitro and prolonged survival of NSG-mice bearing the BCP-ALL cell line REH. Therefore, IgG1-based CD19-TRAIL fusion proteins represent a new potential immunotherapeutic agent against BCP-ALL.

Keywords: BCP-ALL; leukemia; TRAIL; antibody; Fc-engineering; xenograft; CD19

1. Introduction

B-cell precursor acute lymphoblastic leukemia (BCP-ALL) is the most frequent childhood malignancy. Whereas most patients can be cured by chemotherapy, this is associated with severe side effects, and relapse remains a major clinical challenge [1–3]. Immunotherapeutic approaches, especially monoclonal antibodies, exert highly specific anti-tumoral efficacy with lower off-target toxic effects [4]. Accordingly, antibody-based immunotherapy is being introduced into the treatment of B-cell malignancies including BCP-ALL, both in frontline therapy and in the treatment of relapsed and refractory disease [5,6]. An attractive therapeutic target in BCP-ALL is the pan B-lymphocyte antigen CD19, a type I membrane protein of the immunoglobin superfamily that is expressed by the majority of B-lineage lymphoid malignancies [7–10]. To this end, targeting CD19 with novel immunotherapeutic approaches, such as the (CD3 × CD19) bispecific T-cell engager molecule (BiTE) blinatumomab or chimeric antigen receptor (CAR) T-cells, have entered routine clinical care in specific situations [11–13]. CD19 antibody-drug conjugates (ADC) such as coltuximab ravtansine (SAR3419) have shown tolerability but poor clinical response in patients with relapsed or refractory BCP-ALL [14]. Native CD19-IgG1 antibodies displayed only limited efficacy in preclinical models [15,16]. Yet, the therapeutic efficacy of CD19 antibodies can be improved by fragment crystallizable (Fc)-engineering, e.g., through introducing amino acid substitutions into the heavy chain (CH) region 2 or by changing the glycosylation pattern of the antibody. As a result, the affinity to Fcγ receptors on effector cells is increased, leading to enhanced effector cell recruitment and activation [15,17,18]. We previously showed that an Fc-engineered CD19 antibody carrying a S239D/I332E mutation (DE-modification) showed enhanced effector cell-mediated killing of tumor cells and pronounced efficacy in BCP-ALL xenografts in vivo [19]. The DE-modified antibody tafasitamab is currently being tested in BCP-ALL patients (ClinicalTrials.gov identifier NCT01685021).

Another promising antibody modification is the linkage with biological cytotoxic agents such as the tumor necrosis factor (TNF)-related apoptosis-inducing ligand (TRAIL) [20]. TRAIL is a homotrimeric type II transmembrane protein that initiates extrinsic apoptosis by binding its agonistic death receptors TRAIL-Receptor 1 (TRAIL-R1) and TRAIL-R2 on the target cell [21–25]. This results in receptor oligomerization and subsequent assembly of the death-inducing signaling complex (DISC) and activation of a caspase cascade [26]. Of note, TRAIL was shown to induce apoptosis in cancer cells selectively, even in the absence of a high proliferation rate [25,27–29]. Treatment with recombinant TRAIL showed promising results in preclinical studies [30,31]. However, clinical pilot studies with non-small-cell lung cancer and relapsed follicular non-Hodgkin's lymphoma patients found no superior outcomes when adding TRAIL to standard care [32,33]. Proposed reasons for the limited in vivo efficacy are the instability and rapid clearance of TRAIL as well as the apoptosis resistance of tumor cells [31,34]. The latter may be based on the presence of TRAIL-decoy receptors and the widespread TRAIL-R expression in the tumor microenvironment competing for TRAIL ligands, thereby limiting the accumulation of TRAIL on tumor cells [21,35,36]. These limitations can be overcome by fusing TRAIL to tumor-specific antibodies or antibody-fragments, particularly constructs based on IgG structures (IgG-like), which generally harbor a superior pharmacokinetic profile [20,37,38]. These fusion constructs may accumulate on the pre-selected target antigen of tumor cells and lead to the subsequent anchoring of the TRAIL domain on the cell surface promoting increased TRAIL-R engagement. Such constructs may even outperform Fc-less fusion proteins [39,40]. Therefore, we hypothesized that genetic fusion of a monoclonal CD19-directed IgG antibody to monovalent single-chain (sc) TRAIL generates a fusion protein that combines the specificity and beneficial pharmacokinetics of an IgG antibody with the cytotoxic activity of a tumor-cell-specific death ligand.

Here, we report the successful generation of such an IgG fusion protein (CD19-TRAIL) and show that CD19-TRAIL efficiently kills CD19-positive (CD19$^+$) BCP-ALL cell lines in vitro and in vivo and is also effective in BCP-ALL xenograft mouse models. Moreover, we show that the tumor-killing effect of CD19-TRAIL can be synergistically enhanced by dual induction of the extrinsic and intrinsic apoptosis pathways. Our preclinical data suggest that CD19-IgG-antibodies coupled to scTRAIL may be an effective agent to target BCP-ALL cells directly.

2. Materials and Methods

2.1. Cell Culture

The BCP-ALL cell lines REH and NALM-6 and the T-ALL cell line CEM were obtained from the German Collection of Microorganisms and Cell Cultures (DSMZ, Braunschweig, Germany) and cultured in RPMI 1640 Glutamax-I medium containing 10% fetal calf serum (FCS), 100 U/mL penicillin, and 100 µg/mL streptomycin (Thermo Fisher Scientific, Waltham, MA, USA). Chinese hamster ovary (CHO-S) cells were purchased from Thermo Fisher Scientific and cultured in an orbital shaker with serum-free CD-CHO medium containing 1% HT supplement and 2 mM GlutaMax (Thermo Fisher Scientific, Waltham, MA, USA). For culturing of transfected CHO-S cells, the CD OptiCHO medium was supplemented with 1% HT supplement, 2 mM GlutaMax, and 0.1% Pluronic F-68 (Thermo Fisher Scientific, Waltham, MA, USA).

2.2. Antibodies

CD19-TRAIL and HER2-TRAIL were generated by de novo synthesis of the DNA sequences of the variable regions of the antibodies tafasitamab (MOR208) and trastuzumab, respectively, according to published sequences [41,42]. To promote heterodimeric Fc domain pairing, codon exchanges for amino acid substitutions in the CH3 domain (i.e., K392D and K409D for the first HC and E356K and D399K for the second HC) were respectively inserted [43], and a DNA sequence encoding a single chain TRAIL domain containing three TRAIL monomers [44] was genetically fused to the C-terminal part of the first HC.

Sequences were ligated in frame into antibody light chain (LC) expression vector pSECtag2-LC or antibody HC expression vector pSECtag2-HC [17,19]. Validity of the cloned sequences was confirmed by Sanger sequencing, and plasmid DNA was purified with Nucleo Bond 2000 EF (Macherey-Nagel, Düren, Germany). Antibody-TRAIL fusion proteins and a native CD19-IgG1 antibody [19] were produced in CHO-S cells by transient transfection of HC and LC expression vectors using the MaxCyte STX Scalable Transfection System (MaxCyte, Gaithersburg, MD, USA), as previously described [45]. Antibodies were purified from cell culture supernatant with a CaptureSelectTM IgG-CH1 affinity matrix (Thermo Fisher Scientific, Waltham, MA, USA) and size exclusion chromatography (ÄKTA Pure 25 liquid chromatography system; GE Healthcare, Chicago, IL, USA).

2.3. Sodium Dodecyl Sulfate Polyacrylamide Gel Electrophoresis (SDS-PAGE) and Western Blot Analysis

Antibody integrity and concentration were analyzed by SDS-PAGE under reducing conditions and western transfer experiments, as published previously [46].

For detection of human IgG HC, LC, and TRAIL, a goat-anti-human-IgG-HRP conjugate (#AP113P, Sigma Aldrich, St. Louis, MO, USA), a mouse anti-human kappa light chain (#K4377, Sigma Aldrich, St. Louis, MO, USA), and a rabbit anti-human TRAIL antibody (#ab9959, Abcam, Cambridge, UK) were used, respectively.

2.4. CD19 Binding Capacity

Specific binding capacities of CD19-TRAIL, CD19-IgG1, and HER2-TRAIL were analyzed as previously reported using a secondary anti-human IgG Fc F(ab′)2 polyclonal goat antibody conjugated to Fluorescein isothiocyanate (FITC) (Jackson Immuno Research, West Grove, PA, USA) [47]. Flow cytometric analyses were performed with a Navios flow cytometer, and data were analyzed with the Kaluza 1.2 software (Beckman Coulter, Brea, CA, USA).

2.5. Expression of CD19, TRAIL-R1, and TRAIL-R2 on Cell Lines and PDX Samples

Quantification of expression levels of CD19, TRAIL-R1, and TRAIL-R2 on the cell surface was analyzed by flow cytometry using QIFIKIT (Agilent Technologies, Santa Clara, CA, USA) according to the manufacturer´s protocol. Briefly, cells were washed with PBA (phosphate-buffered saline (PBS, Thermo Fisher Scientific, Waltham, MA, USA), 1% bovine serum albumin (BSA, Carl Roth, Karlsruhe, Germany), and 0.1% sodium-azide (Merck,

Darmstadt, Germany). Then, 0.5×10^6 cells were incubated with saturated concentrations of mouse antibodies against CD19 (#392502, Biolegend, San Diego, CA, USA), TRAIL-R1 (#307202, Biolegend, San Diego, CA, USA), and TRAIL-R2 (#307302, Biolegend, San Diego, CA, USA) for 1 h, respectively. After washing with PBA, cells were incubated for 30 min with a FITC-labelled anti-mouse antibody. Fluorescence was measured by flow cytometry using a MACSQuant X Analyzer (Miltenyi Biotec, Bergisch Gladbach, Germany). Antigen density was assessed by generating a standard curve obtained by beads coated with defined amounts of mouse IgG. Data were analyzed by FlowJo software Version 10.7.1 (Becton, Dickinson and Company, Ashland, OR, USA).

2.6. Cell Viability Assay

Direct cytotoxic effects were analyzed by 3-(4,5-Dimethylthiazol-2-yl)2,5-diphenyl tetrazolium bromide (MTT) assay (Roche Diagnostics, Mannheim, Germany). Briefly, 2×10^4 cells per well in 100 µL medium were seeded in flat-bottom 96-well culture plates and treated with serial dilutions of indicated compounds for 72 h. After 4 h incubation with MTT reagent, the assay-solution was added to each well, and absorption at 550 nm (reference 650 nm) was measured after overnight culture. Cell viability was quantified as the percentage of growth inhibition compared to medium control (% relative growth of control). All experimental points were set up in triplicates.

2.7. Analysis of Apoptosis Induction

For analysis of apoptosis induction, cells were treated with 0.5 nM CD19-TRAIL and stained using AnnexinV-APC/PI (Biolegend, San Diego, CA, USA), and early and late apoptotic/necrotic cells were detected by fluorescence measurement using a Navios flow cytometer (Beckman Coulter, Brea, CA, USA). For apoptosis-blocking experiments, cells were pre-incubated with 50 µM of the pan-caspase inhibitor Z-VAD (MedChemExpress, Monmouth Junction, NJ, USA) prior to antibody incubation for 1 h. DMSO-treated cells served as a control. Data were analyzed with the Kaluza 1.2 software (Beckman Coulter, Brea, CA, USA).

2.8. Analysis of Drug Combination Effects

For analysis of the combined treatment effects of CD19-TRAIL with Venetoclax (VTX), 2×10^4 cells were treated with CD19-TRAIL or VTX (LC Laboratories, Woburn, MA, USA) according to the determined EC50 value of either substance (0.06 nM and 6 nM, respectively) as well as increased and decreased concentrations in 5-fold dilution steps and then subjected to MTT assays. Drug synergy was assessed by calculation of the combination index (CI) using CompuSyn 1.0 software (ComboSyn, Inc., Paramus, NJ, USA) after 72 h [48]. Synergism, antagonism, or summation are indicated by CI < 1, CI > 1, or CI = 1, respectively [49]. For western blot analyses, cells were lysed after 48 h and analyzed using an apoptosis antibody sampler kit (#9915, Cell Signaling Technology, Danvers, MA, USA). Tubulin (#ab18251, Abcam, Cambridge, UK) was detected as a loading control.

2.9. Animal Experiments

Xenograft experiments were performed in accordance with governmental regulations (Schleswig-Holstein Ministerium für Energiewende, Landwirtschaft, Umwelt, Natur und Digitalisierung) using NOD.Cg-Prkdcscid Il2rgtm1Wjl/SzJ (NSG) mice bred in our institution.

For these experiments, 0.5×10^6 REH, NALM-6, or 1×10^5 BCP-ALL PDX cells were injected intravenously into 6–10 weeks old female NSG mice (day 0). CD19-TRAIL (1.5 mg/kg) was injected intravenously on day +1, +3, +6, +10, +13 as described previously [19] and every 7 days thereafter. Venetoclax (100 mg/kg) was applied daily by oral gavage [50]. Leukemic engraftment was analyzed via flow cytometric detection of human CD45$^+$/murine CD45$^-$/human CD19$^+$ cells in the peripheral blood, and animals were sacrificed upon detection of >75% leukemic blasts or when showing clinical signs of leukemia (loss of weight or activity, organomegaly, hind-limb paralysis) as published previously [51–53].

2.10. Statistical Analysis

Graphical and statistical analyses were performed using software GraphPad Prism 9.0 (GraphPad, San Diego, CA, USA). If not stated otherwise, *p*-values were calculated using the Mann–Whitney test and repeated measures ANOVA with Bonferroni post-tests. For survival analyses, Kaplan-Meier and log-rank statistics were used. Significance was assumed when $p < 0.05$.

3. Results

3.1. Generation of a CD19-TRAIL Fusion Construct with CD19 Specific Binding Capacity

In order to generate a CD19-TRAIL fusion construct, a single chain TRAIL domain was genetically fused to the 3′-end of one HC of a CD19-IgG1 antibody [17]. As TRAIL-mediated activation of apoptosis relies on the trimerization of death receptors on the target cell surface [26], the TRAIL domain was designed to consist of three TRAIL units as previously reported [44]. To ensure heterodimeric HC pairing, amino acid exchanges were inserted in the CH3 domain: K392D and K409D for the first HC with the TRAIL domain and E356K and D399K for the second HC (Figure 1A). CD19-TRAIL was produced in CHO-S cells and purified by affinity chromatography. Aggregates and Fc homodimers were removed by size exclusion chromatography, resulting in a homogenous protein preparation with a single protein peak with a higher molecular mass compared to CD19-IgG1, indicating the insertion of the TRAIL unit (Figure 1B). SDS-PAGE under reducing conditions followed by Coomassie blue staining of purified CD19-TRAIL revealed three single bands according to the predicted molecular masses of the three different antibody-chains (LC = 25 kDa; HC = 50 kDa; HC + TRAIL = 112 kDa) (Figure 1C). Western blot analysis using a TRAIL-directed antibody further confirmed the successful incorporation of TRAIL into the antibody construct (Figure 1D). Next, CD19-TRAIL was tested for binding specificity to the CD19 antigen. CD19-TRAIL exposed equal binding capacity to the CD19$^+$ BCP-ALL cell lines REH and NALM-6 as compared to the parental CD19-IgG1 antibody, while a HER2-TRAIL control antibody only showed significant binding due to TRAIL-R expression on the HER2-negative/CD19$^+$ tumor cells (Figure 1E, Supplementary Figure S1B). Concordantly, no binding to CD19$^-$ T-ALL CEM cells was observed (Figure 1E). Taken together, these data indicate the successful generation of a fusion construct of CD19-IgG1 and the death receptor ligand TRAIL with a specific binding capacity to CD19.

3.2. CD19-TRAIL Induces Direct Apoptotic Effects in CD19$^+$ BCP-ALL Cells

Next, we characterized the CD19-TRAIL fusion construct with respect to target antigen-specific direct anti-leukemic efficacy. We first confirmed cell surface expression of CD19, TRAIL-R1, and TRAIL-R2 on the BCP-ALL cell lines REH and NALM-6 as compared to the T-ALL cell line CEM by quantitative indirect immunofluorescence analyses. As expected, the CD19 antigen was only expressed on REH and NALM-6 cells (mean specific antibody binding capacity (SABC) = 21,312 and SABC = 27,308, respectively), but not on CEM cells (SABC = 0, Supplementary Figure S1A). Furthermore, cell surface expression of TRAIL-R1 was low or absent (SABC: REH = 65; NALM-6 = 0; CEM = 41), in contrast to a strong TRAIL-R2 expression on all cell lines (SABC: REH = 503; NALM-6 = 2256; CEM = 4720) (Supplementary Figure S1B). We then examined the effect of the antibody on the viability of CD19$^+$ REH and NALM-6 cells and CD19$^-$ CEM cells by MTT assay. Indeed, CD19-TRAIL significantly reduced the viability of REH and NALM-6 cells at low nanomolar concentrations (EC_{50} = 0.0617 nM and EC_{50}= 0.01746 nM, respectively) as compared to a HER2-TRAIL control antibody (Figure 2A,B). In line with higher CD19 and TRAIL-R2 levels on the cell surface, NALM-6 cells showed a response to CD19-TRAIL at lower concentrations as compared to REH cells (Figure 2A,B). As expected, the viability of CEM cells was neither affected by CD19-TRAIL nor HER2-TRAIL (Figure 2C). Of note, pre-incubation of CD19+ target cells with the parental CD19-IgG1 antibody, impeding binding of CD19-TRAIL, rescued the viability of REH and NALM-6 cells, further confirming target-specific effects of CD19-TRAIL (Figure 2D).

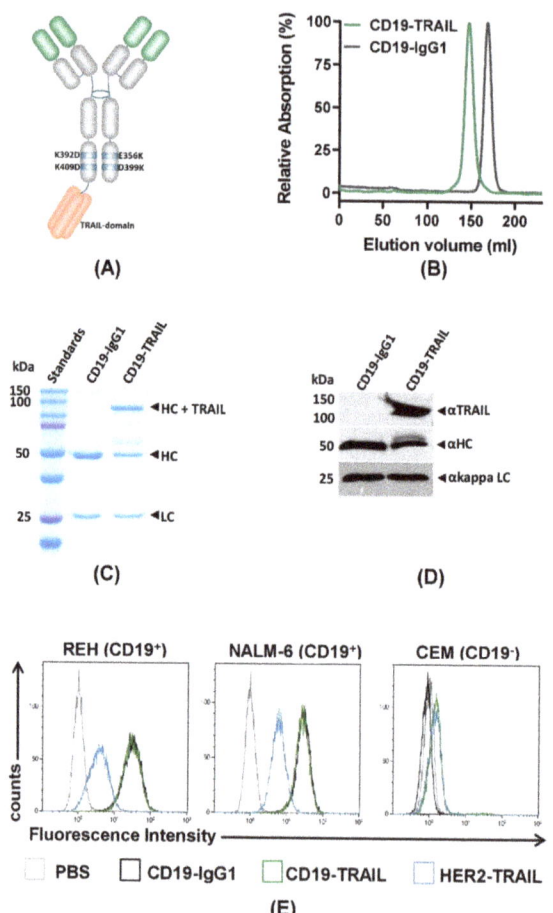

Figure 1. Generation of a target-specific CD19-TRAIL fusion construct: (**A**) Schematic illustration of a CD19-TRAIL fusion construct (CD19-TRAIL) consisting of one heavy chain with two amino acid exchanges (E356K and D399K) and a second heavy chain carrying two amino acid exchanges (K392D and K409D) and a C-terminal fusion of a single chain TRAIL domain, resulting in a heterodimeric antibody promoting TRAIL-receptor trimerization in CD19-positive (CD19+) target cells; (**B**) Purity of CD19-TRAIL and CD19-IgG1 was analyzed by size exclusion chromatography under native buffer conditions, and peak fractions were collected. Representative chromatography image of the isolated and re-analyzed peak fraction (normalized to maximum absorption) is shown; (**C,D**) Purity and molecular masses of CD19-TRAIL and CD19-IgG1 were further validated using SDS-PAGE under reducing conditions followed by staining with Coomassie blue and D) Western blot analyses with immunodetection of TRAIL as well as antibody heavy and light chains. HC = heavy chain, LC = light chain; (**E**) Specificity of the binding capacity of CD19-TRAIL and CD19-IgG1 compared to a HER2-TRAIL control antibody was tested on the CD19+ BCP-ALL cell lines REH and NALM-6 cells and the CD19-negative (CD19−) T-ALL cell line CEM by flow cytometry analyses. Antibodies were detected with a FITC-conjugated anti-human IgG Fc F(ab′)2 secondary antibody. PBS served as control for background staining. Depicted data show representative pictures of $n = 3$ experiments.

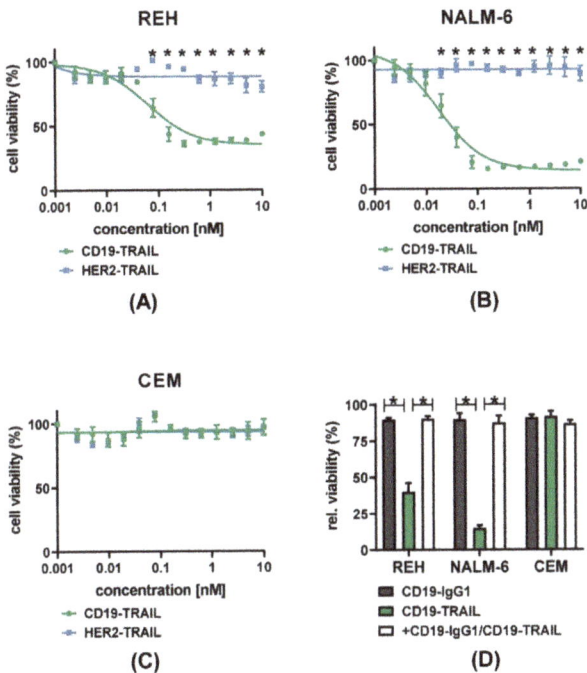

Figure 2. CD19-TRAIL elicits selective anti-proliferative effects in CD19+ ALL-cells: (**A**) CD19+ REH and (**B**) NALM-6 cells as well as (**C**) CD19− CEM cells were treated with escalating concentrations of CD19-TRAIL or HER2-TRAIL for 72 h, and cell viability was analyzed by MTT assay, two-way analysis of variance; (**D**) Specificity of CD19-dependant cell killing was verified by pre-incubating the cell lines REH, NALM-6, and CEM with CD19-IgG1 antibody (100 nM) for 1 h prior to CD19-TRAIL treatment and measuring cell viability by MTT assay after 72 h, one-tailed Mann–Whitney Test. Graphs depict mean values ± SEM of $n = 3$ independent experiments. * $p < 0.05$.

We next investigated whether CD19-TRAIL induces apoptosis in BCP-ALL cells. First, NALM-6 and REH cells were treated with CD19-TRAIL for 24 h, and exposure of phosphatidylserine on the outer cell membrane was assessed by AnnexinV staining at different time points. To distinguish early from late apoptotic or necrotic cells, co-staining with PI was performed. As expected, the progressive increase in AnnexinV-positive/PI-negative REH and NALM-6 cells showed apoptosis induction by CD19-TRAIL compared to untreated control cells (Supplementary Figure S2A,B). To confirm further apoptosis induction as a mechanism of killing, REH and NALM-6 cells were treated with the pan-caspase inhibitor Z-VAD prior to CD19-TRAIL treatment. Indeed, AnnexinV/PI staining revealed a significant reduction in cell death compared to CD19-TRAIL-treated cells ($p = 0.05$, respectively, Figure 3A,B). To confirm further CD19-TRAIL-mediated apoptosis induction, CD19+ REH and NALM-6 cells as well as CD19− CEM cells were treated with CD19-TRAIL, CD19-IgG1, HER2-TRAIL, or a vehicle control, and cell lysates were analyzed for apoptosis-related proteins by western blot. As expected, we observed cleavage of the apoptosis markers Caspases 3, 7, and 9 as well as Poly (ADP-ribose) polymerase (PARP) in REH and NALM-6 cells in response to CD19-TRAIL treatment as compared to CD19-IgG1 and HER2-TRAIL control antibodies. Concomitantly, CD19− CEM cells remained unaffected by CD19-TRAIL treatment (Figure 3C). Together, these data suggest that CD19-TRAIL kills BCP-ALL cells specifically by apoptosis induction.

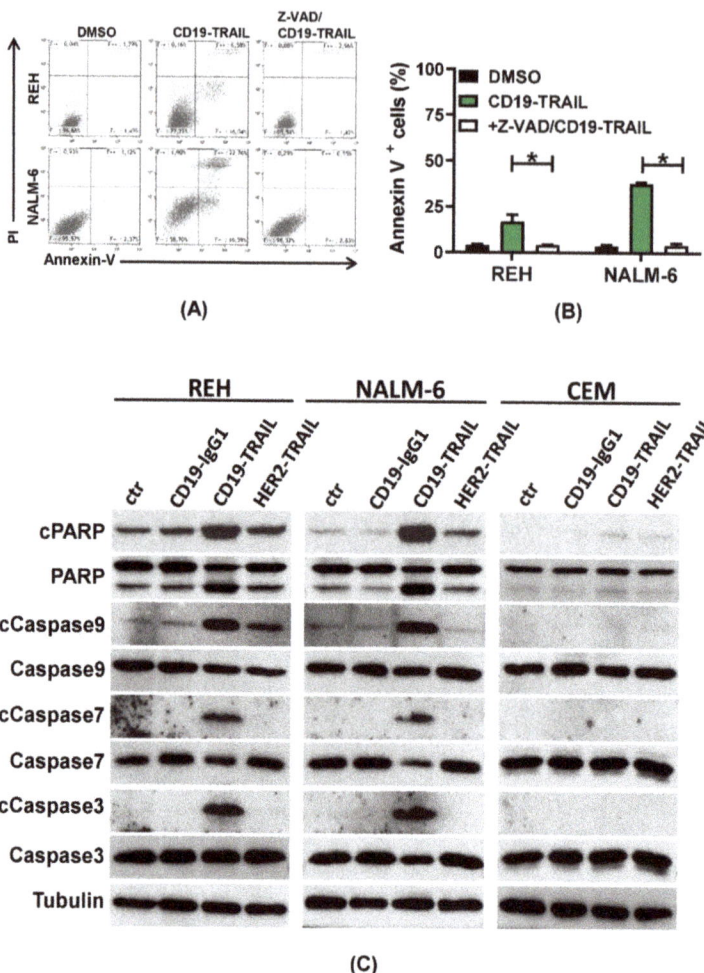

Figure 3. CD19-TRAIL kills ALL-cells via apoptosis induction: (**A,B**) REH and NALM-6 cells were pre-incubated with the pan-caspase inhibitor Z-VAD (50 µM) for 1 h prior to incubation with CD19-TRAIL. DMSO served as negative control; (**A**) Representative histograms of flow cytometric analyses of AnnexinV and PI staining after 24 h and (**B**) mean values ± SEM of $n = 3$ independent experiments are shown, one-tailed Mann–Whitney Test, * $p < 0.05$; (**C**) Representative images of western blot analyses of the pro-apoptotic proteins Caspase 3, Caspase 7, and Caspase 9 and PARP as well as their cleavage (c) products (cCaspase3, cCaspase7, cCaspase9, and cPARP) in the cell lines REH, NALM-6, and CEM after treatment with 0.5 nM of CD19-IgG1, CD19-TRAIL, HER2-TRAIL, or medium (ctr) for 48 h. Tubulin served as loading control.

3.3. CD19-TRAIL Eradicates BCP-ALL Cells In Vivo in Xenograft Models

Encouraged by the potent cell-toxic effects of CD19-TRAIL in vitro, we next investigated the therapeutic effect of CD19-TRAIL in vivo in BCP-ALL xenograft models. REH and NALM-6 cells were injected intravenously into NSG mice and animals treated with CD19-TRAIL on days +1, +3, +6, +10, +13 as published previously [19] and every 7 days thereafter or left untreated ($n = 6$/group). Animals were sacrificed when showing clinical signs of overt leukemia. Indeed, CD19-TRAIL treatment led to a clear prolongation of median mouse survival as compared to control animals in animals transplanted with REH cells (34 vs. 48 days, $p = 0.0009$, Figure 4A) and also in mice bearing NALM-6 cells (19.5 vs. 29 days, $p = 0.0009$, Figure 4B). Moreover, as expected, CD19-TRAIL outperformed CD19-IgG1.

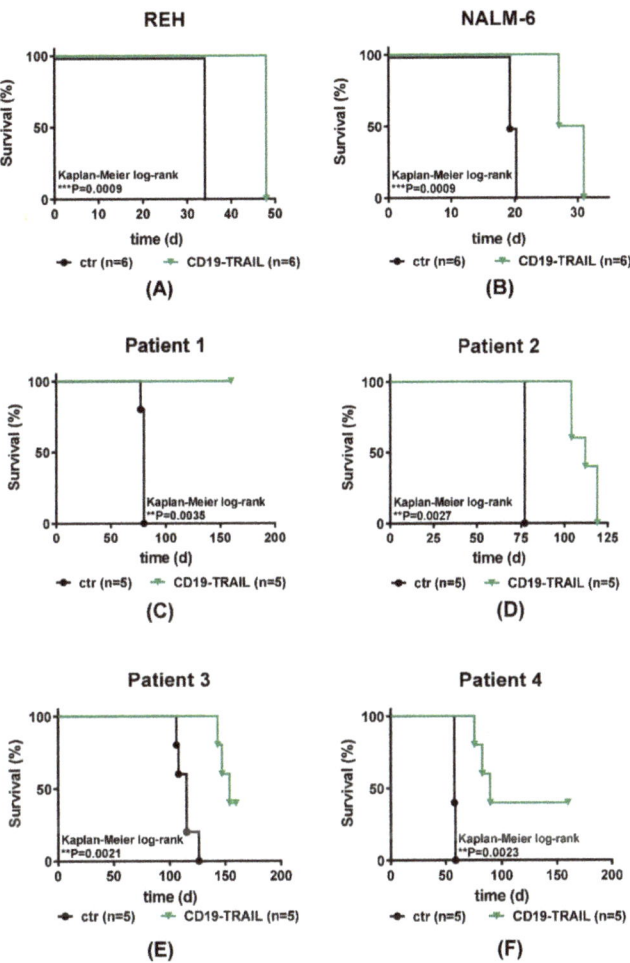

Figure 4. CD19-TRAIL eradicates BCP-ALL cells in vivo. Survival of female NSG-mice intravenously injected with (**A**) 0.5×10^6 REH ($n = 6$ per group); (**B**) 0.5×10^6 NALM-6 ($n = 6$ per group); or (**C–F**) 1×10^5 patient-derived ALL xenograft (PDX; $n = 5$ per group) cells (day 0). On days +1, +3, +6, +10, +13 and every 7 days thereafter, mice were treated with 1.5 mg/kg of CD19-TRAIL intravenously or left untreated (ctr). At signs of overt leukemia (detection of >75% leukemic blasts in the peripheral blood or clinical signs of leukemia including loss of weight or activity, organomegaly, hind-limb paralysis), mice were euthanized. Differences in survival were calculated using Kaplan–Meier log-rank test, ** $p < 0.01$, *** $p < 0.001$.

We found a significant reduction in leukemia engraftment in bone marrow aspirates of animals bearing REH cells and in the peripheral blood of NALM-6-bearing mice that were treated with CD19-TRAIL as compared to animals treated with CD19-IgG1, respectively (38.30% vs. 17.70%, $p = 0.0476$ and 43.5% vs. 24%, $p = 0.0079$, Supplementary Figure S3A,B). In REH cells, bone marrow was analyzed because these cells do not cause leukemia in the peripheral blood of NSG mice.

As in vivo experiments using cell lines do not depict the clinical heterogeneity of BCP-ALL patients, we next tested CD19-TRAIL in patient-derived BCP-ALL xenografts (PDX) from four patients (Patients 1–4, Supplementary Table S1, n = 5 PDX mice/group). All patients exposed cell surface expression of CD19 and TRAIL-R1. One of four patients also exhibited weak TRAIL-R2 expression (Supplementary Figure S3C,D, Supplementary Table S1). Indeed, CD19-TRAIL treatment was efficient in all tested PDX-samples in vivo and significantly prolonged the survival of PDX-animals irrespective of ALL cytogenetics (Supplementary Table S1; Figure 4C–F). For patient 1 (BCR-ABL+), no CD19-TRAIL-treated animal showed clinical signs of leukemia up to day +160, whereas all control animals were sacrificed due to overt leukemia on day +80 (p = 0.0035). Furthermore, CD19-TRAIL-treated mice bearing PDX-cells of patient 2 (BCR-ABL+) showed a median survival prolongation of 35 days as compared to control animals (77 vs. 112 days, p = 0.0027). CD19-TRAIL-treated PDX-mice from patient 3 (E2A-PBX1) showed a median survival prolongation of 39 days (115 vs. 154 days, p = 0.0021). Moreover, PDX-mice of patient 4 (MLL-rearrangement) showed a significant median survival prolongation of 32 days upon CD19-TRAIL treatment as compared to control mice (58 vs. 90 days, p = 0.0023). Of note, 2 out 5 PDX-mice of patient 3 and 4 had not developed leukemia up to day +160, respectively (Figure 4E,F).

These results indicate that CD19-TRAIL efficiently targets CD19$^+$ BCP-ALL cells in vivo in xenograft models.

3.4. The Cytotoxic Effect of CD19-TRAIL Is Synergistically Enhanced by Venetoclax in BCP-ALL Cells

Cancer drugs may initiate apoptosis through activation of the extrinsic or intrinsic pathways [54]. TRAIL acts as an activator of the extrinsic pathway of apoptosis by binding to death receptors [26,54]. On the other hand, Venetoclax (VTX) inhibits BCL-2, thereby inducing the release of the pro-apoptotic BH3-domain family members BAX and BIM, which act as key molecules of the intrinsic apoptosis pathway [54–56]. We hypothesized that the therapeutic efficacy of CD19-TRAIL could be further improved by dual stimulation of different apoptosis pathways. To test this hypothesis, REH cells were treated with CD19-TRAIL or VTX as monotherapies, or with the combination of both. Indeed, we detected a significant and dose-dependent increase in apoptosis induction by co-treatments with CD19-TRAIL and VTX as compared to single and control treatments in REH cells (Figure 5A). Of note, we found that the observed combinatorial pro-apoptotic effects of CD19-TRAIL and VTX were indeed synergistic as determined by synergy analysis according to Chou and Talalay [49] (Supplementary Figure S4A,B). To substantiate further these results, REH cells were treated with DMSO, CD19-TRAIL, VTX, or the combination, and cell lysates were analyzed by western blot. Protein levels of all cleaved apoptotic markers (Caspase 3, 7, 9, and PARP) as well as γH2AX, a marker of DNA-damage, were increased by co-treatment with CD19-TRAIL and VTX as compared to single and control treatments (Figure 5B). The synergy of CD19-TRAIL and VTX was then further investigated in vivo. NSG mice were injected with REH cells and treated with CD19-TRAIL, VTX, or CD19-TRAIL and VTX, as compared to untreated control animals (n = 6/group). Both CD19-TRAIL and VTX treatments as monotherapies significantly prolonged median survival of mice in comparison to untreated control animals by 14 days (34 vs. 48 days for both drugs, p = 0.0009, Figure 5C). Of note, a further prolongation of survival by 29 days was achieved by the combination of CD19-TRAIL and VTX as compared to control (34 vs. 63 days, respectively, p = 0.0009, Figure 5C). Survival prolongation by the combination was also significant compared to the respective monotherapies (48 vs. 63 days, p = 0.0009, respectively, Figure 5C). These data suggest that the efficacy of CD19-TRAIL is enhanced by a combination with the BCL-2 inhibitor VTX, which can be a novel combination strategy for clinical use.

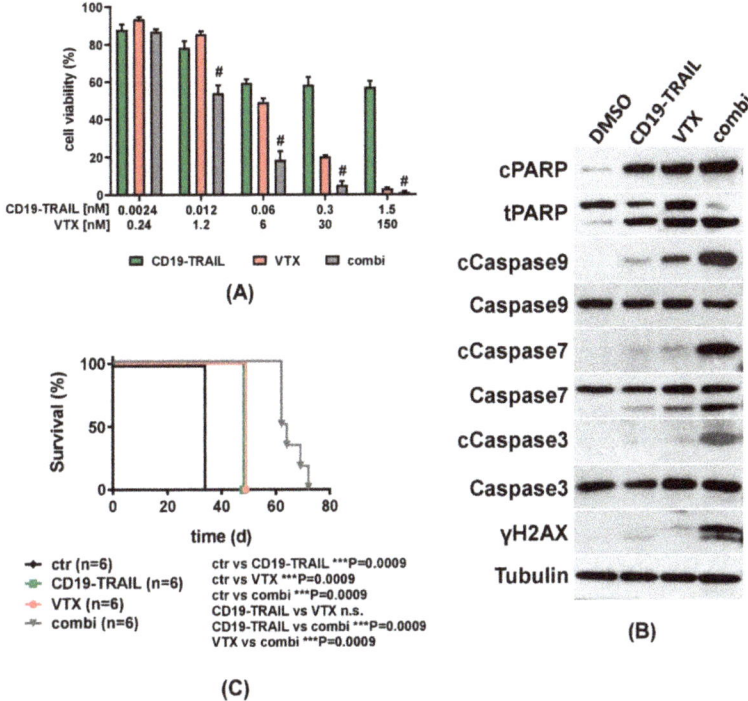

Figure 5. ALL-killing effect of CD19-TRAIL is synergistically enhanced by Venetoclax: (**A**) REH cells were treated with escalating concentrations of CD19-TRAIL, the BCL-2 inhibitor Venetoclax (VTX), or the combination of both (combi). Cell viability was determined by MTT assay after 72 h. Combination Index (CI) was calculated via CompuSyn Software, and synergism (CI < 1) is indicated by (#). Values for CI calculations are noted in Supplementary Figure S4. Data represent mean values ± SEM of n = 3 independent experiments; (**B**) Representative western blot analyses of REH cells treated with DMSO, CD19-TRAIL (0.06 nM), VTX (6 nM), or the combination (combi) for 48 h. Expression levels of indicated proteins were determined in whole-cell protein extracts. Tubulin served as a loading control; (**C**) Female NSG-mice were intravenously injected with 0.5×10^6 REH cells (n = 6 per group) and treated with 1.5 mg/kg of CD19-TRAIL intravenously on days +1, +3, +6, +10, +13 and every 7 days thereafter; 100 mg/kg VTX daily oral gavage; or both (combi). Untreated mice served as control (ctr). When showing signs of overt leukemia (clinical signs of leukemia including loss of weight or activity, organomegaly, hind-limb paralysis), mice were euthanized, and differences in mouse survival were calculated using Kaplan–Meier log-rank test, *** $p < 0.001$.

4. Discussion

Antibody-based immunotherapy is an attractive tool to reduce the toxicity of chemotherapy and to induce target-cell-specific effects either in dependence of the patient's immune system or by directly inducing anti-tumoral effects.

Due to its favorable expression profile, CD19 became a major target for immunotherapy approaches in BCP-ALL. Yet, novel CD19-directed antibodies such as the BiTE molecule blinatumomab harbor a significant toxicity profile due to the side effects of T-cell activation [11]. Native CD19 antibodies reveal a beneficial pharmacokinetic profile with long serum half-lives and low off-target toxicity, but a clinical pilot study using a mouse CD19-IgG2a antibody showed a limited response in B-cell non-Hodgkin's lymphoma patients, probably due to limited effector functions elicited by the native CD19 antibody [16]. Therefore, the current study objective was to generate and characterize a novel CD19-directed antibody therapeutic based on a humanized CD19-IgG1 antibody and fused with the apoptosis-inducing ligand TRAIL, in order to induce BCP-ALL-specific killing. Our data demonstrate that a CD19-TRAIL fusion protein shows potent selective pro-apoptotic activity towards CD19-expressing cells in vitro. Furthermore, CD19-TRAIL significantly prolonged the survival of xenograft mice bearing human BCP-ALL cell lines and PDX cells, and its efficacy could be enhanced by the addition of Venetoclax.

We and others had previously reported that the efficacy of antibodies with low cytolytic capacity can be significantly enhanced by Fc-engineering: For example, the CD19 antibody tafasitamab (MOR208) showed increased FcγR-dependent NK-cell and macrophage recruitment than its wildtype counterpart and has been approved for clinical use [15,57]. Furthermore, we recently showed that a S267E/H268F/S324T/G236A/I332E (EFTAE) Fc-modification equipped a CD19 antibody with enhanced CDC-inducing features. This effect was further improved by reducing the fucose content, which enhanced the affinity of the antibody to FcγRIIIa and thereby increased ADCC [17].

A further option to increase antibody efficacy is to "arm" it with cytotoxic agents. The CD19-ADC loncastuximab tesirine and coltuximab ravtansine (SAR3419) exhibited strong anti-tumoral effects in hematological malignancies in vitro and an acceptable safety profile in patients but only modest efficacy in relapsed/refractory BCP-ALL [14,58].

A previous report showed lower off-target toxicity of a TRAIL antibody construct as compared to a pseudomonas exotoxin A (ETA)-linked counterpart, so that our results indicate that equipping the Fc region of antibodies with a TRAIL ligand may represent a further promising strategy to enhance their direct apoptosis-inducing abilities [59].

TRAIL is a highly potent apoptosis inducer that exists either as a type II membrane protein (memTRAIL) or as a cleaved, soluble protein (sTRAIL) [24,60]. The observations that sTRAIL attacks tumor cells efficiently and selectively and that it is at the same time is well tolerated in patients motivated numerous preclinical and clinical studies testing the effect of sTRAIL in different tumor entities, yet with limited success [30,32,33]. TRAIL-fusion proteins may help to overcome some of the limitations by enhancing the stability of the TRAIL ligand, reducing the formation of detrimental high-molecular weight aggregates as compared to unbound sTRAIL [59], and efficiently promoting the accumulation of TRAIL-R1 and TRAIL-R2 on the surface of target cells [39]. This way, the antibody-TRAIL construct induces the DISC-formation and apoptosis also in cells that lack TRAIL-R1 which responds to sTRAIL and memTRAIL, whereas TRAIL-R2 preferentially responds to memTRAIL [40]. This is particularly valid for the scTRAIL containing three TRAIL protomers of the CD19-construct applied in our study [44]. Accordingly, we found that CD19-TRAIL induced apoptosis in NALM-6 cells, for which we detected no TRAIL-R1 expression. Moreover, CD19-TRAIL induced apoptosis in CD19$^+$ cell lines REH and NALM-6 at nanomolar concentrations. Accordingly, we detected no induction of apoptosis by CD19-TRAIL in CD19$^-$ cells or when using a HER2-TRAIL control antibody, indicating negligible binding of soluble antibody constructs to TRAIL-R1 and TRAIL-R2 via the TRAIL domain. We suspect that CD19-TRAIL potentiates the approximation and oligomerization of TRAIL-R-complexes which strongly enhances the efficiency of TRAIL-R-mediated apoptosis induction and that assembly of multiple CD19-TRAIL-R complexes is needed to induce apoptosis at particularly low concentrations. This is further substantiated by the observation that cell death was arrested after blocking the CD19 epitope with the parental CD19-IgG1 antibody, hampering the crosslinking between the TRAIL-Rs and the CD19 antigen. This is in line with previous studies showing target-specific eradication of tumors cells by TRAIL fusion proteins with a single chain variable fragment (scFv) [37,39,59]. Moreover, antibody-scTRAIL constructs were already shown to spare physiological blood cells from apoptosis induction [37].

The CD19-dependent cytotoxic activities of CD19-TRAIL may be supported by the Fc-modifications that were introduced to promote heterodimeric assembly of the HCs [43] and to generate an antibody carrying only one scTRAIL moiety. In its design, CD19-TRAIL is different to previously reported antibody-scTRAIL constructs, in which scTRAIL was linked to each LC or HC or both, resulting in hexavalent or dodecavalent scTRAIL constructs, respectively [20]. In our design, TRAIL-R activation in the absence of the

CD19 antigen may be reduced further, which may result in superior antigen specificity as compared to multivalent TRAIL constructs.

CD19-TRAIL single treatment was efficient in reducing leukemic burden of BCP-ALL PDX cells from different patients in xenografted NSG-mice and was well tolerated by treated animals, which to our knowledge has not been reported for other CD19 antibody-TRAIL constructs to date. High preclinical efficacy in ALL-PDX-specimen has been reported for TRAIL fused to a CD19-ligand [61]. Comparing different TRAIL-based CD19-targeted therapies would be of high interest on the way to potential clinical application. Yet, the tolerability of CD19-TRAIL constructs would have to be validated in non-human primate models due to the minor interaction of human TRAIL ligands with murine TRAIL-R [62]. Moreover, such models could be used to investigate side effects such as aplasia of normal B cells, which is frequently observed for other CD19-targeted immunotherapies such as blinatumomab and CD19-specific chimeric antigen receptor T-cells [63,64] or cytotoxicity towards other normal blood cells.

Another interesting observation in our study is that the efficacy of CD19-TRAIL was significantly and synergistically enhanced when combined with the BCL-2 inhibitor VTX. VTX has shown promising effects and tolerability in different hematological malignancies including BCP-ALL [50,65]. Whereas CD19-TRAIL induces extrinsic apoptosis via DISC induction, VTX stimulates the intrinsic apoptosis pathway via release of pro-apoptotic BH3-domain family members BAX and BIM [26,54,56]. The concomitant stimulation of both apoptotic pathways may potentiate the efficacy of TRAIL-carrying monoclonal antibodies and may be of general interest for antibody-based immunotherapy.

CD19 loss remains a major challenge in BCP-ALL relapse and a key mechanism of the failure of CD19-directed therapy [10,66]. Our CD19-TRAIL construct may help to overcome this challenge by binding CD19+ cells and concomitantly crosslinking TRAIL receptors on neighboring tumor cells, thereby inducing apoptosis in these cells irrespective of CD19 expression ("bystander killing") [67]. Moreover, the concept of sTRAIL fusion may also be applicable to antibodies targeting other important antigens in hematological malignancies such as CD20 and CD38 for which TRAIL fusion constructs were already described [68,69] or further novel targets such as CD52 and CD79 [53,70]. Furthermore, first antibody-based immunotherapy concepts targeting T-ALL such as daratumumab have shown promising preclinical efficacy [52], which could be enhanced by using TRAIL fusions. To this end, a scFvCD7-TRAIL antibody was already shown to induce T-ALL-specific killing, promoting the view that sTRAIL antibody constructs could also be an interesting option to target T-ALL cells [59].

Taken together, the preclinical data presented here suggest that CD19-TRAIL may represent a promising new tumor cell-specific therapeutic agent in BCP-ALL, warranting further preclinical testing.

Supplementary Materials: The following are available online at https://www.mdpi.com/article/10.3390/jcm10122634/s1, Figure S1: Expression profile of CD19 and TRAIL receptors (TRAILR1/TRAIL-R2) on leukemic cell lines, Figure S2: CD19-TRAIL kills ALL-cells via apoptosis induction, Figure S3: CD19-TRAIL eradicates BCP-ALL cells in vivo, Figure S4: ALL-killing effect of CD19-TRAIL is synergistically enhanced by Venetoclax, Table S1: Clinical characteristics of BCP-ALL patients xenografted in NSG mice.

Author Contributions: D.W. designed and performed experiments, analyzed data, and wrote the manuscript. L.L. analyzed data, discussed the research direction, and wrote the manuscript. M.O., F.V., C.L.G., F.-S.F., K.K., T.R., T.V., and A.T. performed experiments and analyzed data. D.M.S., M.P., and C.K. initiated and designed experiments and discussed the research direction. All authors discussed the manuscript. All authors have read and agreed to the published version of the manuscript.

Funding: D.M.S. and C.K. are funded by the Deutsche José Carreras Leukämie Stiftung (DJCLS 17R/2017, DJCLS 13R/2020) and by the Deutsche Krebshilfe e.V. (70113524). D.M.S. is funded by the

Wilhelm Sander Stiftung (2016.110.1 and 2019.119.1). M.P. was supported by the Deutsche Krebshilfe e. V. (Mildred-Scheel-Professorship program).

Institutional Review Board Statement: The study was conducted according to the guidelines of the Declaration of Helsinki, and approved by the Ethics Committee of the CAU Kiel (D437/17). Animal experiments were approved by the Ministerium für Energiewende, Landwirtschaft, Umwelt, Natur und Digitalisierung Schleswig-Holstein (V 242-30136/2020).

Informed Consent Statement: Informed consent was obtained from all subjects involved in the study in accordance with the declaration of Helsinki.

Data Availability Statement: The data presented in this study are available in the main manuscript or supplementary data.

Acknowledgments: We thank the patients and physicians who contributed samples and data for this study. We thank Britta von Below, Katrin Timm-Richert, Katrin Neumann, Gabriele Riesen, and Anja Muskulus for the excellent technical assistance.

Conflicts of Interest: D.M.S. was an advisory board member for Bayer, SOBI, and Jazz Pharmaceuticals and received research funding from OSE Pharmaceuticals. The other authors declare no competing interest.

References

1. Locatelli, F.; Schrappe, M.; Bernardo, M.E.; Rutella, S. How I treat relapsed childhood acute lymphoblastic leukemia. *Blood* **2012**, *120*, 2807–2816. [CrossRef] [PubMed]
2. Hunger, S.P.; Mullighan, C.G. Acute Lymphoblastic Leukemia in Children. *N. Engl. J. Med.* **2015**, *373*, 1541–1552. [CrossRef]
3. Bhojwani, D.; Pui, C.-H. Relapsed childhood acute lymphoblastic leukaemia. *Lancet Oncol.* **2013**, *14*, e205–e217. [CrossRef]
4. Wedekind, M.F.; Denton, N.L.; Chen, C.-Y.; Cripe, T.P. Pediatric Cancer Immunotherapy: Opportunities and Challenges. *Pediatr. Drugs* **2018**, *20*, 395–408. [CrossRef]
5. Maury, S.; Chevret, S.; Thomas, X.; Heim, D.; Leguay, T.; Huguet, F.; Chevallier, P.; Hunault, M.; Boissel, N.; Escoffre-Barbe, M.; et al. Rituximab in B-Lineage Adult Acute Lymphoblastic Leukemia. *N. Engl. J. Med.* **2016**, *375*, 1044–1053. [CrossRef] [PubMed]
6. Jabbour, E.; O'Brien, S.; Ravandi, F.; Kantarjian, H. Monoclonal antibodies in acute lymphoblastic leukemia. *Blood* **2015**, *125*, 4010–4016. [CrossRef] [PubMed]
7. Hoelzer, D. Novel Antibody-Based Therapies for Acute Lymphoblastic Leukemia. *Hematol. Am. Soc. Hematol. Educ. Program* **2011**, *2011*, 243–249. [CrossRef] [PubMed]
8. Nadler, L.M.; Anderson, K.C.; Marti, G.; Bates, M.; Park, E.; Daley, J.F.; Schlossman, S.F. B4, a human B lymphocyte-associated antigen expressed on normal, mitogen-activated, and malignant B lymphocytes. *J. Immunol.* **1983**, *131*, 244–250.
9. Scheuermann, R.H.; Racila, E. CD19 Antigen in Leukemia and Lymphoma Diagnosis and Immunotherapy. *Leuk. Lymphoma* **1995**, *18*, 385–397. [CrossRef]
10. Mejstríková, E.; Hrusak, O.; Borowitz, M.J.; Whitlock, J.A.; Brethon, B.; Trippett, T.M.; Zugmaier, G.; Gore, L.; Von Stackelberg, A.; Locatelli, F. CD19-negative relapse of pediatric B-cell precursor acute lymphoblastic leukemia following blinatumomab treatment. *Blood Cancer J.* **2017**, *7*, 659. [CrossRef]
11. Kantarjian, H.M.; Stein, A.; Gökbuget, N.; Fielding, A.K.; Schuh, A.C.; Ribera, J.-M.; Wei, A.; Dombret, H.; Foà, R.; Bassan, R.; et al. Blinatumomab versus Chemotherapy for Advanced Acute Lymphoblastic Leukemia. *N. Engl. J. Med.* **2017**, *376*, 836–847. [CrossRef]
12. Locatelli, F.; Zugmaier, G.; Mergen, N.; Bader, P.; Jeha, S.; Schlegel, P.-G.; Bourquin, J.-P.; Handgretinger, R.; Brethon, B.; Rossig, C.; et al. Blinatumomab in pediatric patients with relapsed/refractory acute lymphoblastic leukemia: Results of the RIALTO trial, an expanded access study. *Blood Cancer J.* **2020**, *10*, 1–5. [CrossRef]
13. Anagnostou, T.; Riaz, I.B.; Hashmi, S.K.; Murad, M.H.; Kenderian, S.S. Anti-CD19 chimeric antigen receptor T-cell therapy in acute lymphocytic leukaemia: A systematic review and meta-analysis. *Lancet Haematol.* **2020**, *7*, e816–e826. [CrossRef]
14. Kantarjian, H.M.; Lioure, B.; Kim, S.K.; Atallah, E.; Leguay, T.; Kelly, K.; Marolleau, J.-P.; Escoffre-Barbe, M.; Thomas, X.G.; Cortes, J.; et al. A Phase II Study of Coltuximab Ravtansine (SAR3419) Monotherapy in Patients with Relapsed or Refractory Acute Lymphoblastic Leukemia. *Clin. Lymphoma Myeloma Leuk.* **2016**, *16*, 139–145. [CrossRef] [PubMed]
15. Horton, H.M.; Bernett, M.J.; Pong, E.; Peipp, M.; Karki, S.; Chu, S.Y.; Richards, J.O.; Vostiar, I.; Joyce, P.F.; Repp, R.; et al. Potent In vitro and In vivo Activity of an Fc-Engineered Anti-CD19 Monoclonal Antibody against Lymphoma and Leukemia. *Cancer Res.* **2008**, *68*, 8049–8057. [CrossRef]
16. Hekman, A.; Honselaar, A.; Vuist, W.M.J.; Sein, J.J.; Rodenhuis, S.; Huinink, W.W.T.B.; Somers, R.; Rümke, P.; Melief, C.J.M. Initial experience with treatment of human B cell lymphoma with anti-CD19 monoclonal antibody. *Cancer Immunol. Immunother.* **1991**, *32*, 364–372. [CrossRef] [PubMed]

17. Roßkopf, S.; Eichholz, K.M.; Winterberg, D.; Diemer, K.J.; Lutz, S.; Münnich, I.A.; Klausz, K.; Rösner, T.; Valerius, T.; Schewe, D.M.; et al. Enhancing CDC and ADCC of CD19 Antibodies by Combining Fc Protein-Engineering with Fc Glyco-Engineering. *Antibodies* **2020**, *9*, 63. [CrossRef]
18. Hammer, O. CD19 as an attractive target for antibody-based therapy. *mAbs* **2012**, *4*, 571–577. [CrossRef]
19. Schewe, D.M.; Alsadeq, A.; Sattler, C.; Lenk, L.; Vogiatzi, F.; Cario, G.; Vieth, S.; Valerius, T.; Rosskopf, S.; Meyersieck, F.; et al. An Fc-engineered CD19 antibody eradicates MRD in patient-derived MLL-rearranged acute lymphoblastic leukemia xenografts. *Blood* **2017**, *130*, 1543–1552. [CrossRef]
20. Siegemund, M.; Schneider, F.; Hutt, M.; Seifert, O.; Muller, I.; Kulms, D.; Pfizenmaier, K.; Kontermann, R.E. IgG-single-chain TRAIL fusion proteins for tumour therapy. *Sci. Rep.* **2018**, *8*, 7808. [CrossRef]
21. Pan, G.; Ni, J.; Wei, Y.-F.; Yu, G.-L.; Gentz, R.; Dixit, V.M. An Antagonist Decoy Receptor and a Death Domain-Containing Receptor for TRAIL. *Science* **1997**, *277*, 815–818. [CrossRef] [PubMed]
22. Pan, G.; O'Rourke, K.; Chinnaiyan, A.M.; Gentz, R.; Ebner, R.; Ni, J.; Dixit, V.M. The Receptor for the Cytotoxic Ligand TRAIL. *Science* **1997**, *276*, 111–113. [CrossRef] [PubMed]
23. Walczak, H.; Degli-Esposti, M.A.; Johnson, R.S.; Smolak, P.J.; Waugh, J.Y.; Boiani, N.; Timour, M.S.; Gerhart, M.J.; Schooley, K.A.; Smith, C.A.; et al. TRAIL-R2: A novel apoptosis-mediating receptor for TRAIL. *EMBO J.* **1997**, *16*, 5386–5397. [CrossRef] [PubMed]
24. Pitti, R.M.; Marsters, S.A.; Ruppert, S.; Donahue, C.J.; Moore, A.; Ashkenazi, A. Induction of Apoptosis by Apo-2 Ligand, a New Member of the Tumor Necrosis Factor Cytokine Family. *J. Biol. Chem.* **1996**, *271*, 12687–12690. [CrossRef] [PubMed]
25. Wiley, S.R.; Schooley, K.; Smolak, P.J.; Din, W.S.; Huang, C.-P.; Nicholl, J.K.; Sutherland, G.R.; Smith, T.D.; Rauch, C.; Smith, C.A.; et al. Identification and characterization of a new member of the TNF family that induces apoptosis. *Immunity* **1995**, *3*, 673–682. [CrossRef]
26. Wang, S.; El-Deiry, W.S. TRAIL and apoptosis induction by TNF-family death receptors. *Oncogene* **2003**, *22*, 8628–8633. [CrossRef]
27. Sheridan, J.P.; Marsters, S.A.; Pitti, R.M.; Gurney, A.; Skubatch, M.; Baldwin, D.; Ramakrishnan, L.; Gray, C.L.; Baker, K.; Wood, W.I.; et al. Control of TRAIL-Induced Apoptosis by a Family of Signaling and Decoy Receptors. *Science* **1997**, *277*, 818–821. [CrossRef]
28. Walczak, H.; Miller, R.E.; Ariail, K.; Gliniak, B.; Griffith, T.S.; Kubin, M.; Chin, W.; Jones, J.; Woodward, A.; Le, T.; et al. Tumoricidal activity of tumor necrosis factor–related apoptosis–inducing ligand in vivo. *Nat. Med.* **1999**, *5*, 157–163. [CrossRef]
29. Ashkenazi, A.; Pai, R.C.; Fong, S.; Leung, S.; Lawrence, D.A.; Marsters, S.A.; Blackie, C.; Chang, L.; McMurtrey, A.E.; Hebert, A.; et al. Safety and antitumor activity of recombinant soluble Apo2 ligand. *J. Clin. Investig.* **1999**, *104*, 155–162. [CrossRef]
30. Alves, C.C.; Terziyska, N.; Grunert, M.; Gündisch, S.; Graubner, U.; Quintanilla-Martinez, L.; Jeremias, I. Leukemia-initiating cells of patient-derived acute lymphoblastic leukemia xenografts are sensitive toward TRAIL. *Blood* **2012**, *119*, 4224–4227. [CrossRef]
31. Kelley, S.K.; Harris, L.A.; Xie, D.; Deforge, L.; Totpal, K.; Bussiere, J.; Fox, J.A. Preclinical studies to predict the disposition of Apo2L/tumor necrosis factor-related apoptosis-inducing ligand in humans: Characterization of in vivo efficacy, pharmacokinetics, and safety. *J. Pharmacol. Exp. Ther.* **2001**, *299*, 31–38. [PubMed]
32. Soria, J.-C.; Márk, Z.; Zatloukal, P.; Szima, B.; Albert, I.; Juhász, E.; Pujol, J.-L.; Kozielski, J.; Baker, N.; Smethurst, D.; et al. Randomized phase ii study of dulanermin in combination with paclitaxel, carboplatin, and bevacizumab in advanced non–small-cell lung cancer. *J. Clin. Oncol.* **2011**, *29*, 4442–4451. [CrossRef] [PubMed]
33. Belada, D.; Mayer, J.; Czuczman, M.S.; Flinn, I.W.; Durbin-Johnson, B.; Bray, G.L. Phase II study of dulanermin plus rituximab in patients with relapsed follicular non-Hodgkin's lymphoma (NHL). *J. Clin. Oncol.* **2010**, *28*, 8104. [CrossRef]
34. Herbst, R.S.; Eckhardt, S.G.; Kurzrock, R.; Ebbinghaus, S.; O'Dwyer, P.J.; Gordon, M.S.; Novotny, W.; Goldwasser, M.A.; Tohnya, T.M.; Lum, B.L.; et al. Phase I Dose-Escalation Study of Recombinant Human Apo2L/TRAIL, a Dual Proapoptotic Receptor Agonist, in Patients with Advanced Cancer. *J. Clin. Oncol.* **2010**, *28*, 2839–2846. [CrossRef]
35. Emery, J.G.; McDonnell, P.; Burke, M.B.; Deen, K.C.; Lyn, S.; Silverman, C.; Dul, E.; Appelbaum, E.R.; Eichman, C.; DiPrinzio, R.; et al. Osteoprotegerin Is a Receptor for the Cytotoxic Ligand TRAIL. *J. Biol. Chem.* **1998**, *273*, 14363–14367. [CrossRef]
36. Degli-Esposti, M.A.; Dougall, W.C.; Smolak, P.J.; Waugh, J.Y.; Smith, C.A.; Goodwin, R.G. The Novel Receptor TRAIL-R4 Induces NF-κB and Protects against TRAIL-Mediated Apoptosis, yet Retains an Incomplete Death Domain. *Immunity* **1997**, *7*, 813–820. [CrossRef]
37. Stieglmaier, J.; Bremer, E.; Kellner, C.; Liebig, T.M.; Cate, B.T.; Peipp, M.; Schulze-Koops, H.; Pfeiffer, M.; Bühring, H.-J.; Greil, J.; et al. Selective induction of apoptosis in leukemic B-lymphoid cells by a CD19-specific TRAIL fusion protein. *Cancer Immunol. Immunother.* **2008**, *57*, 233–246. [CrossRef]
38. Unverdorben, F.; Richter, F.; Hutt, M.; Seifert, O.; Malinge, P.; Fischer, N.; Kontermann, R.E. Pharmacokinetic properties of IgG and various Fc fusion proteins in mice. *mAbs* **2016**, *8*, 120–128. [CrossRef]
39. Bremer, E.; Kuijlen, J.; Samplonius, D.; Walczak, H.; De Leij, L.; Helfrich, W. Target cell-restricted and -enhanced apoptosis induction by a scFv:sTRAIL fusion protein with specificity for the pancarcinoma-associated antigen EGP2. *Int. J. Cancer* **2004**, *109*, 281–290. [CrossRef] [PubMed]
40. Wajant, H.; Moosmayer, D.; Wüest, T.; Bartke, T.; Gerlach, E.; Schönherr, U.; Peters, N.; Scheurich, P.; Pfizenmaier, K. Differential activation of TRAIL-R1 and -2 by soluble and membrane TRAIL allows selective surface antigen-directed activation of TRAIL-R2 by a soluble TRAIL derivative. *Oncogene* **2001**, *20*, 4101–4106. [CrossRef]

41. Carter, P.; Presta, L.; Gorman, C.M.; Ridgway, J.B.; Henner, D.; Wong, W.L.; Rowland, A.M.; Kotts, C.; Carver, M.E.; Shepard, H.M. Humanization of an anti-p185HER2 antibody for human cancer therapy. *Proc. Natl. Acad. Sci. USA* **1992**, *89*, 4285–4289. [CrossRef]
42. Amersdorffer, J.; Steidl, S.; Winderlich, M.; Krohn, A.; Rojkjaer, L. Combination Therapy with an Anti-CD19 Antibody and a Purine Analog. U.S. Patent 20140227277, 14 August 2012.
43. Gunasekaran, K.; Pentony, M.; Shen, M.; Garrett, L.; Forte, C.; Woodward, A.; Bin Ng, S.; Born, T.; Retter, M.; Manchulenko, K.; et al. Enhancing antibody Fc heterodimer formation through electrostatic steering effects: Applications to bispecific molecules and monovalent IgG. *J. Biol. Chem.* **2010**, *285*, 19637–19646. [CrossRef]
44. Schneider, B.L.; Munkel, S.; Krippner-Heidenreich, A.; Grunwald, I.; Wels, W.S.; Wajant, H.; Pfizenmaier, K.; Gerspach, J. Potent antitumoral activity of TRAIL through generation of tumor-targeted single-chain fusion proteins. *Cell Death Dis.* **2010**, *1*, e68. [CrossRef] [PubMed]
45. Steger, K.; Brady, J.P.; Wang, W.; Duskin, M.; Donato, K.; Peshwa, M.V. CHO-S antibody titers 1 gram/liter using flow electroporation-mediated transient gene expression followed by rapid migration to high-yield stable cell lines. *J. Biomol. Screen.* **2015**, *20*, 545–551. [CrossRef] [PubMed]
46. Repp, R.; Kellner, C.; Muskulus, A.; Staudinger, M.; Nodehi, S.M.; Glorius, P.; Akramiene, D.; DeChant, M.; Fey, G.H.; Van Berkel, P.H.; et al. Combined Fc-protein- and Fc-glyco-engineering of scFv-Fc fusion proteins synergistically enhances CD16a binding but does not further enhance NK-cell mediated ADCC. *J. Immunol. Methods* **2011**, *373*, 67–78. [CrossRef] [PubMed]
47. Wirt, T.; Rosskopf, S.; Rösner, T.; Eichholz, K.M.; Kahrs, A.; Lutz, S.; Kretschmer, A.; Valerius, T.; Klausz, K.; Otte, A.; et al. An Fc Double-Engineered CD20 Antibody with Enhanced Ability to Trigger Complement-Dependent Cytotoxicity and Antibody-Dependent Cell-Mediated Cytotoxicity. *Transfus. Med. Hemother.* **2017**, *44*, 292–300. [CrossRef] [PubMed]
48. Chou, T.-C. Theoretical basis, experimental design, and computerized simulation of synergism and antagonism in drug combination studies. *Pharmacol. Rev.* **2006**, *58*, 621–681. [CrossRef] [PubMed]
49. Chou, T.-C.; Talalay, P. Quantitative analysis of dose-effect relationships: The combined effects of multiple drugs or enzyme inhibitors. *Adv. Enzym. Regul.* **1984**, *22*, 27–55. [CrossRef]
50. Fischer, U.; Forster, M.; Rinaldi, A.; Risch, T.; Sungalee, S.; Warnatz, H.-J.; Bornhauser, B.; Gombert, M.; Kratsch, C.; Stütz, A.M.; et al. Genomics and drug profiling of fatal TCF3-HLF−positive acute lymphoblastic leukemia identifies recurrent mutation patterns and therapeutic options. *Nat. Genet.* **2015**, *47*, 1020–1029. [CrossRef] [PubMed]
51. Alsadeq, A.; Lenk, L.; Vadakumchery, A.; Cousins, A.; Vokuhl, C.; Khadour, A.; Vogiatzi, F.; Seyfried, F.; Meyer, L.-H.; Cario, G.; et al. IL7R is associated with CNS infiltration and relapse in pediatric B-cell precursor acute lymphoblastic leukemia. *Blood* **2018**, *132*, 1614–1617. [CrossRef]
52. Vogiatzi, F.; Winterberg, D.; Lenk, L.; Buchmann, S.; Cario, G.; Schrappe, M.; Peipp, M.; Richter-Pechanska, P.; Kulozik, A.E.; Lentes, J.; et al. Daratumumab eradicates minimal residual disease in a preclinical model of pediatric T-cell acute lymphoblastic leukemia. *Blood* **2019**, *134*, 713–716. [CrossRef] [PubMed]
53. Lenk, L.; Carlet, M.; Vogiatzi, F.; Spory, L.; Winterberg, D.; Cousins, A.; Vossen-Gajcy, M.; Ibruli, O.; Vokuhl, C.; Cario, G.; et al. CD79a promotes CNS-infiltration and leukemia engraftment in pediatric B-cell precursor acute lymphoblastic leukemia. *Commun. Biol.* **2021**, *4*, 73. [CrossRef] [PubMed]
54. Fulda, S.; Debatin, K.-M. Extrinsic versus intrinsic apoptosis pathways in anticancer chemotherapy. *Oncogene* **2006**, *25*, 4798–4811. [CrossRef] [PubMed]
55. Hockenbery, D.M.; Nuñez, G.; Milliman, C.L.; Schreiber, R.D.; Korsmeyer, S.J. Bcl-2 is an inner mitochondrial membrane protein that blocks programmed cell death. *Nature* **1990**, *348*, 334–336. [CrossRef]
56. Souers, A.J.; Leverson, J.D.; Boghaert, E.R.; Ackler, S.L.; Catron, N.D.; Chen, J.; Dayton, B.D.; Ding, H.; Enschede, S.H.; Fairbrother, W.J.; et al. ABT-199, a potent and selective BCL-2 inhibitor, achieves antitumor activity while sparing platelets. *Nat. Med.* **2013**, *19*, 202–208. [CrossRef]
57. Salles, G.; Duell, J.; Barca, E.G.; Tournilhac, O.; Jurczak, W.; Liberati, A.M.; Nagy, Z.; Obr, A.; Gaidano, G.; André, M.; et al. Tafasitamab plus lenalidomide in relapsed or refractory diffuse large B-cell lymphoma (L-MIND): A multicentre, prospective, single-arm, phase 2 study. *Lancet Oncol.* **2020**, *21*, 978–988. [CrossRef]
58. Jain, N.; Stock, W.; Zeidan, A.; Atallah, E.; McCloskey, J.; Heffner, L.; Tomlinson, B.; Bhatnagar, B.; Feingold, J.; Ungar, D.; et al. Loncastuximab tesirine, an anti-CD19 antibody-drug conjugate, in relapsed/refractory B-cell acute lymphoblastic leukemia. *Blood Adv.* **2020**, *4*, 449–457. [CrossRef]
59. Bremer, E.; Samplonius, D.F.; Peipp, M.; Van Genne, L.; Kroesen, B.-J.; Fey, G.H.; Gramatzki, M.; De Leij, L.F.; Helfrich, W. Target Cell–Restricted Apoptosis Induction of Acute Leukemic T Cells by a Recombinant Tumor Necrosis Factor–Related Apoptosis-Inducing Ligand Fusion Protein with Specificity for Human CD7. *Cancer Res.* **2005**, *65*, 3380–3388. [CrossRef]
60. Mariani, S.M.; Krammer, P.H. Differential regulation of TRAIL and CD95 ligand in transformed cells of the T and B lymphocyte lineage. *Eur. J. Immunol.* **1998**, *28*, 973–982. [CrossRef]
61. Uckun, F.M.; Myers, D.E.; Qazi, S.; Ozer, Z.; Rose, R.; D'Cruz, O.J.; Ma, H. Recombinant human CD19L-sTRAIL effectively targets B cell precursor acute lymphoblastic leukemia. *J. Clin. Investig.* **2015**, *125*, 1006–1018. [CrossRef]
62. Bossen, C.; Ingold, K.; Tardivel, A.; Bodmer, J.-L.; Gaide, O.; Hertig, S.; Ambrose, C.; Tschopp, J.; Schneider, P. Interactions of Tumor Necrosis Factor (TNF) and TNF Receptor Family Members in the Mouse and Human. *J. Biol. Chem.* **2006**, *281*, 13964–13971. [CrossRef]

63. Maude, S.L.; Frey, N.; Shaw, P.A.; Aplenc, R.; Barrett, D.M.; Bunin, N.J.; Chew, A.; Gonzalez, V.E.; Zheng, Z.; Lacey, S.F.; et al. Chimeric antigen receptor T cells for sustained remissions in leukemia. *N. Engl. J. Med.* **2014**, *371*, 1507–1517. [CrossRef] [PubMed]
64. Queudeville, M.; Schlegel, P.; Heinz, A.T.; Lenz, T.; Döring, M.; Holzer, U.; Hartmann, U.; Kreyenberg, H.; von Stackelberg, A.; Schrappe, M.; et al. Blinatumomab in pediatric patients with relapsed/refractory B-cell precursor acute lymphoblastic leukemia. *Eur. J. Haematol.* **2021**, *106*, 473–483. [CrossRef] [PubMed]
65. Khaw, S.L.; Suryani, S.; Evans, K.; Richmond, J.; Robbins, A.; Kurmasheva, R.T.; Billups, C.A.; Erickson, S.W.; Guo, Y.; Houghton, P.J.; et al. Venetoclax responses of pediatric ALL xenografts reveal sensitivity of MLL-rearranged leukemia. *Blood* **2016**, *128*, 1382–1395. [CrossRef] [PubMed]
66. Maude, S.L.; Laetsch, T.W.; Buechner, J.; Rives, S.; Boyer, M.; Bittencourt, H.; Bader, P.; Verneris, M.R.; Stefanski, H.E.; Myers, G.D.; et al. Tisagenlecleucel in Children and Young Adults with B-Cell Lymphoblastic Leukemia. *N. Engl. J. Med.* **2018**, *378*, 439–448. [CrossRef] [PubMed]
67. Bremer, E.; Samplonius, D.; Kroesen, B.-J.; Van Genne, L.; De Leij, L.; Helfrich, W. Exceptionally Potent Anti-Tumor Bystander Activity of an scFv:sTRAIL Fusion Protein with Specificity for EGP2 Toward Target Antigen-Negative Tumor Cells1. *Neoplasia* **2004**, *6*, 636–645. [CrossRef]
68. De Luca, R.; Kachel, P.; Kropivsek, K.; Snijder, B.; Manz, M.G.; Neri, D. A novel dual-cytokine–antibody fusion protein for the treatment of CD38-positive malignancies. *Protein Eng. Des. Sel.* **2018**, *31*, 173–179. [CrossRef]
69. Yan, C.; Li, S.; Li, Z.; Peng, H.; Yuan, X.; Jiang, L.; Zhang, Y.; Fan, N.; Hu, X.; Yang, M.; et al. Human Umbilical Cord Mesenchymal Stem Cells as Vehicles of CD20-Specific TRAIL Fusion Protein Delivery: A Double-Target Therapy against Non-Hodgkin's Lymphoma. *Mol. Pharm.* **2013**, *10*, 142–151. [CrossRef]
70. Wei, G.; Wang, J.; Huang, H.; Zhao, Y. Novel immunotherapies for adult patients with B-lineage acute lymphoblastic leukemia. *J. Hematol. Oncol.* **2017**, *10*, 150. [CrossRef]

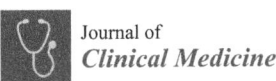

Review

Antibody–Drug Conjugates for the Treatment of Acute Pediatric Leukemia

Jamie L. Stokke [1,*] and Deepa Bhojwani [1,2]

1. Division of Hematology-Oncology, Children's Hospital Los Angeles, Keck School of Medicine, University of Southern California, Los Angeles, CA 90027, USA; dbhojwani@chla.usc.edu
2. Norris Comprehensive Cancer Center, University of Southern California, Los Angeles, CA 90033, USA
* Correspondence: jstokke@chla.usc.edu; Tel.: +1-323-361-2601

Abstract: The clinical development of antibody–drug conjugates (ADCs) has gained momentum in recent years and these agents are gradually moving into frontline regimens for pediatric acute leukemias. ADCs consist of a monoclonal antibody attached to a cytotoxic payload by a cleavable linker. This structure allows for highly cytotoxic agents to be directly delivered to leukemia cells leading to cell death and avoids excessive off-tumor toxicity. Near universal expression on B-cell acute lymphoblastic leukemia (ALL) blasts and the ability of rapid internalization has rendered CD22 an ideal target for ADC in B-ALL. Inotuzumab ozogamicin, the anti-CD22 antibody linked to calicheamicin led to complete remission rates of 60–80% in patients with relapsed/refractory B-ALL. In acute myeloid leukemia (AML), the CD33 targeting gemtuzumab ozogamicin has demonstrated modest improvements in survival and is the only ADC currently licensed in the United States for pediatric patients with de novo AML. Several other ADCs have been developed and tested clinically for leukemia but have achieved limited success to date. The search for additional leukemia-specific targets and optimization of ADC structure and specificity are ongoing efforts to improve their therapeutic window. This review provides a comprehensive overview of ADCs in acute leukemias, with a focus on pediatric ALL and AML.

Keywords: ADC; antibody–drug conjugate; pediatric leukemia; leukemia; ALL; AML; immunotherapy

1. Introduction

The outcome of pediatric patients with leukemia has improved dramatically in recent decades with overall survival exceeding 90% in B-cell acute lymphoblastic leukemia (B-ALL) [1]. Modest improvements have been noted in acute myeloid leukemia (AML) with overall survival of greater than 60% [2]. However, survival for patients with high-risk and relapsed leukemias is much lower, and despite highly toxic, intensified therapies, durable remission is difficult to achieve. In addition, patients suffer significant toxicities related to intensive chemotherapy regimens. Thus, targeted agents are crucial, and several have been developed in the relapsed setting. A few of these agents are now being tested in frontline therapy, with goals of improving outcomes and mitigating short and long-term toxicity. Targeted immunotherapy utilizing antibodies, antibody–drug conjugates (ADCs), immunotoxins, bi-specific antibody T cell engagers (BiTEs), and chimeric antigen receptor (CAR) T cells have changed the treatment landscape for relapsed and high-risk B-ALL. Similar success with targeted therapies has been slower in AML due to disease heterogeneity and the potential for high off-tumor toxicity associated with target antigen expression in normal hematopoietic stem cells resulting in myeloablation.

ADCs are a promising and rapidly expanding repertoire of oncology therapeutics. They offer an effective mechanism of delivering highly cytotoxic agents directly to leukemia cells and avoiding off-target toxicity seen with standard chemotherapy. ADCs consist of a monoclonal antibody bound to chemotherapeutic drugs (payload) via chemical linkers.

Upon antibody binding to its target on a leukemia cell, the ADC is internalized via receptor-mediated endocytosis. The linker is then cleaved, and the cytotoxic drugs are released inside the cell. Depending on the drug delivered, there are multiple mechanisms of action leading to apoptosis and cell death (Figure 1). The cytotoxic agent of the ADCs also has the ability to be cleaved in the tumor microenvironment and cross cell membranes of neighboring tumor cells, known as the "bystander effect".

Multiple generations of ADCs have evolved with improved stability, potency, and internalization kinetics [3,4]. Gemtuzumab ozogamicin (GO) is a first-generation ADC targeting CD33 on myeloid leukemia cells and the first to attain United States Food and Drug Administration (FDA) approval for adult patients with relapsed AML in 2000. Though subsequent development was not straightforward, the indication was extended to newly diagnosed adult patients in 2017, and to newly diagnosed pediatric patients in 2020. At the time of this review, there are six ADCs approved by the US FDA for hematologic malignancies: gemtuzumab ozogamicin (CD33), brentuximab vedotin (CD30), inotuzumab ozogamicin (CD22), polatuzumab vedotin (CD79B), belantamab mafodotin (BCMA) and loncastuximab tesirine (CD19). The first five have also been approved by the European Medicines Agency (EMA); loncastuximab tesirine is awaiting approval [4,5]. This review highlights ADCs developed for clinical use in acute leukemias. Table 1 details ongoing clinical trials.

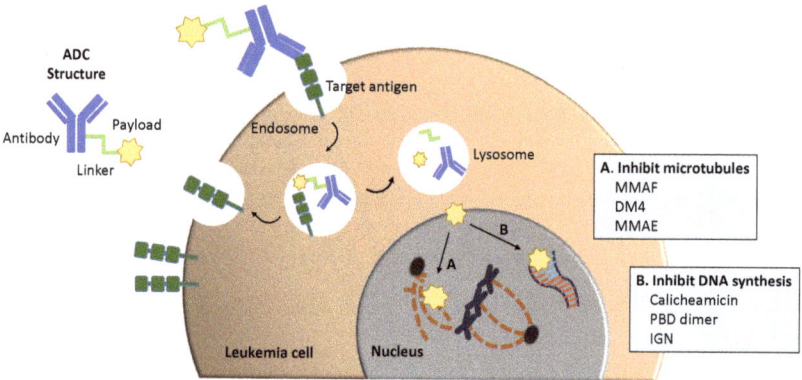

Figure 1. Antibody–drug conjugate structure and mechanisms of action. ADC structure demonstrated on the left consisting of a monoclonal antibody attached to a cytotoxic agent, or payload, by a chemical linker. The ADC binds to the target antigen on the leukemia cell surface, is internalized in an endosome, and then the linker is cleaved from the antibody and payload by chemical or enzymatic reaction in a lysosome. The payload inhibits (**A**) microtubule formation and function or (**B**) DNA synthesis leading to leukemia cell death. The target antigen is recycled back to the cell surface. MMAF, monomethyl auristatin F; DM4, ravtansine; MMAE, monomethyl auristatin E; PBD, pyrrolobenzodiazepine; IGN, indolinobenzodiazepine.

Table 1. Active clinical trials utilizing ADCs for acute leukemia.

ADC	Target	Payload	Cancer Targeted	Phase	Age Group	Trial Design	Identifier
Inotuzumab ozogamicin (InO) Besponsa	CD22	Calicheamicin	R/R B-ALL	I	Adult	ALL.001. InO with 3 and 4 drug augmented BFM	NCT03962465
			R/R B-ALL	I	Adult	InO with DA-EPOCH	NCT03991884
			R/R ALL	I/II	Adult	InO post HSCT	NCT03104491
			Upfront ALL	I/II	Adult	InO with low dose chemotherapy	NCT01371630
			R/R B-ALL	I/II	Adult	InO with liposomal vincristine	NCT03851081
			R/R ALL	I/II	Adult	InO with bosutinib in Ph+ leukemia	NCT02311998
			R/R B-ALL	II	Adult	InO with blinatumomab	NCT03739814
			R/R B-ALL	II	Adult	InO pre and post HSCT	NCT03856216
			R/R B-ALL	II	Adult	InO for MRD positive ALL	NCT03441061
			Upfront ALL	II	Adult	Hyper-CVAD with blinatumomab and inotuzumab	NCT02877303
			Upfront B-ALL	III	Adult	InO with frontline therapy	NCT03150693
			R/R B-ALL	IV	Adult	Varying doses of InO before HSCT	NCT03677596
			Upfront ALL	II	Adult	InO induction followed by conventional chemotherapy	2016-004836-39
			Upfront B-ALL, MPAL, B-LLy	III	Pediatric	AALL1732. InO with standard chemotherapy	NCT03959085
			R/R B ALL	II	Pediatric	InO for MRD positive B ALL	NCT03913559
			Upfront B-ALL	III	Pediatric	ALLTogether1; InO with chemotherapy	NCT04307576
ADCT602 Epratuzumab tesirine	CD22	PBD dimer	R/R ALL	I/II	Adult	Single-agent ADCT602	NCT03698552

Table 1. *Conts.*

ADC	Target	Payload	Cancer Targeted	Phase	Age Group	Trial Design	Identifier
Gemtuzumab ozogamicin (GO) Mylotarg	CD33	Calicheamicin	R/R AML	Ib	Adult	BTCRC-AML17-113; GO and venetoclax	NCT04070768
			R/R AML	I	Adult	CPX-351 and GO	NCT03904251
			FLT3 AML	I	Adult	GO, midostaurin, and chemotherapy	NCT03900949
			Upfront core-binding factor AML, MDS	II	Adult	GO with chemotherapy	NCT00801489
			R/R AML	Ib/II	Adult	OX40 antibody alone or in combination with GO or other agents	NCT03390296
			R/R AML	I/II	Adult	Talazoparib with GO	NCT04207190
			Upfront APL	II	10 years and older	Tretinoin and arsenic with or without GO	NCT01409161
			R/R AML	II	Adult	GO with chemotherapy	NCT04050280
			R/R AML	II	Adult	Liposomal daunorubicin, cytarabine, and GO	NCT03672539
			R/R AML, MDS	II	Adult	Single-agent GO for MRD	NCT03737955
			R/R AML	II	Adult	Mitoxantrone, etoposide with GO	NCT03839446
			Upfront AML	III	Adult	GO with chemotherapy, with or without Clasdegib	NCT04093505
			R/R AML	II	Adult	GO with bortezomib and high dose cytarabine	NCT04173585
			Upfront AML	I	Pediatric	GO with standard chemotherapy	NCT04326439
			Upfront AML	III	Pediatric	AAML1831; GO with standard chemotherapy compared to CPX-351 and/or gilteritinib	NCT04293562
			R/R AML	IV	Pediatric	Single-agent GO	NCT03727750
			Upfront AML	III	Pediatric	Myechild01; GO with chemotherapy	NCT02724163
Brentuximab vedotin	CD30	MMAE	Upfront Adult T cell leukemia and lymphoma	II	Adult	Brentuximab with chemotherapy	NCT03264131
IMGN632	CD123	IGN	R/R AML, ALL, BPDCN	I/II	Adult	IMGN632 as monotherapy	NCT03386513
			R/R AML and upfront	Ib/II	Adult	IMGN643 as monotherapy or in combination with venetoclax and/or azacytidine	NCT04086264
VSL-101	ROR1	MMAE	R/R hematologic malignancies	I	Adult	Single-agent VSL-101	NCT03833180

R/R, relapsed refractory; ALL, acute lymphoblastic leukemia; AML, acute myeloid leukemia; BFM, Berlin-Frankfurt-Munster; Ph+, Philadelphia chromosome-positive; HSCT, hematopoietic stem cell transplant; CVAD, cyclophosphamide, vincristine, doxorubicin, and dexamethasone; MRD, minimal residual disease; MPAL, mixed phenotype acute leukemia; B-LLy, B lymphoblastic lymphoma.; APL, acute promyelocytic leukemia; BPDCN, blastic plasmacytoid dendritic cell neoplasm.

Antibody–Drug Conjugate Design

ADC development requires attention to stability in physiologic conditions and careful consideration for the choice of the target antigen. The target should be sufficiently expressed on the leukemia cell surface, only expressed in low levels on healthy tissues, and rapidly internalized upon antibody binding [6]. The antibody that binds to the antigen must have a suitable affinity to allow for sufficient binding and internalization. Most antibodies used clinically are human IgG to limit immunoreactivity. The linker attaching the antibody to the payload must be stable during circulation. Upon endocytosis, the linker is broken down within the cell by either enzymatic reaction or hydrolyzed by pH conditions, and the cytotoxic drug is released [4]. The cytotoxic agents must also be stable to avoid degeneration prior to reaching their targets. There are two main categories of cytotoxic drugs used in ADCs as payloads: microtubule inhibitors and DNA-damaging drugs. DNA damage can occur via double-stranded DNA breakage (calicheamicin), by alkylating DNA (duocarmycin), or by crosslinking with DNA (pyrrolobenzodiazepine dimers). An example of ADCs that utilize microtubule inhibitors is brentuximab vedotin, and those which induce DNA damage include InO and GO. These cytotoxic agents demonstrate much higher potency than traditional chemotherapeutic agents, and thus, targeted and stable delivery is the key to their clinical success [7].

Despite the benefit of a targeted approach to limit the toxicity of ADCs, there are multiple mechanisms of on and off-target tissue damage. As target antigens may also be expressed in certain healthy tissues, ADCs can result in toxicities from on-target, off-tumor targeting. Also, linker instability can lead to the premature release of the cytotoxic payload into the circulation. Toxicities include those commonly seen with standard chemotherapeutic agents and include anemia, neutropenia, thrombocytopenia, hepatic toxicity, and peripheral neuropathy [8]. For example, both InO and GO are known to cause hepatotoxicity including elevated transaminases, hyperbilirubinemia, and sinusoidal obstructive syndrome (SOS) attributed to calicheamicin. The mechanisms of hepatotoxicity for these agents are multifactorial including on-target, off-tumor antibody binding, nonspecific uptake of the ADCs in the liver, and premature release of the payload into circulation [9]. New generation ADCs are in development with the goals of improved safety and efficacy. For instance, newer antibodies are typically IgG1 subclass to optimize their solubility, target affinity, and half-life. Target selection has improved over time, with the focus placed on higher rates of turnover for increased antitumor activity, and targets that are oncogenic are also being explored. The linker moiety has evolved with the improvement in stability in circulation to limit off-target toxicities. Lastly, the payload itself has undergone engineering improvements. Having a high payload to antibody ratio and utilizing hydrophilic constructs leads to great antitumor activity and avoidance of hepatic clearance [10].

2. Antibody–Drug Conjugates in B-ALL
2.1. Targeting CD22

CD22 is a regulator of B cell signaling and is expressed on 96% of B-ALL blasts [11]. Its B cell-specific expression makes it an ideal target for antibody therapy [12]. In addition, the CD22 receptor is internalized rapidly. Inotuzumab ozogamicin (InO) was approved by the FDA and EMA in 2017 to treat adult patients with relapsed or refractory B-ALL [13]. The structure of InO consists of the antitumor antibiotic calicheamicin, a cleavable linker, and an ant-CD22 IgG4 antibody. Once in the nucleus, calicheamicin causes double-stranded DNA breaks leading to apoptosis and cell death. Additionally, calicheamicin diffuses outside of the cell and into neighboring cancer cells leading to cytotoxicity via the bystander effect [4].

InO has demonstrated excellent efficacy in adults with B-ALL. In the phase III INO-VATE trial comparing single-agent InO to standard chemotherapy for patients with relapsed B-ALL, the rate of complete remission (CR) was significantly higher in the InO group than the chemotherapy group (80% vs. 29%) [14]. In pediatric patients, outcomes have been equally promising. In a compassionate use program, 51 children received InO and 67% of those responders achieve minimal residual disease (MRD) negativity [15]. In the COG study, AALL1621 (NCT02981628), InO was administered in a single-arm phase II trial for patients with multiply relapsed or refractory B-ALL. A CR rate of 58% was achieved [16]. The Innovative Therapies for Children with Cancer (ITCC) Consortium, recently completed a phase I study in multiply relapsed patients with B-ALL. Overall response rate (ORR) after course 1 was 80% and 84% of responders achieved MRD negative remission [17]. To improve on the durability of response and test safety in combination with standard chemotherapy, the ongoing ITCC consortium and the COG trials combine InO with cytotoxic chemotherapy for patients with relapsed/refractory ALL. Additionally, the ongoing COG trial AALL1732 (NCT03959085) for newly diagnosed patients is testing single-agent InO courses between standard chemotherapy phases versus chemotherapy alone. Important adverse events (AEs) of InO include SOS which occurred in 11% of patients in the INO-VATE trial with most cases occurring after hematopoietic stem cell transplant (HSCT) [13,18]. The post-HSCT SOS rate was higher in pediatric patients; a plausible reason is the inclusion of very heavily pretreated patients in the pediatric cohorts [15,16]. Prophylactic therapies such as ursodiol and defibrotide may be warranted for patients who will undergo post-InO HSCT. Other serious AEs of InO include neutropenia, thrombocytopenia, febrile neutropenia, infusion-related reactions, tumor lysis syndrome, and prolonged QT syndrome [13,18]. Despite the high CR rate of InO, the response is suboptimal in those with baseline dim or partial CD22 expression and in patients with *KMT2A* rearrangements [19]. In addition, modulation of CD22 expression and emergence of CD22 negative clones is a mechanism of resistance post InO.

Another ADC targeting CD22, Epratuzumab tesirine, or ADCT 602, composed of an anti-CD22 humanized IgG1 antibody bound to a pyrrolobenzodiazepine (PBD) dimer (a DNA crosslinking agent) via a cleavable linker is currently under investigation in a phase I/II clinical trial in adults with relapsed and refractory B-ALL (NCT03698552) [20].

Immunotoxins are antibody-protein toxin conjugates which, similar to ADCs, utilize the specific binding power of antibodies to deliver toxins derived from bacteria, fungi, and plants. They function by inhibiting protein synthesis, and an antibody fragment is used rather than an entire antibody to allow for improved pharmacokinetics [21]. HA22, Moxetumomab pasudotox is a recombinant CD22 targeting immunotoxin utilizing a pseudomonas exotoxin (PE) [22]. In a phase I trial, approximately 23% of children with relapsed ALL achieved a complete response and toxicities included capillary leak syndrome (CLS) and HUS [23]. In an international Phase 2 study, 28 of 32 enrolled patients were evaluated for a response, and the ORR was 28% with 10% of patients achieving a morphologic CR. However, the study was terminated early as the CR rate was suboptimal and did not achieve the target [24]. In a parallel phase 2 trial administering Moxetumomab to pediatric ALL patients with positive MRD prior to HSCT (12-MOXE), the sole patient enrolled developed fatal CLS and this study was also terminated [25]. Moxetumomab has an acceptable safety profile in adult patients with relapsed/refractory hairy cell leukemia (HCL) and is FDA approved for this indication [26]. Though HUS and CLS are noted in patients with HCL, these toxicities are transient in most patients. It is unclear if the mechanisms of toxicity differ based on the host (pediatric vs. adult patients) or the disease (ALL vs. HCL).

2.2. Targeting CD19

CD19 is expressed on normal and neoplastic B cells and plays a key role in B-cell signaling, activation, and B-cell development. CD19 is ubiquitously expressed on B-ALL cells and has served as an effective target for antibody therapy. However, it is not internalized as rapidly as CD22, thus, is less efficient in drug delivery despite its high cell surface density. Loncastuximab tesirine, or ADCT-402, is an ADC consisting of a humanized anti-CD19 antibody conjugated to SG3199, a PBD dimer-containing toxin [20]. Loncastuximab has demonstrated safety and efficacy in CD19 positive non-Hodgkin lymphomas resulting in an ORR of 45% in the phase I study, and 48% in the phase II study [5,27]. However, in the phase I study of loncasutximab for adults with relapsed or refractory B-ALL, only 3 of

35 patients (8.6%) achieve CR, and the trial closed early due to slow accrual [28]. Common toxicities included nausea, febrile neutropenia, and liver abnormalities [27].

Denintuxumab mafodotin, or SGN-CD19A, is a humanized anti-CD19 monoclonal antibody conjugated to monomethyl auristatin F (MMAF). In vitro studies demonstrated activity against pediatric ALL by delaying progression in eight patient-derived xenografts [29]. A phase I dose-escalation study to assess safety in adult patients with relapsed or refractory B-ALL ended in 2017 and an interim report of this trial noted a 19% CR rate [30]. Phase II studies in combination with chemotherapy for lymphoma were initiated but terminated early due to changes in portfolio prioritization by the sponsor.

Coltuximab ravtansine, or SAR3419, is a humanized CD19 antibody with a maytansoid DM4 payload. Preclinical studies examined SAR3419 alone or in combination with chemotherapy in pediatric patient-derived xenografts and demonstrated an objective response in all but one xenograft prompting its development into a clinical trial [31]. The MYRALL trial was a phase II monotherapy study in 36 adults with relapsed or refractory ALL. At the recommended dose of 70 mg/m^2, 3 of 17 patients attained CR with a duration of response of 1.9 months. The most common toxicities were fever, diarrhea, and nausea. Due to an inadequate response rate, this study was terminated [32].

2.3. Targeting CD25

CD25 is expressed on activated B cells, T cells, and regulatory T cells and is the alpha chain of the IL-2 receptor. Expression on ALL and AML is associated with induction failure, increased risk of relapse, and decreased overall survival [20]. Camidanlumab tesirine, or ADCT-301, is a humanized IgG1 anti-CD25 antibody conjugated to a PBD dimer. In a phase I trial of adult patients with classical Hodgkin lymphoma, the ORR rate was impressive at 81% [33]. Unfortunately, the phase I trial of adults with CD25 positive relapsed or refractory ALL or AML was terminated early due to limited efficacy as only 2 of 35 patients achieved CR. Common toxicities included febrile neutropenia, cytopenias, fatigue, pneumonia, hypophosphatemia, and elevated gamma glutamyltransferase [34,35]. This agent is continuing development as a mechanism to deplete regulatory T cells as a single agent, and in combination with checkpoint inhibitors in solid tumors [36].

2.4. Current Clinical Applications of ADCs in Pediatric B-ALL

The therapeutic approach for relapsed B-ALL varies but most pediatric patients with first relapse B-ALL are treated with a standard four-drug re-induction. Therapy following re-induction is dependent on risk stratification but typically consists of either blinatumomab and chemotherapy for lower-risk patients or chemotherapy followed by HSCT for higher-risk patients [37]. InO has demonstrated efficacy in second or greater relapse (or refractory disease) in both COG trial AALL1621 and the European ITCC trial and is a good option as a bridge to transplant in that patient population [16,17]. InO is also a useful agent as a re-induction regimen for patients with CD19 antigen-negative relapse B-ALL who do not otherwise qualify for CD19 directed CAR T cells or blinatumomab. CD22 targeting CAR T cells and InO demonstrate similar efficacy in relapsed and refractory B-ALL, however, InO is easier to administer as it is available off the shelf and given as a once-weekly IV infusion [38]. CD22 CAR T cells, on the other hand, are still in the early phases of development and are only available in the context of a clinical trial at few centers requiring weeks for manufacturing. Special consideration should be taken when considering salvage InO prior to HSCT due to the risk of SOS which is highest in heavily pre-treated patients. InO is currently being studied as a frontline agent in trials for high-risk B-ALL which combine InO with the standard BFM chemotherapy backbone. Other ADCs in development are currently limited to phase I/II trials in adult patients.

3. Role of Antibody–Drug Conjugates in T-ALL

Development of successful immunotherapy for T-ALL is challenging due to the shared expression of target antigens between normal and leukemic T cells, and toxicities associated with T cell depletion. CAR T cells are currently under development targeting several T cell antigens including CD5, CD7, CD3, and CD4, but ADCs have lagged behind [39]. CD30 expression is noted in 38% of T-ALL cases, with increased expression observed during courses of chemotherapy [40]. Brentuximab vedotin is approved for cutaneous T cell lymphoma, but no studies have been initiated in T-ALL yet. Monoclonal antibodies targeting T-ALL antigens have also shown clinical promise. Daratumumab, an anti-CD38 monoclonal antibody, has demonstrated efficacy in some patients with T-ALL [41]. Other potential targets for ADCs include IL7R which is a transmembrane receptor that plays a role in the maintenance and progression of T-ALL. Preclinical models demonstrated increased steroid sensitivity in lymphoid blasts by targeting IL7R with the ADC A7R-ADC-SN-38, and a clinical trial is in the early stages of development [42].

4. Antibody–Drug Conjugates in AML

4.1. Targeting CD33

CD33 is variably expressed on the majority of leukemic myeloblasts, and high CD33 expression is associated with an inferior outcome [43]. Gemtuzumab ozogamicin (GO) is the first approved ADC for human use [44]. GO is an anti-D33 IgG4 antibody linked to the calicheamicin cytotoxic agent. In the first phase I clinical trial of GO administered to 40 adults with relapsed/refractory AML, a CR rate of 12.5% was achieved [45]. In a follow-up report consisting of three single-arm phase II studies, 270 adult patients in the first relapse were enrolled and 71 (26%) achieved CR with single-agent GO [46]. These results led to the accelerated approval by the FDA in 2000 as a stand-alone treatment of patients over 60 years of age who were not candidates for standard chemotherapy [46]. GO was later withdrawn from the commercial market in October 2010 after a randomized trial examining standard chemotherapy versus chemotherapy with GO in 637 adult patients showed no improvement in survival and increased treatment-related toxicity in the GO arm [47]. However, after additional data including the pivotal ALFA-0701 trial by the Acute Leukemia French Association, the FDA reapproved the use of GO in 2017 [48].

In pediatric patients, the Berlin-Frankfurt-Münster (BFM) group first demonstrated a 4-year overall survival of 18% in a GO compassionate use program followed by a phase II study of GO resulting in a 37% CR/CRi in those with relapsed and refractory AML [49,50]. Subsequently, the UK Medical Research Council (MRC) AML15 trial demonstrated the efficacy of GO in upfront treatment of pediatric AML [51,52]. COG AAML03P1 added GO to standard chemotherapy followed by HSCT if the patient had a matched donor. The CR rate was 83% after 1 course and 87% after 2 courses [52]. The subsequent trial COG AAML0531 compared standard chemotherapy to standard chemotherapy with GO. In this trial, GO significantly improved event-free survival (53% vs. 46% in non-GO arm) but not overall survival [53]. These results supported the FDA approval of GO for pediatric patients aged 1 month and older. Data from the UK MRC15 and ALFA-0701 trials suggest that GO particularly benefits patients with favorable and intermediate-risk cytogenetics [51,54]. Toxicities in the pediatric trials include hyperbilirubinemia, elevated transaminases, SOS, febrile neutropenia, and prolonged neutrophil recovery [52,53,55]. The dosing of GO has evolved over time with infusion-related toxicities and SOS observed at 9 mg/m^2 [56]. Another study demonstrated equivalent CR and less toxicity (including SOS) with a dosing of 3 mg/m^2 compared to 6 mg/m^2 [57]. In combination with chemotherapy, a single dose of 3 mg/m^2 is commonly used in pediatric and adult practice. Several ongoing studies are examining the use of GO with different chemotherapy combinations. MyeChild01 is an ongoing European consortium trial evaluating the optimum tolerated number of 3 mg/m^2 doses of GO to be used in combination with induction chemotherapy in pediatric patients (NCT02724163). AAML1831 (NCT04293562) is the ongoing phase III COG study comparing standard chemotherapy to therapy with CPX-351 in newly diagnosed children with AML. All patients receive GO in the backbone regimen as the standard of care.

To improve upon the efficacy and reduce toxicities of GO, additional ADCs targeting CD33 have been developed, but these continue to face multiple challenges. AVE9633 is an ADC composed of a highly potent maytansinoid derivative, DM4, conjugated to a humanized IgG1 anti-CD33 monoclonal antibody, huMy9-6. In a phase I trial in 54 adults with refractory or relapsed AML, the most common adverse event was an infusion-related reaction. Unfortunately, only two patients had a response; one CR for 8 months and another PR for two months [58]. Vadastuximab talirine, or SGN-CD33A, is an ADC consisting of a PBD dimer linked to an antibody targeting CD33. In a phase I study of 131 adult patients with CD33-positive AML, vadastuximab led to a 28% CR rate [59]. The subsequent phase III CASCADE study assessed vadastuximab in combination with hypomethylating agents (HMAs) compared to HMAs alone. A safety analysis indicated a higher rate of deaths, including fatal infections in the vadastuximab arm compared to the control arm, and the study was closed (NCT02785900). Continued development will incorporate additional safeguards and toxicity monitoring rules. IMGN779 is an anti-CD33 ADC with a DNA-alkylating IGN (indolinobenzodiazepine pseudodimer) payload and a cleavable s-SPDB linker. A phase I trial of IMGN779 enrolled 50 adult patients with relapsed or refractory AML, and the most common toxicities included febrile neutropenia, nausea, diarrhea, and fatigue. Overall, 41% of patients demonstrated a decrease in bone marrow blasts, but it is unclear if the development of this agent will proceed [60].

4.2. Targeting CD123

CD123 is the alpha subunit of the interleukin-3 receptor and is highly expressed in AML, blastic plasmacytoid dendritic cell neoplasm, B-ALL, and early thymic progenitor ALL cases [61,62]. It is rapidly internalized making it an ideal target for antibody therapy [63]. IMGN632 is an ADC consisting of a novel DNA alkylating payload, DGN549 which is an indolinobenzodiazepine pseudodimer (IGN) class, that induces single stranded DNA breaks and a novel peptide linker that confers greater stability in circulation [64]. A phase I study for adult patients with relapsed or refractory CD123 positive leukemia is actively recruiting to assess the safety and tolerability of IMGN632 as monotherapy. Preliminary analysis demonstrated a 33% CR rate, and common toxicities included diarrhea, nausea, febrile neutropenia, peripheral edema, and hypotension (NCT03386513) [65]. A phase Ib/II study for adult patients with CD123-positive AML utilizing IMGN632 as either monotherapy or in combination with venetoclax and/or azacytidine is actively recruiting (NCT04086264).

SGN-CD123A is an anti-CD123 antibody bound to a PBD dimer that was evaluated in a phase I study (NCT02848248) in adult patients with relapsed or refractory AML, however, this study was terminated early at the same time as the CD33 ADC vadastuximab talirine study for safety concerns as it utilized the identical PBD dimer and linker molecules that resulted in excessive toxicities.

4.3. Targeting ROR1

Receptor tyrosine kinase-like orphan receptor 1 (ROR1) is expressed on hematologic malignant cells but not on normal tissues. It is expressed in 35% of AML and in most cases, it is co-expressed with CD34, indicating it is a promising target for leukemia stem cells. The ADC VLS-101 consists of a humanized IgG1 monoclonal antibody (UC-961), and an mc-VC-PAB linker bound to the cytotoxic payload, MMAE [66,67]. An ongoing phase I trial examines the use of VLS-101 in adult patients with relapsed hematologic malignancies including ALL and AML (NCT03833180).

4.4. Targeting Mesothelin

Mesothelin (MSLN) is highly overexpressed in about 33% of pediatric AML cases and not in normal bone marrow making it a viable target [68]. Anetumab ravtensine, or BAY 94-9343, is an ADC consisting of anti-MSLN linked to tubulin polymerase inhibitor DM4. In view of a favorable safety profile for this agent in an adult trial of patients with advanced solid tumors, a COG phase I study is in development for second or greater relapse pediatric patients with mesothelin-positive AML [69,70].

4.5. Targeting CLL-1 (CD371)

C-type lectin-like molecule-1 (CLL-1) is a transmembrane glycoprotein expressed on the surface of AML blasts, AML stem cells, and monocytes but not on hematopoietic stem cells [71]. DCLL9718S is a THIOMAB™ antibody-drug conjugated (TDC) consisting of an IgG1 anti-CLL1 antibody linked to two PBD dimers via a cleavable disulfide linker. THIOMAB™ consists of engineering a recombinant mutation of one or more amino acids to a cysteine which allows the ADC to achieve improved stability of the connection of cytotoxic drug to antibody [72]. A clinical trial examined 18 adult patients with relapsed or refractory AML in a phase I trial of DCLL9718S [73]. Two-thirds of the patients experienced at least one clinically significant AE most commonly including febrile neutropenia and pneumonia. No patients achieved objective CR or PR response. Due to the limited tolerability and efficacy, this drug will not move forward in clinical trials, however, CLL-1 remains a promising target for CAR T-cell therapy and future ADCs [74].

4.6. Additional ADCs with Unclear Clinical Potential in AML

CD30 is a cell membrane protein of the tumor necrosis factor receptor family expressed on activated T and B cells, and also on 36% of high-risk AML/MDS [75]. Brentuximab vedotin is an ADC consisting of an anti-CD30 antibody conjugated to the anti-microtubule compound, MMAE. After licensing in Hodgkin lymphoma and anaplastic large cell lymphoma, brentuximab was studied in other CD30 expressing hematologic malignancies. In a phase I study in adults with AML, brentuximab was combined with re-induction chemotherapy in CD30 expressing relapsed AML [76]. The composite response rate was 36% with a median disease-free survival of 6.8 months [76]. A phase I/II study examining brentuximab with azacytidine in AML was terminated early due to poor accrual (NCT02096042). A phase II study of single-agent brentuximab in CD30 positive non-lymphomatous malignancies enrolled pediatric and adult patients with AML and solid tumors (NCT01461538). According to the preliminary report, 2 of 14 patients with leukemia or high-grade myelodysplastic syndrome (MDS) achieved the objective response [77]. Final results are awaited. CD37 is another transmembrane protein that is highly expressed on myeloid cells and may function as a signaling death receptor. The ADC AGS67E is a humanized monoclonal IgG3 antibody against CD37 conjugated via a protease-cleavable linker to MMAE [78]. In a phase I study, 23 adult patients with AML were enrolled, however, the study was terminated due to business reasons (NCT02610062).

Members of the receptor tyrosine kinase family c-KIT and FLT3 have been amenable to targeting with small molecule inhibitors, and CAR T-cells against these targets are also being developed. Unfortunately, the clinical development of ADCs for c-KIT (CD117) and FLT3 (CD135) has been difficult. LOP628 is a humanized antibody against CD117, conjugated to DM1 via a non-cleavable linker [79]. A phase I study of LOP628 in patients with c-KIT positive solid tumors and AML enrolled three participants and then closed early due to infusion reaction in the first two patients due to mast cell degranulation [80]. AGS62P1 is an ADC consisting of an anti-FLT3 human IgG1 antibody conjugated to a microtubule-disrupting agent (AGL-0182-30) via an alkoxyamine linker [81]. A phase I study enrolled 43 participants with relapsed and/or refractory AML was terminated early due to lack of efficacy (NCT02864290).

4.7. Current Clinical Applications of ADCs in Pediatric AML

GO has demonstrated the highest clinical success among ADCs in AML and is currently used in combination with standard chemotherapy in frontline studies. GO is FDA approved for the treatment of newly diagnosed CD33 positive AML in children ≥ 2 years of age and thus is often utilized with many different standard chemotherapy regimens in pediatric patients with CD33 positive AML. In the relapsed setting, GO is often used in combination with standard chemotherapy as in the frontline setting. In patients with both frontline and relapse use of GO, careful consideration must be used when administering GO prior to HSCT to decrease the risk of SOS. The risk of SOS is decreased when a lower dose (3 mg/m^2) is administered. One question regarding the use of GO is what level of CD33 expression is necessary to achieve survival benefit. In the frontline COG study, AALL1831, all patients receive GO regardless of CD33 expression, however, it may lack clinical benefit in patients with low expression [82]. Other ADCs currently under investigation are available in adult clinical trials but do not yet extend to the pediatric population.

5. Conclusions

Immunotherapy development has increased rapidly in the last decade, and a number of novel and safe and effective therapies are gradually moving to the frontline in pediatric leukemia [83]. The outcome of patients with relapsed B-ALL has considerably improved with CD19 targeting CAR T cells and BiTEs, and the CD22 ADC InO has contributed to this progress. However, other ADC therapies for B-ALL have only shown limited success in comparison, despite promising efficacy in NHL. T-ALL continues to present a challenge for the development of ADC therapy, primarily due to the lack of viable targets. In AML, specific target discovery has been a challenge too, and many tested agents cause unacceptable toxicities. GO experienced a not so straightforward path to FDA approval after concerns of excessive toxicity and limited efficacy, but is now considered a standard component of backbone therapy for de novo AML. Several trials of newer ADCs described above have been abandoned due to a high rate of toxicities and/or lack of clinical response. Despite these setbacks, there continues to be significant interest in ADCs, and refinements of the various components, particularly the linkers and payloads are likely to improve the therapeutic window for these agents. Detailed analyses of the pharmacokinetics and pharmacodynamics of the individual ADCs will guide dosing regimens. The continued search for optimal antigens with greater specificity to the leukemic phenotype compared to normal is leading to preclinical and early clinical studies targeting CD56, CD74, CD276 (B7-H3), CLL1, and FOLR1 among others [84–86]. It remains to be seen whether targeting multiple cell surface antigens will improve cytotoxicity and overcome antigen loss. In addition, the optimal combination with standard chemotherapeutic agents and sequence of therapies to maximize efficacy and minimize overlapping toxicities are areas of continued investigation.

Author Contributions: Conceptualization and preparation of the manuscript: J.L.S. and D.B. All authors have read and agreed to the published version of the manuscript.

Funding: This research received no external funding.

Institutional Review Board Statement: Not applicable.

Informed Consent Statement: Not applicable.

Conflicts of Interest: The authors declare no conflict of interest.

References

1. Pui, C.H.; Yang, J.J.; Hunger, S.P.; Pieters, R.; Schrappe, M.; Biondi, A.; Vora, A.; Baruchel, A.; Silverman, L.B.; Schmiegelow, K.; et al. Childhood Acute Lymphoblastic Leukemia: Progress Through Collaboration. *J. Clin. Oncol.* **2015**, *33*, 2938–2948. [CrossRef] [PubMed]
2. Ward, E.; DeSantis, C.; Robbins, A.; Kohler, B.; Jemal, A. Childhood and adolescent cancer statistics, 2014. *CA Cancer J. Clin.* **2014**, *64*, 83–103. [CrossRef] [PubMed]
3. Beck, A.; Goetsch, L.; Dumontet, C.; Corvaïa, N. Strategies and challenges for the next generation of antibody-drug conjugates. *Nat. Rev. Drug Discov.* **2017**, *16*, 315–337. [CrossRef] [PubMed]

4. Joubert, N.; Beck, A.; Dumontet, C.; Denevault-Sabourin, C. Antibody-Drug Conjugates: The Last Decade. *Pharmaceuticals* **2020**, *13*, 245. [CrossRef]
5. Caimi, P.F.; Ai, W.; Alderuccio, J.P.; Ardeshna, K.M.; Hamadani, M.; Hess, B.; Kahl, B.S.; Radford, J.; Solh, M.; Stathis, A.; et al. Loncastuximab tesirine in relapsed or refractory diffuse large B-cell lymphoma (LOTIS-2): A multicentre, open-label, single-arm, phase 2 trial. *Lancet Oncol.* **2021**, *22*, 790–800. [CrossRef]
6. Zhao, P.; Zhang, Y.; Li, W.; Jeanty, C.; Xiang, G.; Dong, Y. Recent advances of antibody drug conjugates for clinical applications. *Acta Pharm. Sin. B* **2020**, *10*, 1589–1600. [CrossRef]
7. Teicher, B.A.; Chari, R.V. Antibody conjugate therapeutics: Challenges and potential. *Clin. Cancer Res.* **2011**, *17*, 6389–6397. [CrossRef]
8. Masters, J.C.; Nickens, D.J.; Xuan, D.; Shazer, R.L.; Amantea, M. Clinical toxicity of antibody drug conjugates: A meta-analysis of payloads. *Invest. New Drugs* **2018**, *36*, 121–135. [CrossRef]
9. Godwin, C.D.; McDonald, G.B.; Walter, R.B. Sinusoidal obstruction syndrome following CD33-targeted therapy in acute myeloid leukemia. *Blood* **2017**, *129*, 2330–2332. [CrossRef]
10. Drago, J.Z.; Modi, S.; Chandarlapaty, S. Unlocking the potential of antibody-drug conjugates for cancer therapy. *Nat. Rev. Clin. Oncol.* **2021**. [CrossRef]
11. Shah, N.N.; Stevenson, M.S.; Yuan, C.M.; Richards, K.; Delbrook, C.; Kreitman, R.J.; Pastan, I.; Wayne, A.S. Characterization of CD22 expression in acute lymphoblastic leukemia. *Pediatr. Blood Cancer* **2015**, *62*, 964–969. [CrossRef] [PubMed]
12. Piccaluga, P.P.; Arpinati, M.; Candoni, A.; Laterza, C.; Paolini, S.; Gazzola, A.; Sabattini, E.; Visani, G.; Pileri, S.A. Surface antigens analysis reveals significant expression of candidate targets for immunotherapy in adult acute lymphoid leukemia. *Leuk Lymphoma* **2011**, *52*, 325–327. [CrossRef]
13. Kantarjian, H.M.; DeAngelo, D.J.; Stelljes, M.; Martinelli, G.; Liedtke, M.; Stock, W.; Gökbuget, N.; O'Brien, S.; Wang, K.; Wang, T.; et al. Inotuzumab Ozogamicin versus Standard Therapy for Acute Lymphoblastic Leukemia. *N. Engl. J. Med.* **2016**, *375*, 740–753. [CrossRef] [PubMed]
14. Kantarjian, H.M.; DeAngelo, D.J.; Stelljes, M.; Liedtke, M.; Stock, W.; Gökbuget, N.; O'Brien, S.M.; Jabbour, E.; Wang, T.; Liang White, J.; et al. Inotuzumab ozogamicin versus standard of care in relapsed or refractory acute lymphoblastic leukemia: Final report and long-term survival follow-up from the randomized, phase 3 INO-VATE study. *Cancer* **2019**, *125*, 2474–2487. [CrossRef]
15. Bhojwani, D.; Sposto, R.; Shah, N.N.; Rodriguez, V.; Yuan, C.; Stetler-Stevenson, M.; O'Brien, M.M.; McNeer, J.L.; Quereshi, A.; Cabannes, A.; et al. Inotuzumab ozogamicin in pediatric patients with relapsed/refractory acute lymphoblastic leukemia. *Leukemia* **2019**, *33*, 884–892. [CrossRef]
16. O'Brien, M.; Lingyun, J.; Shah, N.; Rheingold, S.; Bhojwani, D.; Yi, J.; Yuan, C.; Harris, A.; Brown, P.; Borowitz, M.; et al. A Phase 2 Trial of Inotuzumab Ozogamicin (InO) in Children and Young Adults with Relapsed or Refractory (R/R) CD22+ B-Acute Lymphoblastic Leukemia (B-ALL): Results from Children's Oncology Group Protocol AALL1621. *Blood* **2019**, *134*, 741. [CrossRef]
17. Brivio, E.; Locatelli, F.; Lopez-Yurda, M.; Malone, A.; Díaz-de-Heredia, C.; Bielorai, B.; Rossig, C.; van der Velden, V.H.J.; Ammerlaan, A.C.J.; Thano, A.; et al. A phase 1 study of inotuzumab ozogamicin in pediatric relapsed/refractory acute lymphoblastic leukemia (ITCC-059 study). *Blood* **2021**, *137*, 1582–1590. [CrossRef]
18. Kebriaei, P.; Cutler, C.; de Lima, M.; Giralt, S.; Lee, S.J.; Marks, D.; Merchant, A.; Stock, W.; van Besien, K.; Stelljes, M. Management of important adverse events associated with inotuzumab ozogamicin: Expert panel review. *Bone Marrow Transplant.* **2018**, *53*, 449–456. [CrossRef] [PubMed]
19. Shah, N.N.; O'Brien, M.M.; Yuan, C.; Ji, L.; Xu, X.; Rheingold, S.R.; Bhojwani, D.; Yi, J.; Harris, A.; Brown, P.A.; et al. Evaluation of CD22 modulation as a mechanism of resistance to inotuzumab ozogamicin (InO): Results from central CD22 testing on the Children's Oncology Group (COG) phase II trial of INO in children and young adults with CD22+ B-acute lymphoblastic leukemia (B-ALL). *J. Clin. Oncol.* **2020**, *38*, 10519.
20. Li, L.; Wang, Y. Recent updates for antibody therapy for acute lymphoblastic leukemia. *Exp. Hematol. Oncol.* **2020**, *9*, 33. [CrossRef]
21. Aruna, G. Immunotoxins: A review of their use in cancer treatment. *J. Stem Cells Regen. Med.* **2006**, *1*, 31–36.
22. Mussai, F.; Campana, D.; Bhojwani, D.; Stetler-Stevenson, M.; Steinberg, S.M.; Wayne, A.S.; Pastan, I. Cytotoxicity of the anti-CD22 immunotoxin HA22 (CAT-8015) against paediatric acute lymphoblastic leukaemia. *Br. J. Haematol.* **2010**, *150*, 352–358. [CrossRef] [PubMed]
23. Wayne, A.S.; Shah, N.N.; Bhojwani, D.; Silverman, L.B.; Whitlock, J.A.; Stetler-Stevenson, M.; Sun, W.; Liang, M.; Yang, J.; Kreitman, R.J.; et al. Phase 1 study of the anti-CD22 immunotoxin moxetumomab pasudotox for childhood acute lymphoblastic leukemia. *Blood* **2017**, *130*, 1620–1627. [CrossRef]
24. Shah, N.N.; Bhojwani, D.; August, K.; Baruchel, A.; Bertrand, Y.; Boklan, J.; Dalla-Pozza, L.; Dennis, R.; Hijiya, N.; Locatelli, F.; et al. Results from an international phase 2 study of the anti-CD22 immunotoxin moxetumomab pasudotox in relapsed or refractory childhood B-lineage acute lymphoblastic leukemia. *Pediatr. Blood Cancer* **2020**, *67*, e28112. [CrossRef] [PubMed]
25. Shah, N.N.; Schneiderman, J.; Kuruvilla, D.; Bhojwani, D.; Fry, T.J.; Martin, P.L.; Schultz, K.R.; Silverman, L.B.; Whitlock, J.A.; Wood, B.; et al. Fatal capillary leak syndrome in a child with acute lymphoblastic leukemia treated with moxetumomab pasudotox for pre-transplant minimal residual disease reduction. *Pediatr. Blood Cancer* **2021**, *68*, e28574. [CrossRef] [PubMed]
26. FDA Approves Moxetumomab Pasudotox-Tdfk for Hairy Cell Leukemia. Available online: https://www.fda.gov/drugs/resources-information-approved-drugs/fda-approves-moxetumomab-pasudotox-tdfk-hairy-cell-leukemia (accessed on 6 May 2021).

27. Hamadani, M.; Radford, J.; Carlo-Stella, C.; Caimi, P.F.; Reid, E.G.; O'Connor, O.A.; Feingold, J.; Ardeshna, K.M.; Townsend, W.M.; Solh, M.; et al. Final Results of a Phase 1 Study of Loncastuximab Tesirine in Relapsed/Refractory B-Cell Non-Hodgkin Lymphoma. *Blood* 2020. [CrossRef]
28. Jain, N.; Stock, W.; Zeidan, A.; Atallah, E.; McCloskey, J.; Heffner, L.; Tomlinson, B.; Bhatnagar, B.; Feingold, J.; Ungar, D.; et al. Loncastuximab tesirine, an anti-CD19 antibody-drug conjugate, in relapsed/refractory B-cell acute lymphoblastic leukemia. *Blood Adv.* 2020, *4*, 449–457. [CrossRef]
29. Jones, L.; McCalmont, H.; Evans, K.; Mayoh, C.; Kurmasheva, R.T.; Billups, C.A.; Houghton, P.J.; Smith, M.A.; Lock, R.B. Preclinical activity of the antibody-drug conjugate denintuzumab mafodotin (SGN-CD19A) against pediatric acute lymphoblastic leukemia xenografts. *Pediatr. Blood Cancer* 2019, *66*, e27765. [CrossRef] [PubMed]
30. Fathi, A.; Borate, U.; DeAngelo, D.J.; O'Brien, M.M.; Trippett, T.; Shah, B.D.; Hale, G.A.; Foran, J.M.; Silverman, L.B.; Tibes, R.; et al. A Phase 1 Study of Denintuzumab Mafodotin (SGN-CD19A) in Adults with Relapsed or Refractory B-Lineage Acute Leukemia (B-ALL) and Highly Aggressive Lymphoma. *Blood* 2015, *126*, 1328. [CrossRef]
31. Carol, H.; Szymanska, B.; Evans, K.; Boehm, I.; Houghton, P.J.; Smith, M.A.; Lock, R.B. The anti-CD19 antibody-drug conjugate SAR3419 prevents hematolymphoid relapse postinduction therapy in preclinical models of pediatric acute lymphoblastic leukemia. *Clin. Cancer Res.* 2013, *19*, 1795–1805. [CrossRef]
32. Kantarjian, H.M.; Lioure, B.; Kim, S.K.; Atallah, E.; Leguay, T.; Kelly, K.; Marolleau, J.P.; Escoffre-Barbe, M.; Thomas, X.G.; Cortes, J.; et al. A Phase II Study of Coltuximab Ravtansine (SAR3419) Monotherapy in Patients With Relapsed or Refractory Acute Lymphoblastic Leukemia. *Clin. Lymphoma Myeloma Leuk.* 2016, *16*, 139–145. [CrossRef] [PubMed]
33. Hamadani, M.; Collins, G.P.; Samaniego, F.; Spira, A.I.; Davies, A.; Radford, J.; Caimi, P.; Menne, T.; Boni, J.; Cruz, H.; et al. Phase 1 Study of Adct-301 (Camidanlumab Tesirine), a Novel Pyrrolobenzodiazepine-Based Antibody Drug Conjugate, in Relapsed/Refractory Classical Hodgkin Lymphoma. *Blood* 2018, *132*, 928. [CrossRef]
34. Flynn, M.J.; Hartley, J.A. The emerging role of anti-CD25 directed therapies as both immune modulators and targeted agents in cancer. *Br. J. Haematol.* 2017, *179*, 20–35. [CrossRef]
35. Goldberg, A.D.; Atallah, E.; Rizzieri, D.; Walter, R.B.; Chung, K.Y.; Spira, A.; Stock, W.; Tallman, M.S.; Cruz, H.G.; Boni, J.; et al. Camidanlumab tesirine, an antibody-drug conjugate, in relapsed/refractory CD25-positive acute myeloid leukemia or acute lymphoblastic leukemia: A phase I study. *Leuk. Res.* 2020, *95*, 106385. [CrossRef] [PubMed]
36. Zammarchi, F.; Havenith, K.; Bertelli, F.; Vijayakrishnan, B.; Chivers, S.; van Berkel, P.H. CD25-targeted antibody-drug conjugate depletes regulatory T cells and eliminates established syngeneic tumors via antitumor immunity. *J. Immunother. Cancer* 2020, *8*. [CrossRef]
37. Hunger, S.P.; Raetz, E.A. How I treat relapsed acute lymphoblastic leukemia in the pediatric population. *Blood* 2020, *136*, 1803–1812. [CrossRef] [PubMed]
38. Fry, T.J.; Shah, N.N.; Orentas, R.J.; Stetler-Stevenson, M.; Yuan, C.M.; Ramakrishna, S.; Wolters, P.; Martin, S.; Delbrook, C.; Yates, B.; et al. CD22-targeted CAR T cells induce remission in B-ALL that is naive or resistant to CD19-targeted CAR immunotherapy. *Nat. Med.* 2018, *24*, 20–28. [CrossRef] [PubMed]
39. Bayón-Calderón, F.; Toribio, M.L.; González-García, S. Facts and Challenges in Immunotherapy for T-Cell Acute Lymphoblastic Leukemia. *Int. J. Mol. Sci* 2020, *21*, 7685. [CrossRef] [PubMed]
40. Zheng, W.; Medeiros, L.J.; Young, K.H.; Goswami, M.; Powers, L.; Kantarjian, H.H.; Thomas, D.A.; Cortes, J.E.; Wang, S.A. CD30 expression in acute lymphoblastic leukemia as assessed by flow cytometry analysis. *Leuk. Lymphoma* 2014, *55*, 624–627. [CrossRef] [PubMed]
41. Ofran, Y.; Ringelstein-Harlev, S.; Slouzkey, I.; Zuckerman, T.; Yehudai-Ofir, D.; Henig, I.; Beyar-Katz, O.; Hayun, M.; Frisch, A. Daratumumab for eradication of minimal residual disease in high-risk advanced relapse of T-cell/CD19/CD22-negative acute lymphoblastic leukemia. *Leukemia* 2020, *34*, 293–295. [CrossRef]
42. Yasunaga, M.; Manabe, S.; Matsumura, Y. Immunoregulation by IL-7R-targeting antibody-drug conjugates: Overcoming steroid-resistance in cancer and autoimmune disease. *Sci. Rep.* 2017, *7*, 10735. [CrossRef] [PubMed]
43. Pollard, J.A.; Alonzo, T.A.; Loken, M.; Gerbing, R.B.; Ho, P.A.; Bernstein, I.D.; Raimondi, S.C.; Hirsch, B.; Franklin, J.; Walter, R.B.; et al. Correlation of CD33 expression level with disease characteristics and response to gemtuzumab ozogamicin containing chemotherapy in childhood AML. *Blood* 2012, *119*, 3705–3711. [CrossRef]
44. Jen, E.Y.; Ko, C.W.; Lee, J.E.; Del Valle, P.L.; Aydanian, A.; Jewell, C.; Norsworthy, K.J.; Przepiorka, D.; Nie, L.; Liu, J.; et al. FDA Approval: Gemtuzumab Ozogamicin for the Treatment of Adults with Newly Diagnosed CD33-Positive Acute Myeloid Leukemia. *Clin. Cancer Res.* 2018, *24*, 3242–3246. [CrossRef] [PubMed]
45. Sievers, E.L.; Appelbaum, F.R.; Spielberger, R.T.; Forman, S.J.; Flowers, D.; Smith, F.O.; Shannon-Dorcy, K.; Berger, M.S.; Bernstein, I.D. Selective ablation of acute myeloid leukemia using antibody-targeted chemotherapy: A phase I study of an anti-CD33 calicheamicin immunoconjugate. *Blood* 1999, *93*, 3678–3684. [CrossRef]
46. Larson, R.A.; Sievers, E.L.; Stadtmauer, E.A.; Löwenberg, B.; Estey, E.H.; Dombret, H.; Theobald, M.; Voliotis, D.; Bennett, J.M.; Richie, M.; et al. Final report of the efficacy and safety of gemtuzumab ozogamicin (Mylotarg) in patients with CD33-positive acute myeloid leukemia in first recurrence. *Cancer* 2005, *104*, 1442–1452. [CrossRef] [PubMed]
47. Petersdorf, S.H.; Kopecky, K.J.; Slovak, M.; Willman, C.; Nevill, T.; Brandwein, J.; Larson, R.A.; Erba, H.P.; Stiff, P.J.; Stuart, R.K.; et al. A phase 3 study of gemtuzumab ozogamicin during induction and postconsolidation therapy in younger patients with acute myeloid leukemia. *Blood* 2013, *121*, 4854–4860. [CrossRef]

48. Appelbaum, F.R.; Bernstein, I.D. Gemtuzumab ozogamicin for acute myeloid leukemia. *Blood* **2017**, *130*, 2373–2376. [CrossRef]
49. Zwaan, C.M.; Reinhardt, D.; Zimmerman, M.; Hasle, H.; Stary, J.; Stark, B.; Dworzak, M.; Creutzig, U.; Kaspers, G.J.; International BFM Study Group on Paediatric AML. Salvage treatment for children with refractory first or second relapse of acute myeloid leukaemia with gemtuzumab ozogamicin: Results of a phase II study. *Br. J. Haematol.* **2010**, *148*, 768–776. [CrossRef]
50. Niktoreh, N.; Lerius, B.; Zimmermann, M.; Gruhn, B.; Escherich, G.; Bourquin, J.P.; Dworzak, M.; Sramkova, L.; Rossig, C.; Creutzig, U.; et al. Gemtuzumab ozogamicin in children with relapsed or refractory acute myeloid leukemia: A report by Berlin-Frankfurt-Münster study group. *Haematologica* **2019**, *104*, 120–127. [CrossRef]
51. Burnett, A.K.; Hills, R.K.; Milligan, D.; Kjeldsen, L.; Kell, J.; Russell, N.H.; Yin, J.A.; Hunter, A.; Goldstone, A.H.; Wheatley, K. Identification of patients with acute myeloblastic leukemia who benefit from the addition of gemtuzumab ozogamicin: Results of the MRC AML15 trial. *J. Clin. Oncol.* **2011**, *29*, 369–377. [CrossRef]
52. Cooper, T.M.; Franklin, J.; Gerbing, R.B.; Alonzo, T.A.; Hurwitz, C.; Raimondi, S.C.; Hirsch, B.; Smith, F.O.; Mathew, P.; Arceci, R.J.; et al. AAML03P1, a pilot study of the safety of gemtuzumab ozogamicin in combination with chemotherapy for newly diagnosed childhood acute myeloid leukemia: A report from the Children's Oncology Group. *Cancer* **2012**, *118*, 761–769. [CrossRef]
53. Gamis, A.S.; Alonzo, T.A.; Meshinchi, S.; Sung, L.; Gerbing, R.B.; Raimondi, S.C.; Hirsch, B.A.; Kahwash, S.B.; Heerema-McKenney, A.; Winter, L.; et al. Gemtuzumab ozogamicin in children and adolescents with de novo acute myeloid leukemia improves event-free survival by reducing relapse risk: Results from the randomized phase III Children's Oncology Group trial AAML0531. *J. Clin. Oncol.* **2014**, *32*, 3021–3032. [CrossRef] [PubMed]
54. Castaigne, S.; Pautas, C.; Terré, C.; Raffoux, E.; Bordessoule, D.; Bastie, J.N.; Legrand, O.; Thomas, X.; Turlure, P.; Reman, O.; et al. Effect of gemtuzumab ozogamicin on survival of adult patients with de-novo acute myeloid leukaemia (ALFA-0701): A randomised, open-label, phase 3 study. *Lancet* **2012**, *379*, 1508–1516. [CrossRef]
55. Arceci, R.J.; Sande, J.; Lange, B.; Shannon, K.; Franklin, J.; Hutchinson, R.; Vik, T.A.; Flowers, D.; Aplenc, R.; Berger, M.S.; et al. Safety and efficacy of gemtuzumab ozogamicin in pediatric patients with advanced CD33+ acute myeloid leukemia. *Blood* **2005**, *106*, 1183–1188. [CrossRef] [PubMed]
56. Sievers, E.L.; Larson, R.A.; Stadtmauer, E.A.; Estey, E.; Löwenberg, B.; Dombret, H.; Karanes, C.; Theobald, M.; Bennett, J.M.; Sherman, M.L.; et al. Efficacy and safety of gemtuzumab ozogamicin in patients with CD33-positive acute myeloid leukemia in first relapse. *J. Clin. Oncol.* **2001**, *19*, 3244–3254. [CrossRef] [PubMed]
57. Burnett, A.; Cavenagh, J.; Russell, N.; Hills, R.; Kell, J.; Jones, G.; Nielsen, O.J.; Khwaja, A.; Thomas, I.; Clark, R.; et al. Defining the dose of gemtuzumab ozogamicin in combination with induction chemotherapy in acute myeloid leukemia: A comparison of 3 mg/m2 with 6 mg/m2 in the NCRI AML17 Trial. *Haematologica* **2016**, *101*, 724–731. [CrossRef] [PubMed]
58. Lapusan, S.; Vidriales, M.B.; Thomas, X.; de Botton, S.; Vekhoff, A.; Tang, R.; Dumontet, C.; Morariu-Zamfir, R.; Lambert, J.M.; Ozoux, M.L.; et al. Phase I studies of AVE9633, an anti-CD33 antibody-maytansinoid conjugate, in adult patients with relapsed/refractory acute myeloid leukemia. *Investig. New Drugs* **2012**, *30*, 1121–1131. [CrossRef]
59. Stein, E.M.; Walter, R.B.; Erba, H.P.; Fathi, A.T.; Advani, A.S.; Lancet, J.E.; Ravandi, F.; Kovacsovics, T.; DeAngelo, D.J.; Bixby, D.; et al. A phase 1 trial of vadastuximab talirine as monotherapy in patients with CD33-positive acute myeloid leukemia. *Blood* **2018**, *131*, 387–396. [CrossRef] [PubMed]
60. Cortes, J.E.; DeAngelo, D.J.; Erba, H.P.; Traer, E.; Papadantonakis, N.; Arana-Yi, C.; Blum, W.; Sloos, C.; Culm-Merdek, K.; Zweidler-Mckay, P.; et al. Maturing Clinical Profile of IMGN779, a Next-Generation CD33-Targeting Antibody-Drug Conjugate, in Patients with Relapsed or Refractory Acute Myeloid Leukemia. *Blood* **2018**, *132*. [CrossRef]
61. Testa, U.; Pelosi, E.; Frankel, A. CD 123 is a membrane biomarker and a therapeutic target in hematologic malignancies. *Biomark Res.* **2014**, *2*, 4. [CrossRef] [PubMed]
62. Angelova, E.; Audette, C.; Kovtun, Y.; Daver, N.; Wang, S.A.; Pierce, S.; Konoplev, S.N.; Khogeer, H.; Jorgensen, J.L.; Konopleva, M.; et al. CD123 expression patterns and selective targeting with a CD123-targeted antibody-drug conjugate (IMGN632) in acute lymphoblastic leukemia. *Haematologica* **2019**, *104*, 749–755. [CrossRef]
63. Han, Y.C.; Kahler, J.; Piché-Nicholas, N.; Hu, W.; Thibault, Y.; Jiang, F.; Leal, M.; Katragadda, M.; Maderna, A.; Dushin, R.; et al. Development of Highly Optimized Antibody-Drug Conjugates against CD33 and CD123 for Acute Myeloid Leukemia. *Clin. Cancer Res.* **2021**, *27*, 622–631. [CrossRef] [PubMed]
64. Kovtun, Y.; Jones, G.E.; Adams, S.; Harvey, L.; Audette, C.A.; Wilhelm, A.; Bai, C.; Rui, L.; Laleau, R.; Liu, F.; et al. A CD123-targeting antibody-drug conjugate, IMGN632, designed to eradicate AML while sparing normal bone marrow cells. *Blood Adv.* **2018**, *2*, 848–858. [CrossRef]
65. Daver, N.G.; Erba, H.P.; Papadantonakis, N.; DeAngelo, D.J.; Wang, E.S.; Konopleva, M.Y.; Sloss, C.M.; Culm-Merdek, K.; Zweidler-McKay, P.A.; Kantarjian, H.M. Phase I, First-in-Human Study Evaluating the Safety and Preliminary Antileukemia Activity of IMGN632, a Novel CD123-Targeting Antibody-Drug Conjugate, in Patients with Relapsed/Refractory Acute Myeloid Leukemia and Other CD123-Positive Hematologic Malignancies. *Blood* **2018**, *132*, 27. [CrossRef]
66. Vaisitti, T.; Arruga, F.; Vitale, N.; Lee, T.T.; Ko, M.; Chadburn, A.; Braggio, E.; Di Napoli, A.; Iannello, A.; Allan, J.; et al. ROR1 targeting with the antibody drug-conjugate VLS-101 is effective in Richter syndrome patient-derived xenograft mouse models. *Blood* **2021**. [CrossRef] [PubMed]
67. Balaian, L.P.D.; Sadarangani, A.; Widhopf, G.F.; Zhong, R.-k.; Prussak, C.; Marra, M.A.; Dick, J.E.; Minden, M.D.; Ball, E.D.; Carson, D.A.; et al. A Highly Selective Anti-ROR1 Monoclonal Antibody Inhibits Human Acute Myeloid Leukemia CD34+ Cell Survival and Self-Renewal. *Blood* **2012**, *120*, 2560. [CrossRef]

68. Tarlock, K.; Alonzo, T.A.; Gerbing, R.B.; Raimondi, S.C.; Hirsch, B.A.; Sung, L.; Pollard, J.A.; Aplenc, R.; Loken, M.R.; Gamis, A.S.; et al. Gemtuzumab Ozogamicin Reduces Relapse Risk in FLT3/ITD Acute Myeloid Leukemia: A Report from the Children's Oncology Group. *Clin. Cancer Res.* **2016**, *22*, 1951–1957. [CrossRef] [PubMed]
69. Hassan, R.; Blumenschein, G.R.; Moore, K.N.; Santin, A.D.; Kindler, H.L.; Nemunaitis, J.J.; Seward, S.M.; Thomas, A.; Kim, S.K.; Rajagopalan, P.; et al. First-in-Human, Multicenter, Phase I Dose-Escalation and Expansion Study of Anti-Mesothelin Antibody-Drug Conjugate Anetumab Ravtansine in Advanced or Metastatic Solid Tumors. *J. Clin. Oncol.* **2020**, *38*, 1824–1835. [CrossRef] [PubMed]
70. Chen, J.; Glasser, C.L. New and Emerging Targeted Therapies for Pediatric Acute Myeloid Leukemia (AML). *Children* **2020**, *7*, 12. [CrossRef]
71. Bakker, A.B.; van den Oudenrijn, S.; Bakker, A.Q.; Feller, N.; van Meijer, M.; Bia, J.A.; Jongeneelen, M.A.; Visser, T.J.; Bijl, N.; Geuijen, C.A.; et al. C-type lectin-like molecule-1: A novel myeloid cell surface marker associated with acute myeloid leukemia. *Cancer Res.* **2004**, *64*, 8443–8450. [CrossRef]
72. Adhikari, P.; Zacharias, N.; Ohri, R.; Sadowsky, J. Site-Specific Conjugation to Cys-Engineered THIOMAB™ Antibodies. *Methods Mol. Biol.* **2020**, *2078*, 51–69. [CrossRef] [PubMed]
73. Daver, N.; Salhotra, A.; Brandwein, J.M.; Podoltsev, N.A.; Pollyea, D.A.; Jurcic, J.G.; Assouline, S.; Yee, K.; Li, M.; Pourmohamad, T.; et al. A Phase I dose-escalation study of DCLL9718S, an antibody-drug conjugate targeting C-type lectin-like molecule-1 (CLL-1) in patients with acute myeloid leukemia. *Am. J. Hematol.* **2021**, *96*, E175–E179. [CrossRef] [PubMed]
74. Zhang, H.; Wang, P.; Li, Z.; He, Y.; Gan, W.; Jiang, H. Anti-CLL1 Chimeric Antigen Receptor T-Cell Therapy in Children with Relapsed/Refractory Acute Myeloid Leukemia. *Clin. Cancer Res.* **2021**, *27*, 3549–3555. [CrossRef] [PubMed]
75. Zheng, W.; Medeiros, L.J.; Hu, Y.; Powers, L.; Cortes, J.E.; Ravandi-Kashani, F.; Kantarjian, H.H.; Wang, S.A. CD30 expression in high-risk acute myeloid leukemia and myelodysplastic syndromes. *Clin. Lymphoma Myeloma Leuk.* **2013**, *13*, 307–314. [CrossRef] [PubMed]
76. Narayan, R.; Blonquist, T.M.; Emadi, A.; Hasserjian, R.P.; Burke, M.; Lescinskas, C.; Neuberg, D.S.; Brunner, A.M.; Hobbs, G.; Hock, H.; et al. A phase 1 study of the antibody-drug conjugate brentuximab vedotin with re-induction chemotherapy in patients with CD30-expressing relapsed/refractory acute myeloid leukemia. *Cancer* **2020**, *126*, 1264–1273. [CrossRef]
77. Brentuximab Vedotin in Patients With CD30-positive Nonlymphomatous Malignancies. Available online: https://www.clinicaltrials.gov/ct2/show/results/NCT01461538?view=results (accessed on 16 April 2021).
78. Pereira, D.S.; Guevara, C.I.; Jin, L.; Mbong, N.; Verlinsky, A.; Hsu, S.J.; Aviña, H.; Karki, S.; Abad, J.D.; Yang, P.; et al. AGS67E, an Anti-CD37 Monomethyl Auristatin E Antibody-Drug Conjugate as a Potential Therapeutic for B/T-Cell Malignancies and AML: A New Role for CD37 in AML. *Mol. Cancer Ther.* **2015**, *14*, 1650–1660. [CrossRef]
79. Abrams, T.; Connor, A.; Fanton, C.; Cohen, S.B.; Huber, T.; Miller, K.; Hong, E.E.; Niu, X.; Kline, J.; Ison-Dugenny, M.; et al. Preclinical Antitumor Activity of a Novel Anti-c-KIT Antibody-Drug Conjugate against Mutant and Wild-type c-KIT-Positive Solid Tumors. *Clin. Cancer Res.* **2018**, *24*, 4297–4308. [CrossRef] [PubMed]
80. L'Italien, L.; Orozco, O.; Abrams, T.; Cantagallo, L.; Connor, A.; Desai, J.; Ebersbach, H.; Gelderblom, H.; Hoffmaster, K.; Lees, E.; et al. Mechanistic Insights of an Immunological Adverse Event Induced by an Anti-KIT Antibody Drug Conjugate and Mitigation Strategies. *Clin. Cancer Res.* **2018**, *24*, 3465–3474. [CrossRef]
81. Rudra-Ganguly, N.; Lowe, C.; Virata, C.; Leavitt, M.; Jin, L.; Mendelsohn, B.; Snyder, J.; Aviña, H.; Zhang, C.; Russell, D.L.; et al. AGS62P1, a Novel Anti-FLT3 Antibody Drug Conjugate, Employing Site Specific Conjugation, Demonstrates Preclinical Anti-Tumor Efficacy in AML Tumor and Patient Derived Xenografts. *Blood* **2015**, *126*, 3806. [CrossRef]
82. Pollard, J.A.; Loken, M.; Gerbing, R.B.; Raimondi, S.C.; Hirsch, B.A.; Aplenc, R.; Bernstein, I.D.; Gamis, A.S.; Alonzo, T.A.; Meshinchi, S. CD33 Expression and Its Association With Gemtuzumab Ozogamicin Response: Results From the Randomized Phase III Children's Oncology Group Trial AAML0531. *J. Clin. Oncol.* **2016**, *34*, 747–755. [CrossRef] [PubMed]
83. McNeer, J.L.; Rau, R.E.; Gupta, S.; Maude, S.L.; O'Brien, M.M. Cutting to the Front of the Line: Immunotherapy for Childhood Acute Lymphoblastic Leukemia. *Am. Soc. Clin. Oncol. Educ. Book* **2020**, *40*, 1–12. [CrossRef] [PubMed]
84. Jiang, Y.P.; Liu, B.Y.; Zheng, Q.; Panuganti, S.; Chen, R.; Zhu, J.; Mishra, M.; Huang, J.; Dao-Pick, T.; Roy, S.; et al. CLT030, a leukemic stem cell-targeting CLL1 antibody-drug conjugate for treatment of acute myeloid leukemia. *Blood Adv.* **2018**, *2*, 1738–1749. [CrossRef]
85. Guery, T.; Roumier, C.; Berthon, C.; Renneville, A.; Preudhomme, C.; Quesnel, B. B7-H3 protein expression in acute myeloid leukemia. *Cancer Med.* **2015**, *4*, 1879–1883. [CrossRef] [PubMed]
86. Yan, H.; Qu, J.; Cao, W.; Liu, Y.; Zheng, G.; Zhang, E.; Cai, Z. Identification of prognostic genes in the acute myeloid leukemia immune microenvironment based on TCGA data analysis. *Cancer Immunol. Immunother.* **2019**, *68*, 1971–1978. [CrossRef] [PubMed]

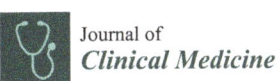

Review

Curing the Curable: Managing Low-Risk Acute Lymphoblastic Leukemia in Resource Limited Countries

Bernice L. Z. Oh [1,2], Shawn H. R. Lee [1,2] and Allen E. J. Yeoh [1,2,*]

1. VIVA-University Children's Cancer Centre, Khoo-Teck Puat-National University Children's Medical Institute, National University Hospital, Singapore 119074, Singapore; paeolzb@nus.edu.sg (B.L.Z.O.); paelhrs@nus.edu.sg (S.H.R.L.)
2. Department of Paediatrics, Yong Loo Lin School of Medicine, National University Singapore, Singapore 119074, Singapore
* Correspondence: allen.yeoh@nus.edu.sg

Abstract: Although childhood acute lymphoblastic leukemia (ALL) is curable, global disparities in treatment outcomes remain. To reduce these global disparities in low-middle income countries (LMIC), a paradigm shift is needed: start with curing low-risk ALL. Low-risk ALL, which accounts for >50% of patients, can be cured with low-toxicity therapies already defined by collaborative studies. We reviewed the components of these low-toxicity regimens in recent clinical trials for low-risk ALL and suggest how they can be adopted in LMIC. In treating childhood ALL, the key is risk stratification, which can be resource stratified. NCI standard-risk criteria (age 1–10 years, WBC < 50,000/uL) is simple yet highly effective. Other favorable features such as *ETV6-RUNX1*, hyperdiploidy, early peripheral blood and bone marrow responses, and simplified flow MRD at the end of induction can be added depending on resources. With limited supportive care in LMIC, more critical than relapse is treatment-related morbidity and mortality. Less intensive induction allows early marrow recovery, reducing the need for intensive supportive care. Other key elements in low-toxicity protocol designs include: induction steroid type; high-dose versus low-dose escalating methotrexate; judicious use of anthracyclines; and steroid pulses during maintenance. In summary, the first effective step in curing ALL in LMIC is to focus on curing low-risk ALL with less intensive therapy and less toxicity.

Keywords: childhood acute lymphoblastic leukemia; low-risk ALL; risk-stratified treatment; treatment related toxicity

1. Introduction

Childhood acute lymphoblastic leukemia (ALL) is curable. Underpinning the cure for ALL is more than half a century of intensive collaborative research [1] that has systematically tested and defined highly effective drug combinations which now form the backbone of contemporary protocols. Although there are minor differences, contemporary ALL protocols are strikingly similar and almost formulaic. However, as the survival of childhood ALL in high-income countries (HIC) surpasses 90% [1], significant disparities in survival have emerged [2]. The high cure rates of ALL achieved in HIC are not seen in low-middle income countries (LMIC) [3]. With 80% of the world childhood ALL burden residing in LMIC [4,5], our success in curing childhood ALL remains limited and geographically restricted [2]. To reduce such glaring disparities, many groups such as the International Pediatric Oncology Society (SIOP), VIVA Foundation for Childhood Cancer, St Jude Global, and the World Health Organization are beginning to tackle the obstacles to widespread adoption of effective treatment. The first steps in improving cures for ALL worldwide, we believe, is for LMIC to focus on curing low-risk ALL as it is highly cost-effective and transformational. In this review, we focus on key components of contemporary trials on curing low-risk ALL, cost-effectively.

2. Causes of Failures in LMIC

We reference the World Bank Income Group classification in defining LMIC (https://datahelpdesk.worldbank.org/knowledgebase/articles/906519-world-bank-country-and-lending-groups accessed on 1 October 2021). Specifically, in 2021, LMIC are defined as countries with gross national income per capita of <USD 12,695. Albeit imperfect and simplistic, this definition is used in the Lancet Oncology Commission on Sustainable Care for Children with Cancer [5], in which we also participated.

In HIC, the main cause of failure in treating childhood ALL is relapse [6]. This fear of relapse is so ingrained that overtreatment is rarely questioned. However, for LMIC, the key reason for failure is treatment toxicity [7]. Treatment toxicity disproportionately inflicts suffering and exponentially increases the cost of treatment [5], which then invariably leads to treatment abandonment [8]. In LMIC, treatment toxicity is further amplified by malnutrition [9], suboptimal supportive care [10], and widespread antibiotic resistance [11]. The Malaysia-Singapore ALL study group (Ma-Spore) is based in Malaysia and Singapore, an example of two countries which have emerged from LMIC status within the past three decades [12]. Given the health resource constraints, the Ma-Spore study group focused on testing cost-effective deintensification of therapy in low-risk ALL patients as one of the main strategies.

3. Identifying Low-Risk Groups in Resource Limited Settings

The key to better cures in ALL is better risk stratification [13]. Specifically, if we can define each patient's risk of relapse early, the optimal intensity of therapy can be given to maximize cure while minimizing side-effects. The two major determinants of relapse are molecular genetics and early response to therapy [6]. Early response to therapy can be measured by (1) widely available peripheral blast counts by light microscopy on day 8; and/or (2) sophisticated minimal residual disease (MRD) quantitation of sub-microscopic disease by flow cytometry or polymerase chain reaction (PCR) [2]. Based on the resources of specific hospitals and the country level of care for ALL and access to tests, we propose various levels for risk assessment of ALL (Table 1).

Table 1. Key stratified strategies discussed in this review on management of low-risk childhood ALL.

	Low-Income Countries (LIC) Setting	Middle-Income Countries (MIC) Setting	High-Income Countries (HIC) Setting
Low-Risk features	NCI SR CNS I No mediastinal mass	NCI SR CNS I Flow T vs. B DNA index Cytogenetics/FISH OFT screening	NCI SR CNS I Flow T vs. B Cytogenetics/FISH OFT screening/RNA-Seq
Early response PB	D8 blast < 1×10^9/L	Day 8 blast < 1×10^9/L	Day 8 blast or PB flow MRD
Early response BM	Day 15 M1/2, EOI M3	Day 15 M1/2, EOI M3 Flow-MRD-lite	Flow MRD or PCR MRD at EOI, EOC
Protocol	One protocol	SR/HR	SR/IR/HR
B-ALL SR	VCR-Dexa	3-drug Dexa-based	3-drug Dexa-based
T-ALL and B-HR	VCR-Dexa	3-drug Dexa-based	4-drug Pred-based
Central Nervous System (CNS) directed Rx	Cranial RT/IT MTX	IT MTX/Cranial RT	IT MTX/HDMTX
Delayed intensification	VCR-Dex-Doxo	VCR-Dex-L-asp + CTX-araC-MP	Protocol II
Maintenance Therapy	4-weekly VCR/Dex pulse	8-weekly VCR/Dex pulse	12-weekly VCR/Dex pulse
TPMT and NUDT15	In sensitive patients	In sensitive patients or routinely	Routine
Clinical Trial Examples	LMIC Examples: RELLA05 [14] ICiCLe ALL 14 [15]	ALL IC-BFM 2002 [16] CCLG-ALL 2008 [17] MS 2003 [18]/ 2010 [19]	AIEOP-BFM ALL 2000 [20] CoALL 07-03 [21] COG AALL 0932 [22]/0331 [23] DCOG ALL10 [24] JACLS ALL-02 [25] St Jude Total XVI [26] UKALL 2003 [27]

In LIC with very limited resources, the only diagnostic facility available may be light microscopy to identify ALL lymphoblasts. Flow cytometry may not be available to subtype ALL into B or T-ALL. Given these limitations, a simple chest X-ray revealing a mediastinal mass [28] may help in differentiating T-ALL from B-ALL. In these resource limited settings, early responses to treatment can be assessed morphologically using day 8 peripheral blast count (>1 × 10^9/L) and day 15 or end-of-induction (EOI) bone marrow morphology [2]. ALL may have to be managed by general pediatricians without access to specialized pediatric oncology nursing care in LIC [10]. Chemotherapy drug availability is also likely to be limited and its supply unreliable [29,30]. Because of these constraints in LIC, it is best to have one simple, common protocol that is minimally myelosuppressive. The SIOP PODC [31] and the Lancet Oncology Asian Consensus Protocol [2] are probably effective stratified regimens.

For MIC, limited panel flow cytometry to diagnose B- and T-ALL may be possible. Working with universities, MIC hospitals can potentially access PCR thermocyclers [12]. With PCR thermocyclers it is possible to run simple oncogene fusion tests to screen for *BCR-ABL1* and *ETV6-RUNX1* fusions [32,33]. In these settings, it is important to put in appropriate positive and negative controls as cross contamination and degraded RNA are common.

The ALL IC-BFM 2002 study group demonstrated the feasibility of a risk stratification approach based on a combination of modified NCI criteria, early morphologic evaluation on days 8, 15, and 33, without PCR-MRD monitoring. The study was successfully implemented in 15 countries across 3 continents in 130 centers. The ALL IC-BFM 2002 [16] study reported an excellent 81% EFS and 90% OS in the standard risk arm. Interestingly, the ALL IC-BFM 2002 standard risk criteria were defined as age 1 to 6 years and lower white blood cell (WBC) count of 20 × 10^9/L. The ALL IC-BFM 2002 protocol was intensive, and treatment administered in national centers with good supportive care.

4. The Importance of the NCI Standard-Risk (SR) Criteria

ALL is a genetically heterogeneous disease [13,34]. The National Cancer Institute (NCI) standard-risk (SR) criteria, presenting age of 1 to 10 years and WBC count < 50 × 10^9/L), are simple yet surprisingly effective risk stratification criteria [35]. Favorable genetic drivers, such as hyperdiploidy and ETV6-RUNX1, form the largest proportion of NCI SR patients [34]. In MS2003 [18], age remained prognostically significant for event-free survival (Figure 1). The NCI criteria can be easily applied even in LMIC settings and should remain one of the mainstays of risk stratification [2].

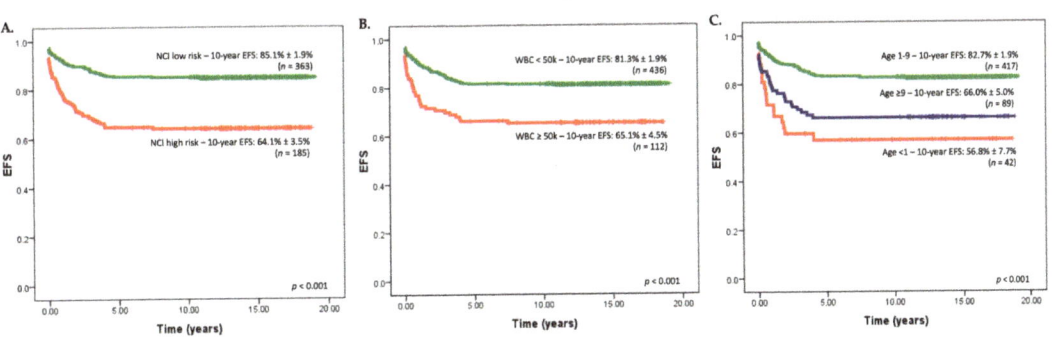

Figure 1. (**A–C**) Kaplan-Meier 10-year event-free-survival (EFS) curves from the Malaysia-Singapore ALL 2003 study cohort: significant differences in outcomes based on features from the National Cancer Institute (NCI) risk criteria such as total white blood cell (WBC) count at diagnosis and age were found; in this study risk stratification was based primarily on end-of-induction PCR-MRD responses. (**A**) 10-year EFS based on the presence of NCI low versus high-risk criteria, (**B**) 10-year EFS based on total white cell count at diagnosis, (**C**) 10-year EFS based on NCI criteria defined age groups. NCI risk criteria has been shown to clearly define groups of patients with clinically significant differences in long term EFS

regardless of MRD response at the end of induction. This is a finding that is especially relevant to children in LMIC settings who may not have access to MRD monitoring and risk stratification during treatment. Children with lower risk ALL can already be defined early at the point of diagnosis based on NCI risk features.

Table 2 summarizes the risk stratification criteria used by various clinical trials to characterize patients with ALL who are at the lowest risk of relapse. Overall, the NCI SR criteria remain a cornerstone of ALL risk stratification for 9 of the 13 clinical trials evaluated in this review. However, the upper age limits for inclusion in these low-risk arms still vary from group to group (Table 2).

Like those of the AIEOP-BFM ALL 2000, the NCI features were not used for risk stratification in MS2003 [18]. However, compared to NCI SR patients, NCI HR patients treated in the MS2003-SR arm did significantly more poorly (Figure 1). Given these findings, in the MS2010 [19], patients aged ≥10 years old were treated in either the intermediate or high-risk arm depending on MRD responses—and not in the lowest risk, SR arm.

In the AIEOP-BFM ALL 2000-SR arm [20], EOI MRD-negative NCI HR patients had poorer outcomes on the less intensive Protocol III compared to standard Protocol II during delayed intensification (DI) (8-y EFS: 82.9% versus 90.4% p = 0.04). In contrast, NCI SR patients did equally well. The AIEOP-BFM ALL 2000 SR study concluded that, despite negative EOI MRD, age >10 years adversely affected outcomes. Taken together, despite EOI MRD negativity, both the MS2003 and ALL AIEOP-BFM ALL 2000 studies suggested that NCI HR patients, specifically teenagers, should *not* be treated with de-intensified treatment.

Table 2. Risk stratification criteria, cumulative chemotherapy dosing and proportions of patients treated in lowest-risk arms.

	B-ALL	T-ALL	Age Criteria	Total White Cell Count at Diagnosis	Central Nervous System (CNS) Status	Specific Cytogenetic Inclusion Criteria	Prednisolone Response	Treatment Responses				Cumulative Cyclophosphamide Dosing (mg/m²)	Cumulative Anthracycline Dosing (mg/m²)	Cumulative L-Asparaginase × 1000 units/m² Dosing ~	% of Study Population Treated in the Lowest-Risk Arms
								D8	D15	End of Induction	Later Timepoints				
AIEOP-BFM ALL 2000	Y	Y	1–17	Any	Any		Y	-	-	PCR MRD NEG	Day 78 PCR MRD NEG	3000	240	80	28
ALL IC-BFM 2002	Y	Y	1–6	<20,000/μL	Any		Y	-	M1/M2	-	-	3000	180	Standard: 80 Expt: 120	31
CCLG-ALL 2008	Y	-	1–10	<50,000/μL	No CNS 3		-	-	M1/M2	PCR MRD NEG or Flow MRD < 0.01%	Week 12 PCR MRD NEG or Flow MRD < 0.01%	2000	125	80	39
CoALL 07-03 LR-R	Y	-	<10	<25,000/μL	Any		-	-	MRD <0.01%	θ MRD < 0.01%	-	900	120	125	13
COG AALL 0331 LR5	Y	-	1.01–9.99	<50,000/μL	CNS 1 only	Triple trisomies of chromosomes 4, 10, and 17 Or ETV6-RUNX1	-	M1 *	M1 *	θ MRD < 0.01%	-	1000	75	80	35
COG AALL 0932 LR-C	Y	-	1.01–9.99	<50,000/μL	CNS 1 only	Triple trisomies of chromosomes 4 and 10 Or ETV6-RUNX1	-	PB MRD < 0.01%	-	θ MRD < 0.01%	-	1000	75	80	3.5
COG AALL 0932 LR-M	Y	-	1.01–9.99	<50,000/μL	CNS 1 only	Triple trisomies of chromosomes 4 and 10 Or ETV6-RUNX1	-	PB MRD < 0.01%	-	θ MRD < 0.01%	-	0	0	40	3.5
DCOG 10	Y	Y	1–18	Any	CNS 1 only		Y	-	-	PCR MRD NEG	Day 80 PCR MRD NEG	2000	120	80	26
JACLS-ALL-02	Y	-	1–9	<10,000/μL	No CNS 3		Y	-	M1/M2	M1	-	1500	^90	72	40
MS 2003	Y	Y	0–18	Any	CNS 1 only		Y	-	-	PCR MRD NEG	Week 8 PCR MRD NEG	3000	120	140	31
MS 2010	Y	-	1–10	Any	CNS 1 only		Y	-	-	PCR MRD NEG	Week 8 PCR MRD NEG	3000	0	167.5	40
RELLA05	Y	-	1–9	<50,000/μL	CNS1/CNS2 Traumatic LP	DNA index of ≥1.16 or ETV6-RUNX1	-	-	** MRD <0.01%	-	-	0	50	160	22
St Jude Total XV	Y	-	1–10	<50,000/μL	Any	DNA index of >/=1.16 or ETV6-RUNX1	-	-	MRD <1%	-	D46 MRD <0.01%	1000	110	208	43
UKALL 2003	Y	Y	1–10	<50,000/μL	Any		Y	-	M1/M2	+ MRD < 0.01%	-	2000	150	64	33

* D8 or 15 M1 marrow; ** Day 19 MRD < 0.01%; + D29 MRD detectable but <0.01% AND undetectable MRD before start of interim maintenance; θ Day 29 responses; ^ Pirarubicin; ~ Where pegylated L-asp was used, 2500 units/m² was calculated to be the equivalent of 40,000 units/m² given over 1 week; DNA Index: (the ratio of DNA content in leukemic cells to that in normal diploid G0/G1 cells).

5. Favorable ALL Genetics: Hyperdiploidy and ETV6-RUNX1

Hyperdiploidy (>50 chromosomes) and *ETV6-RUNX1* ALL are associated with excellent outcomes (5-year EFS >90%). Unfortunately, the karyotyping of lymphoblasts to determine ploidy is technically challenging and different from antenatal karyotyping. Hyperdiploidy is characterized by recurrent, non-random gains in specific chromosomes: 4, 10, 17, and 18. To standardize the diagnosis of hyperdiploid ALL, the Children's Oncology Group (COG) focused on double or triple trisomy fluorescent-in-situ-hybridization (FISH) probes for chromosomes 4, 10, and/or 17 to define these favorable hyperdiploid features.

ETV6-RUNX1 is an oncogene fusion transcript and cannot be defined by conventional karyotyping. UKALL's strategy of low-cost FISH to identify oncogene fusions such as *ETV6-RUNX1, BCR-ABL1* fusion probes and a *KMT2A* break-apart probe in a triple probe FISH screening strategy has been tested in low-resource settings [38,39]. In contrast, Ma-Spore and other groups have used reverse-transcription PCR (RT-PCR) to screen for *ETV6-RUNX1, BCR-ABL1, TCF3-PBX1,* and *KMT2A-AFF1 (AF4)*. RT-PCR can be performed using standard PCR thermocyclers, which are also available in many universities including those in LMIC. Although more expensive, there are also available oncogene fusion screening kits for leukemia, e.g., QuanDx's Leukemia Fusion Gene (Q30) Screening Kit and the HemaVision Screen kit. Given that the instability of mRNA and that PCR reactions may be prone to aerosol contamination, proper positive and negative controls are critical for RT-PCR screening. Referencing and partnering with good laboratories internationally, such as VIVA-NUS CenTRAL and the St Jude Global Alliance, can also be very helpful.

Using a low-intensity protocol, COG AALL0331 [23] demonstrated excellent outcomes in children who achieved EOI MRD negativity with either favorable triple trisomy (38% of population) of chromosomes 4, 10, 17, or ETV6-RUNX1 (62% of population). COG AALL0331 showed that intensification of therapy for these low-risk patients did not improve outcomes. For this low-risk cohort, the successor COG AALL0932 [22] also reported excellent outcomes: 5-year DFS 98.8% and 5-year OS 100% with a P9904-based regimen without alkylating agents or anthracyclines in the LR-M arm. However, only 6.5% of the AALL0932 study population was eligible for this randomization; and only 3.3% of patients were assigned to the P9904-based LR-M arm. Critically, to be able to define this lowest-risk subgroup, there is a requirement for excellent cytogenetics or FISH setup defined hyperdiploidy, oncogene fusion screening for ETV6-RUNX1, and EOI MRD. For LMIC, accurate EOI MRD by flow may not be available.

In the presence of hyperdiploidy and ETV6-RUNX1, poor responses such as high EOI MRD of >1% are fortunately very rare. In MS 2003/2010 and UKALL 2003, only 3% of patients with low-risk genetics had a high EOI MRD of >1% [40]. Hence MRD monitoring for this low-risk genetic group is probably not critical. For MIC, using DNA index >1.16 may be feasible, as demonstrated by the RELLA05 [14] group in low-resource settings in Brazil. FISH for double trisomy 4 and 10 as a surrogate marker for triple trisomy is also feasible.

6. Democratization of Flow Cytometry

Interestingly, it is common for hospitals, even in LMIC, to have a good flow cytometer. The widespread availability of good, multi-color flow cytometers makes it possible to do flow cytometry for diagnosis of ALL. However, not many laboratories are trained to properly perform flow cytometry for the diagnosis of childhood leukemias. Access to a supply chain of good quality fluorochrome-labeled antibodies is also potentially a problem.

While several simple low-cost flow cytometry methodologies to measure MRD have been developed [41,42], they have yet to be widely implemented in Asia. Flow MRD needs to be analyzed and interpreted properly. In the presence of a lot of hematogones, simple, low-cost flow MRD using a limited panel of markers can yield misleading results. Flow MRD-lite end-of-induction assessment has been used in limited resource settings such as the RELLA05 study [43]. Although MRD testing is expensive, its key role in risk assignment would offset costs involved in toxicity related hospitalizations. In addition, it can be cost effective to set up a good flow MRD-lite platform to identify the best responders that can be cured with less therapy.

7. Specific Considerations for T-Lineage ALL

Treatment de-intensification in T-ALL is much less studied and should be undertaken with caution in the context of a clinical trial. Outcomes in T-ALL have only very recently improved significantly, approaching those of B-ALL. This has been achieved with combinations of (1) the use of dexamethasone (Dexa)-based 4 drug induction, (2) a more intensive Berlin-Frankfurt-Munster (BFM) ALL backbone, (3) Capizzi escalating methotrexate, and (4) optimizing the use of L-asparaginase (L-asp). In the MS2003 study [18], which was Dexa-based, 6-year EFS rates of B and T-ALL patients were 80.7% and 80.5%, respectively.

Use of Dexa throughout all phases of therapy, like in the MS2003 [18] and UKALL 2003 [27] studies, has led to better outcomes in children with T-ALL. This better outcome with Dexa could be due to better CNS penetration, given that CNS relapse is more common in T-ALL. T-ALL patients should receive 4-drug Dexa-based induction but will require prolonged inpatient admission throughout the whole period of induction because of high risk of infections and TRM.

The largest T-ALL study, the COG AALL0434 study [44], surprisingly showed superior outcomes with the Capizzi escalating MTX plus L-asp regimen compared to HDMTX regimen (4-y DFS 92.5% ± 1.8% vs. 86.1% ± 2.4%, $p = 0.02$). However, 90% of T-ALL patients on AALL0434 received cranial radiotherapy. AALL0434 also found that addition of 5 days of nelarabine improved outcomes for IR and HR T-ALL (4-y DFS 88.9% vs. 83.3%). However, the high cost and high neurotoxicity of nelarabine will limit its use in LMIC.

8. Delaying the First Intra-Thecal (IT) Chemotherapy

Traumatic lumbar puncture (LP) with blasts is a risk factor for CNS relapse. If the first LP is performed at the time of diagnosis [45], traumatic LP occurs in up to 14%. Delaying the first IT until after clearance of circulating blasts at the end of the first week of induction would reduce incidence of traumatic LP with blasts, an adverse risk feature. This was first described in the Tokyo Children's Cancer Study Group study L89-12 [46]. The TPOG-ALL-2002 study [47] also confirmed that the delay of the first triple IT did not adversely affect survival or CNS control despite omission of cranial irradiation.

Delaying of the first IT also reduces the risk of methotrexate-related kidney injury that may be exacerbated by ongoing tumor lysis syndrome during the induction phase. Reduced need for sedation in the first week of therapy may also be advantageous to patients with large mediastinal masses at diagnosis, given the inherent risks of airway obstruction with procedures requiring sedation in such cases.

9. Prednisolone/Dexamethasone-Based and 3/4-Drug-Based Induction

Pred has historically been used during the BFM ALL induction protocol, while Dexa has been used later during DI (Figure 2). Dexa is more potent than Pred and because of better CNS penetration [48], reduces the rate of CNS relapse. The enduring question of whether Dexa is superior to Pred during induction was tested in the randomized AIEOP-BFM ALL 2000 [36] study in a 4-drug induction including anthracyclines. AIEOP-BFM ALL 2000 showed that patients with a good Pred response who received Dexa during induction had one-third the risk of relapse of those who had received Pred—a remarkable feat. However, these improvements in relapse rates were offset by the higher incidence of life threatening events during induction. Overall, despite the marked reduction in relapse rates in the Dexa arm, there were no differences in OS as relapses in the Dexa arm were less salvageable and more patients died of infections during Dexa-based induction. Subsequently the AIEOP-BFM group reserved 4-drug Dexa-based induction only for a subset of T-ALL patients with good Pred response.

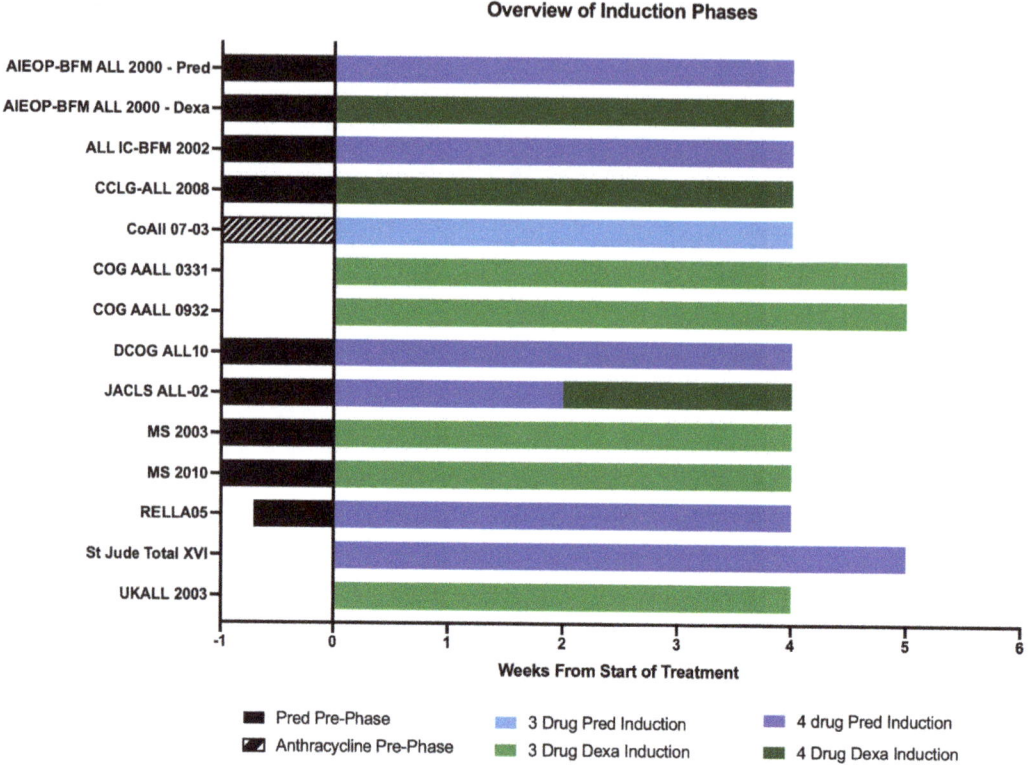

Figure 2. Induction regimens in contemporary ALL studies for low−risk patients. Prednisolone (Pred) prophase allows management of tumor lysis. 3 drug induction refers to induction protocols which include the use of Prednisolone or Dexamethasone (Dexa), Vincristine and L-asp, with the exception of patients treated on the CoALL 07-03 [21] who received 3 drug Prednisolone-based induction consisting of Prednisolone, Vinristine, and either Doxorubicin or Daunorubicin, without L-asp. This included a pre-phase comparing the responses after a single dose of either Doxorubicin or Daunorubicin. 4 drug induction protocols include the use of anthracyclines such as Doxorubicin or Daunorubicin. For LMIC, 3-drug Dexa-based induction is safer. For 4-drug induction, Pred-based induction is probably less toxic than one that is Dexa-based.

The Japanese L95-14 [49] and the Dana-Farber Cancer Institute ALL 91-01P [50] trials also reported a higher rate of infection-related induction deaths in the Dexa arm as compared to those who had received Pred. Infectious deaths also increased during Dexa-based induction in UKALL 97 [51] although there was overall survival benefit.

To use Dexa during induction, a 3-drug induction without anthracyclines is feasible in LMIC. Of note, many groups such as the COG, UKALL, and the Ma-Spore ALL used Dexa-based, 3-drug induction without anthracyclines. COG and UKALL used it for NCI SR induction while Ma-Spore used it for all B-ALL patients. Without anthracyclines, Dexa-based 3-drug induction can be given safely and mainly as outpatient therapy.

Dexa-based 4-drug induction is best reserved for T-ALL patients and used in hospitals with good isolation facilities and ability to treat breakthrough secondary infections including fungal infections. These hospitals should also have good microbiological diagnosis platforms for bacterial, fungal, and viral pathogens. Dexa-based 4-drug induction is toxic, even in the context of HIC where supportive care is good. We do not recommend Dexa-based 4-drug induction for LMIC.

10. L-Asp Doses in Induction and Delayed Intensification

A key drug in treatment of ALL is L-asp. Unlike adult ALL protocols, such as Hyper-CVAD, pediatric-inspired protocols use L-asp as a mainstay drug during induction and DI. L-asp is an enzyme derived from *E. coli* that can cause allergic reactions and silent inactivation. L-asp is moderately myelosuppressive and can cause pancreatitis and thromboembolism, especially in children > 10 years old.

After the first exposure to L-asp during induction therapy for newly diagnosed ALL, the risk of neutralizing antibodies and silent inactivation is low. Because of the lower risk of neutralizing antibodies that have to be overcome with higher doses, Ma-Spore ALL induction starts with a lower dose of L-asp during induction (7500 U/m^2 of Leunase spaced out to twice a week). This lower dose of L-asp during induction also reduces the risk of myelosuppression. During DI, where low levels neutralizing antibodies may already have developed, we use a higher dose of L-asp of 10,000 U/m^2 every 3 days. This high dose allows for sufficient asparagine depletion during DI.

The major brands of L-asp available include: Leunase (Kyowa-Hakko), Kidrolase (Kyowa-Hakko), and Spectrila (Medac, Germany). In addition, L-asp is also manufactured by a few companies in India. The various brands of L-asp have different potencies and different risks of allergic reaction. Pegylated (PEG) L-asp has a much longer half-life than regular L-asp. However, PEG-L-asp is expensive and not registered in most LMICs. Because of these limitations, the Ma-Spore ALL study group focused on using L-asp. Erwinase is given to patients with allergic reactions to L-asp and PEG L-asp. However, Erwinase is less potent and has a much shorter half-life requiring dosing of 20,000 U/m^2 every 2 days to ensure complete asparagine depletion.

The St Jude Total XVI [26] study showed prolonged and more intensive asparagine depletion using higher doses of PEG L-asp (3500 U/m^2 versus 2500 U/m^2) did not improve outcomes. Instead, it was associated with a higher incidence of toxic deaths than in an earlier study (3.2% vs. 1.4%). This prolonged asparagine depletion is also associated with increased risk of pancreatitis and long-term poor pancreatic function with diabetes mellitus.

In MS2010 [52], single doses of vincristine and L-asp were added during DI to maintain treatment intensity during a rest period at day 15. However, this led to more hospitalizations for fever, increased risk of bacteremia, and critical-care admissions, but fortunately without any increase in treatment-related mortality. The DFCI-ALL 05-01 [53] also previously described the myelosuppressive effects of asparaginase.

Because of its high costs, risks of allergy and silent inactivation, we recommend restricting L-asp use to only the induction and DI phases, especially in LMICs. To reduce the risk of allergy, Ma-Spore delayed L-asp until after at least 2 days of steroid cover had been started. We also caution against any additional doses of L-asp given that it causes increased myelosuppression and a higher risk of infections.

11. Anthracycline-Free Regimens

Anthracyclines are most used as part of induction and DI in the BFM-ALL treatment backbone. Although effective, anthracyclines cause severe immediate myelosuppression and long-term cardiotoxicity [54,55]. Because of these side effects, Ma-Spore and other groups have attempted to eliminate or reduce anthracyclines in the treatment of low-risk ALL. The COG AALL0932 [22] and MS2010 are both examples of clinical studies where anthracyclines were completely omitted in their low-risk arms. In terms of toxicity, MS2010-SR [52] revealed excellent results comparable to those of other contemporary protocols, yet with reduced toxicity. As mentioned above, in a highly selected subgroup with low-risk genetics and that were EOI MRD negative, the COG AALL 0932 LR-M arm reported excellent results with 5-year DFS of 98.8% and 5-year OS of 100% with no anthracyclines and alkylating agents.

The CCG-105 [56] study showed that dose dense DI is only critical for *older* children. This is due to residual leukemia cells that persist after induction/consolidation which are relatively resistant to therapy. Anthracyclines, usually doxorubicin, are used with Dexa, vincristine and L-asp (Protocol II) for intensive DI. However, for younger children who have low-risk ALL, the CCG-105 study showed that dose intensive DI is probably not critical.

12. Is High-Dose Methotrexate Really Necessary?

In LMIC, it is difficult to administer high-dose methotrexate (HD MTX) safely. This is because IV MTX > 500 mg/m^2 requires folinic rescue dosing and close MTX level monitoring. Although the adjustment of the start time for administration can allow MTX level monitoring during office hours, this infrequently utilized test is generally not available and not cost-effective in most LMIC settings. Although various groups have devised various strategies [57,58] to overcome challenges of giving HDMTX, we review alternatives to HD-MTX in Table 3.

Table 3. Consolidation and MTX dosing across clinical trials.

	Cumulative Int/High Dose MTX Dose (g/m^2)	Number of Int/High MTX Doses	Dose of Int/High Dose MTX (g/m^2)	Duration of 6MP (weeks)	Daily 6MP Dose (mg/m^2)	Total 6MP Dose (mg/m^2)	Number of Intrathecal Chemotherapy Injections	Other Drugs
AIEOP-BFM ALL 2000 [20,36]	20	4	5	8	25	1400	4	-
ALL IC-BFM 2002 [16]	8	4	2	8	25	1400	4	-
CCLG-ALL 2008 [17]	8	4	2	8	25	1400	4	-
CoAll 07-03 [21]	3	3	1	2	100	1400	3	Teniposide 165 mg/m^2 + Thioguanine (100 mg/m^2/day) for 1 week + L-asp 45,000 units/m^2 + PEG-Asp 5000 units/m^2 + Cytarabine 12,300 mg/m^2
COG AALL 0932 [22] (LR-M)	6	6	1	19	50	6650	6	Dexamethasone 84 mg/m^2 + Vincristine 6 mg/m^2
DCOG 10 [24]	20	4	5	8	25	1400	4	-
JACLS-ALL-02 [25] Arm A	6	2	3	1	50	350	4	Cyclophosphamide 1.5 g/m^2 + Cytarabine 750 mg/m^2
JACLS-ALL-02 [25] Arm B	6	2	3	-	-	-	4	Dexamethasone 50 mg/m^2 + Cyclophosphamide 1 g/m^2 + Cytarabine 500 mg/m^2
MS 2003 [18]	8	4	2	8	25	1400	4	-
MS 2010 [19]	10	4	2.5	8	25	1400	4	Interspersed Cyclophosphamide blocks
RELLA05 [14]	10	4	2.5	8	50	2800	4	-
St Jude Total XVI [26]	10	4	2.5	8	50	2800	4	-
	Total Dose of Dose Escalating MTX (g/m^2)	No. of Dose Escalating MTX	Oral MTX (mg/m^2)	Duration of 6MP (weeks)	Daily 6MP Dose (mg/m^2)	Total 6MP Dose (mg/m^2)	Number of IT Chemotherapy Injections	Other Drugs
COG AALL 0932 [22] (LR-C)	1	5	-	4	75	2100	4	Vincristine 9 mg/m^2
COG AALL 0331 [23,37]	1	5	-	4	75	2100	4	Vincristine 9 mg/m^2 (L-asp intensification arm: 4 additional doses of PEG-Asp (10,000 units/m^2)
UKALL 2003 [27]	-	-	140	4	75	2100	4	Vincristine 4.5 mg/m^2

Differences in MTX dosing strategies are summarized and highlighted in this table, from intermediate to high-dose MTX regimens to low-dose MTX regimens including the characteristic COG dose-escalating MTX. Patients on the **CoALL 07-03** [21] trial were treated with intermediate doses of MTX but were given a combination of other drugs such as Teniposide, L-asp, and Cytarabine as well. In the **COG AALL 0932** [22], low-risk patients were randomized to receive either the P9904 regimen A-based (Arm LR-M) which included 6 courses of intermediate dose (1g/m^2) MTX without any further alkylating agents or anthracyclines, essentially omitting DI entirely and completing therapy with the maintenance phase; or the CCG 1991 regimen-like outpatient-based regimen (Arm LR-C) with standard COG dose-escalating MTX. Patients treated on the **JACLS ALL-02** [25] were randomized to receive either truncated BFM-like consolidation (Arm A) or low-dose Cytarabine containing consolidation (Arm B). Of all the reviewed studies, the **COG AALL 0932** [22] and **COG AALL 0331** [23] studies, together with the **UKALL 2003** [27], included the lowest intensity of MTX treatment. While of interest to LMIC or LIC groups with limited access to serum MTX drug monitoring, the excellent outcomes achieved in these studies were derived from HIC settings with individual protocol-specific caveats such as the more stringent criteria imposed by the COG to be considered as low risk, and later intensification in other parts of the protocol in the UKALL 2003, which have been reported to be toxic even in HIC settings.

For all NCI-SR patients, instead of HDMTX, the COG study used escalating intravenous MTX that started at 100 mg/m^2 and did not require serum MTX level monitoring.

COG AALL0331 [23,37] and COG AALL0932 [22] reported excellent outcomes in NCI SR patients treated without HD MTX. The UKALL 2003 [27] achieved excellent outcomes without use of HDMTX for all patients. Specifically, for EOI MRD negative patients (Regimen A and B), there was no HDMTX or Capizzi MTX-L-asp; while EOI MRD positive patients had two blocks of Capizzi MTX-L-asp.

Although the COG AALL0232 [59] showed that HDMTX was superior to Capizzi MTX, the reported benefits of HDMTX over Capizzi MTX were in fact in *higher risk* B-ALL but not low-risk ALL. The newer UKALL 2011 randomized EOI MRD negative patients to receive HDMTX compared to interim maintenance.

13. Delayed Intensification—Is More Necessarily Better?

Although the importance of DI is clear, a balance between dose intensity and treatment toxicity is paramount. The BFM/COG DI Protocol II is intensive with significant toxicity, thus many groups have focused on deintensification of DI. In SR patients who were MRD negative, DCOG-ALL10 [24] successfully removed doxorubicin, cyclophosphamide, cytarabine, and thioguanine, which were replaced with a single, low-intensity Protocol IV, which consists of Dexamethasone, two doses of Vincristine, and single doses of PEG L-asp and intrathecal chemotherapy; with excellent outcomes (93% 5-y EFS and 99% 5-y OS). The randomized CoALL 07-03 study [21] also successfully de-intensified Protocol II, by removing one dose of doxorubicin and one week of Dexa in SR patients. In contrast, the large, randomized AIEOP-BFM-ALL 2000 study [20] showed that the shortened but dose-dense Protocol III was paradoxically more toxic and less effective in preventing relapse. The AIEOP-BFM ALL Protocol III is shorter and highly compressed DI, resulting in more toxicity and prolonged post-Protocol III delay.

Recent studies have demonstrated that repeated DI blocks might not improve outcomes. Figure 3 summarizes the various strategies and overviews of major clinical trials in childhood ALL. The randomized ALL IC-BFM 2002 study [16] failed to show any improvement in outcomes with additional DI blocks in both standard and medium-risk patients. Similarly, CCG-1991 [60] showed no added benefit with double DI blocks in patients with standard-risk ALL. Instead, escalating MTX during interim maintenance improved outcomes. UKALL2003 randomized EOI MRD negative patients to single versus two blocks of Protocol II; one block of Protocol II was less toxic without compromising outcomes [27].

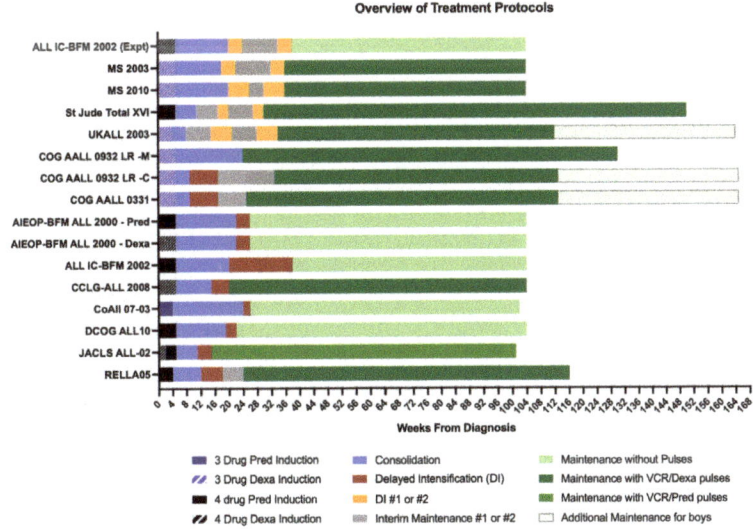

Figure 3. Overview of contemporary ALL protocols for lower-risk ALL: Major differences in protocol

design of delayed intensification (single versus double blocks interspersed with interim maintenance blocks), types of maintenance phases are highlighted. Consolidation phases described in this figure refer to the period following the completion of induction phase and end prior to the start of delayed intensification phase and therefore include HD MTX phases. The experimental arm of the **ALL IC-BFM 2002 study** [16] comprised two shorter DI blocks (Protocol III), split from the original single Protocol II DI. **MS2003** [18] and **MS2010** [19] studies employed a similar dosing strategy with multiple DI blocks with improvements in toxicity following dosing modifications. The **St Jude Total XVI** [26] protocol embeds dual 3 week blocks of DI in interim maintenance phases which start right after the consolidation phase. Similarly, the **UKALL 2003** [27] protocol also comprises two blocks of DI, albeit longer in duration and higher in dose intensity as compared to the abovementioned studies. **COG AALL 0932** [22] randomized low-risk patients to receive either P9904 regimen A-based (Arm LR-M), which is a very low-intensity protocol without alkylating agents or anthracyclines, or the CCG 1991 regimen-like outpatient-based regimen (Arm LR-C) with reduced vincristine/dexamethasone pulses during maintenance phase (every 12 weeks). For patients assigned to Arm LR-M, the total duration of therapy would be $2\frac{1}{2}$ years from diagnosis for both female and male patients. For those assigned to Arm LR-C, the duration of therapy would continue to be gender based: 2 years from the start of interim maintenance for female patients and 3 years from the start of Interim Maintenance I for male patients. In the **COG AALL 0331** [23] study, patients in the lowest defined risk group in the study, the standard risk-low group, were randomized to receive either standard treatment or four additional doses of PEG L-asp at 3 week intervals in an attempt to intensify treatment to improve outcomes in this group of patients. Although intensification failed to improve outcomes, the authors concluded that standard COG therapy without intensification still led to excellent outcomes in this identified low-risk group. **AIEOP-BFM ALL 2000** [36] randomized patients to receive either Prednisolone or Dexamethasone during induction. The **CCLG-ALL 2008** [17] study was based on BFM ALL treatment backbone but modified to reduce toxicity in SR patients by halving the dose intensity of early intensification after induction and before consolidation. DI was modified as per the COG with 25–33% reduction of Dexamethasone and Doxorubicin. Patients were then randomized in the maintenance phase to either receive standard maintenance therapy with vincristine and dexamethasone pulses versus a 1 week rest of mercaptopurine and MTX during the vincristine dexamethasone pulse. The lowest-risk group of patients treated on the **CoALL 07-03** [21] trial was given the reduced intensity LR-R arm with only 1 week of Dexamethasone, two doses of Vincristine and single doses of Doxorubicin with PEG L-asp in a shortened DI protocol. **DCOG ALL10** [24] includes a significantly deintensified DI Protocol IV with only 2 weeks of Dexamethasone, two doses of Vincristine and a single dose of PEG L-asp; this was followed with maintenance therapy consisting only of oral 6-MP and MTX without any pulses. The **JACLS ALL-02** [25] protocol used Prednisolone pulses during maintenance in contrast to most other groups where Dexamethasone was used during pulses with Vincristine during the maintenance phase; Pirarubicin was also used instead of the more commonly used Doxorubicin or Daunorubicin as the anthracycline of choice during induction and DI.

In the MS2003 study [18] SR arm, the DI phase consisted of two blocks of Protocol III like the experimental arms of the ALL IC-BFM 2002 study [16]. Unfortunately, as in the ALL IC-BFM 2002, there was significant toxicity during DI in MS2003 where most of the treatment-related deaths occurred [52]. Although larger randomized clinical trials investigating the effects of DI indicate that a single block of BFM/COG Protocol II is probably sufficient, the Ma-Spore chose to continue with two shorter but further modified DI blocks instead of a single block of Protocol II. In the MS2010, EOI MRD negative patients received two less intensive DI blocks without anthracyclines (Protocol V) with less treatment interruption and toxicity. Toxicity analysis of MS2010 [52] revealed significant reductions in toxicity in terms of infections as well as overall phase delays.

For low-risk ALL, it is not clear whether a strong intensive DI phase is necessary. Taken together, one block of COG Protocol II DI has been shown to be highly effective and is our recommendation for LMIC with good supportive care.

14. The Malaysia Singapore Experience

The Ma-Spore Study Group is a collaborative group of four pediatric oncology units from Malaysia and Singapore. Ma-Spore started with a MRD risk-stratified, Ma-Spore ALL 2003 (MS2003) treatment protocol [12,18]. Because of moderate resources, MS2003 focused on deintensifying therapy in MRD-negative patients.

MS2003 starts with a less myelosuppressive 3-drug Dexa-based induction to reduce the risk of severe infections during induction. The Ma-Spore treatment mantra is "*Patient first, leukemia second.*" The aim was to get the patient to safety first by allowing recovery of marrow function. Depending on MRD response after induction, strength of delayed intensification therapy is tailored later to eliminate residual leukemia. The vast majority of patients with no high-risk genetics and a good day 8 Pred response received 3-drug Dexa-based induction without anthracyclines. In Ma-Spore ALL studies, MRD risk stratification is by using a single PCR MRD marker at EOI and at the end of consolidation (EOC) at week 12. MS2003 focused on intensive DI by adopting the experimental ALL IC-BFM 2002 repeated Protocol III blocks. MS2003 [12] achieved a 6-year EFS of 80%, with an overall survival of 88%.

In addition, a strong collaborative network was forged between the two countries, where bone marrow MRD samples were processed and cryopreserved then couriered weekly on dry ice to the centralized laboratory in Singapore. There was also regular exchange of manpower training and knowledge sharing between the different pediatric oncology centers that extended to regional hospitals in rural areas in Malaysia. An important feature was regular telephone calls to regional hospitals to track count recovery on full blood counts, drug doses, and complications. Regional hospitals were educated on complications such as febrile neutropenia, to be able to reach emergency services in a timely manner should the need arise. Healthcare personnel in rural areas were also educated on the management of neutropenic fever and the importance of up triaging and early administration of antibiotics.

The keys to the success of Ma-Spore are the use of centralized academic molecular laboratories in the National University of Singapore and University Malaya, and a protocol design that is cognizant of moderate access to supportive care. Figure 4 summarizes key networks that have also been used in the Malaysia Singapore experience in establishing a program to treat children with ALL in settings with resource limitations.

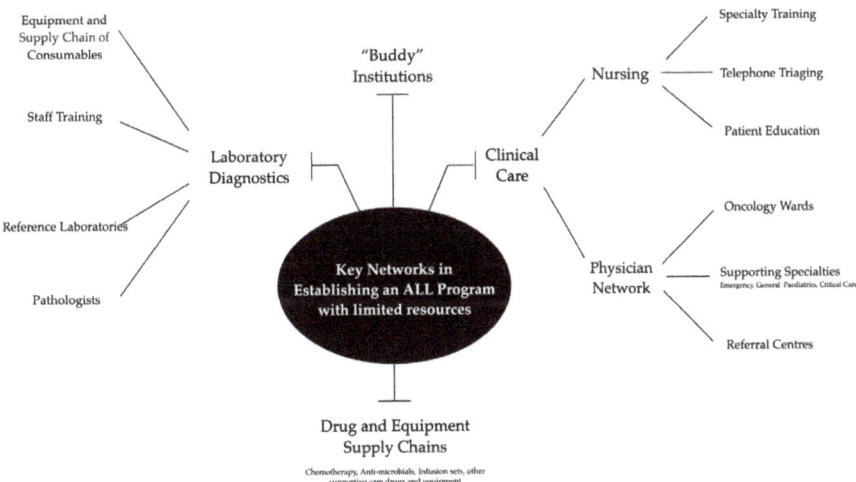

Figure 4. Proposed key networks in establishing an ALL program with limited resources. "Buddy" institutions refer to more established programs that newer growing programs with limited resources can reach out to for help and advice regarding patient care and technical support.

15. Infections

In ALL, given the growing threat of antimicrobial resistance and, more recently, the COVID-19 pandemic, treatment-related infections are a major concern. The risk of infection during ALL treatment is dependent on the treatment phase and its intensity. The induction phase poses the highest risk of infections due to a combination of prolonged myelosuppression from both disease and induction chemotherapy [61,62]. Because of this exquisite vulnerability to sepsis during induction, the Ma-Spore group focused on 3-drug Dexa-based induction, which is less myelosuppressive, yet sufficiently intense to achieve sufficient complete remission to promote marrow recovery.

Although UKALL 2003 [27] had no HDMTX blocks, which made it feasible in limited resource settings, the risk of sepsis during the 4-drug Dexa-based induction protocol was still significant [62]. Given the septic deaths prevalent even in high income settings, these risks may be exponentially higher in limited resource settings. In areas with hygiene concerns and where access to supportive care may be an issue, it may be prudent to keep patients within a closer proximity during such high-risk periods.

In the St Jude Total XV [61] study, the lack of neutrophil surge after Dexa pulse, as a reflection of decreased marrow reserves, was linked to a high risk of sepsis. Dexa suppresses fever. During Dexa pulse, presence of even low-grade fever of >37.3 °C and severe neutropenia (ANC < 0.5×10^9/L) confer increased risk of sepsis. In limited resource settings, neutropenic fever during Dexa-based phases should be prioritized for emergency access to supportive care.

Malnutrition aggravates the risk of infection during cancer treatment [9]. In limited resource settings, training shared-care hospitals and educating families to recognize fever and signs of sepsis is critical. This involves providing clear guidelines to parents and shared-care hospitals on how to treat ALL patients with fever, regardless of neutrophil count. Prediction scoring systems could supplement multidisciplinary efforts specifically involving front line emergency department staff to improve early access to antibiotics and supportive care as a whole. The only problem is that most shared-care hospitals in LMIC settings lack staff who can learn and implement such a prediction score system, given that children with ALL probably only form a minority of cases seen.

Protocol-specific analysis of infections during treatment may help inform positive changes in protocol design. In MS2003 [52], after 2 weeks of Protocol III DI, severe neutropenic fevers were observed. These observations led to the one-week mandatory break after Protocol IIIa, which helped reduced infective complications in the successor MS2010 protocol, unlike the AIEOP-BFM ALL 2000 experience.

16. Improving Supportive Care

Up to now, we have focused on adjusting various aspects of low-risk ALL therapy to the limited supportive care available in LMIC. Good supportive care is the bedrock of our improved cancer outcomes. Without good supportive care, most of what we propose is not possible.

Improving supportive care is cost-effective. Cost-effective measures like setting up appropriate inpatient and outpatient childhood cancer wards is transformational. Cohorting children with cancer who are immunocompromised in a childhood cancer unit reduces cross infections. Common childhood viral infections such as measles and varicella are mild in normal children but can be devastating in immunocompromised ones. With childhood cancer units, both doctors and nurses can be trained to implement life-saving neutropenic fever protocols immediately and give chemotherapy safely. Overcrowding is detrimental. Low-risk ALL can be treated in dedicated outpatient cancer centers where chemotherapy beds can be quickly cleaned and reused after a short IV vincristine or IM L-asp. By recycling outpatient beds, more children can be treated, reducing overcrowding and infections [63].

Setting up a childhood cancer unit must come with improved infectious disease and intensive care unit support. Laboratory tests including FBC and blood cultures, and a safe blood supply, are critical.

17. Overview of Maintenance Therapy

Maintenance therapy is indispensable in the cure of childhood ALL and is universally part of all chemotherapy protocols for ALL [64,65]. However, the exact reason for its essentiality remains unclear. Compared to the intensive prior phases of ALL therapy, MT is only mildly intensive and simple: it comprises a 2 drug "anti-metabolite" backbone of daily oral mercaptopurine (6-MP), and weekly oral/IV/IM MTX. From initial diagnosis, the duration of ALL therapy should exceed 2 years (104 weeks). Attempts to reduce the duration of ALL therapy to 12 months (TCCSG) to 18 months (BFM) have resulted in poorer outcomes. The only times that MT is omitted is after bone marrow transplantation or CAR-T cell therapy.

18. Duration of Maintenance Phase

Although MT is only mildly intensive, toxicities remain and even deaths occur [66]. During MT, patients remained mildly immunocompromised, exposing them to bacterial, fungal, and viral infections. The long duration of MT contributes to the cumulative risk of toxicity. Attempts to intensify MT by adding VCR/Dexa pulses and rotating drug pairs such as cyclophosphamide/cytarabine (SJ Total protocols), can add to the risk of infection (see below).

Historically, for ALL outcomes, boys fared worse compared to girls. However, with modern day risk-stratified therapy, this survival gap between boys and girls has narrowed [67]. In MS2003, which is Dexamethasone-based, boys and girls do equally well. Because of this, boys are not treated differently. However, due to inferior outcome in boys, some groups treated boys with an additional year of maintenance chemotherapy [67]. Thus, most contemporary protocols no longer treat them with separate durations, with very few exceptions (such as the TPOG trial group) [68].

Compared to standard duration of 2 years, a longer duration (i.e., 3 years) of MT confers no overall survival. Although longer MT reduces risk of relapse, it increases toxic deaths which erases the survival advantage [66]. Moreover, relapse on therapy is less salvageable. Numerous attempts have been made to shorten the duration of MT down to as little as 6 months, mostly with significantly poorer results [69–71]. However, certain small subsets of patients were cured despite shorter treatment. In the Tokyo Children's Cancer Study Group's L92-13 study, where MT was truncated to 6 months, patients with *TCF3-PBX1* or *ETV6-RUNX1* fusion had favorable survival [69]. Surprisingly, hyperdiploid ALL, which is low genetic risk group, fared the worst with shortened MT. However, these analyses are based on retrospective data of failed attempts to reduce duration of therapy. A shortened duration of MT generally resulted in a higher overall rate of late relapses. Therefore, 2-year ALL therapy including MT remains the current de facto strategy.

An intriguing model to reduce the risk of immunosuppression and infectious toxicity is the Brazilian Childhood Cooperative Group for ALL Treatment's (GBTLI) use of an intermittent schedule of 6-MP and MTX [72]. Children were randomized to receive either continuous therapy (i.e., continuous oral 6-MP 50 mg/m^2 daily and intramuscular MTX 25 mg/m^2/week) or intermittent therapy (i.e., intermittent 6-MP 100 mg/m^2 daily for 10 days and 11 days' rest, plus MTX 200 mg/m^2 as 6 h IV infusion every 3 weeks, with leucovorin rescue). Here, they found that children with LR ALL treated with the intermittent schedule had improved survival than those receiving the standard continuous schedule. Significantly, there was lower severe toxicity even though the overall cumulative MTX dose was higher in the intermittent group. Notably, boys allocated to the intermittent regimen had significantly better EFS than those receiving the continuous schedule.

19. VCR/Steroid Pulses

The addition of vincristine plus steroid (VCR/steroid) pulses during maintenance therapy significantly improved EFS by at least 10% in multiple clinical trials in the 1980s [66,73]. This was subsequently adopted by all major study groups. However, the benefits of these VCR/steroid pulses in contemporary more intensive protocols are increasingly questioned. The International BFM (I-BFM) Study Group prospective randomized multi-protocols study found that IR patients who received intensive ALL BFM-backbone protocols did not benefit from six pulses of VCR/Dexa during MT [74]. A recent large randomized trial from China showed that omitting these pulses in LR patients did not impact survival outcomes [75]. However, the EORTC ALL 58951-trial showed better survival [76]. With the contemporary intensive BFM-ALL protocol, LR or IR patients probably do not need VCR/steroid pulses during MT. However, for HR patients, the role of VCR/steroid pulses during MT is still unclear.

For the lower-risk groups, reduction of VCR/steroid pulses has been studied. The COG AALL0932 for NCI-SR B-ALL found that reducing the intensity of VCR/steroid pulses from 4 weekly to 12 weekly maintained the same excellent outcomes (OS 98%), although this was not performed in the context of a non-inferiority trial [77]. In the Ma-Spore trials, VCR/steroid pulses in the SR and IR arms were also given 10 weekly (MS2003) and 12 weekly (MS2010), with excellent outcomes [18,19]. Taken together, reduction or removal of these pulses might be applicable to those with the most favorable risk groups; i.e., favorable molecular subtypes with negative minimal residual disease (MRD) throughout [78]. MS2020 will continue VCR/Dexa pulses during MT every 12 weeks for SR/IR patients and 4 weeks for HR patients.

It is important to remember a successful ALL protocol is tested as one protocol with many phases. The intensity of all the phases contributes to the successful outcome. Currently, most contemporary protocols in HIC utilize sustained and highly intensive induction and reintensification blocks. This intensive ALL-BFM and augmented BFM backbone have been highly effective. In HIC, it is feasible for families to focus on an intensive 1 year of therapy and then a lower-intensity MT. With an intensive first year of therapy, the subsequent use of VCR/steroid pulses in MT is probably less important [73]. Whether a similar finding will result from a less intensive initial backbone, such as earlier trials that showed that VCR/Dexa pulses were useful, remains to be determined. In countries with limited resources for supportive care, a more spaced out and moderate intensity protocol during the first year followed by a slightly more intensive MT (with VCR/steroid pulses) might be more manageable. However, it is to be noted that these monthly VCR/Dexa pulses during maintenance can cause severe infections, especially with prolonged Dexa pulses of 2 weeks. VCR/Dexa pulses during MT may be complicated by varicella, measles, multi-resistant bacteria, and fungal infections. For low-risk ALL in LMIC, starting with less intensive upfront phases, shorter blocks of dexamethasone (6 mg/m^2/day for 5–7 days without tailing) and one dose of VCR every 4-6 weeks, is recommended. To further mitigate risk of infections, some groups have even stopped MP/MTX during the weeks of VCR/Dexa pulses with no significant issues.

20. TPMT and NUDT15 Variants on 6-MP Metabolism

Mercaptopurine (6-MP), the main anti-metabolite medication used in MT, exhibits wide interpatient variability in its efficacy and toxicity. In dosing of 6-MP, the two actionable pharmacogenetic variants are TPMT and NUDT15. TPMT variants are common in Caucasians (10%) while NUDT15 variants occur more frequently in 20% of Asians.

TPMT methylates 6-MP and thioguanine, reducing their efficacy. Low TPMT activity increases the levels of active metabolites of thiopurines (TGNs), causing myelosuppression [79,80]. NUDT15 encodes a nucleoside diphosphatase which degrades thioguanine triphosphates by dephosphorylation. This dephosphorylation of thioGTP reduces its incorporation into DNA and protecting cells from apoptosis [81,82]. TPMT and NUDT15 variants have low enzymatic activities and these act in a co-dominant manner. Specifically, heterozygosity of TPMT and NUDT15 variants reduces the levels of TPMT and NUDT15 activities, causing mild sensitivity to 6-MP. Yang et al. proposed a thiopurine genetic score incorporating both TPMT and NUDT15 variants. In the MS2010 study [19], score 1 patients who carried either the TPMT or NUDT15 variant tolerated a reduced dose of 6-MP at 40 mg/m^2/day. The frequency and type of variants affecting both enzymes vary significantly by ethnicity [83,84].

Pre-emptive testing of both TPMT and NUDT15 for possible dose modification is now standard care, with carefully established guidelines [85]. This is because doses that are customized based on TPMT or NUDT15 status reduce the likelihood of acute and severe toxicities (e.g., myelosuppression), without compromising disease control. Therefore, the risk-benefit ratio of pre-emptive genotyping is favorable and should be implemented in regions likely to have a high allelic frequency of these variants, and where testing resources are available.

21. Conclusions

Taken together, NCI SR features, low-risk genetics (hyperdiploidy, ETV6-RUNX1) and a rapid early response identify a group of patients who can be cured with low-intensity ALL therapy. Even in LMIC settings, these low-risk patients can be identified and cured cost-effectively with low-intensity protocols. Low-intensity protocols are based on two principles of (1) starting slow, with a 3-drug, anthracycline-free induction, delaying first IT to day 8, and (2) keeping safe, with low-intensity DI and uninterrupted metronomic MP/MTX maintenance. Setting up the appropriate supportive care to support the treatment protocol is as important. Adapting and testing therapy appropriate to resource-constrained supportive care and testing for TPMT/NUDT15 variants in high-frequency areas can be cost-effective. To appropriately adapt the best standards of care, partnering aspirant institutions through St Jude Global and SIOP is key. As a community caring for children with cancer, we have been fortunate. Realizing that childhood cancer is rare and we cannot do it alone make sharing experience and working together the guiding principles. By learning how to better treat low-risk ALL cost-effectively, LMIC could potentially contribute to the global ALL knowledge of how to cure with less. We are hopeful that HIC, in the near future, can learn from LMIC on "curing the curable" with less. As teachers, we learn best from our students.

Author Contributions: B.L.Z.O., S.H.R.L., and A.E.J.Y.: data curation, conceptualization, formal analysis, and writing—review and editing of the final manuscript. All authors have read and agreed to the published version of the manuscript.

Funding: Supported by the Singapore National Medical Research Council Clinician Scientist Investigator (NMRC/CSA/0053/2008, NMRC/CSA/0053/2013 and NMRC/CSA/MOH/000227) and Research Training Fellowships (NMRC/RTF/MOH/000616 and Cancer Science Institute, Singapore, and Centre Grant No. NMRC/CG/NCIS/2010, Goh Foundation, Children's Cancer Foundation, Singapore Totalisator Board, and VIVA Foundation for Children with Cancer.

Institutional Review Board Statement: The studies involving human participants in the Malaysia -Singapore (MS) ALL 2003 and 2010 clinical trials were reviewed and approved by Domain Specific Review Board (DSRB ref: 2004/00275, 2008/00081 and 2015/00164).

Acknowledgments: We would like to thank Edwynn Chiew and Tai Si Ting for their kind assistance with administration and data curation in the writing of this paper.

Conflicts of Interest: The authors have no conflict of interest to disclose.

References

1. Pui, C.H.; Yang, J.J.; Hunger, S.P.; Pieters, R.; Schrappe, M.; Biondi, A.; Vora, A.; Baruchel, A.; Silverman, L.B.; Schmiegelow, K.; et al. Childhood Acute Lymphoblastic Leukemia: Progress Through Collaboration. *J. Clin. Oncol.* **2015**, *33*, 2938–2948. [CrossRef] [PubMed]
2. Yeoh, A.E.J.; Tan, D.; Li, C.-K.; Hori, H.; Tse, E.; Pui, C.-H. Management of adult and paediatric acute lymphoblastic leukaemia in Asia: Resource-stratified guidelines from the Asian Oncology Summit 2013. *Lancet Oncol.* **2013**, *14*, e508–e523. [CrossRef]

3. Rodriguez-Galindo, C.; Friedrich, P.; Alcasabas, P.; Antillon, F.; Banavali, S.; Castillo, L.; Israels, T.; Jeha, S.; Harif, M.; Sullivan, M.J.; et al. Toward the Cure of All Children With Cancer Through Collaborative Efforts: Pediatric Oncology As a Global Challenge. *J. Clin. Oncol.* **2015**, *33*, 3065–3073. [CrossRef]
4. Bhakta, N.; Force, L.M.; Allemani, C.; Atun, R.; Bray, F.; Coleman, M.P.; Steliarova-Foucher, E.; Frazier, A.L.; Robison, L.L.; Rodriguez-Galindo, C.; et al. Childhood cancer burden: A review of global estimates. *Lancet Oncol.* **2019**, *20*, e42–e53. [CrossRef]
5. Atun, R.; Bhakta, N.; Denburg, A.; Frazier, A.L.; Friedrich, P.; Gupta, S.; Lam, C.G.; Ward, Z.J.; Yeh, J.M.; Allemani, C.; et al. Sustainable care for children with cancer: A Lancet Oncology Commission. *Lancet Oncol.* **2020**, *21*, e185–e224. [CrossRef]
6. Locatelli, F.; Schrappe, M.; Bernardo, M.E.; Rutella, S. How I treat relapsed childhood acute lymphoblastic leukemia. *Blood* **2012**, *120*, 2807–2816. [CrossRef]
7. Arora, R.S.; Challinor, J.M.; Howard, S.C.; Israels, T. Improving Care for Children With Cancer in Low- and Middle-Income Countries—A SIOP PODC Initiative. *Pediatr. Blood Cancer* **2016**, *63*, 387–391. [CrossRef]
8. Suarez, A.; Pina, M.; Nichols-Vinueza, D.X.; Lopera, J.; Rengifo, L.; Mesa, M.; Cardenas, M.; Morrissey, L.; Veintemilla, G.; Vizcaino, M.; et al. A strategy to improve treatment-related mortality and abandonment of therapy for childhood ALL in a developing country reveals the impact of treatment delays. *Pediatr. Blood Cancer* **2015**, *62*, 1395–1402. [CrossRef]
9. Ladas, E.J.; Arora, B.; Howard, S.C.; Rogers, P.C.; Mosby, T.T.; Barr, R.D. A Framework for Adapted Nutritional Therapy for Children With Cancer in Low- and Middle-Income Countries: A Report From the SIOP PODC Nutrition Working Group. *Pediatr. Blood Cancer* **2016**, *63*, 1339–1348. [CrossRef] [PubMed]
10. Israels, T.; Renner, L.; Hendricks, M.; Hesseling, P.; Howard, S.; Molyneux, E.; Paediatric Oncology in Developing Countries. SIOP PODC: Recommendations for supportive care of children with cancer in a low-income setting. *Pediatr. Blood Cancer* **2013**, *60*, 899–904. [CrossRef] [PubMed]
11. Ariffin, H.; Navaratnam, P.; Kee, T.K.; Balan, G. Antibiotic resistance patterns in nosocomial gram-negative bacterial infections in units with heavy antibiotic usage. *J. Trop. Pediatr.* **2004**, *50*, 26–31. [CrossRef] [PubMed]
12. Ariffin, H.; Ab Rahman, S.; Leong, S.H.; Chiew, E.K.-H.; Lin, H.P.; Quah, T.C.; Yeoh, A.E.-J. Malaysia-Singapore (MASPORE) leukaemia study group: From common history to successful collaboration. *Pediatr. Hematol. Oncol. J.* **2020**, *5*, 11–16. [CrossRef]
13. Inaba, H.; Mullighan, C.G. Pediatric acute lymphoblastic leukemia. *Haematologica* **2020**, *105*, 2524–2539. [CrossRef]
14. Pedrosa, F.; Coustan-Smith, E.; Zhou, Y.; Cheng, C.; Pedrosa, A.; Lins, M.M.; Pedrosa, M.; Lucena-Silva, N.; Ramos, A.M.L.; Vinhas, E.; et al. Reduced-dose intensity therapy for pediatric lymphoblastic leukemia: Long-term results of the Recife RELLA05 pilot study. *Blood* **2020**, *135*, 1458–1466. [CrossRef]
15. Narula, G.; Prasad, M.; Jatia, S.; Subramanian, P.G.; Patkar, N.; Tembhare, P.; Shetty, D.; Khanna, N.; Laskar, S.; Shet, T.; et al. Clinicoepidemiological profiles, clinical practices, and the impact of holistic care interventions on outcomes of pediatric hematolymphoid malignancies—A 7-year audit of the pediatric hematolymphoid disease management group at Tata Memorial Hospital. *Indian J. Cancer* **2017**, *54*, 609–615. [CrossRef]
16. Stary, J.; Zimmermann, M.; Campbell, M.; Castillo, L.; Dibar, E.; Donska, S.; Gonzalez, A.; Izraeli, S.; Janic, D.; Jazbec, J.; et al. Intensive chemotherapy for childhood acute lymphoblastic leukemia: Results of the randomized intercontinental trial ALL IC-BFM 2002. *J. Clin. Oncol.* **2014**, *32*, 174–184. [CrossRef]
17. Cui, L.; Li, Z.G.; Chai, Y.H.; Yu, J.; Gao, J.; Zhu, X.F.; Jin, R.M.; Shi, X.D.; Zhang, L.P.; Gao, Y.J.; et al. Outcome of children with newly diagnosed acute lymphoblastic leukemia treated with CCLG-ALL 2008: The first nation-wide prospective multicenter study in China. *Am. J. Hematol.* **2018**, *93*, 913–920. [CrossRef]
18. Yeoh, A.E.; Ariffin, H.; Chai, E.L.; Kwok, C.S.; Chan, Y.H.; Ponnudurai, K.; Campana, D.; Tan, P.L.; Chan, M.Y.; Kham, S.K.; et al. Minimal residual disease-guided treatment deintensification for children with acute lymphoblastic leukemia: Results from the Malaysia-Singapore acute lymphoblastic leukemia 2003 study. *J. Clin. Oncol.* **2012**, *30*, 2384–2392. [CrossRef] [PubMed]
19. Yeoh, A.E.J.; Lu, Y.; Chin, W.H.N.; Chiew, E.K.H.; Lim, E.H.; Li, Z.; Kham, S.K.Y.; Chan, Y.H.; Abdullah, W.A.; Lin, H.P.; et al. Intensifying Treatment of Childhood B-Lymphoblastic Leukemia With IKZF1 Deletion Reduces Relapse and Improves Overall Survival: Results of Malaysia-Singapore ALL 2010 Study. *J. Clin. Oncol.* **2018**, *36*, 2726–2735. [CrossRef] [PubMed]
20. Schrappe, M.; Bleckmann, K.; Zimmermann, M.; Biondi, A.; Moricke, A.; Locatelli, F.; Cario, G.; Rizzari, C.; Attarbaschi, A.; Valsecchi, M.G.; et al. Reduced-Intensity Delayed Intensification in Standard-Risk Pediatric Acute Lymphoblastic Leukemia Defined by Undetectable Minimal Residual Disease: Results of an International Randomized Trial (AIEOP-BFM ALL 2000). *J. Clin. Oncol.* **2018**, *36*, 244–253. [CrossRef]
21. Schramm, F.; Zur Stadt, U.; Zimmermann, M.; Jorch, N.; Pekrun, A.; Borkhardt, A.; Imschweiler, T.; Christiansen, H.; Faber, J.; Schmid, I.; et al. Results of CoALL 07-03 study childhood ALL based on combined risk assessment by in vivo and in vitro pharmacosensitivity. *Blood Adv.* **2019**, *3*, 3688–3699. [CrossRef]
22. Schore, R.J.; Angiolillo, A.J.; Kairalla, J.A.; Devidas, M.; Rabin, K.R.; Zweidler-McKay, P.A.; Borowitz, M.J.; Wood, B.L.; Carroll, A.J.; Heerema, N.A.; et al. Outcomes with reduced intensity therapy in a low-risk subset of children with National Cancer Institute (NCI) standard-risk (SR) B-lymphoblastic leukemia (B-ALL): A report from Children's Oncology Group (COG) AALL0932. *J. Clin. Oncol.* **2020**, *38*, 10509. [CrossRef]
23. Mattano, L.A., Jr.; Devidas, M.; Maloney, K.W.; Wang, C.; Friedmann, A.M.; Buckley, P.; Borowitz, M.J.; Carroll, A.J.; Gastier-Foster, J.M.; Heerema, N.A.; et al. Favorable Trisomies and ETV6-RUNX1 Predict Cure in Low-Risk B-Cell Acute Lymphoblastic Leukemia: Results From Children's Oncology Group Trial AALL0331. *J. Clin. Oncol.* **2021**, *39*, 1540–1552. [CrossRef] [PubMed]

24. Pieters, R.; de Groot-Kruseman, H.; Van der Velden, V.; Fiocco, M.; van den Berg, H.; de Bont, E.; Egeler, R.M.; Hoogerbrugge, P.; Kaspers, G.; Van der Schoot, E.; et al. Successful Therapy Reduction and Intensification for Childhood Acute Lymphoblastic Leukemia Based on Minimal Residual Disease Monitoring: Study ALL10 From the Dutch Childhood Oncology Group. *J. Clin. Oncol.* **2016**, *34*, 2591–2601. [CrossRef]
25. Hasegawa, D.; Imamura, T.; Yumura-Yagi, K.; Takahashi, Y.; Usami, I.; Suenobu, S.I.; Nishimura, S.; Suzuki, N.; Hashii, Y.; Deguchi, T.; et al. Risk-adjusted therapy for pediatric non-T cell ALL improves outcomes for standard risk patients: Results of JACLS ALL-02. *Blood Cancer J.* **2020**, *10*, 23. [CrossRef] [PubMed]
26. Jeha, S.; Pei, D.; Choi, J.; Cheng, C.; Sandlund, J.T.; Coustan-Smith, E.; Campana, D.; Inaba, H.; Rubnitz, J.E.; Ribeiro, R.C.; et al. Improved CNS Control of Childhood Acute Lymphoblastic Leukemia Without Cranial Irradiation: St Jude Total Therapy Study 16. *J. Clin. Oncol.* **2019**, *37*, 3377–3391. [CrossRef]
27. Vora, A.; Goulden, N.; Wade, R.; Mitchell, C.; Hancock, J.; Hough, R.; Rowntree, C.; Richards, S. Treatment reduction for children and young adults with low-risk acute lymphoblastic leukaemia defined by minimal residual disease (UKALL 2003): A randomised controlled trial. *Lancet Oncol.* **2013**, *14*, 199–209. [CrossRef]
28. Attarbaschi, A.; Mann, G.; Dworzak, M.; Wiesbauer, P.; Schrappe, M.; Gadner, H. Mediastinal mass in childhood T-cell acute lymphoblastic leukemia: Significance and therapy response. *Med. Pediatr. Oncol.* **2002**, *39*, 558–565. [CrossRef]
29. Pommert, L.; Tasian, S.K. Chemotherapy Drug Shortages in Pediatric Oncology: A Global Public Health Crisis Threatening Our Children. *Hematologist* **2021**. [CrossRef]
30. Cohen, P.; Friedrich, P.; Lam, C.; Jeha, S.; Metzger, M.L.; Qaddoumi, I.; Naidu, P.; Faughnan, L.; Rodriguez-Galindo, C.; Bhakta, N. Global Access to Essential Medicines for Childhood Cancer: A Cross-Sectional Survey. *J. Glob. Oncol.* **2018**, *4*, 1–11. [CrossRef]
31. Howard, S.C.; Davidson, A.; Luna-Fineman, S.; Israels, T.; Chantada, G.; Lam, C.G.; Hunger, S.P.; Bailey, S.; Ribeiro, R.C.; Arora, R.S.; et al. A framework to develop adapted treatment regimens to manage pediatric cancer in low- and middle-income countries: The Pediatric Oncology in Developing Countries (PODC) Committee of the International Pediatric Oncology Society (SIOP). *Pediatr. Blood Cancer* **2017**, *64* (Suppl. S5), e26879. [CrossRef]
32. Loh, L.H.; Chen, S.P.; Quah, T.C.; Yeoh, A.E.; Ariffin, H. Real-time quantitative polymerase chain reaction (RQ-PCR) using the LightCycler: A rapid, high-throughput method for detecting and quantifying fusion transcripts in childhood leukaemias for disease stratification and prognostication. *Ann. Acad. Med. Singap.* **2003**, *32*, S18–S21. [PubMed]
33. Ibrahim, K.; Daud, S.S.; Seah, Y.L.; Yeoh, A.; Ariffin, H.; Malaysia-Singapore Leukemia Study, G. Rapid detection of prognostically important childhood acute lymphoblastic leukemia chimeric transcripts using multiplex SYBR green real-time reverse transcription PCR. *Ann. Clin. Lab. Sci.* **2008**, *38*, 338–343.
34. Lee, S.H.R.; Li, Z.; Tai, S.T.; Oh, B.L.Z.; Yeoh, A.E.J. Genetic Alterations in Childhood Acute Lymphoblastic Leukemia: Interactions with Clinical Features and Treatment Response. *Cancers* **2021**, *13*, 4068. [CrossRef]
35. Smith, M.; Arthur, D.; Camitta, B.; Carroll, A.J.; Crist, W.; Gaynon, P.; Gelber, R.; Heerema, N.; Korn, E.L.; Link, M.; et al. Uniform approach to risk classification and treatment assignment for children with acute lymphoblastic leukemia. *J. Clin. Oncol.* **1996**, *14*, 18–24. [CrossRef]
36. Moricke, A.; Zimmermann, M.; Valsecchi, M.G.; Stanulla, M.; Biondi, A.; Mann, G.; Locatelli, F.; Cazzaniga, G.; Niggli, F.; Arico, M.; et al. Dexamethasone vs prednisone in induction treatment of pediatric ALL: Results of the randomized trial AIEOP-BFM ALL 2000. *Blood* **2016**, *127*, 2101–2112. [CrossRef]
37. Maloney, K.W.; Devidas, M.; Wang, C.; Mattano, L.A.; Friedmann, A.M.; Buckley, P.; Borowitz, M.J.; Carroll, A.J.; Gastier-Foster, J.M.; Heerema, N.A.; et al. Outcome in Children With Standard-Risk B-Cell Acute Lymphoblastic Leukemia: Results of Children's Oncology Group Trial AALL0331. *J. Clin. Oncol.* **2020**, *38*, 602–612. [CrossRef]
38. Parihar, M.; Singh, M.K.; Islam, R.; Saha, D.; Mishra, D.K.; Saha, V.; Krishnan, S. A triple-probe FISH screening strategy for risk-stratified therapy of acute lymphoblastic leukaemia in low-resource settings. *Pediatr. Blood Cancer* **2018**, *65*, e27366. [CrossRef] [PubMed]
39. Sharma, P.; Rana, S.; Sreedharanunni, S.; Gautam, A.; Sachdeva, M.U.S.; Naseem, S.; Varma, N.; Jain, R.; Bansal, D.; Trehan, A. An Evaluation of a Fluorescence In Situ Hybridization Strategy Using Air-dried Blood and Bone-marrow Smears in the Risk Stratification of Pediatric B-Lineage Acute Lymphoblastic Leukemia in Resource-limited Settings. *J. Pediatr. Hematol. Oncol.* **2021**, *43*, e481–e485. [CrossRef]
40. O'Connor, D.; Moorman, A.V.; Wade, R.; Hancock, J.; Tan, R.M.; Bartram, J.; Moppett, J.; Schwab, C.; Patrick, K.; Harrison, C.J.; et al. Use of Minimal Residual Disease Assessment to Redefine Induction Failure in Pediatric Acute Lymphoblastic Leukemia. *J. Clin. Oncol.* **2017**, *35*, 660–667. [CrossRef] [PubMed]
41. Coustan-Smith, E.; Ribeiro, R.C.; Stow, P.; Zhou, Y.; Pui, C.H.; Rivera, G.K.; Pedrosa, F.; Campana, D. A simplified flow cytometric assay identifies children with acute lymphoblastic leukemia who have a superior clinical outcome. *Blood* **2006**, *108*, 97–102. [CrossRef]
42. Vinhas, E.; Lucena-Silva, N.; Pedrosa, F. Implementation of a simplified flow cytometric assays for minimal residual disease monitoring in childhood acute lymphoblastic leukemia. *Cytometry B Clin. Cytom.* **2018**, *94*, 94–99. [CrossRef]
43. Sidhom, I.; Shaaban, K.; Youssef, S.H.; Ali, N.; Gohar, S.; Rashed, W.M.; Mehanna, M.; Salem, S.; Soliman, S.; Yassin, D.; et al. Reduced-intensity therapy for pediatric lymphoblastic leukemia: Impact of residual disease early in remission induction. *Blood* **2021**, *137*, 20–28. [CrossRef] [PubMed]

44. Winter, S.S.; Dunsmore, K.P.; Devidas, M.; Wood, B.L.; Esiashvili, N.; Chen, Z.; Eisenberg, N.; Briegel, N.; Hayashi, R.J.; Gastier-Foster, J.M.; et al. Improved Survival for Children and Young Adults With T-Lineage Acute Lymphoblastic Leukemia: Results From the Children's Oncology Group AALL0434 Methotrexate Randomization. *J. Clin. Oncol.* **2018**, *36*, 2926–2934. [CrossRef] [PubMed]
45. Pui, C.H.; Campana, D.; Pei, D.; Bowman, W.P.; Sandlund, J.T.; Kaste, S.C.; Ribeiro, R.C.; Rubnitz, J.E.; Raimondi, S.C.; Onciu, M.; et al. Treating childhood acute lymphoblastic leukemia without cranial irradiation. *N. Engl. J. Med.* **2009**, *360*, 2730–2741. [CrossRef] [PubMed]
46. Manabe, A.; Tsuchida, M.; Hanada, R.; Ikuta, K.; Toyoda, Y.; Okimoto, Y.; Ishimoto, K.; Okawa, H.; Ohara, A.; Kaneko, T.; et al. Delay of the diagnostic lumbar puncture and intrathecal chemotherapy in children with acute lymphoblastic leukemia who undergo routine corticosteroid testing: Tokyo Children's Cancer Study Group study L89-12. *J. Clin. Oncol.* **2001**, *19*, 3182–3187. [CrossRef] [PubMed]
47. Yeh, T.C.; Liang, D.C.; Hou, J.Y.; Jaing, T.H.; Lin, D.T.; Yang, C.P.; Peng, C.T.; Hung, I.J.; Lin, K.H.; Hsiao, C.C.; et al. Treatment of childhood acute lymphoblastic leukemia with delayed first intrathecal therapy and omission of prophylactic cranial irradiation: Results of the TPOG-ALL-2002 study. *Cancer* **2018**, *124*, 4538–4547. [CrossRef]
48. Teuffel, O.; Kuster, S.P.; Hunger, S.P.; Conter, V.; Hitzler, J.; Ethier, M.C.; Shah, P.S.; Beyene, J.; Sung, L. Dexamethasone versus prednisone for induction therapy in childhood acute lymphoblastic leukemia: A systematic review and meta-analysis. *Leukemia* **2011**, *25*, 1232–1238. [CrossRef]
49. Igarashi, S.; Manabe, A.; Ohara, A.; Kumagai, M.; Saito, T.; Okimoto, Y.; Kamijo, T.; Isoyama, K.; Kajiwara, M.; Sotomatsu, M.; et al. No advantage of dexamethasone over prednisolone for the outcome of standard- and intermediate-risk childhood acute lymphoblastic leukemia in the Tokyo Children's Cancer Study Group L95-14 protocol. *J. Clin. Oncol.* **2005**, *23*, 6489–6498. [CrossRef]
50. Hurwitz, C.A.; Silverman, L.B.; Schorin, M.A.; Clavell, L.A.; Dalton, V.K.; Glick, K.M.; Gelber, R.D.; Sallan, S.E. Substituting dexamethasone for prednisone complicates remission induction in children with acute lymphoblastic leukemia. *Cancer* **2000**, *88*, 1964–1969. [CrossRef]
51. Mitchell, C.D.; Richards, S.M.; Kinsey, S.E.; Lilleyman, J.; Vora, A.; Eden, T.O.; Medical Research Council Childhood Leukaemia Working Party. Benefit of dexamethasone compared with prednisolone for childhood acute lymphoblastic leukaemia: Results of the UK Medical Research Council ALL97 randomized trial. *Br. J. Haematol.* **2005**, *129*, 734–745. [CrossRef]
52. Oh, B.L.Z.; Lee, S.H.R.; Foo, K.M.; Chiew, K.H.; Seeto, Z.Z.L.; Chen, Z.W.; Neoh, C.C.C.; Liew, G.S.M.; Eng, J.J.; Lam, J.C.M.; et al. Successful toxicity reduction during delayed intensification in the non-high-risk arm of Malaysia-Singapore Acute Lymphoblastic Leukaemia 2010 study. *Eur. J. Cancer* **2021**, *142*, 92–101. [CrossRef] [PubMed]
53. Merryman, R.; Stevenson, K.E.; Gostic, W.J., 2nd; Neuberg, D.; O'Brien, J.; Sallan, S.E.; Silverman, L.B. Asparaginase-associated myelosuppression and effects on dosing of other chemotherapeutic agents in childhood acute lymphoblastic leukemia. *Pediatr. Blood Cancer* **2012**, *59*, 925–927. [CrossRef] [PubMed]
54. Bhakta, N.; Liu, Q.; Ness, K.K.; Baassiri, M.; Eissa, H.; Yeo, F.; Chemaitilly, W.; Ehrhardt, M.J.; Bass, J.; Bishop, M.W.; et al. The cumulative burden of surviving childhood cancer: An initial report from the St Jude Lifetime Cohort Study (SJLIFE). *Lancet* **2017**, *390*, 2569–2582. [CrossRef]
55. Suh, E.; Stratton, K.L.; Leisenring, W.M.; Nathan, P.C.; Ford, J.S.; Freyer, D.R.; McNeer, J.L.; Stock, W.; Stovall, M.; Krull, K.R.; et al. Late mortality and chronic health conditions in long-term survivors of early-adolescent and young adult cancers: A retrospective cohort analysis from the Childhood Cancer Survivor Study. *Lancet Oncol.* **2020**, *21*, 421–435. [CrossRef]
56. Tubergen, D.G.; Gilchrist, G.S.; O'Brien, R.T.; Coccia, P.F.; Sather, H.N.; Waskerwitz, M.J.; Hammond, G.D. Improved outcome with delayed intensification for children with acute lymphoblastic leukemia and intermediate presenting features: A Childrens Cancer Group phase III trial. *J. Clin. Oncol.* **1993**, *11*, 527–537. [CrossRef]
57. Khera, S.; Kapoor, R.; Pramanik, S.K. Solitary serum methotrexate level 36 hours post high-dose methotrexate: A safe, efficacious, and cost-effective strategy to monitor methotrexate toxicities in childhood leukemia in resource-limited centers. *Pediatr. Blood Cancer* **2020**, *67*, e28387. [CrossRef]
58. Dhingra, H.; Kalra, M.; Mahajan, A. Safe administration of high-dose methotrexate with minimal drug level monitoring: Experience from a center in north India. *Pediatr. Blood Cancer* **2020**, *67*, e28394. [CrossRef]
59. Larsen, E.C.; Devidas, M.; Chen, S.; Salzer, W.L.; Raetz, E.A.; Loh, M.L.; Mattano, L.A., Jr.; Cole, C.; Eicher, A.; Haugan, M.; et al. Dexamethasone and High-Dose Methotrexate Improve Outcome for Children and Young Adults With High-Risk B-Acute Lymphoblastic Leukemia: A Report From Children's Oncology Group Study AALL0232. *J. Clin. Oncol.* **2016**, *34*, 2380–2388. [CrossRef]
60. Matloub, Y.; Bostrom, B.C.; Hunger, S.P.; Stork, L.C.; Angiolillo, A.; Sather, H.; La, M.; Gastier-Foster, J.M.; Heerema, N.A.; Sailer, S.; et al. Escalating intravenous methotrexate improves event-free survival in children with standard-risk acute lymphoblastic leukemia: A report from the Children's Oncology Group. *Blood* **2011**, *118*, 243–251. [CrossRef]
61. Inaba, H.; Pei, D.; Wolf, J.; Howard, S.C.; Hayden, R.T.; Go, M.; Varechtchouk, O.; Hahn, T.; Buaboonnam, J.; Metzger, M.L.; et al. Infection-related complications during treatment for childhood acute lymphoblastic leukemia. *Ann. Oncol.* **2017**, *28*, 386–392. [CrossRef] [PubMed]

62. O'Connor, D.; Bate, J.; Wade, R.; Clack, R.; Dhir, S.; Hough, R.; Vora, A.; Goulden, N.; Samarasinghe, S. Infection-related mortality in children with acute lymphoblastic leukemia: An analysis of infectious deaths on UKALL2003. *Blood* **2014**, *124*, 1056–1061. [CrossRef] [PubMed]
63. Vora, A. *Childhood Acute Lymphoblastic Leukemia, Chapter: Developing World Perspective*; Springer: Cham, Switzerland, 2017; pp. 323–336. [CrossRef]
64. Schmiegelow, K. Maintenance therapy of childhood acute lymphoblastic leukemia: Do all roads lead to Rome? *Pediatr. Blood Cancer* **2020**, *67*, e28418. [CrossRef] [PubMed]
65. Hunger, S.P.; Mullighan, C.G. Acute Lymphoblastic Leukemia in Children. *N. Engl. J. Med.* **2015**, *373*, 1541–1552. [CrossRef] [PubMed]
66. Duration and intensity of maintenance chemotherapy in acute lymphoblastic leukaemia: Overview of 42 trials involving 12,000 randomised children. *Lancet* **1996**, *347*, 1783–1788. [CrossRef]
67. Teachey, D.T.; Hunger, S.P.; Loh, M.L. Optimizing therapy in the modern age: Differences in length of maintenance therapy in acute lymphoblastic leukemia. *Blood* **2021**, *137*, 168–177. [CrossRef] [PubMed]
68. Liang, D.C.; Yang, C.P.; Lin, D.T.; Hung, I.J.; Lin, K.H.; Chen, J.S.; Hsiao, C.C.; Chang, T.T.; Peng, C.T.; Lin, M.T.; et al. Long-term results of Taiwan Pediatric Oncology Group studies 1997 and 2002 for childhood acute lymphoblastic leukemia. *Leukemia* **2010**, *24*, 397–405. [CrossRef] [PubMed]
69. Kato, M.; Ishimaru, S.; Seki, M.; Yoshida, K.; Shiraishi, Y.; Chiba, K.; Kakiuchi, N.; Sato, Y.; Ueno, H.; Tanaka, H.; et al. Long-term outcome of 6-month maintenance chemotherapy for acute lymphoblastic leukemia in children. *Leukemia* **2017**, *31*, 580–584. [CrossRef]
70. Toyoda, Y.; Manabe, A.; Tsuchida, M.; Hanada, R.; Ikuta, K.; Okimoto, Y.; Ohara, A.; Ohkawa, Y.; Mori, T.; Ishimoto, K.; et al. Six months of maintenance chemotherapy after intensified treatment for acute lymphoblastic leukemia of childhood. *J. Clin. Oncol.* **2000**, *18*, 1508–1516. [CrossRef]
71. Moricke, A.; Zimmermann, M.; Reiter, A.; Henze, G.; Schrauder, A.; Gadner, H.; Ludwig, W.D.; Ritter, J.; Harbott, J.; Mann, G.; et al. Long-term results of five consecutive trials in childhood acute lymphoblastic leukemia performed by the ALL-BFM study group from 1981 to 2000. *Leukemia* **2010**, *24*, 265–284. [CrossRef]
72. Brandalise, S.R.; Pinheiro, V.R.; Aguiar, S.S.; Matsuda, E.I.; Otubo, R.; Yunes, J.A.; Pereira, W.V.; Carvalho, E.G.; Cristofani, L.M.; Souza, M.S.; et al. Benefits of the intermittent use of 6-mercaptopurine and methotrexate in maintenance treatment for low-risk acute lymphoblastic leukemia in children: Randomized trial from the Brazilian Childhood Cooperative Group-protocol ALL-99. *J. Clin. Oncol.* **2010**, *28*, 1911–1918. [CrossRef] [PubMed]
73. Eden, T.; Pieters, R.; Richards, S.; Childhood Acute Lymphoblastic Leukaemia Collaborative Group. Systematic review of the addition of vincristine plus steroid pulses in maintenance treatment for childhood acute lymphoblastic leukaemia—An individual patient data meta-analysis involving 5659 children. *Br. J. Haematol* **2010**, *149*, 722–733. [CrossRef] [PubMed]
74. Conter, V.; Valsecchi, M.G.; Silvestri, D.; Campbell, M.; Dibar, E.; Magyarosy, E.; Gadner, H.; Stary, J.; Benoit, Y.; Zimmermann, M.; et al. Pulses of vincristine and dexamethasone in addition to intensive chemotherapy for children with intermediate-risk acute lymphoblastic leukaemia: A multicentre randomised trial. *Lancet* **2007**, *369*, 123–131. [CrossRef]
75. Yang, W.; Cai, J.; Shen, S.; Gao, J.; Yu, J.; Hu, S.; Jiang, H.; Fang, Y.; Liang, C.; Ju, X.; et al. Pulse therapy with vincristine and dexamethasone for childhood acute lymphoblastic leukaemia (CCCG-ALL-2015): An open-label, multicentre, randomised, phase 3, non-inferiority trial. *Lancet Oncol.* **2021**, *29*, 1322–1332. [CrossRef]
76. De Moerloose, B.; Suciu, S.; Bertrand, Y.; Mazingue, F.; Robert, A.; Uyttebroeck, A.; Yakouben, K.; Ferster, A.; Margueritte, G.; Lutz, P.; et al. Improved outcome with pulses of vincristine and corticosteroids in continuation therapy of children with average risk acute lymphoblastic leukemia (ALL) and lymphoblastic non-Hodgkin lymphoma (NHL): Report of the EORTC randomized phase 3 trial 58,951. *Blood* **2010**, *116*, 36–44. [CrossRef]
77. Angiolillo, A.L.; Schore, R.J.; Kairalla, J.A.; Devidas, M.; Rabin, K.R.; Zweidler-McKay, P.; Borowitz, M.J.; Wood, B.; Carroll, A.J.; Heerema, N.A.; et al. Excellent Outcomes With Reduced Frequency of Vincristine and Dexamethasone Pulses in Standard-Risk B-Lymphoblastic Leukemia: Results From Children's Oncology Group AALL0932. *J. Clin. Oncol.* **2021**, *39*, 1437–1447. [CrossRef]
78. Jeha, S.; Choi, J.; Roberts, K.G.; Pei, D.; Coustan-Smith, E.; Inaba, H.; Rubnitz, J.E.; Ribeiro, R.C.; Gruber, T.A.; Raimondi, S.C.; et al. Clinical significance of novel subtypes of acute lymphoblastic leukemia in the context of minimal residual disease-directed therapy. *Blood Cancer Discov.* **2021**, *2*, 326–337. [CrossRef]
79. Relling, M.V.; Hancock, M.L.; Rivera, G.K.; Sandlund, J.T.; Ribeiro, R.C.; Krynetski, E.Y.; Pui, C.H.; Evans, W.E. Mercaptopurine therapy intolerance and heterozygosity at the thiopurine S-methyltransferase gene locus. *J. Natl. Cancer Inst.* **1999**, *91*, 2001–2008. [CrossRef] [PubMed]
80. Evans, W.E.; Hon, Y.Y.; Bomgaars, L.; Coutre, S.; Holdsworth, M.; Janco, R.; Kalwinsky, D.; Keller, F.; Khatib, Z.; Margolin, J.; et al. Preponderance of thiopurine S-methyltransferase deficiency and heterozygosity among patients intolerant to mercaptopurine or azathioprine. *J. Clin. Oncol.* **2001**, *19*, 2293–2301. [CrossRef]
81. Cai, J.-P.; Ishibashi, T.; Takagi, Y.; Hayakawa, H.; Sekiguchi, M. Mouse MTH2 protein which prevents mutations caused by 8-oxoguanine nucleotides. *Biochem. Biophys. Res. Commun.* **2003**, *305*, 1073–1077. [CrossRef]
82. Takagi, Y.; Setoyama, D.; Ito, R.; Kamiya, H.; Yamagata, Y.; Sekiguchi, M. Human MTH3 (NUDT18) protein hydrolyzes oxidized forms of guanosine and deoxyguanosine diphosphates: Comparison with MTH1 and MTH2. *J. Biol. Chem.* **2012**, *287*, 21541–21549. [CrossRef]

83. Saiz-Rodriguez, M.; Ochoa, D.; Belmonte, C.; Roman, M.; Martinez-Ingelmo, C.; Ortega-Ruiz, L.; Sarmiento-Iglesias, C.; Herrador, C.; Abad-Santos, F. Influence of thiopurine S-methyltransferase polymorphisms in mercaptopurine pharmacokinetics in healthy volunteers. *Basic Clin. Pharmacol. Toxicol.* **2019**, *124*, 449–455. [CrossRef] [PubMed]
84. Yang, J.J.; Landier, W.; Yang, W.; Liu, C.; Hageman, L.; Cheng, C.; Pei, D.; Chen, Y.; Crews, K.R.; Kornegay, N.; et al. Inherited NUDT15 variant is a genetic determinant of mercaptopurine intolerance in children with acute lymphoblastic leukemia. *J. Clin. Oncol.* **2015**, *33*, 1235–1242. [CrossRef] [PubMed]
85. Relling, M.V.; Schwab, M.; Whirl-Carrillo, M.; Suarez-Kurtz, G.; Pui, C.H.; Stein, C.M.; Moyer, A.M.; Evans, W.E.; Klein, T.E.; Antillon-Klussmann, F.G.; et al. Clinical Pharmacogenetics Implementation Consortium Guideline for Thiopurine Dosing Based on TPMT and NUDT15 Genotypes: 2018 Update. *Clin. Pharmacol. Ther.* **2019**, *105*, 1095–1105. [CrossRef] [PubMed]

Review

Pediatric Acute Myeloid Leukemia—Past, Present, and Future

Dirk Reinhardt *,†, Evangelia Antoniou † and Katharina Waack †

Pediatrics III, Department of Pediatric Hematology, Oncology and Stem Cell Therapy, University Children's Hospital, University Duisburg, 45147 Essen, Germany; Evangelia.Antoniou@uk-essen.de (E.A.); katharina.waack@uk-essen.de (K.W.)
* Correspondence: dirk.reinhardt@uk-essen.de
† AML-BFM Study Group—German Society of Pediatric Oncology/Hematology (GPOH).

Abstract: This review reports about the main steps of development in pediatric acute myeloid leukemia (AML) concerning diagnostics, treatment, risk groups, and outcomes. Finally, a short overview of present and future approaches is given.

Keywords: acute myeloid leukemia; children; treatment; prognosis

1. Introduction

The treatment of pediatric acute myeloid leukemia (AML) is a success story in improving prognosis. Whereas, in the 1980s, almost all children suffering from AML died, today, up to 75% of the children survive. However, this is only feasible in a well-structured setting of comprehensive diagnostics, intensive therapy, and effective supportive care. This has been achieved by the cooperative study groups in Europe, North America, and Japan. By contrast, even within Europe, the prognosis of children with AML shows an unacceptable level of inequality of survival rates, ranging from less than 50% to 80% [1].

The incidence of pediatric AML is about seven per million, with only minor differences between continents or countries. The malignant blasts originate from early hematopoietic progenitors as an evolution from (pre-)leukemia stem cells. External/environmental factors could explain only a tiny percentage. In addition, predisposing syndromes or germline mutations are associated with less than 10% of pediatric AML. During childhood and adolescence, infants less than two years old and adolescents have the highest incidence. Whereas MLL-rearranged leukemia dominates during infancy, the frequency of core-binding leukemia (CBL) and AML associated with mutations, such as NPM 1 or FLT3-ITD, increases by age [2].

Except for acute promyeloblastic leukemia (APL), improved survival has been achieved by using long-known conventional drugs, mainly cytarabine and anthracyclines. Scheduling risk group stratification, modifications of allogeneic stem cell transplant (alloHSCT), and management of complications allowed for curing most children (Figure 1) [3,4].

The only new approach within the most recent 20 years was the targeted CD33 antibody gemtuzumab ozogamicin (GO), which showed some advantages in at least one randomized trial, but GO is only approved in North America [5].

The successful therapy of APL with all-trans retinoic acid and arsenic-trioxide is a rare example of curing leukemia targeting specifically leukemia-inducing molecular mechanisms and eradicating the leukemic stem cell [5,6].

Liposomal drug formulation of daunoribiicn allowed treatment intensification without increasing toxicities, but this has disappeared due to economic reasons, such as a limited pediatric market. The actual approach with a liposomal nanoscale co-formulation of cytarabine and daunorubicin seems to be promising but needs confirmatory trials in pediatric AML and marketing approval thereof.

Although stem cell transplantation is still an unspecific treatment option with severe acute and long-term side effects, combined with a better risk group stratification, alloHSCT significantly improved survival in children with high-risk (HR) AML [7,8].

There are a broad number of new compounds explicitly targeting signaling pathways. However, it is not confirmed in children to what extent these approaches will contribute to curing or be able to reduce toxicities by allowing reduction of treatment intensity of conventional drugs.

A fast-growing field are immune and cellular therapies, which show promising results in preclinical and early phase clinical trials (mainly in adults).

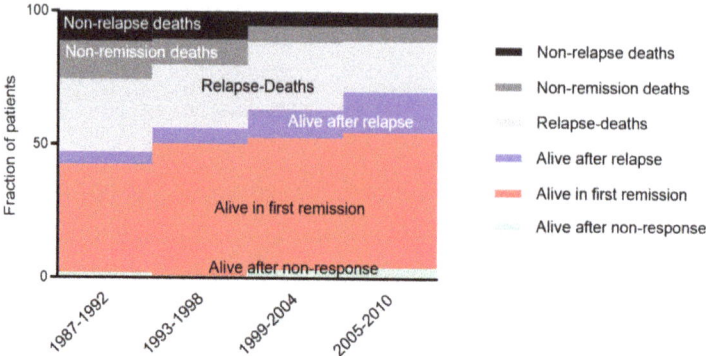

Figure 1. Improvement of outcome in pediatric AML. Continuous increase of survival in first remission (red), following initial non-response (green), and after relapse (blue). In parallel, the treatment-related mortality (black, non-relapse deaths) and non-remission deaths (grey) decreased significantly. This supported the hypothesis that the improved overall survival is based on better treatment and improved supportive care.

2. Past

Although pediatric AML has been described since the 1900s, a formal classification was established, such as in adults, in 1976 by the French-American-British (FAB)-Classification [9]. There are already six subtypes of AML that have been established and described. The regular introduction of immunophenotyping modified this morphology and cytochemistry-based classification during the 1990s [10–13]. In the WHO classification in 2001, a shift from morphology to a primarily genetically-based classification has been released and continuously extended.

Until 1968, the remission rate was inferior, and the median survival was about 1.5 months [14]. With the implementation of an intensified block therapy, including cyclophosphamide and cytarabine, a survival of 9.5 months was achieved, in 1976 [15].

Since 1975 the first clinical trials for pediatric patients with AML were initiated [16–18]. Cooperative Study groups have been established: AIEOP (Associazione Italiana di Ematologia e Oncologia Pediatrica), AML-BFM (Berlin, Frankfurt, Münster), NOPHO (Nordic Society for Pediatric Hematology and Oncology), MRC (Medical Research Council), and EORTC (European Organization of Research and Treatment of Cancer), CCG (Childhood Cancer Group), POG (Pediatric Oncology Group; merged in 2000 to COG (Children's Oncology Group); and SJCRH (St. Jude Children's Research Hospital). Whereas the MRC conducted combined pediatric and adult trials [19], the AML-BFM 78 study (1978–1983) was a pure pediatric trial to examine the application of two to six courses of daunorubicin, cytarabine, and 6-thioguanine (DAT) after a first induction of the same course [17]. In the AML 10 trial of the MRC group, the comparison of etoposide with thioguanine, as randomization from ADE versus DAT, showed no significant difference [20]. Significant progress in pediatric AML was made by the AML-BFM 83 trial, based on the introduction of block-scheduling. Within this trial, the favorable risk groups of AML with t(8; 21) and, inv(16) have been identified and confirmed in children. The same favorable cytogenetic criteria were confirmed in the MRC AML 10. As adverse characteristics, -5, -7, del(5q), abn(3q), and complex karyotype were documented [20,21].

Although most patients were defined just by morphology, due to the high correlation between FAB M2 with Auer rods and t(8;21), the presence of atypical eosinophils in FAB M4 Eo with inv(16) or, later, FAB M2 and NPM1-mutated AML allowed event-free survival (EFS) rates of 70% and more [22,23]. Interestingly, despite further intensification, this has not changed until today. In the LAME90/91 study, patients were classified into two groups dependent on whole blood count (WBC) and cytogenetics [24]. The standard risk group included t(8;21), inv(16), t(15;17) (defined as FAB M2, M4, and M3), and also patients with <100 000/µL leukocytes, initially. The AML BFM Study Group described hyperleukocytosis as a poor prognostic marker but was not used for risk stratification [25].

Within the 20th century, the relevance of anthracycline analogs has been discussed. Randomized trials, such as AML-BFM 98 and MRC 12/15, tested idarubicin versus daunorubicin or mitoxantrone. Significant achievements were the identification of idarubicin as the most effective anthracycline if applied in a 1 to 5 conversion rate compared to daunorubicin [26,27].

In the NOPHO-93, all the patients initially underwent the same treatment (ATE-Dox), but, dependent on the response after the first induction, an extra AM (cytarabine, Mitoxantrone) induction was recommended [28]. Those patients with excess blasts after the AM course received an HA2E course.

The tested antileukemic drug in the NOPHO 2004 trial was GO and did not show any significant effect on the recurrence rate of leukemia or overall survival (OS) [29]. An extra criterium of this study was the presence of mixed lineage leukemia (MLL) rearrangements other than t(9;11), suppoeritng for the first time the independent involvement of cytogenetics in the risk stratification. During this study, especially in 2009, the criteria for the high-risk (HR) patients were restricted to the poor response [7].

The St. Jude AML02 Study stratified the patients into two subgroups according to morphologic and genetic characteristics. Patients were randomized to receive daunorubicin (50 mg/m^2 on days 2, 4, and 6) and etoposide (100 mg/m^2 on days 2–6), and high-dose cytarabine (3 g/m^2 every 12 hours) [30].

The Japanese AML99 study (JPLSG) implemented a risk stratification of three groups. The initial stratification was made for the low-risk patients, and including the HR group criteria of WBC (>100.000 µL) and the age of the patients (<2 years). Additionally, the response after the first induction and the karyotype led to the allocation of the patients in the final stratification group. An alloHSCT was indicated only for the intermediate and HR groups, especially for the last group; a "not familiar" donor was suggested [31].

In the AML05 study (JPLSG), the reduced cumulative anthracycline dose (<300 mg/m^2) was tested in the low and intermediate-risk patients. At the same time, 50% of the etoposide dose was used in the AML99 protocol. A higher incidence of relapse was noticed, but the OS was not influenced [32].

In the early 2000s, international cooperative projects, analyzing a larger cohort of patients, finally defined further prognostic factors [4]. This also led to a harmonization of risk group definition worldwide. All major study groups agreed on AML with t(8;21) and inv(16) as a favorable prognostic group that could be cured with chemotherapy only [23,31]. There are still controversies about the definition and post-remission therapy of the patients belonging to the intermediate-risk group. Some groups recommend alloHSCT, while others stick to chemotherapy. In addition, the HR group was not finally defined, hence remaining heterogenous. In addition, in that period, large treatment groups failed to demonstrate the advantage of alloHSCT in the HR group [33–35].

2.1. Hematopoietic Stem Cell Transplantation

AlloHSCT was introduced in the 1980s as post-consolidation therapy in pediatric AML. Although effective in some cases, it never achieved the status as a general standard in contrast to adults. This is explained by the relevant side and long-term effects and the effective chemotherapy in children, which already allowed in the 1990s a long-term survival of about 60% [36,37]. Finally, the improved risk group stratification allowed the identification of those children who benefit. Nevertheless, it is an ongoing process to identify the pediatric AML subgroups who finally benefit from alloHSCT. This includes all associated issues, such as donor selection, prevention and treatment of graft versus host disease, management of virus reactivation, and immune reconstitution.

Between the mid-1980s and the 1990s, progress in pediatric AML was limited. Autologous HSCT or alloHSCT from a matched sibling donor have been introduced to the therapy [38,39]. Although there was a reduction of relapses, this could not be translated to improved OS. Transplant-related mortality counterbalanced the potentially increased antileukemic effect [40]. Considering the significantly higher risk of post-transplant late sequelae, long-lasting controversies about the relevance and importance of alloHSCT in first complete remission occurred [33,40–44].

In the AML-BFM 87 study and the MRC AML 12 trial, the response on day 15 after the first induction was added as a criterium for stratification [27,45]. Whereas alloHSCT was not generally recommended in the AML-BFM trial, the British study group limited alloHSCT to the intermediate and poor-risk group [27].

2.2. CNS Prophylaxis and Treatment

A monotherapy with intrathecal cytarabine was used as prophylactic therapy in the CCG-2891 and as a treatment twice a week in a total of six doses for the central nervous system (CNS) positive patients [46]. In Italy, the VAPA protocol, the first conducted study in children, also included monotherapy with cytarabine with 12 doses for all included patients [47]. Triple intrathecal therapy with methotrexate, cytarabine, and hydrocortisone was administered in the MCR AML10 and NOPHO 2004 twice a week by CNS positive patients until cerebrospinal fluid (CSF) clearance. The difference was the clearance duration after the extra intrathecal inductions, one and two weeks, respectively, for the MRC and NOPHO treatment groups [29].

In the AML-BFM-87 study, prophylactic irradiation was randomized. However, an increased rate of relapses in children without cranial irradiation led to a premature stop [45]. Since then, the AML-BFM studies have included cranial irradiation as a mandatory treatment for all patients, except those who received alloHSCT [48]. In contrast, the CCG and MRC group applied cranial irradiation only if the CSF was not cleared after the intrathecal therapy [35,49]. The standard therapy in the AML02 study of the JPLSG included triple intrathecal therapy in each course but no prophylactic cranial irradiation [31]. Based on the more intensive and CNS-effective chemotherapy, since 2012 the AML-BFM group no longer applied prophylactic cranial irradiation. Only in patients with CNS involvement is irradiation still recommended [50].

To summarize, different intrathecal therapies, such as monotherapy or triple treatment, were administered from the studies mentioned above. Cranial irradiation was excluded from the standard treatment and is now only recommended for children with CNS involvement.

2.3. Development of Minimal Residual Disease (MRD) Diagnostics

In parallel to the intensified therapy, the relevance of genetic risk groups and treatment response became obvious. Improved techniques, such as multicolor immunophenotyping and quantitative PCR, allowed a more precise response detection.

Detection of MRD by multicolor flow cytometric immunophenotyping started during the 1990s. The leukemic blasts were selected via different antigens (CD45 and CD34, CD117, CD13, CD15, CD33, etc.).

Langebrake et al. defined different response measurements within AML subtypes, including the prognostics relevance [51]. In contrast, in the SJCRH AML02 study, a higher incidence of relapse was noticed in patients with MRD 1% after the first induction and

>0.1% after the second induction. MRD was characterized as a poor prognostic factor EFS and OS [52].

In the NOPHO 2004 study, a difference in the EFS, but not in OS, comparing the MRD positive with the morphologic positive patients was noticed [53].

Within the Dutch Childhood Oncology Group (DCOG) ANLL, 97, and the MRC 12 trials, MRD levels measured by flow were prognostically favorable for the patients achieving MRD negativity after the first/second induction [54].

Polymerase chain reaction (PCR) is also used to detect MRD for different fusion transcripts. The correlation of expression with the clinical progress of the patients is supported in many studies. The data presented are promising for using this method as a sensitive diagnostic tool. The studies include a small number of patients for the specific subpopulations in the pediatric population, such as t(8;21), in(16) [55].

3. Present

The cooperative trial groups achieved significant improvements in overall survival. Table A1 (Appendix A) summarizes recent results, showing similar despite different chemotherapy schemes.

The analysis of the AML-BFM trials between 1993 and 2010 revealed a continuous improvement of OS but limited progress of EFS [50]. This suggests that 2nd line treatment plays a relevant role in explaining the increasing gap between EFS and OS [56].

Treatment regimens include initial double induction and 2- or 3-consolidation blocks. Even if the definitions vary, it is evident that about 60% of children with AML can be cured by chemotherapy only. On the other hand, a significant achievement within the ongoing trials was the establishment of a risk group dependent indication for alloHSCT in the 1st CR [4].

Along with the improvements in the transplant procedure and the option to rescue refractory AML, EFS improved [8]. A condition is supportive care to prevent and manage expected complications and more precise diagnostics to allow a genetic and response-based stratification [4].

3.1. alloHSCT

The AML-BFM Study group and the NOPHO proved that alloHSCT in the 1st CR of high-risk pediatric AML improves EFS, which is not significantly lower than intermediate-risk (IR) or standard risk (SR) [7,8]. However, due to the intensified therapy, including alloHSCT, the salvage treatment is ineffective, compared to IR/SR, resulting in a still inferior OS.

In case of relapse, all patients indicate alloHSCT in the 2nd CR. Although the prognostic characteristics of relapsed AML are impaired, the survival rate has been maintained or improved [56,57].

This allows treating the "right" patient group with the "right" intensity. In particular, the precise definition of the high-risk group by genetics and response associated with the indication of alloHSCT in the 1st CR eliminated significant differences in EFS.

To achieve this, the results of the AML-BFM 2004 trial have been re-analyzed. Based on the genetic characteristics and augmented by the treatment response to the 1st and 2nd induction, three risk groups could be defined [58].

In the AML-BFM 2012 Registry, this risk group stratification has been implemented. The NOPHO Group and others have published similar reports [7].

Figure 2 shows the improvement of the HR Group in the AML-BFM 2012 Registry, including the suspension of significant differences between the risk groups.

In addition to the improved risk group stratification, the selection of conditioning regimens, preparation of the transplanted stem cells, the donor identification and availability, and the graft-versus-host prophylaxis significantly contributed to a better outcome in the 1st/2nd CR but also in children with a refractory AML [59]. Within the de-novo AML patients who were transplanted in the 1st CR, the OS increased continuously between 1981 and 2019, documenting the improvement of the treatment approach over time (Figure 3).

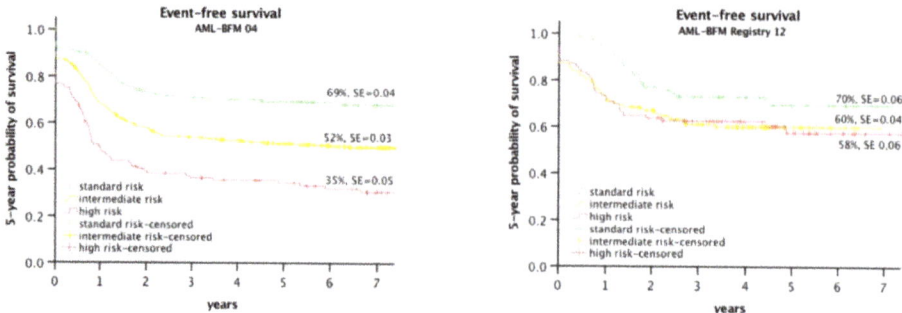

Figure 2. EFS of risk groups in Study AML-BFM 2004 [58] and AML-BFM registry 2012 [8].

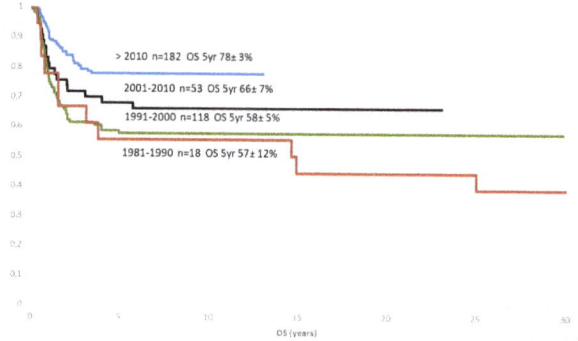

Figure 3. Increase of overall survival of children with AML and HSCT in CR1 (any donor/conditioning) since 1981; 10 year-periods (AML-BFM trials).

Most groups have accepted the standard for myeloablative conditioning with busulfan, melphalan, and cyclophosphamide. Earlier studies with less intensive conditioning (busulfan/cyclophosphamide) resulted in unacceptably high relapses [37]. However, concerns about severe acute toxicities, especially in adolescents, supported the application of alternative regimens, such as treosulfan, fludarabine, and thiotepa [60,61]. Other regiments include clofarabine, busulfan, and fludarabine [59].

Regarding stem cell selection, the CD3/CD19-depleted graft transplantation of bone marrow or apheresis cells is the most widely used approach. The donor selection included matched sibling donors (MSD) or matched unrelated donors (MUD), defined as a 9/10 or 10/10 allele match for the HLA loci A, B, C, DR, and DQ, as determined by molecular 4-digit high-resolution typing. For the HR patients without a matched donor, a haploidentical donor is accepted [59].

An unexpected, good outcome has been achieved in children with refractory AML, who got fludarabine/amsacrine (FLAMSA) and reduced conditioning (TBI/DLI). The reported 4-years EFS of 41% seems to be promising because, in the past, almost all patients of this cohort died [59].

3.2. Diagnostics

The diagnostic of pediatric AML requires morphology, immunophenotyping, and comprehensive cyto- and molecular genetics of the leukemic blasts. All available methods, such as multicolor flow with at least eight colors, panel-next-generation sequencing (NGS), and RNA seq, must be integrated. In general, the risk groups definition can be based mainly on genetics augmented by response measurement by flow and morphology (AIEOP/AML-

BFM/FRANCE/UK/COG/Japan), or visa-versa, preferentially MRD-driven augmented by genetics (NOPHO) [62].

Table 1 shows the definition of risk groups according to genetics aberrations and response. The rarity and, in several cases, cryptic translocations require high qualification of the reference laboratories to provide reliable results within a short time frame.

Table 1. Risk Group definition by genetics and response, an example from the AIEOP-BFM AML 2020 Study.

Risk Group	Genetic Risk Criteria	Response Criteria
Standard Risk (SR)	<ul><li>CBFβ abnormalities<ul><li>t(8;21)(q22;q22) with adequate (≥2 log) reduction by qPCR at IND2</li><li>inv(16)(p13q22)/t(16;16)(p13;q22)</li></ul></li><li>Biallelic CEBPα aberrations</li><li>t(16;21) CBFA2T3/RUNX1 *and* FLT3-ITD negative</li></ul>	Genetic standard risk and<ul><li>MRD < 0.1% at IND 2</li></ul>t(8;21) and<ul><li>MRD > 2 log reduction at IND 2 (qPCR)</li></ul>
Intermediate Risk (IR)	<ul><li>NON SR and NON HR patients</li></ul>	Genetic standard or intermediate risk and<ul><li>MRD at IND 1 ≥ 0.1% and <1% and MRD at IND 2 < 0.1%</li></ul>
High Risk (HR)	<ul><li>Complex karyotype (≥3 aberrations including at least one structural aberration) *excluding those with recurrent translocations*</li><li>Monosomal Karyotype, i.e., -7, -5/del(5q)</li><li>11q23/KMT2A rearrangements involving:<ul><li>t(4;11)(q21;q23) KMT2A/AFF1</li><li>t(6;11)(q27;q23) KMT2A/AFDN</li><li>t(10;11)(p12;q23) KMT2A/MLLT10</li><li>t(9;11)(p21;q23) KMT2A/MLLT3 with other cytogenetic aberrations</li></ul></li><li>t(16;21)(p11;q22) FUS/ERG</li><li>t(9;22)(q34;q11.2) BCR/ABL1</li><li>t(6;9)(p22;q34) DEK/NUP214</li><li>t(7;12)(q36;p13) MNX1/ETV6</li><li>inv3(q21q26)/t(3;3)(q21;q26) RPN1/MECOM</li><li>12p abnormalities</li><li>FLT3-ITD with AR ≥ 0.5 not in combination with other recurrent abnormalities or NPM1 mutations</li><li>WT1 mutation and FLT3-ITD</li><li>inv(16)(p13q24) CBFA2T3/GLIS2</li><li>t(5;11)(q35;p15.5) NUP98/NSD1 and t(11;12)(p15;p13) NUP98/KDM5A</li><li>Pure Erythroid leukemia</li></ul>	<ul><li>MRD ≥ 1% at IND 1 or ≥0.1% at IND 2 or (only if FLOW-result not available/informative) blast count ≥5% at IND 1</li></ul>

Today, measurement of residual disease by immunophenotyping is the most appropriate method to define initial treatment response. The ongoing treatment protocols use residual disease detection either by immunophenotyping only or in combination with morphology for treatment stratification. The different response kinetics of fusion genes (KMT2A; AML1/Eto, CBL/M) and mutations (NPM1, FLT3-ITD, WT1), measured by quantitative PCR, makes this approach suitable and prognostically relevant only in some subgroups, such as PML/RARA. However, continuous monitoring after remission allows the early detection of molecular relapse. Although it is not entirely proven yet, the treatment of molecular relapse might be feasible with less intensive chemotherapy as bridge to transplant option. The international AmoRe 2017 trial (conducted by GPOH as sponsor) should allow alloHSCT without toxic re-induction in children with a molecular relapse by applying the epigenetically-effective low dose azacytidine. A reduction of MRD-levels to less than 10^{-3} should allow direct alloHSCT.

3.3. Myeloid Leukemia of Down Syndrome (ML-DS)

Until almost the end of the 20th century, patients with AML and Down syndrome (DS) were treated identically with the whole group of pediatric AML [63]. In the NOPHO

AML-93, after the same treatment, a better 5-year survival was obsereved [64]. In CCG Studies 2861 and 2981, a significantly better 4-year-EFS and no benefit of the BMT was achieved in the patients with DS [65]. A significantly lower relapse rate was noticed in the MRC AML10 study and the BFM-83 and 98 studies [66,67]. Consequently, the therapeutic schema was modified to minimize the toxicities for this favorable group. In the AML02 Trial (JCCSG) patients with ML-DS were treated separately, and a stratification depended on the response after the inductions were implemented [68,69]. In the MRC AML 12, they were allocated for only four courses of chemotherapy and were not eligible for alloHSCT [70]. In the AML-BFM-93 study, the treatment of the DS patients included reduced doses of anthracycline and no high-dose cytarabine/mitoxantrone or cranial irradiation [71]. Since then, these patients have been treated with lower doses of chemotherapy. No maintenance therapy is recommended. Contrary to the excellent response and survival in the case newly diagnosed ML-DS, the overall survival after a relapse, which affects less than 10% of those patients, remains disappointing [65,72].

3.4. Supportive Care

All the improvements of the recent decades would be impossible without the progress in supportive care. The introduction of prophylactic antimycotic and, effective antibiotic regimens as well as improved intensive care, including sufficient, sensitive, and specific microbiologic diagnostics, enables intensive treatment with a limited rate of treatment-related death and toxicity [73–75]. In addition, recent data confirmed that strict separation of children under immunosuppressive therapy might not be required. The best strategy could be to react immediately with a very high level of awareness and structures in pediatric oncology sites [76]. Unfortunately, these structures are only given in some developed countries.

3.5. Long-Term Toxicities

Pediatric AML and intensive treatment are associated with relevant long-term sequelae. All organ systems could be involved. Although much attention has been spent on cardiotoxicities, especially anthracycline-induced cardiomyopathy, severe damages of the liver, renal function, and endocrinology must be considered. Recent data showed the increased risk of early-onset cardiovascular diseases, neurology, and mental diseases [68]. In addition, treatment-induced malignancies occur in 2 to 5% within 10 to 20 years post-treatment. Unfortunately, to date, there is no plateau of the cumulative incidence [77].

4. Future

The therapy of pediatric AML is still based on intensive chemotherapy and, if necessary, alloHSCT. Despite significantly improved survival chances, this therapy has severe acute and long-term side effects [68,78,79]. Therapy-related toxicity is also relatively high at 2 to 4% [75] The aim of new, innovative therapies must be a more targeted treatment, presumably with fewer side effects, without jeopardizing achieved the results. Another aspect is that cure has a the highest priority. While, in adult disease with an age peak above 70 years, it may be beneficial to gain control of the disease for several years, cure must remain the primary aim in children.

Early deaths from AML in children and adolescents continue to be a significant problem [80–82]. While, in some cases, the course is fateful due to the disease dynamics, on the other hand, a higher awareness of pediatricians, general practitioners, and pediatric hospitals could rescue some children. This is especially true for APL and monoblastic leukemia. These must be considered acute emergencies and treated immediately in cooperation with an experienced pediatric oncology center. Effective, quality-assuring structures (central consultation, reference laboratories), as established in some European countries, improve the chances of survival [83].

Several achievements will allow more reliable and precise diagnostics, mainly based on NGS, genome mapping, RNA seq, acetylation/methylation assays, and molecular single-cell characterization [84–86]. The challenge will be to integrate the complex data into meaningful results, allowing clinical decisions, better stratification, and more precise treatments. The reliable measurement of MRD by NGS-based approaches will cover all patients and give better insights into the fate of leukemic stem cells, clonal hierarchies, and evolution [86–89].

Regarding more precise treatment options, the differentiating therapies with all-trans retinoic acid (ATRA) and arsenic trioxide (ATO) in APL are already in use. For the first time, this allows the cure without chemotherapy and with significantly reduced side effects [90].

The use of antigen-mediated therapies was successful, especially with the CD33-specific and ozogamicin-coupled antibody GO (Mylotarg) [91]. However, even the positive randomized trials in adults and children have not yet led to a general marketing authorization in pediatric AML [5]. Other specific-acting agents, such as FLT3 or IDH1/2 inhibitors, have also shown efficacy in children and adolescents. Still, it has not been conclusively investigated whether this improves the chances of a cure or only means an effective but transient blast reduction [61]. The same is probably true for epigenetic approaches, which have been used very successfully in older adults. Combining BCL-2 inhibitors (venetoclax) with low-dose, mainly epigenetically active chemotherapy (e.g.azacytidine) modifies the clinical course of myelodysplastic syndromes/AML, especially with low proliferation activity, very positively with significantly improved survival [92]. Other approaches combined venetoclax with MDM2 or FLT3-ITD inhibitors; however, experience in children is lacking. The addition of venetoclax to high-dose cytarabine with or without idarubicin revealed a promising overall response of 69% [93]. Nevertheless, the contribution of venetoclax to this response rate needs to be evaluated. In summary, the relevance of venetoclax in pediatric AML needs to be confirmed in further trials (such as planned within the LLS-PedAL initiative).

Another complex area of AML therapy includes various immunotherapies. One approach will be post-HSCT immunomodulation. The effectiveness has already been shown in post-HSCT treatment with donor-lymphocyte infusions (DLI) but definitively provides more options. Cytokine-induced killer (CIK) cells have already been introduced to clinical trials [94]. Other approaches use activated NK-cells [95]. In particular, the combination with immunomodulatory agents that optimize cellular treatments shows promising efficacy in preclinical and initial clinical studies. Directly related to these approaches are the current research findings on the importance of the microenvironment [96], its interaction with leukemic blasts, and the effects it induces on the selective proliferation of malignant cells, support of escape mechanism of leukemic stem cells, and inhibition of immunocompetence of effector cells, such as T/NK cells [97].

The successful cellular therapy approaches in B-cell lymphocytic leukemia/lymphomas raise high hopes for myeloid neoplasms [98]. However, the challenge in pediatric AML is more complex, while it is relatively easy to compensate for B lymphocyte eradication with antibody substitution, the reconstitution of myelopoiesis is only feasible with alloHSCT. Accordingly, to date, these therapeutic options must be viewed primarily as "bridge-to-transplant" regime. Nevertheless, cellular treatment options, such as gene-engineered T-CAR or NK-CAR cells, are promising approaches to enable more precise and hopefully less side-effective therapy in the future [99–101] Several targets have been addressed so far (CD33, CD123, CLL1, and others) [101–103].

Overall, it is unlikely that there will be "the one" effective therapy for a heterogeneous disease like AML. Only the optimized combination of all available options will allow a further, significant improvement of cure rates so that likely different treatments adapted to the AML subtype are needed. This underlines the need for further comprehensive research into the mechanisms of leukemogenesis, specific therapies, and, above all, systematic clinical research to develop scientifically-validated treatments, despite the small number of cases. This will only be possible if the international collaboration between the study groups will be further improved on a global level. It is important to learn more about small subgroups and more precise treatment, as well as reducing inequalities between countries and continents. The recently established Leukemia & Lymphoma Society (LLS), Pediatric Acute Leukemia (PedAL) initiative and the European Pediatric Acute Leukemia (EuPAL) foundation are on the way to launching such a platform in North America, Europe, Australia, and, hopefully, in Japan [3,104].

In this context, the therapies of AML in children, even if they have low economic impact, should not be considered exclusively as a "waste product" of adult medicine but should have a right to their own, child-specific therapy development. This applies to both, research on pediatric therapies and the timely establishment of therapies that have been successfully used in adult AML.

Author Contributions: Conceptualization: D.R. and K.W.; resources: D.R., E.A. and K.W.; writing and original draft preparation: D.R., E.A. and K.W.; writing, review and editing: D.R., E.A. and K.W.; visualization: D.R.; supervision: D.R.; project administration: D.R.; funding acquisition: D.R. and K.W. All authors have read and agreed to the published version of the manuscript.

Funding: This research received no external funding.

Institutional Review Board Statement: Not applicable.

Informed Consent Statement: Not applicable.

Conflicts of Interest: The authors declare no conflict of interest.

Appendix A

Table A1. The outcome of pediatric AML. Clinical trials by the Cooperative Study Groups.

Study Group	Study	Periode	Patients (N)	EFS (%)	OS (%)	Relapse (%)	Source
AIEOP	AML2002/01	2002–2011	482	8-years 55.0 ± 2.6	8-years 67.7 ± 2.4	24	Pession et al. 2013 [105]
AML-BFM	AML-BFM 2012	2012–2018	324	5-years 65 ± 3	5-years 82 ± 3	22	Waack et al. 2020 [106]
	AML-BFM 2004	2004–2010	521	5-years 55 ± 2	5-years 74 ± 2	29	Creutzig et al. 2013 [107]
	AAML03P1	2003–2005	340	3-years 53 ± 6	3-years 66 ± 5	33 ± 6	Cooper et al. 2012 [108]
COG	AAML0531	2006–2010	1022	3-years 53.1 vs. 46.9	3-years 69.4 vs. 65.4	32.8 vs. 41.3	Gamis et al. 2014 [109]
	AAML1031	2011–2016	1097	3-years 45.9 ± 3	3-years 65.4 ± 3	47.2	Aplenc et al. 2020 [110]
JACLS	AML99	2000–2002	240	5-years 61.6 ± 6.5	5-years 75.6 ± 5.3	32.2	Tsukimoto et al. 2009 [31]
JPLSG	AML05	2006–2010	443	3-years 54.3 ± 2.4	3-years 73.2 ± 2.3	30.3	Tomizawa et al. 2013 [32]
MRC	MRC AML12	1995–2002	564	10-years 54	10-years 63	32	Gibson et al. 2011 [27]
	MRC AML 17	2010–2014			5-years 74		Burnett et al. [111]
NOPHO	NOPHO AML 2004	2004–2009	151	3-years 57 ± 5	3-years 69 ± 5	30	Abrahamsson et al. 2011 [7] Hasle et al. 2012 [29]
99PPLLSG	PPLLSG AML-98	1998–2002	195	5-years 46 ± 5	5-years 53 ± 5	24	Dluzniewska et al. 2010 [112]
	AML-BFM 2012	2015–2019	131	3-years 67 ± 5	3 years 75 ± 5	27 17	Czogala et al. 2021 [113]
SJCRH	AML02	2002–2008	216	3-years 61	3-years 71	21	Rubnitz et al. 2010 [30]
	AML08	2008–2017	285	3-years 52.9	3-years 74.8		Rubnitz et al. 2019 [114]

AIEOP (Associazione Italiana di Ematologia e Oncologia Pediatrica), AML-BFM (Berlin, Frankfurt, Münster), COG (Childhood Oncology Group), JACLS (Japanese Association of Childhood Leukemia Study), JPLSG (Japanese Pediatric Leukemia Study Group), NOPHO (Nordic Society for Pediatric Hematology and Oncology), MRC (Medical Research Council), PPLLSG (Polish Pediatric Leukemia/Lymphoma Study Group), SJCRH (St. Jude Children's Research Hospital).

References

1. Bonaventure, A.; Harewood, R.; Stiller, C.A.; Gatta, G.; Clavel, J.; Stefan, D.C.; Carreira, H.; Spika, D.; Marcos-Gragera, R.; Peris-Bonet, R.; et al. Worldwide comparison of survival from childhood leukaemia for 1995–2009, by subtype, age, and sex (CONCORD-2): A population-based study of individual data for 89,828 children from 198 registries in 53 countries. *Lancet Haematol.* **2017**, *4*, e202–e217. [CrossRef]
2. Elgarten, C.W.; Aplenc, R. Pediatric acute myeloid leukemia: Updates on biology, risk stratification, and therapy. *Curr. Opin. Pediatr.* **2020**, *32*, 57–66. [CrossRef]
3. Plana, A.; Furner, B.; Palese, M.; Dussault, N.; Birz, S.; Graglia, L.; Kush, M.; Nicholson, J.; Hecker-Nolting, S.; Gaspar, N.; et al. Pediatric Cancer Data Commons: Federating and Democratizing Data for Childhood Cancer Research. *JCO Clin. Cancer Inform.* **2021**, *5*, 1034–1043. [CrossRef] [PubMed]
4. Zwaan, C.M.; Kolb, E.A.; Reinhardt, D.; Abrahamsson, J.; Adachi, S.; Aplenc, R.; de Bont, E.S.J.M.; de Moerloose, B.; Dworzak, M.; Gibson, B.E.S.; et al. Collaborative Efforts Driving Progress in Pediatric Acute Myeloid Leukemia. *J. Clin. Oncol.* **2015**, *33*, 2949–2962. [CrossRef]

5. Creutzig, U.; van den Heuvel-Eibrink, M.M.; Gibson, B.; Dworzak, M.N.; Adachi, S.; de Bont, E.; Harbott, J.; Hasle, H.; Johnston, D.; Kinoshita, A.; et al. Diagnosis and management of acute myeloid leukemia in children and adolescents: Recommendations from an international expert panel. *Blood* **2012**, *120*, 3187–3205. [CrossRef]
6. Pollard, J.A.; Guest, E.; Alonzo, T.A.; Gerbing, R.B.; Loken, M.R.; Brodersen, L.E.; Kolb, E.A.; Aplenc, R.; Meshinchi, S.; Raimondi, S.C.; et al. Gemtuzumab Ozogamicin Improves Event-Free Survival and Reduces Relapse in Pediatric KMT2A-Rearranged AML: Results From the Phase III Children's Oncology Group Trial AAML0531. *J. Clin. Oncol.* **2021**, *39*, 3149–3160. [CrossRef]
7. Gurnari, C.; Voso, M.T.; Girardi, K.; Mastronuzzi, A.; Strocchio, L. Acute Promyelocytic Leukemia in Children: A Model of Precision Medicine and Chemotherapy-Free Therapy. *Int. J. Mol. Sci.* **2021**, *22*, 642. [CrossRef]
8. Abrahamsson, J.; Forestier, E.; Heldrup, J.; Jahnukainen, K.; Jónsson, O.G.; Lausen, B.; Palle, J.; Zeller, B.; Hasle, H. Response-guided induction therapy in pediatric acute myeloid leukemia with excellent remission rate. *J. Clin. Oncol.* **2011**, *29*, 310–315. [CrossRef]
9. Rasche, M.; Steidel, E.; Kondryn, D.; von Neuhoff, N.; Sramkova, L.; Creutzig, U.; Dworzak, M.; Reinhardt, D. Impact of a Risk-Adapted Treatment Approach in Pediatric AML: A Report of the AML-BFM Registry 2012. *Blood* **2019**, *134*, 293. [CrossRef]
10. Bennett, J.M.; Catovsky, D.; Daniel, M.T.; Flandrin, G.; Galton, D.A.; Gralnick, H.R.; Sultan, C. Proposals for the classification of the acute leukaemias. French-American-British (FAB) co-operative group. *Br. J. Haematol.* **1976**, *33*, 451–458. [CrossRef] [PubMed]
11. Bennett, J.M.; Catovsky, D.; Daniel, M.T.; Flandrin, G.; Galton, D.A.; Gralnick, H.R.; Sultan, C. Proposed revised criteria for the classification of acute myeloid leukemia. A report of the French-American-British Cooperative Group. *Ann. Intern. Med.* **1985**, *103*, 620–625. [CrossRef] [PubMed]
12. Bennett, J.M.; Catovsky, D.; Daniel, M.T.; Flandrin, G.; Galton, D.A.; Gralnick, H.R.; Sultan, C. Proposal for the recognition of minimally differentiated acute myeloid leukaemia (AML-M0). *Br. J. Haematol.* **1991**, *78*, 325–329. [CrossRef] [PubMed]
13. Bloomfield, C.D.; Brunning, R.D. FAB M7: Acute megakaryoblastic leukemia–beyond morphology. *Ann. Intern. Med.* **1985**, *103*, 450–452. [CrossRef] [PubMed]
14. Lee, E.J.; Pollak, A.; Leavitt, R.D.; Testa, J.R.; Schiffer, C.A. Minimally differentiated acute nonlymphocytic leukemia: A distinct entity. *Blood* **1987**, *70*, 1400–1406. [CrossRef] [PubMed]
15. Boiron, M.; Jacquillat, C.; Weil, M.; Tanzer, J.; Levy, D.; Sultan, C.; Bernard, J. DAUNORUBICIN IN THE TREATMENT OF ACUTE MYELOCYTIC LEUKÆMIA. *Lancet* **1969**, *293*, 330–333. [CrossRef]
16. Pizzo, P.A.; Henderson, E.S.; Leventhal, B.G. Acute myelogenous leukemia in children: A preliminary report of combination chemotherapy. *J. Pediatr.* **1976**, *88*, 125–130. [CrossRef]
17. Wells, R.J.; Feusner, J.; Devney, R.; Woods, W.G.; Provisor, A.J.; Cairo, M.S.; Odom, L.F.; Nachman, J.; Jones, G.R.; Ettinger, L.J. Sequential high-dose cytosine arabinoside-asparaginase treatment in advanced childhood leukemia. *J. Clin. Oncol.* **1985**, *3*, 998–1004. [CrossRef] [PubMed]
18. Creutzig, U.; Ritter, J.; Langermann, H.J.; Riehm, H.; Henze, G.; Niethammer, D.; Jürgens, H.; Stollmann, B.; Lasson, U.; Kabisch, H.; et al. Acute myelogenous leukemia in children: Results of the cooperative BFM-78 therapy study after 3 3/4 years. *Klin. Pädiatr.* **1983**, *195*, 152–160. [CrossRef]
19. Steuber, C.P.; Humphrey, G.B.; McMillan, C.W.; Vietti, T.J. Remission induction in acute myelogenous leukemia using cytosine arabinoside synchronization: A Southwest Oncology Group Study. *Med. Pediatr. Oncol.* **1978**, *4*, 337–342. [CrossRef]
20. Rees, J. Principal results of the medical research council's 8th acute myeloid leukaemia trial. *Lancet* **1986**, *328*, 1236–1241. [CrossRef]
21. Stevens, R.F.; Hann, I.M.; Wheatley, K.; Gray, R. Intensive chemotherapy with or without additional bone marrow transplantation in paediatric AML: Progress report on the MRC AML 10 trial. Medical Research Council Working Party on Childhood Leukaemia. *Leukemia* **1992**, *6* (Suppl. 2), 55–58.
22. Swirsky, D.M.; Li, Y.S.; Matthews, J.G.; Flemans, R.J.; Rees, J.K.; Hayhoe, F.G. 8;21 translocation in acute granulocytic leukaemia: Cytological, cytochemical and clinical features. *Br. J. Haematol.* **1984**, *56*, 199–213. [CrossRef] [PubMed]
23. Creutzig, U.; Ritter, J.; Niederbiermann-Koczy, G.; Harbott, J.; Schellong, G. Prognostische Bedeutung der Eosinophilie bei Kindern mit akuter myeloischer Leukämie in den Studien AML-BFM-78 und -83. *Klin. Pädiatr.* **1989**, *201*, 220–226. [CrossRef]
24. Creutzig, U.; Ritter, J.; Schellong, G. Identification of two risk groups in childhood acute myelogenous leukemia after therapy intensification in study AML-BFM-83 as compared with study AML-BFM-78. AML-BFM Study Group. *Blood* **1990**, *75*, 1932–1940. [CrossRef] [PubMed]
25. Perel, Y.; Auvrignon, A.; Leblanc, T.; Michel, G.; Reguerre, Y.; Vannier, J.-P.; Dalle, J.-H.; Gandemer, V.; Schmitt, C.; Méchinaud, F.; et al. Treatment of childhood acute myeloblastic leukemia: Dose intensification improves outcome and maintenance therapy is of no benefit–multicenter studies of the French LAME (Leucémie Aiguë Myéloblastique Enfant) Cooperative Group. *Leukemia* **2005**, *19*, 2082–2089. [CrossRef]
26. Creutzig, U.; Zimmermann, M.; Reinhardt, D.; Rasche, M.; von Neuhoff, C.; Alpermann, T.; Dworzak, M.; Perglerová, K.; Zemanova, Z.; Tchinda, J.; et al. Changes in cytogenetics and molecular genetics in acute myeloid leukemia from childhood to adult age groups. *Cancer* **2016**, *122*, 3821–3830. [CrossRef]
27. Creutzig, U.; Ritter, J.; Zimmermann, M.; Hermann, J.; Gadner, H.; Sawatzki, D.B.; Niemeyer, C.M.; Schwabe, D.; Selle, B.; Boos, J.; et al. Idarubicin improves blast cell clearance during induction therapy in children with AML: Results of study AML-BFM 93. AML-BFM Study Group. *Leukemia* **2001**, *15*, 348–354. [CrossRef]

28. Gibson, B.E.S.; Webb, D.K.H.; Howman, A.J.; de Graaf, S.S.N.; Harrison, C.J.; Wheatley, K. Results of a randomized trial in children with Acute Myeloid Leukaemia: Medical research council AML12 trial. *Br. J. Haematol.* **2011**, *155*, 366–376. [CrossRef]
29. Lie, S.O.; Abrahamsson, J.; Clausen, N.; Forestier, E.; Hasle, H.; Hovi, L.; Jonmundsson, G.; Mellander, L.; Siimes, M.A.; Yssing, M.; et al. Long-term results in children with AML: NOPHO-AML Study Group–report of three consecutive trials. *Leukemia* **2005**, *19*, 2090–2100. [CrossRef] [PubMed]
30. Hasle, H.; Abrahamsson, J.; Forestier, E.; Ha, S.-Y.; Heldrup, J.; Jahnukainen, K.; Jónsson, Ó.G.; Lausen, B.; Palle, J.; Zeller, B. Gemtuzumab ozogamicin as postconsolidation therapy does not prevent relapse in children with AML: Results from NOPHO-AML 2004. *Blood* **2012**, *120*, 978–984. [CrossRef] [PubMed]
31. Rubnitz, J.E.; Inaba, H.; Dahl, G.; Ribeiro, R.C.; Bowman, W.P.; Taub, J.; Pounds, S.; Razzouk, B.I.; Lacayo, N.J.; Cao, X.; et al. Minimal residual disease-directed therapy for childhood acute myeloid leukaemia: Results of the AML02 multicentre trial. *Lancet Oncol.* **2010**, *11*, 543–552. [CrossRef]
32. Tsukimoto, I.; Tawa, A.; Horibe, K.; Tabuchi, K.; Kigasawa, H.; Tsuchida, M.; Yabe, H.; Nakayama, H.; Kudo, K.; Kobayashi, R.; et al. Risk-stratified therapy and the intensive use of cytarabine improves the outcome in childhood acute myeloid leukemia: The AML99 trial from the Japanese Childhood AML Cooperative Study Group. *J. Clin. Oncol.* **2009**, *27*, 4007–4013. [CrossRef] [PubMed]
33. Tomizawa, D.; Tawa, A.; Watanabe, T.; Saito, A.M.; Kudo, K.; Taga, T.; Iwamoto, S.; Shimada, A.; Terui, K.; Moritake, H.; et al. Appropriate dose reduction in induction therapy is essential for the treatment of infants with acute myeloid leukemia: A report from the Japanese Pediatric Leukemia/Lymphoma Study Group. *Int. J. Hematol.* **2013**, *98*, 578–588. [CrossRef]
34. Creutzig, U.; Reinhardt, D. Current controversies: Which patients with acute myeloid leukaemia should receive a bone marrow transplantation?—A European view. *Br. J. Haematol.* **2002**, *118*, 365–377. [CrossRef] [PubMed]
35. Creutzig, U.; Diekamp, S.; Zimmermann, M.; Reinhardt, D. Longitudinal evaluation of early and late anthracycline cardiotoxicity in children with AML. *Pediatr. Blood Cancer* **2007**, *48*, 651–662. [CrossRef] [PubMed]
36. Gibson, B.E.S.; Wheatley, K.; Hann, I.M.; Stevens, R.F.; Webb, D.; Hills, R.K.; de Graaf, S.S.N.; Harrison, C.J. Treatment strategy and long-term results in paediatric patients treated in consecutive UK AML trials. *Leukemia* **2005**, *19*, 2130–2138. [CrossRef]
37. Klingebiel, T.; Ritter, J.; Schellong, G.; Creutzig, U.; Riehm, H.; Henze, G.; Bender-Götze, C.; Dopfer, R.; Ebell, W.; Friedrich, W. Role and perspectives of BMT in AML: The BFM experience. *Bone Marrow Transplant.* **1991**, *7* (Suppl. 3), 66–70.
38. Klusmann, J.-H.; Reinhardt, D.; Zimmermann, M.; Kremens, B.; Vormoor, J.; Dworzak, M.; Creutzig, U.; Klingebiel, T. The role of matched sibling donor allogeneic stem cell transplantation in pediatric high-risk acute myeloid leukemia: Results from the AML-BFM 98 study. *Haematologica* **2012**, *97*, 21–29. [CrossRef] [PubMed]
39. Locatelli, F.; Masetti, R.; Rondelli, R.; Zecca, M.; Fagioli, F.; Rovelli, A.; Messina, C.; Lanino, E.; Bertaina, A.; Favre, C.; et al. Outcome of children with high-risk acute myeloid leukemia given autologous or allogeneic hematopoietic cell transplantation in the aieop AML-2002/01 study. *Bone Marrow Transplant.* **2015**, *50*, 181–188. [CrossRef]
40. Lonetti, A.; Pession, A.; Masetti, R. Targeted Therapies for Pediatric AML: Gaps and Perspective. *Front. Pediatr.* **2019**, *7*, 463. [CrossRef]
41. Woods, W.G.; Neudorf, S.; Gold, S.; Sanders, J.; Buckley, J.D.; Barnard, D.R.; Dusenbery, K.; DeSwarte, J.; Arthur, D.C.; Lange, B.J.; et al. A comparison of allogeneic bone marrow transplantation, autologous bone marrow transplantation, and aggressive chemotherapy in children with acute myeloid leukemia in remission. *Blood* **2001**, *97*, 56–62. [CrossRef] [PubMed]
42. Goldman, F.D.; Rumelhart, S.L.; DeAlarcon, P.; Holida, M.D.; Lee, N.F.; Miller, J.; Trigg, M.; Giller, R. Poor outcome in children with refractory/relapsed leukemia undergoing bone marrow transplantation with mismatched family member donors. *Bone Marrow Transplant.* **2000**, *25*, 943–948. [CrossRef]
43. Sung, L.; Buckstein, R.; Doyle, J.J.; Crump, M.; Detsky, A.S. Treatment options for patients with acute myeloid leukemia with a matched sibling donor: A decision analysis. *Cancer* **2003**, *97*, 592–600. [CrossRef]
44. Chen, A.R.; Alonzo, T.A.; Woods, W.G.; Arceci, R.J. Current controversies: Which patients with acute myeloid leukaemia should receive a bone marrow transplantation?—An American view. *Br. J. Haematol.* **2002**, *118*, 378–384. [CrossRef] [PubMed]
45. Wheatley, K. Current controversies: Which patients with acute myeloid leukaemia should receive a bone marrow transplantation? A statistician's view. *Br. J. Haematol.* **2002**, *118*, 351–356. [CrossRef]
46. Creutzig, U.; Ritter, J.; Zimmermann, M.; Schellong, G. Does cranial irradiation reduce the risk for bone marrow relapse in acute myelogenous leukemia? Unexpected results of the Childhood Acute Myelogenous Leukemia Study BFM-87. *J. Clin. Oncol.* **1993**, *11*, 279–286. [CrossRef] [PubMed]
47. Woods, W.G.; Kobrinsky, N.; Buckley, J.D.; Lee, J.W.; Sanders, J.; Neudorf, S.; Gold, S.; Barnard, D.R.; DeSwarte, J.; Dusenbery, K.; et al. Timed-sequential induction therapy improves postremission outcome in acute myeloid leukemia: A report from the Children's Cancer Group. *Blood* **1996**, *87*, 4979–4989. [CrossRef] [PubMed]
48. Pession, A.; Rondelli, R.; Basso, G.; Rizzari, C.; Testi, A.M.; Fagioli, F.; de Stefano, P.; Locatelli, F. Treatment and long-term results in children with acute myeloid leukaemia treated according to the AIEOP AML protocols. *Leukemia* **2005**, *19*, 2043–2053. [CrossRef] [PubMed]
49. Creutzig, U.; Büchner, T.; Sauerland, M.C.; Zimmermann, M.; Reinhardt, D.; Döhner, H.; Schlenk, R.F. Significance of age in acute myeloid leukemia patients younger than 30 years: A common analysis of the pediatric trials AML-BFM 93/98 and the adult trials AMLCG 92/99 and AMLSG HD93/98A. *Cancer* **2008**, *112*, 562–571. [CrossRef]

50. Wells, R.J.; Woods, W.G.; Buckley, J.D.; Odom, L.F.; Benjamin, D.; Bernstein, I.; Betcher, D.; Feig, S.; Kim, T.; Ruymann, F. Treatment of newly diagnosed children and adolescents with acute myeloid leukemia: A Childrens Cancer Group study. *J. Clin. Oncol.* **1994**, *12*, 2367–2377. [CrossRef]
51. Rasche, M.; Zimmermann, M.; Borschel, L.; Bourquin, J.-P.; Dworzak, M.; Klingebiel, T.; Lehrnbecher, T.; Creutzig, U.; Klusmann, J.-H.; Reinhardt, D. Successes and challenges in the treatment of pediatric acute myeloid leukemia: A retrospective analysis of the AML-BFM trials from 1987 to 2012. *Leukemia* **2018**, *32*, 2167–2177. [CrossRef]
52. Langebrake, C.; Creutzig, U.; Dworzak, M.; Hrusak, O.; Mejstrikova, E.; Griesinger, F.; Zimmermann, M.; Reinhardt, D. Residual disease monitoring in childhood acute myeloid leukemia by multiparameter flow cytometry: The MRD-AML-BFM Study Group. *J. Clin. Oncol.* **2006**, *24*, 3686–3692. [CrossRef]
53. Rubnitz, J.E.; Crews, K.R.; Pounds, S.; Yang, S.; Campana, D.; Gandhi, V.V.; Raimondi, S.C.; Downing, J.R.; Razzouk, B.I.; Pui, C.-H.; et al. Combination of cladribine and cytarabine is effective for childhood acute myeloid leukemia: Results of the St Jude AML97 trial. *Leukemia* **2009**, *23*, 1410–1416. [CrossRef]
54. Tierens, A.; Bjørklund, E.; Siitonen, S.; Marquart, H.V.; Wulff-Juergensen, G.; Pelliniemi, T.-T.; Forestier, E.; Hasle, H.; Jahnukainen, K.; Lausen, B.; et al. Residual disease detected by flow cytometry is an independent predictor of survival in childhood acute myeloid leukaemia; results of the NOPHO-AML 2004 study. *Br. J. Haematol.* **2016**, *174*, 600–609. [CrossRef]
55. van der Velden, V.H.J.; van der Sluijs-Geling, A.; Gibson, B.E.S.; te Marvelde, J.G.; Hoogeveen, P.G.; Hop, W.C.J.; Wheatley, K.; Bierings, M.B.; Schuurhuis, G.J.; de Graaf, S.S.N.; et al. Clinical significance of flowcytometric minimal residual disease detection in pediatric acute myeloid leukemia patients treated according to the DCOG ANLL97/MRC AML12 protocol. *Leukemia* **2010**, *24*, 1599–1606. [CrossRef] [PubMed]
56. Inaba, H.; Coustan-Smith, E.; Cao, X.; Pounds, S.B.; Shurtleff, S.A.; Wang, K.Y.; Raimondi, S.C.; Onciu, M.; Jacobsen, J.; Ribeiro, R.C.; et al. Comparative analysis of different approaches to measure treatment response in acute myeloid leukemia. *J. Clin. Oncol.* **2012**, *30*, 3625–3632. [CrossRef]
57. Rasche, M.; Zimmermann, M.; Steidel, E.; Alonzo, T.; Aplenc, R.; Bourquin, J.-P.; Boztug, H.; Cooper, T.; Gamis, A.S.; Gerbing, R.B.; et al. Survival Following Relapse in Children with Acute Myeloid Leukemia: A Report from AML-BFM and COG. *Cancers* **2021**, *13*, 2336. [CrossRef] [PubMed]
58. Rasche, M.; Steidel, E.; Zimmermann, M.; Bourquin, J.-P.; Boztug, H.; Janotova, I.; Kolb, E.A.; Lehrnbecher, T.; von Neuhoff, N.; Niktoreh, N.; et al. Second Relapse of Pediatric Patients with Acute Myeloid Leukemia: A Report on Current Treatment Strategies and Outcome of the AML-BFM Study Group. *Cancers* **2021**, *13*, 789. [CrossRef]
59. Reinhardt, D.; von Neuhoff, C.; Sander, A.; Creutzig, U. Prognostische Relevanz genetischer Aberrationen der akuten myeloischen Leukämie bei Kindern und Jugendlichen. *Klin. Padiatr.* **2012**, *224*, 372–376. [CrossRef]
60. Sauer, M.G.; Lang, P.J.; Albert, M.H.; Bader, P.; Creutzig, U.; Eyrich, M.; Greil, J.; Gruhn, B.; Holter, W.; Klingebiel, T.; et al. Hematopoietic stem cell transplantation for children with acute myeloid leukemia-results of the AML SCT-BFM 2007 trial. *Leukemia* **2020**, *34*, 613–624. [CrossRef] [PubMed]
61. Kalwak, K.; Mielcarek, M.; Patrick, K.; Styczynski, J.; Bader, P.; Corbacioglu, S.; Burkhardt, B.; Sykora, K.W.; Drabko, K.; Gozdzik, J.; et al. Treosulfan-fludarabine-thiotepa-based conditioning treatment before allogeneic hematopoietic stem cell transplantation for pediatric patients with hematological malignancies. *Bone Marrow Transplant.* **2020**, *55*, 1996–2007. [CrossRef] [PubMed]
62. Inaba, H.; Rubnitz, J.E.; Coustan-Smith, E.; Li, L.; Furmanski, B.D.; Mascara, G.P.; Heym, K.M.; Christensen, R.; Onciu, M.; Shurtleff, S.A.; et al. Phase I pharmacokinetic and pharmacodynamic study of the multikinase inhibitor sorafenib in combination with clofarabine and cytarabine in pediatric relapsed/refractory leukemia. *J. Clin. Oncol.* **2011**, *29*, 3293–3300. [CrossRef]
63. de Rooij, J.D.E.; Branstetter, C.; Ma, J.; Li, Y.; Walsh, M.P.; Cheng, J.; Obulkasim, A.; Dang, J.; Easton, J.; Verboon, L.J.; et al. Pediatric non-Down syndrome acute megakaryoblastic leukemia is characterized by distinct genomic subsets with varying outcomes. *Nat. Genet.* **2017**, *49*, 451–456. [CrossRef] [PubMed]
64. Abildgaard, L.; Ellebaek, E.; Gustafsson, G.; Abrahamsson, J.; Hovi, L.; Jonmundsson, G.; Zeller, B.; Hasle, H. Optimal treatment intensity in children with Down syndrome and myeloid leukaemia: Data from 56 children treated on NOPHO-AML protocols and a review of the literature. *Ann. Hematol.* **2006**, *85*, 275–280. [CrossRef] [PubMed]
65. Hitzler, J.K.; He, W.; Doyle, J.; Cairo, M.; Camitta, B.M.; Chan, K.W.; Diaz Perez, M.A.; Fraser, C.; Gross, T.G.; Horan, J.T.; et al. Outcome of transplantation for acute myelogenous leukemia in children with Down syndrome. *Biol. Blood Marrow Transplant.* **2013**, *19*, 893–897. [CrossRef]
66. Flasinski, M.; Scheibke, K.; Zimmermann, M.; Creutzig, U.; Reinhardt, K.; Verwer, F.; de Haas, V.; van der Velden, V.H.J.; von Neuhoff, C.; Zwaan, C.M.; et al. Low-dose cytarabine to prevent myeloid leukemia in children with Down syndrome: TMD Prevention 2007 study. *Blood Adv.* **2018**, *2*, 1532–1540. [CrossRef]
67. Rao, A.; Hills, R.K.; Stiller, C.; Gibson, B.E.; de Graaf, S.S.N.; Hann, I.M.; O'Marcaigh, A.; Wheatley, K.; Webb, D.K.H. Treatment for myeloid leukaemia of Down syndrome: Population-based experience in the UK and results from the Medical Research Council AML 10 and AML 12 trials. *Br. J. Haematol.* **2006**, *132*, 576–583. [CrossRef] [PubMed]
68. Bhatt, N.S.; Baassiri, M.J.; Liu, W.; Bhakta, N.; Chemaitilly, W.; Ehrhardt, M.J.; Inaba, H.; Krull, K.; Ness, K.K.; Rubnitz, J.E.; et al. Late outcomes in survivors of childhood acute myeloid leukemia: A report from the St. Jude Lifetime Cohort Study. *Leukemia* **2021**, *35*, 2258–2273. [CrossRef]

69. Mast, K.J.; Taub, J.W.; Alonzo, T.A.; Gamis, A.S.; Mosse, C.A.; Mathew, P.; Berman, J.N.; Wang, Y.-C.; Jones, H.M.; Campana, D.; et al. Pathologic Features of Down Syndrome Myelodysplastic Syndrome and Acute Myeloid Leukemia: A Report From the Children's Oncology Group Protocol AAML0431. *Arch. Pathol. Lab. Med.* **2020**, *144*, 466–472. [CrossRef]
70. Sussman, R.T.; Manning, B.; Ackerman, D.; Bigdeli, A.; Pammer, P.; Velu, P.D.; Luger, S.M.; Bagg, A.; Carroll, M.; Morrissette, J.J.D. Interpretative differences of combined cytogenetic and molecular profiling highlights differences between MRC and ELN classifications of AML. *Cancer Genet.* **2021**, *256–257*, 68–76. [CrossRef] [PubMed]
71. Creutzig, U.; Reinhardt, D.; Diekamp, S.; Dworzak, M.; Stary, J.; Zimmermann, M. AML patients with Down syndrome have a high cure rate with AML-BFM therapy with reduced dose intensity. *Leukemia* **2005**, *19*, 1355–1360. [CrossRef]
72. Uffmann, M.; Rasche, M.; Zimmermann, M.; von Neuhoff, C.; Creutzig, U.; Dworzak, M.; Scheffers, L.; Hasle, H.; Zwaan, C.M.; Reinhardt, D.; et al. Therapy reduction in patients with Down syndrome and myeloid leukemia: The international ML-DS 2006 trial. *Blood* **2017**, *129*, 3314–3321. [CrossRef]
73. Bochennek, K.; Hassler, A.; Perner, C.; Gilfert, J.; Schöning, S.; Klingebiel, T.; Reinhardt, D.; Creutzig, U.; Lehrnbecher, T. Infectious complications in children with acute myeloid leukemia: Decreased mortality in multicenter trial AML-BFM 2004. *Blood Cancer J.* **2016**, *6*, e382. [CrossRef]
74. Lehrnbecher, T.; Kaiser, J.; Varwig, D.; Ritter, J.; Groll, A.H.; Creutzig, U.; Klingebiel, T.; Schwabe, D. Antifungal usage in children undergoing intensive treatment for acute myeloid leukemia: Analysis of the multicenter clinical trial AML-BFM 93. *Eur. J. Clin. Microbiol. Infect. Dis.* **2007**, *26*, 735–738. [CrossRef]
75. Lehrnbecher, T.; Varwig, D.; Kaiser, J.; Reinhardt, D.; Klingebiel, T.; Creutzig, U. Infectious complications in pediatric acute myeloid leukemia: Analysis of the prospective multi-institutional clinical trial AML-BFM 93. *Leukemia* **2004**, *18*, 72–77. [CrossRef]
76. Tramsen, L.; Salzmann-Manrique, E.; Bochennek, K.; Klingebiel, T.; Reinhardt, D.; Creutzig, U.; Sung, L.; Lehrnbecher, T. Lack of Effectiveness of Neutropenic Diet and Social Restrictions as Anti-Infective Measures in Children With Acute Myeloid Leukemia: An Analysis of the AML-BFM 2004 Trial. *J. Clin. Oncol.* **2016**, *34*, 2776–2783. [CrossRef] [PubMed]
77. Bhakta, N.; Liu, Q.; Ness, K.K.; Baassiri, M.; Eissa, H.; Yeo, F.; Chemaitilly, W.; Ehrhardt, M.J.; Bass, J.; Bishop, M.W.; et al. The cumulative burden of surviving childhood cancer: An initial report from the St Jude Lifetime Cohort Study (SJLIFE). *Lancet* **2017**, *390*, 2569–2582. [CrossRef]
78. Molgaard-Hansen, L.; Glosli, H.; Jahnukainen, K.; Jarfelt, M.; Jónmundsson, G.K.; Malmros-Svennilson, J.; Nysom, K.; Hasle, H. Quality of health in survivors of childhood acute myeloid leukemia treated with chemotherapy only: A NOPHO-AML study. *Pediatr. Blood Cancer* **2011**, *57*, 1222–1229. [CrossRef] [PubMed]
79. Stefanski, K.J.; Anixt, J.S.; Goodman, P.; Bowers, K.; Leisenring, W.; Scott Baker, K.; Burns, K.; Howell, R.; Davies, S.; Robison, L.L.; et al. Long-Term Neurocognitive and Psychosocial Outcomes After Acute Myeloid Leukemia: A Childhood Cancer Survivor Study Report. *JNCI J. Natl. Cancer Inst.* **2021**, *113*, 481–495. [CrossRef]
80. Lins, M.M.; Mello, M.J.G.; Ribeiro, R.C.; de Camargo, B.; de Fátima Pessoa Militão Albuquerque, M.; Thuler, L.C.S. Survival and risk factors for mortality in pediatric patients with acute myeloid leukemia in a single reference center in low-middle-income country. *Ann. Hematol.* **2019**, *98*, 1403–1411. [CrossRef]
81. Creutzig, U.; Zimmermann, M.; Reinhardt, D.; Dworzak, M.; Stary, J.; Lehrnbecher, T. Early deaths and treatment-related mortality in children undergoing therapy for acute myeloid leukemia: Analysis of the multicenter clinical trials AML-BFM 93 and AML-BFM 98. *J. Clin. Oncol.* **2004**, *22*, 4384–4393. [CrossRef]
82. Abla, O.; Angelini, P.; Di Giuseppe, G.; Kanani, M.F.; Lau, W.; Hitzler, J.; Sung, L.; Naqvi, A. Early Complications of Hyperleukocytosis and Leukapheresis in Childhood Acute Leukemias. *J. Pediatr. Hematol. Oncol.* **2016**, *38*, 111–117. [CrossRef]
83. Klein, K.; van Litsenburg, R.R.L.; de Haas, V.; Dors, N.; van den Heuvel-Eibrink, M.M.; Knops, R.R.G.; Tissing, W.J.E.; Versluys, B.A.; Zwaan, C.M.; Kaspers, G.J.L. Causes of early death and treatment-related death in newly diagnosed pediatric acute myeloid leukemia: Recent experiences of the Dutch Childhood Oncology Group. *Pediatr. Blood Cancer* **2020**, *67*, e28099. [CrossRef]
84. Velten, L.; Story, B.A.; Hernández-Malmierca, P.; Raffel, S.; Leonce, D.R.; Milbank, J.; Paulsen, M.; Demir, A.; Szu-Tu, C.; Frömel, R.; et al. Identification of leukemic and pre-leukemic stem cells by clonal tracking from single-cell transcriptomics. *Nat. Commun.* **2021**, *12*, 1366. [CrossRef] [PubMed]
85. Walter, C.; Pozzorini, C.; Reinhardt, K.; Geffers, R.; Xu, Z.; Reinhardt, D.; von Neuhoff, N.; Hanenberg, H. Single-cell whole exome and targeted sequencing in NPM1/FLT3 positive pediatric acute myeloid leukemia. *Pediatr. Blood Cancer* **2018**, *65*. [CrossRef]
86. Thol, F.; Gabdoulline, R.; Liebich, A.; Klement, P.; Schiller, J.; Kandziora, C.; Hambach, L.; Stadler, M.; Koenecke, C.; Flintrop, M.; et al. Measurable residual disease monitoring by NGS before allogeneic hematopoietic cell transplantation in AML. *Blood* **2018**, *132*, 1703–1713. [CrossRef] [PubMed]
87. Bertuccio, S.N.; Anselmi, L.; Masetti, R.; Lonetti, A.; Cerasi, S.; Polidori, S.; Serravalle, S.; Pession, A. Exploiting Clonal Evolution to Improve the Diagnosis and Treatment Efficacy Prediction in Pediatric AML. *Cancers* **2021**, *13*, 1995. [CrossRef]
88. Chen, X.; Zhu, H.; Qiao, C.; Zhao, S.; Liu, L.; Wang, Y.; Jin, H.; Qian, S.; Wu, Y. Next-generation sequencing reveals gene mutations landscape and clonal evolution in patients with acute myeloid leukemia. *Hematology* **2021**, *26*, 111–122. [CrossRef] [PubMed]
89. Onecha, E.; Rapado, I.; Luz Morales, M.; Carreño-Tarragona, G.; Martinez-Sanchez, P.; Gutierrez, X.; Sáchez Pina, J.M.; Linares, M.; Gallardo, M.; Martinez-López, J.; et al. Monitoring of clonal evolution of acute myeloid leukemia identifies the leukemia subtype, clinical outcome and potential new drug targets for post-remission strategies or relapse. *Haematologica* **2021**, *106*, 2325–2333. [CrossRef]

90. Creutzig, U.; Dworzak, M.; von Neuhoff, N.; Rasche, M.; Reinhardt, D. Akute Promyelozyten-Leukämie: Neue Behandlungsstrategien mit ATRA und ATO-AML-BFM-Empfehlungen. *Klin. Padiatr.* **2018**, *230*, 299–304. [CrossRef]
91. Zwaan, C.M.; Meshinchi, S.; Radich, J.P.; Veerman, A.J.P.; Huismans, D.R.; Munske, L.; Podleschny, M.; Hählen, K.; Pieters, R.; Zimmermann, M.; et al. FLT3 internal tandem duplication in 234 children with acute myeloid leukemia: Prognostic significance and relation to cellular drug resistance. *Blood* **2003**, *102*, 2387–2394. [CrossRef]
92. Winters, A.C.; Maloney, K.W.; Treece, A.L.; Gore, L.; Franklin, A.K. Single-center pediatric experience with venetoclax and azacitidine as treatment for myelodysplastic syndrome and acute myeloid leukemia. *Pediatr. Blood Cancer* **2020**, *67*, e28398. [CrossRef]
93. Karol, S.E.; Alexander, T.B.; Budhraja, A.; Pounds, S.B.; Canavera, K.; Wang, L.; Wolf, J.; Klco, J.M.; Mead, P.E.; Das Gupta, S.; et al. Venetoclax in combination with cytarabine with or without idarubicin in children with relapsed or refractory acute myeloid leukaemia: A phase 1, dose-escalation study. *Lancet Oncol.* **2020**, *21*, 551–560. [CrossRef]
94. Merker, M.; Salzmann-Manrique, E.; Katzki, V.; Huenecke, S.; Bremm, M.; Bakhtiar, S.; Willasch, A.; Jarisch, A.; Soerensen, J.; Schulz, A.; et al. Clearance of Hematologic Malignancies by Allogeneic Cytokine-Induced Killer Cell or Donor Lymphocyte Infusions. *Biol. Blood Marrow Transplant.* **2019**, *25*, 1281–1292. [CrossRef] [PubMed]
95. Nguyen, R.; Wu, H.; Pounds, S.; Inaba, H.; Ribeiro, R.C.; Cullins, D.; Rooney, B.; Bell, T.; Lacayo, N.J.; Heym, K.; et al. A phase II clinical trial of adoptive transfer of haploidentical natural killer cells for consolidation therapy of pediatric acute myeloid leukemia. *J. Immunother. Cancer* **2019**, *7*, 81. [CrossRef] [PubMed]
96. Sendker, S.; Waack, K.; Reinhardt, D. Far from Health: The Bone Marrow Microenvironment in AML, A Leukemia Supportive Shelter. *Children* **2021**, *8*, 371. [CrossRef]
97. Sendker, S.; Reinhardt, D.; Niktoreh, N. Redirecting the Immune Microenvironment in Acute Myeloid Leukemia. *Cancers* **2021**, *13*, 1423. [CrossRef] [PubMed]
98. Maude, S.L.; Laetsch, T.W.; Buechner, J.; Rives, S.; Boyer, M.; Bittencourt, H.; Bader, P.; Verneris, M.R.; Stefanski, H.E.; Myers, G.D.; et al. Tisagenlecleucel in Children and Young Adults with B-Cell Lymphoblastic Leukemia. *N. Engl. J. Med.* **2018**, *378*, 439–448. [CrossRef]
99. Morgan, M.A.; Kloos, A.; Lenz, D.; Kattre, N.; Nowak, J.; Bentele, M.; Keisker, M.; Dahlke, J.; Zimmermann, K.; Sauer, M.; et al. Improved Activity against Acute Myeloid Leukemia with Chimeric Antigen Receptor (CAR)-NK-92 Cells Designed to Target CD123. *Viruses* **2021**, *13*, 1365. [CrossRef]
100. Tang, X.; Yang, L.; Li, Z.; Nalin, A.P.; Dai, H.; Xu, T.; Yin, J.; You, F.; Zhu, M.; Shen, W.; et al. First-in-man clinical trial of CAR NK-92 cells: Safety test of CD33-CAR NK-92 cells in patients with relapsed and refractory acute myeloid leukemia. *Am. J. Cancer Res.* **2018**, *8*, 1083–1089. [PubMed]
101. Zhang, H.; Wang, P.; Li, Z.; He, Y.; Gan, W.; Jiang, H. Anti-CLL1 Chimeric Antigen Receptor T-Cell Therapy in Children with Relapsed/Refractory Acute Myeloid Leukemia. *Clin. Cancer Res.* **2021**, *27*, 3549–3555. [CrossRef]
102. Epperly, R.; Gottschalk, S.; Velasquez, M.P. Harnessing T Cells to Target Pediatric Acute Myeloid Leukemia: CARs, BiTEs, and Beyond. *Children* **2020**, *7*, 14. [CrossRef]
103. Pizzitola, I.; Anjos-Afonso, F.; Rouault-Pierre, K.; Lassailly, F.; Tettamanti, S.; Spinelli, O.; Biondi, A.; Biagi, E.; Bonnet, D. Chimeric antigen receptors against CD33/CD123 antigens efficiently target primary acute myeloid leukemia cells in vivo. *Leukemia* **2014**, *28*, 1596–1605. [CrossRef] [PubMed]
104. Pearson, A.D.J.; Zwaan, C.M.; Kolb, E.A.; Karres, D.; Guillot, J.; Kim, S.Y.; Marshall, L.; Tasian, S.K.; Smith, M.; Cooper, T.; et al. Paediatric Strategy Forum for medicinal product development for acute myeloid leukaemia in children and adolescents: ACCELERATE in collaboration with the European Medicines Agency with participation of the Food and Drug Administration. *Eur. J. Cancer* **2020**, *136*, 116–129. [CrossRef] [PubMed]
105. Pession, A.; Masetti, R.; Rizzari, C.; Putti, M.C.; Casale, F.; Fagioli, F.; Luciani, M.; Lo Nigro, L.; Menna, G.; Micalizzi, C.; et al. Results of the AIEOP AML 2002/01 multicenter prospective trial for the treatment of children with acute myeloid leukemia. *Blood* **2013**, *122*, 170–178. [CrossRef] [PubMed]
106. Waack, K. Improved Outcome in Pediatric AML—THe AML-BFM 2012 Study. *Blood* **2020**, *136*, 12–14. [CrossRef]
107. Creutzig, U.; Zimmermann, M.; Bourquin, J.-P.; Dworzak, M.N.; Fleischhack, G.; Graf, N.; Klingebiel, T.; Kremens, B.; Lehrnbecher, T.; von Neuhoff, C.; et al. Randomized trial comparing liposomal daunorubicin with idarubicin as induction for pediatric acute myeloid leukemia: Results from Study AML-BFM 2004. *Blood* **2013**, *122*, 37–43. [CrossRef] [PubMed]
108. Cooper, T.M.; Franklin, J.; Gerbing, R.B.; Alonzo, T.A.; Hurwitz, C.; Raimondi, S.C.; Hirsch, B.; Smith, F.O.; Mathew, P.; Arceci, R.J.; et al. AAML03P1, a pilot study of the safety of gemtuzumab ozogamicin in combination with chemotherapy for newly diagnosed childhood acute myeloid leukemia: A report from the Children's Oncology Group. *Cancer* **2012**, *118*, 761–769. [CrossRef]
109. Gamis, A.S.; Alonzo, T.A.; Meshinchi, S.; Sung, L.; Gerbing, R.B.; Raimondi, S.C.; Hirsch, B.A.; Kahwash, S.B.; Heerema-McKenney, A.; Winter, L.; et al. Gemtuzumab ozogamicin in children and adolescents with de novo acute myeloid leukemia improves event-free survival by reducing relapse risk: Results from the randomized phase III Children's Oncology Group trial AAML0531. *J. Clin. Oncol.* **2014**, *32*, 3021–3032. [CrossRef]
110. Aplenc, R.; Meshinchi, S.; Sung, L.; Alonzo, T.; Choi, J.; Fisher, B.; Gerbing, R.; Hirsch, B.; Horton, T.; Kahwash, S.; et al. Bortezomib with standard chemotherapy for children with acute myeloid leukemia does not improve treatment outcomes: A report from the Children's Oncology Group. *Haematologica* **2020**, *105*, 1879–1886. [CrossRef]

111. Burnett, A.K.; Hills, R.K.; Russell, N. Twenty five years of UK trials in acute myeloid leukaemia: What have we learned? *Br. J. Haematol.* **2020**, *188*, 86–100. [CrossRef] [PubMed]
112. Dłuzniewska, A.; Balwierz, W.; Balcerska, A.; Chybicka, A.; Kamieńska, E.; Karolczyk, G.; Karpińska-Derda, I.; Krawczuk-Rybak, M.; Kowalczyk, J.R.; Lewandowska, D.; et al. Niepowodzenia leczenia w ostrej białaczce szpikowej u dzieci: Ponad 25-letnie doświadczenia Polskiej Pediatrycznej Grupy ds. Leczenia Białaczek i Chłoniaków. *Przegl. Lek.* **2010**, *67*, 366–370. [PubMed]
113. Czogała, M.; Balwierz, W.; Pawińska-Wąsikowska, K.; Książek, T.; Bukowska-Strakova, K.; Czogała, W.; Sikorska-Fic, B.; Matysiak, M.; Skalska-Sadowska, J.; Wachowiak, J.; et al. Advances in the First Line Treatment of Pediatric Acute Myeloid Leukemia in the Polish Pediatric Leukemia and Lymphoma Study Group from 1983 to 2019. *Cancers* **2021**, *13*, 4356. [CrossRef] [PubMed]
114. Rubnitz, J.E.; Lacayo, N.J.; Inaba, H.; Heym, K.; Ribeiro, R.C.; Taub, J.; McNeer, J.; Degar, B.; Schiff, D.; Yeoh, A.E.-J.; et al. Clofarabine Can Replace Anthracyclines and Etoposide in Remission Induction Therapy for Childhood Acute Myeloid Leukemia: The AML08 Multicenter, Randomized Phase III Trial. *J. Clin. Oncol.* **2019**, *37*, 2072–2081. [CrossRef] [PubMed]

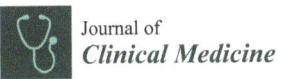

Review

Current Treatment of Juvenile Myelomonocytic Leukemia

Christina Mayerhofer [1], Charlotte M. Niemeyer [1,2] and Christian Flotho [1,2,*]

[1] Division of Pediatric Hematology and Oncology, Department of Pediatrics and Adolescent Medicine, Medical Center, Faculty of Medicine, University of Freiburg, 79106 Freiburg, Germany; christina.mayerhofer@uniklinik-freiburg.de (C.M.); charlotte.niemeyer@uniklinik-freiburg.de (C.M.N.)

[2] German Cancer Consortium (DKTK), 79106 Freiburg, Germany

* Correspondence: christian.flotho@uniklinik-freiburg.de

Abstract: Juvenile myelomonocytic leukemia (JMML) is a rare pediatric leukemia characterized by mutations in five canonical RAS pathway genes. The diagnosis is made by typical clinical and hematological findings associated with a compatible mutation. Although this is sufficient for clinical decision-making in most JMML cases, more in-depth analysis can include DNA methylation class and panel sequencing analysis for secondary mutations. *NRAS*-initiated JMML is heterogeneous and adequate management ranges from watchful waiting to allogeneic hematopoietic stem cell transplantation (HSCT). Upfront azacitidine in *KRAS* patients can achieve long-term remissions without HSCT; if HSCT is required, a less toxic preparative regimen is recommended. Germline *CBL* patients often experience spontaneous resolution of the leukemia or exhibit stable mixed chimerism after HSCT. JMML driven by *PTPN11* or *NF1* is often rapidly progressive, requires swift HSCT and may benefit from pretransplant therapy with azacitidine. Because graft-versus-leukemia alloimmunity is central to cure high risk patients, the immunosuppressive regimen should be discontinued early after HSCT.

Keywords: juvenile myelomonocytic leukemia; RAS signaling; hematopoietic stem cell transplantation; 5-azacitidine; myelodysplastic/myeloproliferative disorders; targeted therapy

1. Introduction

JMML is a pediatric leukemia with shared features of myelodysplastic and myeloproliferative neoplasms, usually manifesting during early childhood with leukocytosis, thrombocytopenia, pronounced monocytosis, splenomegaly, immature precursors on peripheral blood (PB) smear, and bone marrow (BM) blast count below 20% [1–3]. Its clinical and hematological picture, as well as natural history and outcome, are remarkably diverse [4]. The common molecular denominator of JMML is the deregulation of the intracellular Ras signal transduction pathway, caused in >90% of cases by mutations in one (or, rarely, more than one) of five primordial genes (*PTPN11*, *NRAS*, *KRAS*, *NF1*, or *CBL*) [5]. For most patients, allogeneic hematopoietic stem cell transplantation (HSCT) is the only curative treatment option, in contrast to a smaller percentage of children who survive long-term without HSCT and eventually experience spontaneous clinical remissions [6,7]. Clinical and molecular risk factors were established to help predict the disease course and guide therapeutic decisions, including age at diagnosis, percentage of fetal hemoglobin (HbF), platelet count, and aberrant DNA methylation patterns [8,9]. In this article, we review the current knowledge of genetic and epigenetic properties of JMML and provide detailed recommendations for the clinical management of children diagnosed with this challenging disorder.

2. The Origin of JMML: The Ras Pathway

The Ras pathway is a sequence of kinases in the cell that serves as a chain of communication between extracellular mitogens and the cell nucleus [10]. External cytokine signals, relayed through receptor tyrosine kinases and intracellular adapter proteins, lead to guanosine exchange factor-mediated transformation of Ras proteins into their active guanosine triphosphate (GTP)-bound state (reviewed in more detail in [11,12]). The Ras signal is terminated by intrinsic Ras phosphatase activity, which converts Ras back to an inactive guanosine diphosphate (GDP)-bound configuration. An additional layer of regulation is provided by GTPase activating proteins (GAPs). Effects of Ras activation include the subsequent phosphorylation of Raf, Mek, and Erk kinases [13–17], activation of the mammalian target of rapamycin (mTOR) axis via phosphoinositide 3-kinase (PI3K) [18], and others [19]. Among nuclear targets are the transcription factors Jun and Fos [20].

Genetic mutations in specific Ras pathway components (PTPN11, NRAS, KRAS, NF1, or CBL), resulting in net hyperactivation of the Ras-GTP-GDP loop, are present in hematopoietic cells of >90% of children diagnosed with JMML [4,21–26]. These can be traced back to early myeloid stem/progenitor cell compartments [27–29], and they are found in patient cord blood samples [24], substantiating their role as initiating events and suggesting the inception of the leukemogenic sequence before birth [30].

Somatic mutations in exons 3 or 13 of the PTPN11 gene are present in ~35% of JMML cases [22,31], resulting in a gain-of-function of the nonreceptor tyrosine phosphatase Shp2 [32]. Somatic mutations in NRAS or KRAS codons 12, 13, or 61, accounting for ~25% of JMML cases [4,25,33], freeze Ras in its active GTP-bound form by inhibition of GTPase activity or resistance to GAPs [4]. Somatic PTPN11, NRAS, and KRAS mutations occur in heterozygous form in JMML, indicating strong cell-transforming capacity already in monoallelic fashion.

Two congenital developmental disorders predispose to JMML: NF-1 and CBL syndrome [26,34–36]. Here, the germline of the patient carries a monoallelic loss-of-function mutation of the NF1 or CBL gene, which may have been inherited or arisen de novo. JMML develops after somatic biallelic inactivation of the respective gene in hematopoietic progenitor cells, predominantly by mitotic gene recombination resulting in uniparental isodisomy [21,37]. NF1 functions as a Ras-GAP and thus negatively regulates the Ras pathway [38,39]. Indicative features in children with JMML/NF-1 are the presence of ≥6 cutaneous café au lait spots and/or the family history; other characteristics of NF-1, such as neurofibromas, optic pathway gliomas, bone lesions and neurological abnormalities, usually manifest only later. Overall, 10–15% of JMML cases are driven by NF1 [33,40]. CBL is a E3 ubiquitin ligase mediating the decay of receptor tyrosine kinases in the Ras pathway. Mutations targeting exons 8 or 9account for ~15% of JMML cases [26,33]. CBL syndrome, a Noonan-like rasopathy, has a wide phenotypic spectrum. Features include impaired growth, facial anomalies, developmental delay, cryptorchidism, autoimmune phenomena, and notably, neurovasculitis [26,37]. However, it is not rare for patients with JMML and CBL germline mutation to display no abnormalities at all [26,41,42].

Noonan syndrome (NS), the most common rasopathy with an incidence of 1 in 1000–2500 children [43], bears clinical similarities with Turner syndrome. Patients with NS exhibit a short statue, facial dysmorphism, congenital heart defects, skeletal defects, a webbed neck, mental retardation, and cryptorchidism. The genetic basis is a germline mutation in PTPN11 (around 50% of NS cases), SOS1, RAF1, KRAS, BRAF, NRAS or other members of the RAS pathway [5,22,44,45]. Children with NS may experience a polyclonal myeloproliferative disorder (MPD) at a very young age, sometimes shortly after birth [4,46]. Although the condition is indistinguishable from JMML by clinical and hematological features, it has a self-limiting course in the vast majority of cases. Only a small fraction of children with NS/MPD progress to JMML, presumably after the acquisition of additional genetic changes [5,47]. Although the landscape of PTPN11 mutations is not identical in JMML and NS/MPD [31], there is considerable overlap, and it is not well understood how the same mutation elicits a transient disorder when present in the germline and a fatal disorder when acquired somatically. Obviously, the occurrence of germline and somatic Ras pathway mutations in the same clinical context requires analysis of non-hematopoietic tissue (e.g., hair follicles or skin fibroblasts) to differentiate these conditions [9].

Systematic exome sequencing studies revealed that JMML is generally characterized by a paucity of somatic mutations in the neoplastic clone when compared to most other types of cancer [48]. However, subclonal secondary gene mutations can be found in up to half of the cases [23,24,48]. These mutations primarily target the *SETBP1, JAK3, SH2B3,* or *ASXL1* genes. Not infrequently, the secondary mutations affect the Ras pathway itself ("Ras double mutants"). In addition, a role for subclonal mutations in the Polycomb Repressive Complex 2 network was highlighted [23]. Several studies have linked the presence of secondary mutations with an aggressive clinical course or disease progression [23,49]. Furthermore, an association with an increased risk of recurrence after allogeneic HSCT was demonstrated [23,49].

Less than 10% of JMML cases are negative for the five canonical driver mutations. Rarely, these children harbor germline or somatic activating *RRAS* mutations [23,50]. Recently, a *CCDC88C-FLT3* fusion responsive to sorafenib was described in a pediatric patient with clinical features of JMML and monosomy 7 [51]. Other fusions detected in children with myeloproliferative disease include *ALK* [52,53], *ROS1* [52,53], *FIP1L1-RARA* [54], *HCMOGT-1-PDGFRB* [55], *NDEL1-PDGFRB* [56], and *NUP98-HOXA11* [57]. Although kinase fusion-positive cases without Ras pathway mutation may fulfill the clinical and diagnostic criteria of JMML, they likely represent a genetically distinct myeloproliferative neoplasm in childhood. When identified, these tyrosine kinase fusions offer an attractive target for personalized therapies [51,53].

3. Clinical and Hematological Features of JMML

JMML occurs in 1.2 children per million per year, accounting for 2% of pediatric hematopoietic malignancies [58]. One half of the children with JMML are diagnosed below the age of two years and two-thirds are male [59]. Clinical signs at diagnosis include non-specific symptoms such as infections, fatigue, or failure to thrive. Splenomegaly is noted in nearly all cases, often accompanied by hepatomegaly and lymphadenopathy. Pulmonary infiltration by leukemic cells manifests with dry cough, tachypnea and, radiologically, interstitial infiltrates [59,60]. Abdominal symptoms may arise in patients with intestinal infiltration [59]. Variable cutaneous features may be present, ranging from eczematous lesions to erythematous papules or nodules and/or petechiae [60]. In contrast to other pediatric leukemias, JMML does not usually invade the central nervous system. As a substantial proportion of JMML cases arise on the basis of an underlying predisposition syndrome, the clinician needs to examine the patient carefully, paying attention to growth, facial dysmorphism, congenital heart defects, skeletal anomalies, developmental status, and skin lesions such as café-au-lait macules or juvenile xanthogranulomas [45,61–63].

The PB smear typically shows mild to pronounced leukocytosis with monocytosis without a significantly increased number of blasts (median 2% myeloblasts) [60,64]. Immature precursor cells of the granulocytic lineage (myelocytes, metamyelocytes), immature monocytes and nucleated erythropoietic cells are found, giving the blood film examination a pivotal diagnostic role [59]. Platelet and erythrocyte counts are usually decreased, whereas the absolute monocyte count is increased to $>1 \times 10^9$ G/L in all but exceptional cases [1]. Bone marrow examination is necessary to exclude acute leukemia, but is per se insufficient to confirm a suspected diagnosis of JMML. BM findings in JMML include hypercellularity from myelomonocytic proliferation, reduction of megakaryocytes and moderate increase of blasts (<20% myeloblasts) [59].

The combination of young age, splenomegaly, skin lesions, appearance of myeloid and erythroid precursors in the PB, and/or elevated levels of HbF should prompt the pediatric oncologist to suspect JMML and initiate specific tests. First of all, this involves the molecular analysis of driver mutations in the *PTPN11, KRAS, NRAS,* and *CBL* genes, and a meticulous search for features of NF-1 including family history. Genetic analysis of *NF1* can be added, but it is laborious, and the interpretation of findings is not always straightforward. On cytogenetics, two-thirds of cases exhibit a normal karyotype. Monosomy 7 is the most frequent aberration [33,53,65], occurring in combination with *PTPN11* and *KRAS* mutations, but rarely with *NF1*, *NRAS*, or *CBL*. A traditional hallmark of clonogenic JMML cells is their hypersensitivity to GM-CSF in vitro [66,67]. However, laboratory tests of this feature are poorly standardized and not widely available. In the era of efficient mutational analysis, GM-CSF hypersensitivity has become largely dispensable, but may potentially be helpful in occasional cases without a canonical driver mutation. The direct antiglobulin test may come back positive due to autoantibodies, but this is usually not accompanied by clinical or laboratory hemolysis [59]. Similarly, increased levels of IgG, IgM and IgA can be observed [59]. It was suggested that flow cytometric analysis of STAT5 hyperphosphorylation after stimulation with GM-CSF may aid in distinguishing JMML from other conditions [68].

Bacterial [69] and viral (e.g., Epstein–Barr virus [70], cytomegalovirus [71], and herpesvirus 6 [72]) infections can mimic the clinical and laboratory findings of JMML in infants, including fever, splenomegaly, leukocytosis with monocytosis, hypersensitivity to GM-CSF, and STAT5 hyperphosphorylation. Genetic or non-leukemic hematological disorders, such as infantile malignant osteopetrosis, leukocyte adhesion deficiency, Wiskott–Aldrich syndrome, or Ras-related autoimmune lymphoproliferative disease (RALD), must also be differentiated from JMML [69,73,74]. The latter is a non-malignant, chronic condition induced by an apoptosis defect in lymphocytes [74,75]. RALD is characterized by monocytosis, lymphoproliferation and autoimmune phenomena. Blood leukocytes exhibit similar somatic *NRAS* and *KRAS* mutations as in JMML [74], but these patients do not require aggressive treatment. Two cases of JMML evolving from RALD were described in the literature [75,76], highlighting the need for close observation. Differentiation of both entities can be difficult in the absence of monosomy 7. Functional apoptosis assays might be helpful to diagnose RALD [75].

4. The Emerging Role of Epigenetics

The genetic subtypes discussed above account for the phenotypic diversity of JMML only incompletely. For example, long-identified prognostic parameters, such as age of the patient, sex, platelet count, or elevated levels of fetal hemoglobin [6,40,59], do not correspond to a specific Ras genotype. Further molecular factors related to the course of the disease were observed in JMML, including micro and long non-coding RNA expression [77,78], AML-like expression profile [79], secondary mutations [48,49] and alterations of the fetal hematopoietic regulator gene *LIN28B* [80]. In addition, the previous observation of epigenetic dysregulation during Ras-mediated transformation suggested aberrant DNA methylation as a potential disease modifier [81,82].

The first study examining the role DNA methylation changes in a large European series of 127 children with JMML revealed CpG island hypermethylation of a candidate gene set in up to half of the cases [81]. Importantly, CpG hypermethylation at diagnosis was an independent risk factor for poor overall survival (OS) and risk of relapse after HSCT [81]. The conclusions were largely confirmed in a Japanese study investigating a similar candidate gene set [83]. Both studies observed that hypermethylation in JMML affected a narrow subset of gene promoters, as opposed to broad random distribution across all genetic regions examined, suggesting that high-risk JMML is characterized by a CpG island hypermethylation phenotype, as discovered previously in other specific cancer types [82–84]. Several follow-up studies corroborated this concept at the candidate gene level [85–87].

Extending these findings to a genome-wide scope using array-based methods, study groups in Europe [33], Japan [53] and United States [65] analyzed independent JMML cohorts with the aim to establish a methylation based risk-stratification. Comparing the methylome patterns of 167 children with JMML, the European Working Group of Myelodysplastic Syndromes in Childhood (EWOG-MDS) discriminated 3 distinct methylation groups, again highlighting epigenetic dysregulation as a strong prognostic risk factor [33]. Factors associated with hypermethylation were repressed chromatin, Ras pathway double mutants and upregulation of methyltransferases DNMT1 and DNMT3B.

This supported the emergence of DNA hypermethylation as a consequence of hyperactive Ras signaling [81,83]. Several associations between genetic driver mutation and DNA methylation pattern were noted. The group of patients with highest hypermethylation was dominated by somatic *PTPN11* mutation and older children, both known factors for inferior clinical course, whereas the low-methylation group was enriched for patients with NS/MPD, CBL cases, and young children with somatic *NRAS* mutations. The group with intermediate hypermethylation was characterized by somatic *KRAS* mutations and occurrence of monosomy 7 [33]. The Japanese cohort, consisting of 106 JMML cases, was split into two methylation groups [53]. In addition to known clinical risk factors, the high-methylation group involved cases with *NF1* or *PTPN11* mutations, secondary mutations, *LIN28B* overexpression and AML-like expression profile [53]. The North American study defined three similar methylation classes in 39 patients [65]. Interestingly, some JMML patients with good transplantation-free outcome and all patients with NS/MPD exhibited a DNA methylation signature closer to healthy controls than to other JMML cases [65,88], again underlining the significance of disrupted epigenetic control for the biology of JMML. The fact that all three methylome studies had used a comparable technical platform provided the unique opportunity for a comprehensive overarching meta-analysis. These collaborative efforts succeeded in developing and validating an international standard classifier of three different methylation categories matching those above and correlating with disease biology and outcome [88]. The prospective use of methylation analysis as a biomarker in JMML will aid in adapting treatment strategies, e.g., use of pretransplant therapy or low-intensity graft-versus-host disease (GVHD) prophylaxis, and support the generation of internationally comparable JMML study data.

5. Current Recommendations for the Management of JMML

With extensive molecular diagnostic work-up of JMML established in major international study groups and large centers around the world, it has become evident that there can no longer be a uniform one-size-fits-all approach for this disorder (Table 1). The authors recommend that therapeutic decisions in a newly diagnosed case of JMML be based on the following diagnostic information (Figure 1):

- Level of fetal hemoglobin (measured in a blood sample taken prior to erythrocyte transfusion; levels far above the age-adjusted reference value are also meaningful if sampled after transfusion)
- Panel sequence analysis of the five primordial Ras pathway genes (*PTPN11, NF1, KRAS, NRAS, CBL*)
- Presence of the primordial mutation in non-hematopoietic tissue (indicating germline status)
- Where available, the following additional information will aid in clinical decision-making, though it is not indispensable for adequate management in most cases:
- DNA methylation class
- Panel sequence analysis of recurrent secondary mutations. The assessment should include *SETBP1, JAK3, RRAS, RRAS2*, and *ASXL1*; other targets are rare.

5.1. Somatic NRAS Mutation

The disease course in this group is remarkably heterogeneous. In older children with severe thrombocytopenia, increased HbF and high methylation class, a rapidly progressive course with a considerable risk of recurrence after HSCT is to be expected, likening the disorder to *PTPN11*- or *NF1*-driven JMML. On the other hand, a group of patients exist who are clinically well and have low HbF. Here, spontaneous clinical regression of the disease can occur in the long run without therapy. The search for an unrelated stem cell donor may be deferred in these cases. In between these two ends of the spectrum, the prospective identification of patients who benefit from watchful waiting is the real challenge. Factors suggesting surveillance without therapy include infant age, clinical status, age-appropriate levels of HbF, and low methylation class [41,89,90]. However, this must be balanced with the concern that delaying HSCT may compromise the outcome in some patients. EWOG-MDS data shows that the survival curve of JMML patients without HSCT keeps dropping during the first ten years and then plateaus at 25%.

Table 1. Management of JMML according to driver mutation. HSCT, hematopoietic stem cell transplantation; GVHD, graft-versus-host disease; DLI, donor lymphocyte infusions; NF-1, neurofibromatosis 1.

Ras Pathway Mutation	Frequency in JMML	Features	DNA Methylation Profile	Recommendations for Treatment
Somatic NRAS	10–15%	Diverse	Mostly low, occasional IM or HM	HSCT for many, careful selection of candidates for watch-and-wait
Somatic KRAS	10–15%	Frequent monosomy 7, autoimmune phenomena	Intermediate or low	Azacitidine and/or HSCT
Somatic PTPN11	35%	Compromised clinical status at diagnosis, highest risk of unfavorable outcome	Mostly high	Swift HSCT (+pretransplant azacitidine) with low intensity GVHD prophylaxis, in absence of GVHD early withdrawal of prophylaxis, consider azacitidine plus DLI posttransplant
Germline NF1	10–15%	Café-au-lait spots, possibly positive family history, older age at diagnosis, less severe thrombocytopenia	High or intermediate	Swift HSCT (+pretransplant azacitidine) with low intensity GVHD prophylaxis, in absence of GVHD early withdrawal of prophylaxis
Germline CBL	15%	Syndromic rasopathy features, autoimmunity and vasculitis	Low	Watch-and-wait. HSCT if disease progresses, patients after HSCT often revert to stable mixed chimerism
All negative	5–10%	Rarely activating kinase fusions in RNA sequencing	Low or intermediate	Differentiate non-neoplastic disease, perform extended work-up for rasopathies. Most patients require HSCT

It is very rare for a germline *NRAS* or *KRAS* mutation to be detected in a suspected JMML case. Most of these children have additional syndromic features of the rasopathy spectrum [91,92] or correspond in phenotype to Noonan syndrome [93]. Anecdotal observations contradict the paradigm that the canonical tumor-associated Ras mutations in codons 12, 13 or 61 are not tolerated in the germline; such cases are sometimes based on mosaicism [94,95]. Because of their rarity, no general recommendation can be given for the treatment of these highly individual cases.

5.2. Somatic KRAS Mutation

Children diagnosed with *KRAS*-JMML are typically very young, often infants. Concurrent monosomy 7 in the neoplastic clone is often observed (see below). Autoimmune phenomena (hyperimmunoglobulinemia, autoantibodies) should be searched for, and a diagnostic differentiation from RALD [74,96,97] should be kept in mind. The clinical presentation of *KRAS*-driven JMML tends to be aggressive, requiring rapid intervention. In the past, long-term survival without HSCT has not been reported for this group, but the picture is now changing with the introduction of azacitidine. *KRAS*-mutated JMML responds particularly well to low-dose azacitidine with long-lasting clinical and molecular remissions [98,99]. Regimens use 100 mg/m^2/day on five consecutive days or 75 mg/m^2/day on seven consecutive days, repeated every 28 days; due to instability, immediate intravenous or subcutaneous application of the cold reconstituted solution must be observed.

Azacitidine has a favorable toxicity profile in children with JMML, mainly including lower-grade cytopenias, gastrointestinal discomfort, and infections [64,98]. It is variable how many cycles of azacitidine are necessary to achieve a response; between 6 and 9 cycles are usually administered. Frequently, the earliest sign of response to azacitidine is the improvement of thrombocytopenia. The spleen size diminishes after three to six cycles. Possibly, long-term cure with azacitidine alone will be achievable in *KRAS*-mutated JMML with a low risk profile.

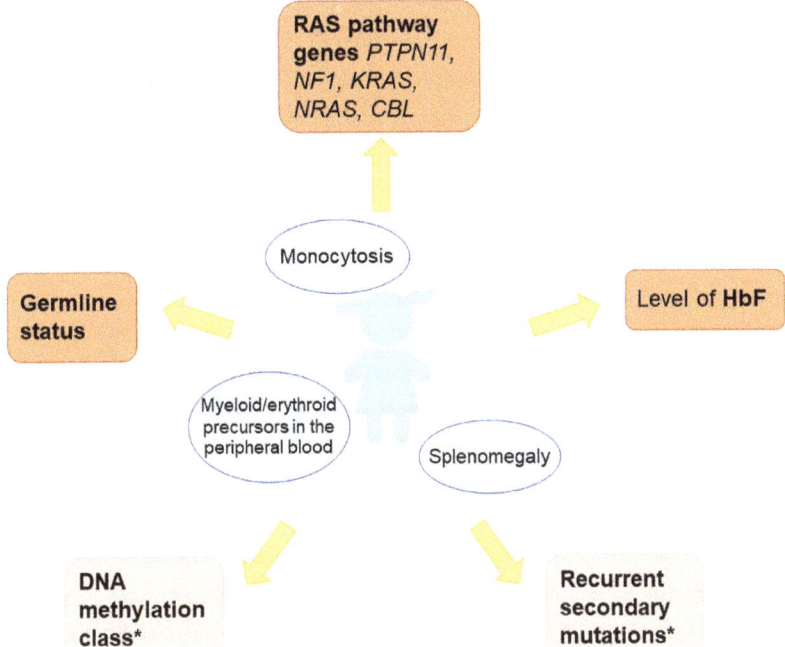

Figure 1. Diagnostic approach for children with JMML. * Helpful for clinical decision making, but not mandatory.

5.3. Somatic PTPN11 Mutation

This is the numerically largest group that also carries the highest risk of rapid progression and early death. As no curative chemotherapy regimen is known, expeditious planning of allogeneic HSCT is mandatory. Within this group, risk factors for an unfavorable course are: age at diagnosis ≥2 years, significantly increased level of HbF, presence of secondary mutations, and/or high methylation class. In these cases, the aim should be to perform HSCT within a period of 3 months after diagnosis (recommendations for implementation see below). Low-dose azacitidine is the preferable option for upfront therapy until HSCT in non-high risk cases, with the goal to achieve a more favorable biological status of the leukemia. In many affected children, this treatment leads to a clinical partial remission or at least sufficient disease control until HSCT [64,98–100] However, high-risk cases carry the potential of immediate progression under azacitidine and may therefore be better off with more instant cytoreduction using 6-mercaptopurine (50 mg/m^2/day, to be adjusted according to clinical course) and/or cytarabine (40 mg/m^2/day × 5 days) [7]. If a patient presents in a critically ill condition that requires rapid reduction of tumor burden, the use of intensive chemotherapy with cytarabine (2 g/m^2/day × 5 days) and fludarabine (30 mg/m^2/day × 5 days) may also be considered [7]. However, this involves a substantial risk of organ toxicity and life-threatening infections. Removal of the spleen, which is often grossly enlarged, can be justified in individual cases to control respiratory impairment. A systematic beneficial effect of splenectomy on the further course of the disease has not been proven [40,101]. It is not yet clear whether treatment with azacitidine before HSCT also improves the long-term prognosis in this patient group. A recent non-randomized prospective study using a matched historical cohort as control group supports this assumption [98]. Until more precise evidence is available, the authors emphasize that treatment with azacitidine must not delay urgent HSCT in patients with *PTPN11* mutation.

5.4. Germline Mutation in PTPN11

Germline mutations in *PTPN11* cause Noonan syndrome, a condition of the rasopathy spectrum predisposing to a myeloproliferative disorder imitating JMML. For this reason, genetic diagnostics in suspected cases of JMML must always be carried out in both hematopoietic and non-hematopoietic material. Cultivated fibroblasts from a skin biopsy are ideal; hair follicles are less invasive, but more challenging to analyze. An oral mucous membrane swab has a high probability of contamination with hematopoietic cells, even if it is macroscopically not bloody, and should therefore only be scored if the result is negative.

In cases of suspected JMML in very young patients or with clinical evidence of Noonan syndrome, the diagnostic test for *PTPN11* should not just encompass the hotspot exons 3 and 13 because Noonan syndrome mutations may also be found in exons 4 or 8. The spectrum of somatic *PTPN11* mutations in nonsyndromic JMML and germline *PTPN11* mutations in Noonan-associated MPD overlaps to a great extent but not completely [31].

The distinction between non-syndromic JMML and Noonan-associated MPD is important, as the latter is usually self-limiting. However, these patients must be monitored carefully, as there can be relevant clinical compromise from cell infiltrates, making it necessary to begin cytoreductive therapy. In individual cases, a clonal development towards a bona fide neoplastic disease is possible [47,102,103].

5.5. Neurofibromatosis Type 1

If not already recognized in the patient, the syndrome can usually be diagnosed clinically and/or through family history at the time of onset of JMML. In younger children, only café-au-lait spots but not the other typical signs of neurofibromatosis may be present. Six or more café-au-lait spots as stipulated in the NIH criteria are noted in the majority of children, but in exceptional cases there may be none or fewer. Genetic analysis of *NF1* usually confirms the clinical diagnosis in children with JMML/NF-1 [104]. The typical finding is an *NF1*-inactivating heterozygous variation in the germline of the patient that arose de novo (~50% of cases) or was inherited. These lesions are often, but not always, deletions or truncating missense mutations reported as recurrent aberrations in the NF-1 literature. In addition, the neoplastic clone exhibits somatic loss of heterozygosity at the *NF1* locus or an independent second *NF1* mutation, leading to biallelic *NF1* inactivation [21,104,105]. The judgment is more difficult if no clinical signs of neurofibromatosis are present and the genetic findings correspond to the above paradigm only incompletely (for example, in case of monoallelic lesions, variants of unclear significance, no germline findings or low allelic frequency). In such cases, a myeloid disorder with a secondary *NF1* lesion, but driven by an unrelated event, may be present. With careful work-up, however, such dilemmas are rare.

JMML on the basis of NF-1 manifests more frequently at an older age than the other groups and typically does not involve a drastically reduced platelet count. Some children initially show little clinical impairment. However, long-term survival without HSCT has not yet been observed in this group, so that proceeding to transplant and inception of therapy with azacitidine is advisable as in patients with somatic *PTPN11* mutation. Consistent with this recommendation, JMML/NF-1 cases almost always have an intermediate or high methylation profile [88].

5.6. CBL Mutation

The typical configuration of *CBL* mutations in JMML is a heterozygous missense point mutation in *CBL* exons 8 or 9 in the germline, accompanied by uniparental isodisomy of the 11q chromosome arm as a somatic event in hematopoietic cells, leading to loss of heterozygosity [26,36,37]. Many, but not all, children show syndromic rasopathy features, such as facial dysmorphia and growth retardation. A particular phenomenon in this patient group is the frequent occurrence of autoimmunity and vasculitis. Some children with CBL-JMML have massive organ enlargement and may require splenectomy for symptom relief. Most patients do not require swift HSCT but can be managed with watchful waiting; many of these experience spontaneous resolution of the myeloproliferation. The homozygous *CBL*-mutant status in hematopoietic cells may persist until adulthood even in the absence of hematologic abnormalities [106]. Patients who undergo transplant often revert to stable mixed chimerism with sufficient disease control [6,26,36]. It is still unclear if the allograft also prevents the later development of symptoms related to autoimmune vasculitis. A recent report highlighted the role of somatic-only *CBL* inactivation in five patients with a clinical course that required HSCT [42], again illustrating the need for proper germline analysis in the diagnostic evaluation of JMML.

5.7. None of the Above

Suspected cases of JMML with negative panel sequencing for all five primordial genes and no clinical evidence of NF-1 are called "quintuple-negative" or "all-negative". In a third of these cases, in-depth multimodal genetic analysis uncovered a driving role of the *NF1* gene in the absence of clinical NF-1 features [104]. In other cases, RNA sequencing identified activating fusions involving *ALK*, *ROS1*, or *FLT3* [51,53]. Some authors argue in favor of diagnosing such myeloproliferative disorders as JMML due to the indistinguishable clinical and hematologic presentation. Excluding non-neoplastic causes of myelomonocytic proliferation, a maximum of 5–10% of suspected JMML cases remain genetically unexplained. It is advisable to refer these patients to an extended rasopathy work-up, especially if additional syndromic stigmata are present.

5.8. Monosomy 7

The significance of monosomy 7 for the biology of JMML is unclear, and there seems to be no association with clinical features or relevance for outcome [40]. Interestingly, monosomy 7 is observed more frequently in European compared to Japanese patients with JMML [33]. In a large international series, all patients with monosomy 7 and intermediate methylation class carried *KRAS* mutations, in contrast to an association between monosomy 7 and *PTPN11* or *NF1* in the high methylation group, and the absence of monosomy 7 in patients with low methylation pattern [88]. The mechanistic connection between this particular chromosomal lesion and aberrant DNA methylation patterns is not understood. Overall, it is likely that the presence of monosomy 7 plays a supportive role in JMML rather than being an independent pathogenetic factor [107]. This concept is also supported by the observation of secondary monosomy 7 in a watch-and-wait patient with Noonan syndrome and neonatal myeloproliferative disorder [102].

5.9. Allogeneic HSCT

Busulfan-based myeloablative conditioning regimens are commonly chosen and achieve 55–73% OS with a moderate 10–15% rate of transplant-related mortality but significant probability of leukemia relapse in the order of 25–35% [7,40,101,108–112]. The EWOG-MDS currently recommends a three-alkylator regimen consisting of busulfan (0.8–1.2 mg/kg/dose given 4 doses per day, day 7 to day 4), cyclophosphamide (60 mg/kg/d, day 3 to day 2), and melphalan (125–140 mg/m^2/d on day 1) [40]. In an attempt to reduce toxicity, a recent prospective randomized trial compared busulfan, cyclophosphamide, and melphalan with busulfan and fludarabine alone but terminated early due to excessive disease recurrence in the latter arm [113]. Matched sibling donors

(MSD) or matched/1-antigen-disparate unrelated donors (MUD) are considered the most suitable stem cell sources [40]. Matched cord blood units are a viable alternative, especially for smaller patients [114–117]. Although haploidentical relatives are readily available for urgent transplant and highly motivated, this should still be viewed as an approach with limited experience [101,112,118]. A recent study from China in 47 JMML patients suggested a lower relapse incidence in mismatched/haploidentical donor transplants compared to matched donors with similar rates of acute/chronic graft-versus-host disease and non-relapse mortality [101].

The North American group noted better post-HSCT outcome of patients with JMML who experienced molecular response to pretransplant chemotherapy [119], similar to other pediatric leukemias [120,121]. However, a limitation was that only a minority of patients responded to chemotherapy, conceivably those with favorable disease biology. Biomarkers predicting response to chemotherapy are lacking. Therefore, it cannot be generalized that pretransplant chemotherapy benefits survival in JMML, and the risk of unwarranted organ damage remains a concern [122].

Beside the leukemia biology factors discussed above, the way the transplant procedure is handled significantly influences the risk of relapse. It is likely that it is not so much the conditioning regimen but rather the establishment of a graft-versus-leukemia effect that is decisive for the success of allogeneic HSCT in JMML [101,109–111]. For this reason, EWOG-MDS recommends keeping immunosuppressive therapy with cyclosporine A at low levels (trough levels around 80 µg/L) and tapering early (from day +40 in the absence of grade II-IV GVHD). It is advisable to determine the recipient-donor chimerism at very close intervals (up to weekly in high-risk patients), as the reappearance of even small autologous cell populations mandates immediate withdrawal of the immunosuppressive therapy [123–125].

Age at diagnosis ≥ 2 years, *NF1* or somatic *PTPN11* mutation, and high DNA methylation define a patient group whose risk of JMML recurrence after HSCT is even higher than 50%, bringing up the question of post-transplant prophylaxis. On the basis of favorable data for other myeloid neoplasms [126–131] and in the absence of better alternatives, the authors consider it appropriate to recommend azacitidine (started as soon as safe and tolerable after engraftment; 32 mg/m^2/day for five consecutive days, every 28 days) plus donor lymphocyte infusions (started after 3 cycles of azacitidine and 4 weeks after discontinuation of immunosuppressive prophylaxis, CD3$^+$ cell dose 1–5 $\times$ 10^6/kg, repeated every 8 weeks with increasing cell dose up to 1–5 $\times$ 10^7/kg). However, we emphasize that there are no systematic data for this approach in JMML.

5.10. Experimental Agents and Targeted Therapy

Despite the prominent role of the Ras/MAPK network, attempts to target this complex signal cascade have shown limited therapeutic benefit in JMML [10,132]. The Children's Oncology Group is currently recruiting patients for a phase II trial to examine the safety and efficacy of oral trametinib, a MEK1/2 inhibitor, in refractory or relapsed JMML (NCT03190915). In vitro data from induced pluripotent stem cell lines suggests mutation-specific sensitivity to kinase inhibition, with a preferential sensitivity of *PTPN11*-driven JMML to trametinib [133]. BCL2 inhibition gave impressive results when combined with azacitidine in elderly AML patients [134,135] and early results argue for a benefit in pediatric patients with advanced MDS/AML [136,137]. With an upregulation of the macrophage immune checkpoint CD47 in myeloid malignancies, ongoing preclinical and clinical trials test CD47-directed agents in MDS/AML, with encouraging efficacy results in combination with azacitidine [138–140].

Author Contributions: Conceptualization, C.M., C.M.N. and C.F.; writing—original draft preparation, C.M.; writing—review and editing, C.M.N. and C.F.; funding acquisition, C.M.N. and C.F. All authors have read and agreed to the published version of the manuscript.

Funding: This manuscript was supported by Bundesministerium für Bildung und Forschung MyPred 01GM1911A (to C.M.N. and C.F.) and Deutsche Forschungsgemeinschaft CRC992-C05 (to C.F.).

Institutional Review Board Statement: Not applicable.

Informed Consent Statement: Not applicable.

Acknowledgments: The authors wish to thank all physicians and scientists collaborating in the European Working Group of Myelodysplastic Syndromes in Childhood for their valuable contributions.

Conflicts of Interest: C.M.N. has a consultancy with Bristol-Myers Squibb. The other authors declare no conflict of interest. The funders had no role in the writing of the manuscript.

References

1. Arber, D.A.; Orazi, A.; Hasserjian, R.; Thiele, J.; Borowitz, M.J.; Le Beau, M.M.; Bloomfield, C.D.; Cazzola, M.; Vardiman, J.W. The 2016 revision to the World Health Organization classification of myeloid neoplasms and acute leukemia. *Blood* **2016**, *127*, 2391–2405. [CrossRef]
2. Harris, N.L.; Jaffe, E.S.; Diebold, J.; Flandrin, G.; Muller-Hermelink, H.K.; Vardiman, J.; Lister, T.A.; Bloomfield, C.D. World Health Organization classification of neoplastic diseases of the hematopoietic and lymphoid tissues: Report of the Clinical Advisory Committee meeting-Airlie House, Virginia, November 1997. *J. Clin. Oncol.* **1999**, *17*, 3835–3849. [CrossRef]
3. Vardiman, J.W.; Thiele, J.; Arber, D.A.; Brunning, R.D.; Borowitz, M.J.; Porwit, A.; Harris, N.L.; Le Beau, M.M.; Hellström-Lindberg, E.; Tefferi, A.; et al. The 2008 revision of the World Health Organization (WHO) classification of myeloid neoplasms and acute leukemia: Rationale and important changes. *Blood* **2009**, *114*, 937–951. [CrossRef] [PubMed]
4. Niemeyer, C.M. JMML genomics and decisions. *Hematol. Am. Soc. Hematol. Educ. Prog.* **2018**, *2018*, 307–312. [CrossRef]
5. Niemeyer, C.M. RAS diseases in children. *Haematologica* **2014**, *99*, 1653–1662. [CrossRef]
6. Locatelli, F.; Niemeyer, C.M. How I treat juvenile myelomonocytic leukemia. *Blood* **2015**, *125*, 1083–1090. [CrossRef]
7. Dvorak, C.C.; Loh, M.L. Juvenile myelomonocytic leukemia: Molecular pathogenesis informs current approaches to therapy and hematopoietic cell transplantation. *Front. Pediatr.* **2014**, *2*, 25. [CrossRef]
8. Loh, M.L. Recent advances in the pathogenesis and treatment of juvenile myelomonocytic leukaemia. *Br. J. Haematol.* **2011**, *152*, 677–687. [CrossRef]
9. Niemeyer, C.M.; Flotho, C. Juvenile myelomonocytic leukemia: Who's the driver at the wheel? *Blood* **2019**, *133*, 1060–1070. [CrossRef]
10. Stephen, A.G.; Esposito, D.; Bagni, R.K.; McCormick, F. Dragging ras back in the ring. *Cancer Cell* **2014**, *25*, 272–281. [CrossRef]
11. Ward, A.F.; Braun, B.S.; Shannon, K.M. Targeting oncogenic Ras signaling in hematologic malignancies. *Blood* **2012**, *120*, 3397–3406. [CrossRef]
12. Brummer, T.; McInnes, C. RAF kinase dimerization: Implications for drug discovery and clinical outcomes. *Oncogene* **2020**, *39*, 4155–4169. [CrossRef]
13. Warne, P.H.; Viciana, P.R.; Downward, J. Direct interaction of Ras and the amino-terminal region of Raf-1 in vitro. *Nature* **1993**, *364*, 352–355. [CrossRef]
14. Pelech, S.L.; Sanghera, J.S. MAP kinases: Charting the regulatory pathways. *Science* **1992**, *257*, 1355–1356. [CrossRef]
15. Boulton, T.G.; Nye, S.H.; Robbins, D.J.; Ip, N.Y.; Radzlejewska, E.; Morgenbesser, S.D.; DePinho, R.A.; Panayotatos, N.; Cobb, M.H.; Yancopoulos, G.D. ERKs: A family of protein-serine/threonine kinases that are activated and tyrosine phosphorylated in response to insulin and NGF. *Cell* **1991**, *65*, 663–675. [CrossRef]
16. Khosravi-Far, R.; White, M.A.; Westwick, J.K.; Solski, P.A.; Chrzanowska-Wodnicka, M.; van Aelst, L.; Wigler, M.H.; Der, C.J. Oncogenic Ras activation of Raf/mitogen-activated protein kinase-independent pathways is sufficient to cause tumorigenic transformation. *Mol. Cell. Biol.* **1996**, *16*, 3923–3933. [CrossRef] [PubMed]
17. Joneson, T.; White, M.A.; Wigler, M.H.; Bar-Sagi, D. Stimulation of membrane ruffling and MAP kinase activation by distinct effectors of RAS. *Science* **1996**, *271*, 810–812. [CrossRef]
18. Dinner, S.; Platanias, L.C. Targeting the mTOR Pathway in Leukemia. *J. Cell. Biochem.* **2016**, *117*, 1745–1752. [CrossRef]
19. Simanshu, D.K.; Nissley, D.V.; McCormick, F. RAS Proteins and Their Regulators in Human Disease. *Cell* **2017**, *170*, 17–33. [CrossRef]
20. Yordy, J.S.; Muise-Helmericks, R.C. Signal transduction and the Ets family of transcription factors. *Oncogene* **2000**, *19*, 6503–6513. [CrossRef]
21. Steinemann, D.; Arning, L.; Praulich, I.; Stuhrmann, M.; Hasle, H.; Stary, J.; Schlegelberger, B.; Niemeyer, C.M.; Flotho, C. Mitotic recombination and compound-heterozygous mutations are predominant NF1-inactivating mechanisms in children with juvenile myelomonocytic leukemia and neurofibromatosis type 1. *Haematologica* **2010**, *95*, 320–323. [CrossRef]
22. Tartaglia, M.; Niemeyer, C.M.; Fragale, A.; Song, X.; Buechner, J.; Jung, A.; Hählen, K.; Hasle, H.; Licht, J.D.; Gelb, B.D. Somatic mutations in PTPN11 in juvenile myelomonocytic leukemia, myelodysplastic syndromes and acute myeloid leukemia. *Nat. Genet.* **2003**, *34*, 148–150. [CrossRef]

23. Caye, A.; Strullu, M.; Guidez, F.; Cassinat, B.; Gazal, S.; Fenneteau, O.; Lainey, E.; Nouri, K.; Nakhaei-Rad, S.; Dvorsky, R.; et al. Juvenile myelomonocytic leukemia displays mutations in components of the RAS pathway and the PRC2 network. *Nat. Genet.* **2015**, *47*, 1334–1340. [CrossRef]
24. Stieglitz, E.; Taylor-Weiner, A.N.; Chang, T.Y.; Gelston, L.C.; Wang, Y.-D.; Mazor, T.; Esquivel, E.; Yu, A.; Seepo, S.; Olsen, S.; et al. The genomic landscape of juvenile myelomonocytic leukemia. *Nat. Genet.* **2015**, *47*, 1326–1333. [CrossRef] [PubMed]
25. Flotho, C.; Valcamonica, S.; Mach-Pascual, S.; Schmahl, G.; Corral, L.; Ritterbach, J.; Hasle, H.; Aricò, M.; Biondi, A.; Niemeyer, C.M. RAS mutations and clonality analysis in children with juvenile myelomonocytic leukemia (JMML). *Leukemia* **1999**, *13*, 32–37. [CrossRef]
26. Niemeyer, C.M.; Kang, M.W.; Shin, D.H.; Furlan, I.; Erlacher, M.; Bunin, N.J.; Bunda, S.; Finklestein, J.Z.; Gorr, T.A.; Mehta, P.; et al. Germline CBL mutations cause developmental abnormalities and predispose to juvenile myelomonocytic leukemia. *Nat. Genet.* **2010**, *42*, 794–800. [CrossRef]
27. Caye, A.; Rouault-Pierre, K.; Strullu, M.; Lainey, E.; Abarrategi, A.; Fenneteau, O.; Arfeuille, C.; Osman, J.; Cassinat, B.; Pereira, S.; et al. Despite mutation acquisition in hematopoietic stem cells, JMML-propagating cells are not always restricted to this compartment. *Leukemia* **2020**, *34*, 1658–1668. [CrossRef]
28. Louka, E.; Povinelli, B.; Rodriguez-Meira, A.; Buck, G.; Wen, W.X.; Wang, G.; Sousos, N.; Ashley, N.; Hamblin, A.; Booth, C.A.G.; et al. Heterogeneous disease-propagating stem cells in juvenile myelomonocytic leukemia. *J. Exp. Med.* **2021**, *218*. [CrossRef]
29. Busque, L.; Gilliland, D.G.; Prchal, J.T.; Sieff, C.A.; Weinstein, H.J.; Sokol, J.M.; Belickova, M.; Wayne, A.S.; Zuckerman, K.S.; Sokol, L. Clonality in juvenile chronic myelogenous leukemia. *Blood* **1995**, *85*, 21–30. [CrossRef]
30. Matsuda, K.; Sakashita, K.; Taira, C.; Tanaka-Yanagisawa, M.; Yanagisawa, R.; Shiohara, M.; Kanegane, H.; Hasegawa, D.; Kawasaki, K.; Endo, M.; et al. Quantitative assessment of PTPN11 or RAS mutations at the neonatal period and during the clinical course in patients with juvenile myelomonocytic leukaemia. *Br. J. Haematol.* **2010**, *148*, 593–599. [CrossRef]
31. Kratz, C.P.; Niemeyer, C.M.; Castleberry, R.P.; Cetin, M.; Bergsträsser, E.; Emanuel, P.D.; Hasle, H.; Kardos, G.; Klein, C.; Kojima, S.; et al. The mutational spectrum of PTPN11 in juvenile myelomonocytic leukemia and Noonan syndrome/myeloproliferative disease. *Blood* **2005**, *106*, 2183–2185. [CrossRef] [PubMed]
32. Tartaglia, M.; Mehler, E.L.; Goldberg, R.; Zampino, G.; Brunner, H.G.; Kremer, H.; van der Burgt, I.; Crosby, A.H.; Ion, A.; Jeffery, S.; et al. Mutations in PTPN11, encoding the protein tyrosine phosphatase SHP-2, cause Noonan syndrome. *Nat. Genet.* **2001**, *29*, 465–468. [CrossRef] [PubMed]
33. Lipka, D.B.; Witte, T.; Toth, R.; Yang, J.; Wiesenfarth, M.; Nöllke, P.; Fischer, A.; Brocks, D.; Gu, Z.; Park, J.; et al. RAS-pathway mutation patterns define epigenetic subclasses in juvenile myelomonocytic leukemia. *Nat. Commun.* **2017**, *8*, 2126. [CrossRef]
34. Stiller, C.A.; Chessells, J.M.; Fitchett, M. Neurofibromatosis and childhood leukaemia/lymphoma: A population-based UKCCSG study. *Br. J. Cancer* **1994**, *70*, 969–972. [CrossRef] [PubMed]
35. Shannon, K.M.; O'Connell, P.; Martin, G.A.; Paderanga, D.; Olson, K.; Dinndorf, P.; McCormick, F. Loss of the normal NF1 allele from the bone marrow of children with type 1 neurofibromatosis and malignant myeloid disorders. *N. Engl. J. Med.* **1994**, *330*, 597–601. [CrossRef]
36. Pérez, B.; Mechinaud, F.; Galambrun, C.; Ben Romdhane, N.; Isidor, B.; Philip, N.; Derain-Court, J.; Cassinat, B.; Lachenaud, J.; Kaltenbach, S.; et al. Germline mutations of the CBL gene define a new genetic syndrome with predisposition to juvenile myelomonocytic leukaemia. *J. Med. Genet.* **2010**, *47*, 686–691. [CrossRef]
37. Loh, M.L.; Sakai, D.S.; Flotho, C.; Kang, M.; Fliegauf, M.; Archambeault, S.; Mullighan, C.G.; Chen, L.; Bergstraesser, E.; Bueso-Ramos, C.E.; et al. Mutations in CBL occur frequently in juvenile myelomonocytic leukemia. *Blood* **2009**, *114*, 1859–1863. [CrossRef]
38. Bollag, G.; Clapp, D.W.; Shih, S.; Adler, F.; Zhang, Y.Y.; Thompson, P.; Lange, B.J.; Freedman, M.H.; McCormick, F.; Jacks, T.; et al. Loss of NF1 results in activation of the Ras signaling pathway and leads to aberrant growth in haematopoietic cells. *Nat. Genet.* **1996**, *12*, 144–148. [CrossRef]
39. Largaespada, D.A.; Brannan, C.I.; Jenkins, N.A.; Copeland, N.G. Nf1 deficiency causes Ras-mediated granulocyte/macrophage colony stimulating factor hypersensitivity and chronic myeloid leukaemia. *Nat. Genet.* **1996**, *12*, 137–143. [CrossRef] [PubMed]
40. Locatelli, F.; Nöllke, P.; Zecca, M.; Korthof, E.; Lanino, E.; Peters, C.; Pession, A.; Kabisch, H.; Uderzo, C.; Bonfim, C.S.; et al. Hematopoietic stem cell transplantation (HSCT) in children with juvenile myelomonocytic leukemia (JMML): Results of the EWOG-MDS/EBMT trial. *Blood* **2005**, *105*, 410–419. [CrossRef]
41. Matsuda, K.; Yoshida, N.; Miura, S.; Nakazawa, Y.; Sakashita, K.; Hyakuna, N.; Saito, M.; Kato, F.; Ogawa, A.; Watanabe, A.; et al. Long-term haematological improvement after non-intensive or no chemotherapy in juvenile myelomonocytic leukaemia and poor correlation with adult myelodysplasia spliceosome-related mutations. *Br. J. Haematol.* **2012**, *157*, 647–650. [CrossRef]
42. Hecht, A.; Meyer, J.A.; Behnert, A.; Wong, E.; Chehab, F.; Olshen, A.; Hechmer, A.; Aftandilian, C.; Bhat, R.; Choi, S.W.; et al. Molecular and phenotypic diversity of CBL-mutated juvenile myelomonocytic leukemia. *Haematologica* **2020**. [CrossRef]
43. Mendez, H.M.; Opitz, J.M. Noonan syndrome: A review. *Am. J. Med. Genet.* **1985**, *21*, 493–506. [CrossRef]
44. Aoki, Y.; Niihori, T.; Inoue, S.; Matsubara, Y. Recent advances in RASopathies. *J. Hum. Genet.* **2016**, *61*, 33–39. [CrossRef]
45. Roberts, A.E.; Allanson, J.E.; Tartaglia, M.; Gelb, B.D. Noonan syndrome. *Lancet* **2013**, *381*, 333–342. [CrossRef]
46. Bader-Meunier, B.; Tchernia, G.; Miélot, F.; Fontaine, J.L.; Thomas, C.; Lyonnet, S.; Lavergne, J.M.; Dommergues, J.P. Occurrence of myeloproliferative disorder in patients with Noonan syndrome. *J. Pediatr.* **1997**, *130*, 885–889. [CrossRef]

47. Hofmans, M.; Schröder, R.; Lammens, T.; Flotho, C.; Niemeyer, C.; van Roy, N.; Decaluwe, W.; Philippé, J.; de Moerloose, B. Noonan syndrome-associated myeloproliferative disorder with somatically acquired monosomy 7: Impact on clinical decision making. *Br. J. Haematol.* **2019**, *187*, E83–E86. [CrossRef]
48. Sakaguchi, H.; Okuno, Y.; Muramatsu, H.; Yoshida, K.; Shiraishi, Y.; Takahashi, M.; Kon, A.; Sanada, M.; Chiba, K.; Tanaka, H.; et al. Exome sequencing identifies secondary mutations of SETBP1 and JAK3 in juvenile myelomonocytic leukemia. *Nat. Genet.* **2013**, *45*, 937–941. [CrossRef] [PubMed]
49. Stieglitz, E.; Troup, C.B.; Gelston, L.C.; Haliburton, J.; Chow, E.D.; Yu, K.B.; Akutagawa, J.; Taylor-Weiner, A.N.; Liu, Y.L.; Wang, Y.-D.; et al. Subclonal mutations in SETBP1 confer a poor prognosis in juvenile myelomonocytic leukemia. *Blood* **2015**, *125*, 516–524. [CrossRef] [PubMed]
50. Flex, E.; Jaiswal, M.; Pantaleoni, F.; Martinelli, S.; Strullu, M.; Fansa, E.K.; Caye, A.; de Luca, A.; Lepri, F.; Dvorsky, R.; et al. Activating mutations in RRAS underlie a phenotype within the RASopathy spectrum and contribute to leukaemogenesis. *Hum. Mol. Genet.* **2014**, *23*, 4315–4327. [CrossRef]
51. Chao, A.K.; Meyer, J.A.; Lee, A.G.; Hecht, A.; Tarver, T.; van Ziffle, J.; Koegel, A.K.; Golden, C.; Braun, B.S.; Sweet-Cordero, E.A.; et al. Fusion driven JMML: A novel CCDC88C-FLT3 fusion responsive to sorafenib identified by RNA sequencing. *Leukemia* **2020**, *34*, 662–666. [CrossRef] [PubMed]
52. Röttgers, S.; Gombert, M.; Teigler-Schlegel, A.; Busch, K.; Gamerdinger, U.; Slany, R.; Harbott, J.; Borkhardt, A. ALK fusion genes in children with atypical myeloproliferative leukemia. *Leukemia* **2010**, *24*, 1197–1200. [CrossRef] [PubMed]
53. Murakami, N.; Okuno, Y.; Yoshida, K.; Shiraishi, Y.; Nagae, G.; Suzuki, K.; Narita, A.; Sakaguchi, H.; Kawashima, N.; Wang, X.; et al. Integrated molecular profiling of juvenile myelomonocytic leukemia. *Blood* **2018**, *131*, 1576–1586. [CrossRef] [PubMed]
54. Buijs, A.; Bruin, M. Fusion of FIP1L1 and RARA as a result of a novel t(4;17)(q12;q21) in a case of juvenile myelomonocytic leukemia. *Leukemia* **2007**, *21*, 1104–1108. [CrossRef]
55. Morerio, C.; Acquila, M.; Rosanda, C.; Rapella, A.; Dufour, C.; Locatelli, F.; Maserati, E.; Pasquali, F.; Panarello, C. HCMOGT-1 is a novel fusion partner to PDGFRB in juvenile myelomonocytic leukemia with t(5;17)(q33;p11.2). *Cancer Res.* **2004**, *64*, 2649–2651. [CrossRef] [PubMed]
56. Byrgazov, K.; Kastner, R.; Gorna, M.; Hoermann, G.; Koenig, M.; Lucini, C.B.; Ulreich, R.; Benesch, M.; Strenger, V.; Lackner, H.; et al. NDEL1-PDGFRB fusion gene in a myeloid malignancy with eosinophilia associated with resistance to tyrosine kinase inhibitors. *Leukemia* **2017**, *31*, 237–240. [CrossRef]
57. Mizoguchi, Y.; Fujita, N.; Taki, T.; Hayashi, Y.; Hamamoto, K. Juvenile myelomonocytic leukemia with t(7;11)(p15;p15) and NUP98-HOXA11 fusion. *Am. J. Hematol.* **2009**, *84*, 295–297. [CrossRef]
58. Hasle, H.; Kerndrup, G.; Jacobsen, B.B. Childhood myelodysplastic syndrome in Denmark: Incidence and predisposing conditions. *Leukemia* **1995**, *9*, 1569–1572.
59. Niemeyer, C.M.; Arico, M.; Basso, G.; Biondi, A.; Rajnoldi, A.C.; Creutzig, U.; Haas, O.; Harbott, J.; Hasle, H.; Kerndrup, G.; et al. Chronic myelomonocytic leukemia in childhood: A retrospective analysis of 110 cases. European Working Group on Myelodysplastic Syndromes in Childhood (EWOG-MDS). *Blood* **1997**, *89*, 3534–3543.
60. Castro-malaspina, H.; Schaison, G.; Passe, S.; Pasquier, A.; Berger, R.; Bayle-Weisgerber, C.; Miller, D.; Seligmann, M.; Bernard, J. Subacute and chronic myelomonocytic leukemia in children (juvenile CML). Clinical and hematologic observations, and identification of prognostic factors. *Cancer* **1984**, *54*, 675–686. [CrossRef]
61. So, N.; Liu, R.; Hogeling, M. Juvenile xanthogranulomas: Examining single, multiple, and extracutaneous presentations. *Pediatr. Dermatol.* **2020**, *37*, 637–644. [CrossRef]
62. Tidyman, W.E.; Rauen, K.A. The RASopathies: Developmental syndromes of Ras/MAPK pathway dysregulation. *Curr. Opin. Genet. Dev.* **2009**, *19*, 230–236. [CrossRef]
63. Aoki, Y.; Matsubara, Y. Ras/MAPK syndromes and childhood hemato-oncological diseases. *Int. J. Hematol.* **2013**, *97*, 30–36. [CrossRef] [PubMed]
64. Cseh, A.; Niemeyer, C.M.; Yoshimi, A.; Dworzak, M.; Hasle, H.; van den Heuvel-Eibrink, M.M.; Locatelli, F.; Masetti, R.; Schmugge, M.; Groß-Wieltsch, U.; et al. Bridging to transplant with azacitidine in juvenile myelomonocytic leukemia: A retrospective analysis of the EWOG-MDS study group. *Blood* **2015**, *125*, 2311–2313. [CrossRef] [PubMed]
65. Stieglitz, E.; Mazor, T.; Olshen, A.B.; Geng, H.; Gelston, L.C.; Akutagawa, J.; Lipka, D.B.; Plass, C.; Flotho, C.; Chehab, F.F.; et al. Genome-wide DNA methylation is predictive of outcome in juvenile myelomonocytic leukemia. *Nat. Commun.* **2017**, *8*, 2127. [CrossRef]
66. Bagby, G.C.; Dinarello, C.A.; Neerhout, R.C.; Ridgway, D.; McCall, E. Interleukin 1-dependent paracrine granulopoiesis in chronic granulocytic leukemia of the juvenile type. *J. Clin. Investig.* **1988**, *82*, 1430–1436. [CrossRef] [PubMed]
67. Emanuel, P.D.; Bates, L.J.; Castleberry, R.P.; Gualtieri, R.J.; Zuckerman, K.S. Selective hypersensitivity to granulocyte-macrophage colony-stimulating factor by juvenile chronic myeloid leukemia hematopoietic progenitors. *Blood* **1991**, *77*, 925–929. [CrossRef]
68. Hasegawa, D.; Bugarin, C.; Giordan, M.; Bresolin, S.; Longoni, D.; Micalizzi, C.; Ramenghi, U.; Bertaina, A.; Basso, G.; Locatelli, F.; et al. Validation of flow cytometric phospho-STAT5 as a diagnostic tool for juvenile myelomonocytic leukemia. *Blood Cancer J.* **2013**, *3*, e160. [CrossRef]
69. Karow, A.; Baumann, I.; Niemeyer, C.M. Morphologic differential diagnosis of juvenile myelomonocytic leukemia—Pitfalls apart from viral infection. *J. Pediatr. Hematol. Oncol.* **2009**, *31*, 380. [CrossRef]

70. Herrod, H.G.; Dow, L.W.; Sullivan, J.L. Persistent epstein-barr virus infection mimicking juvenile chronic myelogenous leukemia: Immunologic and hematologic studies. *Blood* **1983**, *61*, 1098–1104. [CrossRef]
71. Nishio, N.; Takahashi, Y.; Tanaka, M.; Xu, Y.; Yoshida, N.; Sakaguchi, S.; Doisaki, S.; Hama, A.; Muramatsu, H.; Shimada, A.; et al. Aberrant phosphorylation of STAT5 by granulocyte-macrophage colony-stimulating factor in infant cytomegalovirus infection mimicking juvenile myelomonocytic leukemia. *Leuk. Res.* **2011**, *35*, 1261–1264. [CrossRef]
72. Lorenzana, A.; Lyons, H.; Sawaf, H.; Higgins, M.; Carrigan, D.; Emanuel, P.D. Human herpesvirus 6 infection mimicking juvenile myelomonocytic leukemia in an infant. *J. Pediatr. Hematol. Oncol.* **2002**, *24*, 136–141. [CrossRef]
73. Yoshimi, A.; Kamachi, Y.; Imai, K.; Watanabe, N.; Nakadate, H.; Kanazawa, T.; Ozono, S.; Kobayashi, R.; Yoshida, M.; Kobayashi, C.; et al. Wiskott-Aldrich syndrome presenting with a clinical picture mimicking juvenile myelomonocytic leukaemia. *Pediatr. Blood Cancer* **2013**, *60*, 836–841. [CrossRef] [PubMed]
74. Calvo, K.R.; Price, S.; Braylan, R.C.; Oliveira, J.B.; Lenardo, M.; Fleisher, T.A.; Rao, V.K. JMML and RALD (Ras-associated autoimmune leukoproliferative disorder): Common genetic etiology yet clinically distinct entities. *Blood* **2015**, *125*, 2753–2758. [CrossRef]
75. Neven, Q.; Boulanger, C.; Bruwier, A.; de Ville Goyet, M.; Meyts, I.; Moens, L.; van Damme, A.; Brichard, B. Clinical Spectrum of Ras-Associated Autoimmune Leukoproliferative Disorder (RALD). *J. Clin. Immunol.* **2021**, *41*, 51–58. [CrossRef] [PubMed]
76. Lanzarotti, N.; Bruneau, J.; Trinquand, A.; Stolzenberg, M.-C.; Neven, B.; Fregeac, J.; Levy, E.; Jeremiah, N.; Suarez, F.; Mahlaoui, N.; et al. RAS-associated lymphoproliferative disease evolves into severe juvenile myelo-monocytic leukemia. *Blood* **2014**, *123*, 1960–1963. [CrossRef]
77. Hofmans, M.; Lammens, T.; Helsmoortel, H.H.; Bresolin, S.; Cavé, H.; Flotho, C.; Hasle, H.; van den Heuvel-Eibrink, M.M.; Niemeyer, C.; Stary, J.; et al. The long non-coding RNA landscape in juvenile myelomonocytic leukemia. *Haematologica* **2018**, *103*, e501–e504. [CrossRef]
78. Leoncini, P.P.; Bertaina, A.; Papaioannou, D.; Flotho, C.; Masetti, R.; Bresolin, S.; Menna, G.; Santoro, N.; Zecca, M.; Basso, G.; et al. MicroRNA fingerprints in juvenile myelomonocytic leukemia (JMML) identified miR-150-5p as a tumor suppressor and potential target for treatment. *Oncotarget* **2016**, *7*, 55395–55408. [CrossRef]
79. Bresolin, S.; Zecca, M.; Flotho, C.; Trentin, L.; Zangrando, A.; Sainati, L.; Stary, J.; de Moerloose, B.; Hasle, H.; Niemeyer, C.M.; et al. Gene expression-based classification as an independent predictor of clinical outcome in juvenile myelomonocytic leukemia. *J. Clin. Oncol.* **2010**, *28*, 1919–1927. [CrossRef]
80. Helsmoortel, H.H.; Bresolin, S.; Lammens, T.; Cavé, H.; Noellke, P.; Caye, A.; Ghazavi, F.; de Vries, A.; Hasle, H.; Labarque, V.; et al. LIN28B overexpression defines a novel fetal-like subgroup of juvenile myelomonocytic leukemia. *Blood* **2016**, *127*, 1163–1172. [CrossRef] [PubMed]
81. Olk-Batz, C.; Poetsch, A.R.; Nöllke, P.; Claus, R.; Zucknick, M.; Sandrock, I.; Witte, T.; Strahm, B.; Hasle, H.; Zecca, M.; et al. Aberrant DNA methylation characterizes juvenile myelomonocytic leukemia with poor outcome. *Blood* **2011**, *117*, 4871–4880. [CrossRef] [PubMed]
82. Issa, J.-P.J.; Kantarjian, H.M.; Kirkpatrick, P. Azacitidine. *Nat. Rev. Drug Discov.* **2005**, *4*, 275–276. [CrossRef]
83. Abe, M.; Ohira, M.; Kaneda, A.; Yagi, Y.; Yamamoto, S.; Kitano, Y.; Takato, T.; Nakagawara, A.; Ushijima, T. CpG island methylator phenotype is a strong determinant of poor prognosis in neuroblastomas. *Cancer Res.* **2005**, *65*, 828–834. [PubMed]
84. Toyota, M.; Ahuja, N.; Ohe-Toyota, M.; Herman, J.G.; Baylin, S.B.; Issa, J.P. CpG island methylator phenotype in colorectal cancer. *Proc. Natl. Acad. Sci. USA* **1999**, *96*, 8681–8686. [CrossRef]
85. Fluhr, S.; Boerries, M.; Busch, H.; Symeonidi, A.; Witte, T.; Lipka, D.B.; Mücke, O.; Nöllke, P.; Krombholz, C.F.; Niemeyer, C.M.; et al. CREBBP is a target of epigenetic, but not genetic, modification in juvenile myelomonocytic leukemia. *Clin. Epigenet.* **2016**, *8*, 50. [CrossRef]
86. Poetsch, A.R.; Lipka, D.B.; Witte, T.; Claus, R.; Nöllke, P.; Zucknick, M.; Olk-Batz, C.; Fluhr, S.; Dworzak, M.; de Moerloose, B.; et al. RASA4 undergoes DNA hypermethylation in resistant juvenile myelomonocytic leukemia. *Epigenetics* **2014**, *9*, 1252–1260. [CrossRef] [PubMed]
87. Wilhelm, T.; Lipka, D.B.; Witte, T.; Wierzbinska, J.A.; Fluhr, S.; Helf, M.; Mücke, O.; Claus, R.; Konermann, C.; Nöllke, P.; et al. Epigenetic silencing of AKAP12 in juvenile myelomonocytic leukemia. *Epigenetics* **2016**, *11*, 110–119. [CrossRef] [PubMed]
88. Schönung, M.; Meyer, J.; Nöllke, P.; Olshen, A.B.; Hartmann, M.; Murakami, N.; Wakamatsu, M.; Okuno, Y.; Plass, C.; Loh, M.L.; et al. International Consensus Definition of DNA Methylation Subgroups in Juvenile Myelomonocytic Leukemia. *Clin. Cancer Res.* **2021**, *27*, 158–168. [CrossRef]
89. Matsuda, K.; Shimada, A.; Yoshida, N.; Ogawa, A.; Watanabe, A.; Yajima, S.; Iizuka, S.; Koike, K.; Yanai, F.; Kawasaki, K.; et al. Spontaneous improvement of hematologic abnormalities in patients having juvenile myelomonocytic leukemia with specific RAS mutations. *Blood* **2007**, *109*, 5477–5480. [CrossRef] [PubMed]
90. Flotho, C.; Kratz, C.P.; Bergsträsser, E.; Hasle, H.; Starý, J.; Trebo, M.; van den Heuvel-Eibrink, M.M.; Wójcik, D.; Zecca, M.; Locatelli, F.; et al. Genotype-phenotype correlation in cases of juvenile myelomonocytic leukemia with clonal RAS mutations. *Blood* **2008**, *111*, 966–967. [CrossRef]
91. De Filippi, P.; Zecca, M.; Lisini, D.; Rosti, V.; Cagioni, C.; Carlo-Stella, C.; Radi, O.; Veggiotti, P.; Mastronuzzi, A.; Acquaviva, A.; et al. Germ-line mutation of the NRAS gene may be responsible for the development of juvenile myelomonocytic leukaemia. *Br. J. Haematol.* **2009**, *147*, 706–709. [CrossRef]
92. Kratz, C.P.; Schubbert, S.; Bollag, G.; Niemeyer, C.M.; Shannon, K.M.; Zenker, M. Germline mutations in components of the Ras signaling pathway in Noonan syndrome and related disorders. *Cell Cycle* **2006**, *5*, 1607–1611. [CrossRef] [PubMed]

93. Kratz, C.P.; Franke, L.; Peters, H.; Kohlschmidt, N.; Kazmierczak, B.; Finckh, U.; Bier, A.; Eichhorn, B.; Blank, C.; Kraus, C.; et al. Cancer spectrum and frequency among children with Noonan, Costello, and cardio-facio-cutaneous syndromes. *Br. J. Cancer* **2015**, *112*, 1392–1397. [CrossRef] [PubMed]
94. Bourdeaut, F.; Hérault, A.; Gentien, D.; Pierron, G.; Ballet, S.; Reynaud, S.; Paris, R.; Schleiermacher, G.; Baumann, C.; Philippe-Chomette, P.; et al. Mosaicism for oncogenic G12D KRAS mutation associated with epidermal nevus, polycystic kidneys and rhabdomyosarcoma. *J. Med. Genet.* **2010**, *47*, 859–862. [CrossRef] [PubMed]
95. Hafner, C.; Toll, A.; Real, F.X. HRAS mutation mosaicism causing urothelial cancer and epidermal nevus. *N. Engl. J. Med.* **2011**, *365*, 1940–1942. [CrossRef]
96. Niemela, J.E.; Lu, L.; Fleisher, T.A.; Davis, J.; Caminha, I.; Natter, M.; Beer, L.A.; Dowdell, K.C.; Pittaluga, S.; Raffeld, M.; et al. Somatic KRAS mutations associated with a human nonmalignant syndrome of autoimmunity and abnormal leukocyte homeostasis. *Blood* **2011**, *117*, 2883–2886. [CrossRef]
97. Takagi, M.; Piao, J.; Lin, L.; Kawaguchi, H.; Imai, C.; Ogawa, A.; Watanabe, A.; Akiyama, K.; Kobayashi, C.; Mori, M.; et al. Autoimmunity and persistent RAS-mutated clones long after the spontaneous regression of JMML. *Leukemia* **2013**, *27*, 1926–1928. [CrossRef]
98. Niemeyer, C.M.; Flotho, C.; Lipka, D.B.; Stary, J.; Rössig, C.; Baruchel, A.; Klingebiel, T.; Micalizzi, C.; Michel, G.; Nysom, K.; et al. Response to upfront azacitidine in juvenile myelomonocytic leukemia in the AZA-JMML-001 trial. *Blood Adv.* **2021**, in press..
99. Furlan, I.; Batz, C.; Flotho, C.; Mohr, B.; Lübbert, M.; Suttorp, M.; Niemeyer, C.M. Intriguing response to azacitidine in a patient with juvenile myelomonocytic leukemia and monosomy 7. *Blood* **2009**, *113*, 2867–2868. [CrossRef]
100. Fabri, O.; Horakova, J.; Bodova, I.; Svec, P.; Laluhova Striezencova, Z.; Bubanska, E.; Cermak, M.; Galisova, V.; Skalicka, K.; Vaska, L.; et al. Diagnosis and treatment of juvenile myelomonocytic leukemia in Slovak Republic: Novel approaches. *Neoplasma* **2019**, *66*, 818–824. [CrossRef]
101. Lin, Y.-C.; Luo, C.-J.; Miao, Y.; Wang, J.-M.; Luo, C.-Y.; Qin, X.; Cai, J.-Y.; Li, B.-S.; Chen, J. Human leukocyte antigen disparities reduce relapse after hematopoietic stem cell transplantation in children with juvenile myelomonocytic leukemia: A single-center retrospective study from China. *Pediatr. Transplant.* **2020**, *25*, e13825. [CrossRef]
102. O'Halloran, K.; Ritchey, A.K.; Djokic, M.; Friehling, E. Transient juvenile myelomonocytic leukemia in the setting of PTPN11 mutation and Noonan syndrome with secondary development of monosomy 7. *Pediatr. Blood Cancer* **2017**, *64*. [CrossRef]
103. Strullu, M.; Caye, A.; Lachenaud, J.; Cassinat, B.; Gazal, S.; Fenneteau, O.; Pouvreau, N.; Pereira, S.; Baumann, C.; Contet, A.; et al. Juvenile myelomonocytic leukaemia and Noonan syndrome. *J. Med. Genet.* **2014**, *51*, 689–697. [CrossRef] [PubMed]
104. Ramamoorthy, S.; Lebrecht, D.; Schanze, D.; Schanze, I.; Wieland, I.; Albert, M.H.; Borkhardt, A.; Bresters, D.; Büchner, J.; Catala, A.; et al. NF1 Tumor Suppressor Gene Inactivation in Juvenile Myelomonocytic Leukemia: New Genetic Evidence and Consequences for Diagnostic Work-up. *Blood* **2020**, *136*, 2181. [CrossRef]
105. Flotho, C.; Steinemann, D.; Mullighan, C.G.; Neale, G.; Mayer, K.; Kratz, C.P.; Schlegelberger, B.; Downing, J.R.; Niemeyer, C.M. Genome-wide single-nucleotide polymorphism analysis in juvenile myelomonocytic leukemia identifies uniparental disomy surrounding the NF1 locus in cases associated with neurofibromatosis but not in cases with mutant RAS or PTPN11. *Oncogene* **2007**, *26*, 5816–5821. [CrossRef] [PubMed]
106. Becker, H.; Yoshida, K.; Blagitko-Dorfs, N.; Claus, R.; Pantic, M.; Abdelkarim, M.; Niemöller, C.; Greil, C.; Hackanson, B.; Shiraishi, Y.; et al. Tracing the development of acute myeloid leukemia in CBL syndrome. *Blood* **2014**, *123*, 1883–1886. [CrossRef]
107. Inaba, T.; Honda, H.; Matsui, H. The enigma of monosomy 7. *Blood* **2018**, *131*, 2891–2898. [CrossRef] [PubMed]
108. Yabe, M.; Sako, M.; Yabe, H.; Osugi, Y.; Kurosawa, H.; Nara, T.; Tokuyama, M.; Adachi, S.; Kobayashi, C.; Yanagimachi, M.; et al. A conditioning regimen of busulfan, fludarabine, and melphalan for allogeneic stem cell transplantation in children with juvenile myelomonocytic leukemia. *Pediatr. Transplant.* **2008**, *12*, 862–867. [CrossRef]
109. Manabe, A.; Okamura, J.; Yumura-Yagi, K.; Akiyama, Y.; Sako, M.; Uchiyama, T.; Kojima, S.; Koike, K.; Saito, T.; Nakahata, T. Allogeneic hematopoietic stem cell transplantation for 27 children with juvenile myelomonocytic leukemia diagnosed based on the criteria of the International JMML Working Group. *Leukemia* **2002**, *16*, 645–649. [CrossRef]
110. Smith, F.O.; King, R.; Nelson, G.; Wagner, J.E.; Robertson, K.A.; Sanders, J.E.; Bunin, N.; Emauel, P.D.; Davies, S.M. Unrelated donor bone marrow transplantation for children with juvenile myelomonocytic leukaemia. *Br. J. Haematol.* **2002**, *116*, 716–724. [CrossRef]
111. Yoshida, N.; Sakaguchi, H.; Yabe, M.; Hasegawa, D.; Hama, A.; Hasegawa, D.; Kato, M.; Noguchi, M.; Terui, K.; Takahashi, Y.; et al. Clinical Outcomes after Allogeneic Hematopoietic Stem Cell Transplantation in Children with Juvenile Myelomonocytic Leukemia: A Report from the Japan Society for Hematopoietic Cell Transplantation. *Biol. Blood Marrow Transplant.* **2020**, *26*, 902–910. [CrossRef]
112. Yabe, M.; Ohtsuka, Y.; Watanabe, K.; Inagaki, J.; Yoshida, N.; Sakashita, K.; Kakuda, H.; Yabe, H.; Kurosawa, H.; Kudo, K.; et al. Transplantation for juvenile myelomonocytic leukemia: A retrospective study of 30 children treated with a regimen of busulfan, fludarabine, and melphalan. *Int. J. Hematol.* **2015**, *101*, 184–190. [CrossRef] [PubMed]
113. Dvorak, C.C.; Satwani, P.; Stieglitz, E.; Cairo, M.S.; Dang, H.; Pei, Q.; Gao, Y.; Wall, D.; Mazor, T.; Olshen, A.B.; et al. Disease burden and conditioning regimens in ASCT1221, a randomized phase II trial in children with juvenile myelomonocytic leukemia: A Children's Oncology Group study. *Pediatr. Blood Cancer* **2018**, *65*, e27034. [CrossRef] [PubMed]

114. Locatelli, F.; Crotta, A.; Ruggeri, A.; Eapen, M.; Wagner, J.E.; MacMillan, M.L.; Zecca, M.; Kurtzberg, J.; Bonfim, C.; Vora, A.; et al. Analysis of risk factors influencing outcomes after cord blood transplantation in children with juvenile myelomonocytic leukemia: A EUROCORD, EBMT, EWOG-MDS, CIBMTR study. *Blood* **2013**, *122*, 2135–2141. [CrossRef] [PubMed]
115. Eapen, M.; Klein, J.P.; Ruggeri, A.; Spellman, S.; Lee, S.J.; Anasetti, C.; Arcese, W.; Barker, J.N.; Baxter-Lowe, L.A.; Brown, M.; et al. Impact of allele-level HLA matching on outcomes after myeloablative single unit umbilical cord blood transplantation for hematologic malignancy. *Blood* **2014**, *123*, 133–140. [CrossRef]
116. Locatelli, F. Improving cord blood transplantation in children. *Br. J. Haematol.* **2009**, *147*, 217–226. [CrossRef] [PubMed]
117. Flotho, C.; Vraetz, T.; Lang, P.; Niemeyer, C.M.; Strahm, B. Successful double umbilical cord blood transplantation for relapsed juvenile myelomonocytic leukemia. *Leukemia* **2013**, *27*, 988–989. [CrossRef] [PubMed]
118. Peng, Z.; Xiaoqin, F.; Yuelin, H.; Yuchen, L.; Jianyun, L.; Xuedong, W.; Jiaqi, C.; Chunfu, L. Hypomethylation of Decitabine Improved Outcomes of Hematopoietic Stem Cell Transplantation in Children with Juvenile Myelomonocytic Leukemia. *Blood* **2017**, *130*, 3232. [CrossRef]
119. Hecht, A.; Meyer, J.; Chehab, F.F.; White, K.L.; Magruder, K.; Dvorak, C.C.; Loh, M.L.; Stieglitz, E. Molecular assessment of pretransplant chemotherapy in the treatment of juvenile myelomonocytic leukemia. *Pediatr. Blood Cancer* **2019**, *66*, e27948. [CrossRef] [PubMed]
120. Bader, P.; Kreyenberg, H.; Henze, G.H.R.; Eckert, C.; Reising, M.; Willasch, A.; Barth, A.; Borkhardt, A.; Peters, C.; Handgretinger, R.; et al. Prognostic value of minimal residual disease quantification before allogeneic stem-cell transplantation in relapsed childhood acute lymphoblastic leukemia: The ALL-REZ BFM Study Group. *J. Clin. Oncol.* **2009**, *27*, 377–384. [CrossRef]
121. van der Velden, V.H.J.; van der Sluijs-Geling, A.; Gibson, B.E.S.; te Marvelde, J.G.; Hoogeveen, P.G.; Hop, W.C.J.; Wheatley, K.; Bierings, M.B.; Schuurhuis, G.J.; de Graaf, S.S.N.; et al. Clinical significance of flowcytometric minimal residual disease detection in pediatric acute myeloid leukemia patients treated according to the DCOG ANLL97/MRC AML12 protocol. *Leukemia* **2010**, *24*, 1599–1606. [CrossRef] [PubMed]
122. Bergstraesser, E.; Hasle, H.; Rogge, T.; Fischer, A.; Zimmermann, M.; Noellke, P.; Niemeyer, C.M. Non-hematopoietic stem cell transplantation treatment of juvenile myelomonocytic leukemia: A retrospective analysis and definition of response criteria. *Pediatr. Blood Cancer* **2007**, *49*, 629–633. [CrossRef] [PubMed]
123. Inagaki, J.; Fukano, R.; Nishikawa, T.; Nakashima, K.; Sawa, D.; Ito, N.; Okamura, J. Outcomes of immunological interventions for mixed chimerism following allogeneic stem cell transplantation in children with juvenile myelomonocytic leukemia. *Pediatr. Blood Cancer* **2013**, *60*, 116–120. [CrossRef]
124. Yoshimi, A.; Niemeyer, C.M.; Bohmer, V.; Duffner, U.; Strahm, B.; Kreyenberg, H.; Dilloo, D.; Zintl, F.; Claviez, A.; Wössmann, W.; et al. Chimaerism analyses and subsequent immunological intervention after stem cell transplantation in patients with juvenile myelomonocytic leukaemia. *Br. J. Haematol.* **2005**, *129*, 542–549. [CrossRef]
125. Locatelli, F.; Lucarelli, B. Treatment of disease recurrence after allogeneic hematopoietic stem cell transplantation in children with juvenile myelomonocytic leukemia: A great challenge still to be won. *Pediatr. Blood Cancer* **2013**, *60*, 1–2. [CrossRef]
126. Guillaume, T.; Malard, F.; Magro, L.; Labopin, M.; Tabrizi, R.; Borel, C.; Chevallier, P.; Vigouroux, S.; Peterlin, P.; Garnier, A.; et al. Prospective phase II study of prophylactic low-dose azacitidine and donor lymphocyte infusions following allogeneic hematopoietic stem cell transplantation for high-risk acute myeloid leukemia and myelodysplastic syndrome. *Bone Marrow Transplant.* **2019**, *54*, 1815–1826. [CrossRef]
127. Craddock, C.; Slade, D.; de Santo, C.; Wheat, R.; Ferguson, P.; Hodgkinson, A.; Brock, K.; Cavenagh, J.; Ingram, W.; Dennis, M.; et al. Combination Lenalidomide and Azacitidine: A Novel Salvage Therapy in Patients Who Relapse After Allogeneic Stem-Cell Transplantation for Acute Myeloid Leukemia. *J. Clin. Oncol.* **2019**, *37*, 580–588. [CrossRef]
128. Craddock, C.; Jilani, N.; Siddique, S.; Yap, C.; Khan, J.; Nagra, S.; Ward, J.; Ferguson, P.; Hazlewood, P.; Buka, R.; et al. Tolerability and Clinical Activity of Post-Transplantation Azacitidine in Patients Allografted for Acute Myeloid Leukemia Treated on the RICAZA Trial. *Biol. Blood Marrow Transplant.* **2016**, *22*, 385–390. [CrossRef]
129. Schmid, C.; Labopin, M.; Schaap, N.; Veelken, H.; Schleuning, M.; Stadler, M.; Finke, J.; Hurst, E.; Baron, F.; Ringden, O.; et al. Prophylactic donor lymphocyte infusion after allogeneic stem cell transplantation in acute leukaemia—A matched pair analysis by the Acute Leukaemia Working Party of EBMT. *Br. J. Haematol.* **2019**, *184*, 782–787. [CrossRef] [PubMed]
130. Oran, B.; de Lima, M.; Garcia-Manero, G.; Thall, P.F.; Lin, R.; Popat, U.; Alousi, A.M.; Hosing, C.; Giralt, S.; Rondon, G.; et al. A phase 3 randomized study of 5-azacitidine maintenance vs. observation after transplant in high-risk AML and MDS patients. *Blood Adv.* **2020**, *4*, 5580–5588. [CrossRef]
131. Schroeder, T.; Rautenberg, C.; Haas, R.; Germing, U.; Kobbe, G. Hypomethylating agents for treatment and prevention of relapse after allogeneic blood stem cell transplantation. *Int. J. Hematol.* **2018**, *107*, 138–150. [CrossRef]
132. Stieglitz, E.; Ward, A.F.; Gerbing, R.B.; Alonzo, T.A.; Arceci, R.J.; Liu, Y.L.; Emanuel, P.D.; Widemann, B.C.; Cheng, J.W.; Jayaprakash, N.; et al. Phase II/III trial of a pre-transplant farnesyl transferase inhibitor in juvenile myelomonocytic leukemia: A report from the Children's Oncology Group. *Pediatr. Blood Cancer* **2015**, *62*, 629–636. [CrossRef] [PubMed]
133. Tasian, S.K.; Casas, J.A.; Posocco, D.; Gandre-Babbe, S.; Gagne, A.L.; Liang, G.; Loh, M.L.; Weiss, M.J.; French, D.L.; Chou, S.T. Mutation-specific signaling profiles and kinase inhibitor sensitivities of juvenile myelomonocytic leukemia revealed by induced pluripotent stem cells. *Leukemia* **2019**, *33*, 181–190. [CrossRef] [PubMed]

134. DiNardo, C.D.; Pratz, K.; Pullarkat, V.; Jonas, B.A.; Arellano, M.; Becker, P.S.; Frankfurt, O.; Konopleva, M.; Wei, A.H.; Kantarjian, H.M.; et al. Venetoclax combined with decitabine or azacitidine in treatment-naive, elderly patients with acute myeloid leukemia. *Blood* **2019**, *133*, 7–17. [CrossRef] [PubMed]
135. Pollyea, D.A.; Pratz, K.; Letai, A.; Jonas, B.A.; Wei, A.H.; Pullarkat, V.; Konopleva, M.; Thirman, M.J.; Arellano, M.; Becker, P.S.; et al. Venetoclax with azacitidine or decitabine in patients with newly diagnosed acute myeloid leukemia: Long term follow-up from a phase 1b study. *Am. J. Hematol.* **2021**, *96*, 208–217. [CrossRef] [PubMed]
136. Winters, A.C.; Maloney, K.W.; Treece, A.L.; Gore, L.; Franklin, A.K. Single-center pediatric experience with venetoclax and azacitidine as treatment for myelodysplastic syndrome and acute myeloid leukemia. *Pediatr. Blood Cancer* **2020**, *67*, e28398. [CrossRef]
137. Karol, S.E.; Alexander, T.B.; Budhraja, A.; Pounds, S.B.; Canavera, K.; Wang, L.; Wolf, J.; Klco, J.M.; Mead, P.E.; Das Gupta, S.; et al. Venetoclax in combination with cytarabine with or without idarubicin in children with relapsed or refractory acute myeloid leukaemia: A phase 1, dose-escalation study. *Lancet Oncol.* **2020**, *21*, 551–560. [CrossRef]
138. Chao, M.P.; Takimoto, C.H.; Feng, D.D.; McKenna, K.; Gip, P.; Liu, J.; Volkmer, J.-P.; Weissman, I.L.; Majeti, R. Therapeutic Targeting of the Macrophage Immune Checkpoint CD47 in Myeloid Malignancies. *Front. Oncol.* **2019**, *9*, 1380. [CrossRef]
139. Zeidan, A.M.; DeAngelo, D.J.; Palmer, J.M.; Seet, C.S.; Tallman, M.S.; Wei, X.; Li, Y.F.; Hock, N.; Burgess, M.R.; Hege, K.; et al. A Phase I Study of CC-90002, a Monoclonal Antibody Targeting CD47, in Patients with Relapsed and/or Refractory (R/R) Acute Myeloid Leukemia (AML) and High-Risk Myelodysplastic Syndromes (MDS): Final Results. *Blood* **2019**, *134*, 1320. [CrossRef]
140. Sallman, D.A.; Asch, A.S.; Al Malki, M.M.; Lee, D.J.; Donnellan, W.B.; Marcucci, G.; Kambhampati, S.; Daver, N.G.; Garcia-Manero, G.; Komrokji, R.S.; et al. The First-in-Class Anti-CD47 Antibody Magrolimab (5F9) in Combination with Azacitidine Is Effective in MDS and AML Patients: Ongoing Phase 1b Results. *Blood* **2019**, *134*, 569. [CrossRef]

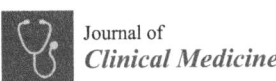

Review

Chronic Myeloid Leukemia in Children: Immune Function and Vaccinations

Meinolf Suttorp [1,*], Andrea Webster Carrion [2] and Nobuko Hijiya [2]

1. Hematology and Oncology, Medical Faculty, Technical University, D-01307 Dresden, Germany
2. Division of Pediatric Hematology, Oncology and Stem Cell Transplantation, Columbia University Medical Center, New York, NY 10032, USA; aw3240@cumc.columbia.edu (A.W.C.); nh2636@cumc.columbia.edu (N.H.)
* Correspondence: Meinolf.suttorp@uniklinikum-dresden.de

Abstract: Children with CML need TKI treatment for many years, and the lack of knowledge about immune dysfunction with TKI has hindered routine immunizations. This review attempts to provide an overview of the effects of TKIs licensed for children (e.g., imatinib, dasatinib, and nilotinib) on immune function, as well as its implications on immunizations. We discuss surveillance strategies (e.g., immunoglobulin blood serum levels and hepatitis B reactivation) and immunizations. All inactivated vaccines (e.g., influenza, pneumococcal, and streptococcal) can be given during the treatment of CML in the chronic phase, although their efficacy may be lower. As shown in single cases of children and adults with CML, live vaccines (e.g., varicella, measles, mumps, rubella, and yellow fever) may be administered under defined circumstances with great precautions. We also highlight important aspects of COVID-19 in this patient population (e.g., the outcome of COVID-19 infection in adults with CML and in children with varying hemato-oncological diseases) and discuss the highly dynamic field of presently available different vaccination options. In conclusion, TKI treatment for CML causes humoral and cellular immune dysfunction, which is mild in most patients, and thus infectious complications are rare. Routine immunizations are important for health maintenance of children, but vaccinations for children with CML on TKI therapy should be carefully considered.

Keywords: chronic myeloid leukemia; CML; tyrosine kinase inhibitor; immunizations; COVID-19

1. Introduction

Chronic myeloid leukemia (CML) is a clonal myeloproliferative malignancy characterized by the presence of a BCR-ABL1 fusion gene as a consequence of the t(9;22)(q34.1;q11.2) reciprocal chromosomal translocation. CML is a rare disease in children and adolescents, with an estimated annual incidence of 2.5 cases per million in children and young adults and accounting for 2–3% of all childhood leukemia cases and ~9% of leukemia cases in adolescents between 15 and 19 years of age [1–3]. The current standard of care for patients with CML is indefinite tyrosine kinase inhibitor (TKI) treatment, while discontinuing TKI treatment is possible in a subset of patients [4]. TKIs function by blocking the activity of BCR-ABL1. The introduction of TKIs has dramatically increased the survival of patients with CML. However, TKIs inhibit not only BCR-ABL1 but also many other targets, and they cause various side effects via off-target effects, including impaired immune function [5]. Children with CML need TKI treatment for many years, and the lack of knowledge about immune dysfunction with TKIs has hindered routine immunizations.

In this review, we provide an overview of the effects of TKIs on immune function that have emerged to date, as well as its implications for immunizations. We discuss surveillance strategies and immunizations. We also highlight important aspects of COVID-19 in this patient population and discuss the different vaccination options.

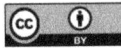

2. Effect of TKI on Immune Function

BCR-ABL1-specific TKIs that are used for the treatment of CML are not entirely BCR-ABL1-specific and inhibit other targets (e.g., c-KIT, TEC, SRC, FLT3, Lck, and mitogen-activated kinases (MAPK)). This "off-target" effect causes various adverse events and alters immune responses. The immunosuppressive effects of TKIs have been demonstrated in vitro and in animal models by modulating the differentiation of dendritic cells (DCs) as well as by impeding proper T-cell responses and macrophage functions [6,7]. Patients with CML have impaired innate and adaptive immunity at diagnosis, and patients on TKI treatment are considered to be clinically vulnerable. While data on the immune function in children receiving TKIs for CML are lacking, opportunistic infections or serious infectious complications are not reported in large pediatric CML trials [8–10]. Rohon et al. investigated the immunoprofile at diagnosis of CML and during therapy with imatinib and dasatinib in adult patients ($N = 54$) [11]. A lower proportion of B cells and dendritic cells and an increased number of NKT-like cells were observed in the BM at diagnosis. With imatinib therapy, all these changes returned to normal, and the immunoprofile was similar to the healthy controls. Among patients receiving dasatinib, however, two groups were identified. One group resembled healthy controls, while the other group showed activation of immune functions characterized by significant elevations of CD8+ and NK- and NKT-like cells. Data on immune functions in patients on other TKIs are sparse [12].

2.1. Altered Humoral and Cellular Immune Function

The plasma immunoglobulin levels were measured in adult patients with CML at diagnosis and after 12 months of treatment with imatinib ($N = 20$), dasatinib ($N = 16$), nilotinib ($N = 8$), and bosutinib ($N = 12$) [13]. The proportion of patients with IgA, IgG, and IgM levels below the lower limit of normal was 0%, 11%, and 6%, respectively, at diagnosis; however, at 12 months, they increased to 6% ($p = 0.13$), 31% ($p = 0.042$), and 28% ($p = 0.0078$), respectively. Low IgG levels in imatinib-treated patients were associated with higher percentages of immature bone marrow B cells, and IgG levels in the low-to-normal range at diagnosis in patients predisposed them to hypogammaglobinemia during the treatment with TKIs. Patients who had low immunoglobulin levels during the TKI therapy experienced significantly more frequent minor infections during the follow-up compared with the patients with normal levels (33% vs. 3%, $p = 0.0016$). Another study showed that TKIs, particularly second-generation TKIs with greater off-target kinase inhibition, inhibited B-lymphocyte functioning and the antibody response [14].

Similar findings were reported in a pediatric cohort with CML ($N = 30$, mean age: 16.4 years, range: 9–23 years) where they were treated with imatinib at a median dose of 287.5 mg/m^2 (IQR: 267.3, 345.0) for a median duration of 6 years [15]. The IgG, IgA, and IgM plasma levels decreased in 9 (30%), 8 (27%), and 10 (33%) patients, respectively. In 5 (17%) patients, pan-hypogammaglobulinemia was detected. Thus, if patients with CML on imatinib experience recurrent or unusual infections, measuring the immunoglobulin levels should be considered.

In general, infectious complications are rare in patients with CML of all ages who are on TKI treatment. Routine prophylaxis for opportunistic infections (e.g., pneumocystis jirovecii) is not recommended [16]. However, during the first months after diagnosis, leukopenia as a side effect of TKI treatment is observed commonly in children. In this situation, short-term pneumocystis prophylaxis may be considered in addition to temporary interruption of TKI treatment. TKIs may cause reactivation of CMV infections, with a particularly higher risk for dasatinib treatment [17,18]. Depending on the geographic region, patients may also benefit from screening for tuberculosis and treatment of latent infections [19,20].

A risk of hepatitis B reactivation in patients with CML on TKI therapy has been reported, while hepatitis C infections have not been reported so far [21]. However, there are no clear guidelines or recommendations regarding the screening and monitoring of hepatitis B virus (HBV). Atteya et al. reviewed the literature to estimate the risk of chronic

HBV reactivation associated with TKI treatment and addressed the following unanswered questions: (1) is there a need to screen all patients who will receive TKIs; (2) how long should patients with CML be on HBV prophylaxis, and (3) which are the best antiviral agents to use for prophylaxis against HBV for patients on TKIs [22]? The authors concluded that (1) it is advisable to screen all patients scheduled for TKI treatment by testing with ALT, a complete hepatitis B serology panel (including HBsAg, anti-HBs antibodies, anti-HBc antibodies, HBeAg, anti-HBe antibodies), and HBV DNA, (2) in HBsAg positive patients, prophylaxis against HBV reactivation should be started, as reactivation may happen any time after the commencement of TKIs with a median time of 9–10 months (range: 1–69 months), and (3) there was no clear answer from the literature as to which antiviral drug should be used.

2.2. Immunizations

Very little data are available about the safety and efficacy of vaccinations for immunosuppressed patients [23]. As a consequence, immunocompromised children are under-vaccinated and vulnerable to vaccine-preventable infections. It is very difficult to study the efficacy of vaccinations for rare diseases such as pediatric CML due to the very small sample size. Biological parameters demonstrating a protective effect in healthy individuals may not be extrapolated to immunocompromised individuals. Lower responses to vaccination in immunosuppressed individuals compared with healthy people are expected, and little data exist on the durability of the response. Concerning live vaccines, with a few exceptions, these are generally considered to be contraindicated in immunosuppressed individuals because of safety concerns.

The prevalence of children with CML is constantly increasing as the disease becomes more curable. Stem cell transplantation is associated with a high risk for morbidity but has become a third line option, and it is performed for very few children. TKI treatment may be needed for many years, and that makes the timing of vaccination crucial. Two different goals must be achieved by vaccination in immunosuppressed children: (1) protect the patient against specific infections whose risks are evidently increased by the treatment in comparison with healthy individuals and (2) offer an individual patient the same protection as the healthy community (e.g., against measles or influenza) [24].

2.2.1. Inactivated (Killed) Vaccines

Inactivated vaccines are generally safe in immunosuppressed patients, but it must be considered to what extent they are efficacious. Mild adverse events, mostly local reactions at the injection site, may be observed, but they are similar to immunocompetent hosts. Data in the literature regarding vaccination in immunosuppressed patients are scarce. However, the guidelines from the 2017 European Conference on Infections in Leukaemia (ECIL 7) for patients with hematological malignancies including CML have recently been published [24]. In the guidelines, TKIs inhibiting BCR-ABL1 are categorized as only mildly immunosuppressive, and all inactivated vaccines can be given during treatment, although their efficacy may be lower.

Vaccination with an inactivated influenza vaccine is recommended annually. It was demonstrated in adults that the proportion of patients exhibiting a protective immune response (antibody titer 1:32 or more) was slightly inferior in patients with CML (85%) compared with the healthy controls (100%). However, T-cell responses to the H1N1 vaccine were not significantly different between the patients and controls [25].

Patients with CML should also be vaccinated against *Streptococcus pneumoniae*. It has been demonstrated that TKIs impair B-cell responses through off-target inhibition of the kinases involved in cell signaling. Adult patients with CML on TKIs achieved lower pneumococcal IgG and IgM titer responses (75% versus 100% in the healthy controls) after vaccination with PPSV23 [14]. The immunogenicity of pneumococcal conjugate vaccines (PCVs) is higher than PPSV23 because of the T-cell dependent response induced by the conjugation with the diphtheria protein. While there are no data on PCV in patients with

CML, one may reasonably deduce from data in other immunocompromised populations to recommend one dose of PCV, followed at least 2 months later by one dose of PPSV23 [24].

Other inactivated vaccines should be administered according to the guidelines in each country. Current issues concerning vaccination against COVID-19 (all developed vaccines thus far are killed vaccines) are discussed below in a separate section. It must be kept in mind that immunoglobulin titers are low in a considerable proportion of children on TKI treatment. In the pre-TKI era, it was demonstrated that 18% of patients were not immune to tetanus [26]. Thus, it may be prudent to check the titers against inactivated vaccines regularly and to perform a booster vaccination in children with non-protective levels of titers. It should be also considered that the expected response rates to vaccines may be lower when on dasatinib or bosutinib (not yet licensed in children) treatment than with imatinib or nilotinib [14].

2.2.2. Live Attenuated Vaccines

According to current recommendations, vaccinations with live vaccines are completed by the age of 4–6 years in most countries. As CML is rarely seen in children below that age, only very few children face the issue of live vaccine administration during TKI treatment [27–29]. A problem exists for older children who missed their booster vaccinations, as well as an increasing number of children whose parents generally have refused vaccination (e.g., the measles vaccine) [27,28,30].

Live vaccines are typically contraindicated in immunosuppressed individuals in general. While the degree of immunosuppression may vary among patients receiving antineoplastic treatment, emerging data support the safety and effectiveness of live vaccines in certain immunocompromised individuals. In Swiss travel clinics, 197 patients on immunosuppressive treatments including corticosteroids, mesalazine, methotrexate, and TNF-alpha inhibitors received live vaccines against yellow fever, measles/mumps/rubella (MMR), varicella, or oral typhoid vaccines. In this cohort, no serious side effects or infections by the attenuated vaccine strain occurred [31].

For children with CML on TKI therapy, live attenuated vaccines should be administered with great caution. For patients who are in deep molecular response, a window for vaccination can be created by interrupting the TKI therapy [27]. Experience in children with and without interruption of TKI treatment is limited so far to vaccinations against MMR and VZV in four patients [30]. When a patient is on treatment with imatinib (no experience exists with the other TKIs), live vaccines may be considered on an individual basis if the following prerequisites are fulfilled: (1) the patient lives in or is traveling to an area where a vaccine-preventable infection is endemic, (2) the patient is in the chronic phase of CML and in an overall stable situation (a complete cytogenetic response has been achieved with a BCR-ABL1/ABL1 ratio of 1% or lower (expressed on the international scale), peripheral blood lymphocyte counts stable at >1500/µL, and changes in the full blood count caused by imatinib treatment or switching to another TKI not expected), (3) a prior vaccination with an inactivated vaccine has resulted in an adequate immune response, and (4) the benefits and risks of the planned live attenuated vaccination are discussed in depth with the patient and his or her legal guardians [30].

Attenuated Varicella Virus Live Vaccine

The natural course of a varicella zoster virus infection has been described in a cohort of adult patients on imatinib, in which 16 out of 771 patients (2%) developed VZV infections (15 episodes of herpes zoster and 1 of varicella). All patients received and responded well to therapy with antiviral agents. The authors concluded that imatinib therapy in CML is associated with a low incidence of VZV infection, does not disseminate, responds well to therapy, and does not mandate a recommendation for herpes zoster prophylaxis in patients with CML [32]. In pediatric trials of imatinib, no unusual cases of VZV infection were reported [8,9,33]. This is in contrast to the experience with other pediatric cancers or other diseases requiring immunosuppressive therapies, which have the risk for a potentially fatal course of VZV infection. A varicella live attenuated vaccine may be given to patients with CML [30]. Our own very limited experience with attenuated live VZV vaccination stems from two girls aged 14 and 15 years with CML-CP and under imatinib treatment for 2 years and 3 years, respectively, having achieved major molecular response when vaccinated. Both patients tolerated the vaccination well without any side effects, but only one girl developed protective serological VZV titers [30]. As a word of caution, the zoster live attenuated vaccine, which contains 15–20-fold higher titers of attenuated viruses than the varicella live attenuated vaccine, should not be used, as no experience with the zoster live vaccine has been published thus far.

Attenuated Measles Mumps Rubella Live Vaccine

The measles virus is considered to be one of the most highly contagious known human pathogens [34]. The World Health Organization's (WHO's) goal of global elimination of measles by vaccination successfully prevented an estimated 21 million deaths worldwide since the year 2000. However, despite this achievement, there is concern of a new increase in the number of measles cases reported globally [35]. The growing number of travel-related infections and local outbreaks in industrialized countries due to vaccine refusal is alarming. Endemic measles has now been reestablished in several European countries where transmission was previously dormant. Additionally, with more than 1000 reported measles cases from 1 January 2019 to 20 June 2019, the United States experienced the largest number of measles cases per annum since the disease was eliminated in the year 2000 [36]. Aside from North America and Europe, the seriousness of the problem is highlighted by the WHO's report of 207,500 measles deaths worldwide in 2019, the highest annual number of deaths since 1996, occurring mostly in countries with weak health systems [37,38]. For the last few years, the priority has shifted to handling the current pandemic of COVID-19, and millions of children are at risk of not receiving measles vaccines [39]. Thus, patients with CML undoubtedly will need protective serum titers not only when traveling to countries where measles are endemic but also when a local outbreak occurs in their area.

As outlined before, most children diagnosed with pediatric CML are at school age, and protective serum titers against measles should be the same as in the age-matched general population. In Germany, 88.8% of the children were MMR-vaccinated at least once, and a study with more than 13,000 children and adolescents aged 0–17 years found that 76.8% of them showed evidence of antibodies to MMR [40].

To what extent pediatric patients with malignancies lose their humoral immunity against vaccine-preventable diseases was investigated in a German single-center study comprising 195 children (122 male) with ALL ($N = 80$), AML ($N = 15$), non-Hodgkin's lymphoma ($N = 18$), Hodgkin's disease ($N = 22$), and various solid tumors ($N = 60$). Overall, 27%, 47%, 19%, and 17% of the patients lost their humoral immunity against measles, mumps, rubella, and VZV, respectively [41]. To the best of our knowledge, no such analysis has been performed for CML under TKI treatment so far.

Bettoni da Cunha-Riehm et al. published their very limited experience with live attenuated vaccines for pediatric CML, including four patients aged 12–15 years who were on imatinib treatment for 1–3 years and had missing protective measles titers during local outbreaks of measles in Germany [30]. After careful consideration of the risks and benefits, three patients were vaccinated while receiving TKI therapy, while imatinib treatment was interrupted in the fourth patient for 1 week prior and 2 weeks after vaccination. No acute or late adverse events from vaccination were observed in any of the four patients. While patients 1 and 3 developed stable long-term seroconversions, a serum titer conversion against measles and varicella could not be demonstrated in patient 2. However, MMR revaccination, given 3 years later, did not result in the development of a protective measles titer or the titer was lost again. Patient 4 also had lost protective titers against measles when assessed 10 months after the first vaccination, but revaccination resulted in stable seroprotective titers that were stable for over 12 months during a follow-up. Of note, no clear conclusions should be drawn from these four cases until more experience from a larger number of patients demonstrates that live attenuated vaccines are safe and that stable protective titers are achieved. Whether or not TKI impedes the seroconversion by blocking attenuated virus proliferation via a blockade of the virus' release from an infected cell (see below in "Putative Antiviral Action of TKIs") should also be investigated in more detail [38,42,43].

Yellow Fever Live Attenuated Vaccine

Yellow fever (YF) is endemic in the tropical regions of Africa and South America. The course of an infection is serious, with case fatality rates of 20–50%. A very effective live attenuated vaccine was developed in the 1930s, and a single vaccination providing lifelong immunity has proven to be critical in the control of the disease [44]. An international certificate of vaccination may even be required when entering a country from another region where yellow fever is endemic [45]. Travel medicine authorities may advise immunosuppressed patients to avoid yellow fever endemic regions altogether or provide letters of exception when there is an entry requirement but little or no actual risk of exposure [46].

Vaccination against YF is recommended in children from the age of 9–12 months onward. However, a decline in specific immune response has been observed as a consequence of a lower seroconversion rate observed in infants compared with adults. Booster regimens should be performed to guarantee the long-term persistence of immune protection for children living in areas with a high risk of YF transmission [47].

Concerning patients on immunosuppressive treatment, the question arises as to what extent the protection achieved against YF by vaccination is maintained. One smaller study examined 35 healthy individuals as controls and 40 immunosuppressed adult patients (autoimmune diseases and organ transplantation), all having received YF vaccination prior to the onset of their immunosuppression [48]. With a median follow-up interval of 21.1 years (interquartile range: 14.4–31.3) after YF vaccination and while taking immunosuppressive drugs, no statistical difference was found, exhibiting a total of 35 seropositive immunosuppressed patients (88%) compared with 31 patients (89%) in the control group.

Another report focused on the side effects of vaccination with a YF live attenuated vaccine when it was administered inadvertently to 19 immunosuppressed patients (prednisone, azathioprine, cyclosporine, mycophenolate, sirolimus, or tacrolimus) following solid organ transplantation (kidneys N = 14, heart N = 3, and liver N = 2). Transplantation had been performed at a median interval of 65 months (range: 3–340) prior to vaccination [49]. None of the 19 patients experienced side effects except for slight reactions at the injection site in one case.

The largest data set on immunosuppressed patients receiving YF vaccines stems from a report describing when, in 2016, the largest outbreak in several decades of YF occurred in a previously transmission-free area in southeast Brazil and expanded to previously YF-free areas in highly populated areas near Espirito Santo, Rio de Janeiro, and Sao Paulo. YF vaccination was expanded to the entire population living in areas without prior vaccine recommendations in which the outbreaks took place. Given the high risk of YF transmission, experts standardized the criteria for YF vaccination to include immunocompromised patients in Sao Paulo. Low-grade immunosuppression was defined by single-drug therapy with hydroxychloroquine or sulfasalazine (any dosage), corticosteroids in a prednisone equivalence dosage of ≤ 2 mg/kg or ≤ 20 mg daily, methotrexate ≤ 0.4 mg/kg or ≤ 20 mg weekly, or leflunomide ≤ 20 mg/day. The YF vaccine was defined as contraindicated for persons taking methylprednisolone pulse therapy, mycophenolate mofetil, cyclosporine, cyclophosphamide, azathioprine, JAK inhibitors, or biological immunomodulators [50], and 381 immunosuppressed individuals (median age: 50.8 years, range: 1.4–89.3 years) without prior YF vaccination were vaccinated with a full dose of the YF 17DD vaccine. Although more details are not explicitly listed in the report, among these were 12 patients with hematological malignancies, including patients with CML, of whom 5 were on imatinib treatment and 2 were on dasatinib. From the total cohort of immunocompromised vaccinees, at least one adverse event was reported by 32.6% of patients, with no statistically significant difference in the spectrum of complaints according to the vaccine producer report. Four severe events, including 3 deaths, were observed but did not occur in patients with CML and were classified to be not related to the vaccination. The authors concluded that the YF attenuated live vaccine may be administered to mildly immunocompromised, clinically stable persons living in high-risk areas, always preceded by a careful individual assessment weighing the benefits and risks of vaccination.

To the best of our knowledge, no further data on YF vaccination in CML are available at this time. Therefore, we consider it desirable to put efforts on this issue in countries with emerging financial resources, where YF is endemic and where patients with CML have access to TKI treatment. In addition, data from YF vaccination in patients on TKI might support approaches with other live attenuated vaccinations such as MMR and varicella.

2.3. COVID-19

2.3.1. Putative Antiviral Action of TKIs

During the COVID-19 pandemic, data reported from Italy and China pointed to a lower prevalence in patients under TKI treatment. Some authors argued that this finding might demonstrate a protective effect of TKI therapy [51–53]. Earlier in vitro experiments had demonstrated that the tyrosine kinase ABL1 is involved in controlling the protein arrangement of the cytoskeleton. If inhibited by imatinib in infected cells, the syncytia formation induced by the corona virus spike protein is blocked [54,55]. Using quantitative assessment of the torque teno virus (TTV) viremia as a model for virus replication in immunosuppressed patients and patients with CML on imatinib, it was shown that in contrast to other immunosuppressive drugs, the TTV load did not increase while on TKI treatment [56–58]. From a clinical viewpoint, two trials, one in the Netherlands and one in France, will evaluate the benefits of early imatinib therapy to prevent severe COVID-19 disease in adult patients (COUNTER-COVID, ClinicalTrials.gov (accessed on 31 August 2021) Identifier NCT04357613) [59,60].

2.3.2. COVID-19 Infection in Patients with CML

In China, 530 patients with CML at a median age of 44 years (range: 6–89 years) were studied by questionnaire during the COVID-19 epidemic in Hubei Province [61]. Five patients with COVID-19 were identified (confirmed $N = 4$, probable $N = 1$), and thus the prevalence of COVID-19 in these subjects was calculated to be 0.9% (95% CI, 0.1–1.8%). This was ninefold higher than that reported in healthy persons (0.1%) but lower than 10% as reported in hospitalized persons with other hematological cancers or in healthcare providers (7%, CI 4–12%). Subjects from that cohort exhibited an increased risk of developing COVID-19 if diagnosed with advanced phases of CML ($p = 0.004$), even if they had achieved a complete cytogenetic response or major molecular response at the time of exposure to COVID-19. Covariates such as age and TKI therapy duration were not significantly associated with an increased risk of developing COVID-19.

The largest global cohort study so far characterizing COVID-19 in adult patients with CML was recently reported in an abstract form by the international CML foundation (iCMLf), which is a charitable foundation established to improve the outcomes of patients with CML globally [62]. One hundred ten cases of COVID-19 (median age: 54 years; range: 18–89) were collected from 20 countries. Among these, 91/110 cases were reported by physicians out of a total of 12,236 CML patients that they were treating (prevalence: 0.7%). COVID-19 was diagnosed by PCR or serology in 93 patients (85%) and clinically suspected in 17 patients (15%) while patients were under treatment (median duration: 7 years; range: 0–25) for CML with TKIs in most cases (hydroxyurea 1%, TKI 70%, 16% untreated at the time of COVID-19 diagnosis, 13% lacking information). During COVID-19 infection, 33 patients (30%) interrupted their TKI treatment, and 8/110 (7%) cases with COVID-19 were asymptomatic. In the 102 symptomatic patients (93%), the course of COVID-19 was considered to be mild (no hospitalization) in 49 cases (45%), moderate (hospitalization) in 19 cases (17%), severe (intensive care) in 19 cases (17%), and of unknown severity in

15 cases (14%). As of 1 July 2020, COVID-19 was still active in 14 patients (13%), and the outcome was unknown in 9 patients (8%), favorable in 75 patients (68%), and fatal in 12 patients (14%). The authors could show that factors associated with a higher mortality rate were older age and imatinib therapy. However, imatinib may represent a confounder effect, as a strong link between imatinib treatment and advanced age was identified.

An observational cohort study was conducted in the Netherlands during the COVID-19 pandemic [63] that assessed differences in susceptibility for COVID-19 and the severity of the disease's course in adult CML patients ($N = 148$, median age: 57.5 years; range: 26–82), with their adult housemates ($N = 123$, median age: 60 years; range: 24–88) serving as the controls. In a preliminary report, no significantly increased prevalence of COVID-19 in adult CML patients was observed, and only one patient (0.7%) tested positive and required inpatient care.

In comparison with adults, the proportion of children without underlying diseases who are affected by COVID-19 is smaller. Reports so far have demonstrated that the severity of the infection's course is mild, presenting as self-limiting symptoms of the upper respiratory tract in most children [64]. Only a very small number of children developed a rare multisystem inflammatory syndrome (MIS) or died from COVID-19. Data specifically in relation to outcomes in the pediatric oncology population are limited. An analysis of 33 studies from single centers and from national reports from different countries comprising a total of 226 children were comprehensively reviewed in a recent publication. The incidence of COVID-19 was found to be higher in children with neoplastic diseases than in the general pediatric population [65]. More children with hematological malignancies ($N = 120$) were affected than those with solid tumors ($N = 76$). As there was no analysis conducted with subgroups of hematological malignancies, it is unclear how many children with CML were included. In the entire cohort, the male gender and children in intensive treatment were affected more significantly, with fever as the leading symptom. The course of COVID-19 was asymptomatic or mild in 48% and severe in 9.6% of the children. Thirty-two percent needed oxygen support, 10% were admitted to the intensive care unit, and 4.9% died from COVID-19. In general, the severity, morbidity, and mortality of the infection in children with malignancies were more or less comparable to the general pediatric population. However, it must be kept in mind that the data sets are still small and heterogenous, and the findings in these studies vary as they are from different countries with diverse health infrastructures and policies. Thus far, there is no report on the course of COVID-19 in a child treated for CML.

2.3.3. Vaccines against COVID-19

In the COVID-19 pandemic, various vaccines have been developed rapidly in different countries of the world (Table 1). Among these new types are mRNA-based vaccines (Comirnaty®, BioNTech/Pfizer, Mainz, Germany; Moderna COVID-19 Vaccine®, Moderna, Norwood, MA, USA) which had not been used in humans prior to the pandemic. Another new approach to vaccination in humans is represented by vector-based vaccines (COVID-19 Vaccine Janssen®, Janssen-Cilag, Beerse, Belgium; COVID-19 SARS-CoV2 Vaccine, Johnson & Johnson, New Brunswick, NJ, USA; Gam-COVID-Vac®/Sputnik V, Biocad, Moscow, Russia; Vaxzevria®, AstraZeneca, Nijmegen, The Netherlands). Both m-RNA and vector-based vaccines have been classified as inactivated vaccines.

The classical way of challenging the immune system with inactivated vaccines is represented by using either protein components (in this case, the spike (S)-protein of the COVID-19 virus) in conjunction with an adjuvant (NVX-CoV2372, Novavax, Gaithersburg, MD, USA) or by using inactivated strains (CN02, HB02) of SARS-CoV-2 in conjunction with Al(OH)$_3$ as an adjuvant as produced and applied first as vaccines (CoronaVac, Sinovac Biotech, Being, China; BBIBP-CorV, Sinopharm $\frac{1}{2}$) in China and also in India (Covaxin, Bharat Biotech, Genome Valley, Hyderabad, India).

Table 1. SARS-CoV-2 vaccines developed and currently under emergency use application, modified from and, for more details, see [66].

Vaccine	Company	Vaccine Type	Antigen	Dose	Licensed or Emergency Use Application (EUA, as of 12 March 2021) in
Comirnaty® Tozinameran BNT162b2	BioNtech (Germany). Pfizer (USA)	mRNA	Full-length spike (S) protein with proline substitutions of the SARS-CoV-2 virus	2 doses, each 30 µg, 21 days apart	Canada, EU, Japan, UK, USA *
Covid-19 Vaccine Moderna, (mRNA-1273)	Moderna (USA)	mRNA	Full-length spike (S) protein with proline substitutions of the SARS-CoV-2 virus	2 doses, each 100 µg, 28 days apart	Canada, EU, UK, USA
CVnCoV	Curevac (Germany), Bayer (Germany), Glaxo-Smith-Kline (UK)	mRNA	Prefusion stabilized full-length spike (S) protein with proline substitutions of the SARS-CoV-2 virus	2 doses, each 12 µg, 28 days apart	(under a rolling review in the EU)
Covid-19 Vaccine Astra-Zeneca, ChAdOx1, AZD1222	Astra-Zeneca (UK, Sweden)	Viral vector	Replication-deficient chimpanzee adenoviral vector with the SARS-CoV-2S protein	2 doses, each containing 5×10^{10} virus particles 28 days apart	Canada, EU, India, Mexico, UK
Covid-19 Vaccine Janssen, Ad26.CoV2.S	Janssen (Belgium), Johnson & Johnson (USA)	Viral vector	Recombinant replication incompetent human adenovirus-vector serotype 26, encoding a full-length, stabilized SARS-CoV-2 spike (S)-protein with proline-substitutions	1 dose containing 5×10^{10} virus particles	Canada, EU, USA

Table 1. Cont.

Vaccine	Company	Vaccine Type	Antigen	Dose	Licensed or Emergency Use Application (EUA, as of 12 March 2021) in
Gam-Covid-Vac, Sputnik V	Gamaleya National Research Center for Epidemiology and Microbiology (Russia)	Viral vector	Full-length recombinant spike (S) protein with proline substitutions of the SARS-CoV-2 virus, carried by each replication-incompetent human adenovirus vector serotype 5 or 26	2 doses (first with rAd26, second with rAd5), each containing 10^{11} virus particles 21 days apart	Algeria, Argentina, Belarus, Egypt, Palestina, Russia, Serbia (under a rolling review in the EU)
NVX-CoV2373	Novavax (USA)	Protein subunit	Recombinant full-length prefusion stabilized spike (S) protein	2 doses each, both containing 5 µg protein plus 50 µg matrix protein as adjuvants	(under a rolling review in the EU)
CoronaVac	Sinovac Biotech (China)	Inactivated virus	Inactivated strain CN02 of SARS-CoV-2, produced in Vero cells	2 doses, each containing 3 µg plus $Al(OH)_3$ as adjuvants 14 days apart	Azerbaijan, Bolivia, Brazil, China, Chile, Columbia, Indonesia, Uruguay, Turkey
BBIBP-CorV	Sinopharm 1/2 (China)	Inactivated virus	Inactivated strain HB02 of SARS-CoV-2, produced in Vero cells	2 doses, each containing 4 µg plus $Al(OH)_3$ as adjuvants 21 days apart	Bahrain, China, Peru, Serbia, Zimbabwe
Covaxin	Bharat Biotech (India)	Inactivated virus	Inactivated strain NIV-2020-770 of SARS-CoV-2, produced in Vero cells	2 doses, each containing 6 µg plus $(Al(OH)_3$ as adjuvants at least 28 days apart	Guyana, India, Iran, Mauritius, Mexico, Nepal, Paraguay, the Philippines, Zimbabwe

* Note added during the reviewing process of the manuscript: Comirnaty™ received full approval by the FDA for individuals over 16 years old as of 23 August 2021.

The vaccines developed by different companies thus far are listed below (see Table 1). For a more detailed overview, we kindly refer the reader to an article by Creech et al. [66].

As of April 2021, trials for COVID-19 vaccines are also underway for children. For children with CML, the rarity of this type of leukemia represents an additional hurdle when trying to assess the benefit of a given vaccine. In the USA, the FDA approved the Comirnaty® vaccine (Pfizer) for ages 12–15 on 20 May 2021. In ongoing trials, both Pfizer and Moderna started testing their COVID-19 vaccines in children aged 6 months to 11 years back in March 2021. This will further help to protect the community from passing the infection inadvertently at school and at home. In adults with CML, data are emerging that robust memory T-cell responses develop in patients with CML following infection with severe acute respiratory syndrome coronavirus-2 [67]. In a recent publication it was also shown in adults that COVID-19 vaccination induces immunity [68]. Sixteen patients with CML (median age: 48 years; range: 21–75 years) all developed neutralizing antibody responses, and 14/16 patients (87%) developed T-cell responses against SARS-CoV-2 infection 21 days following a single first dose of the Pfizer-BioNTech BNT162b2 vaccine. The vaccine was safe in this cohort, and tolerable side effects consisted of localized inflammation in 9 patients (56%) and a transient flu-like illness in 4 patients (25%). Four patients each were on treatment with imatinib, nilotinib, and ponatinib, with 2 patients each undergoing treatment with bosutinib and dasatinib. However, these encouraging preliminary results must be confirmed in further prospective trials.

3. Conclusions

TKI treatment for CML causes humoral and cellular immune dysfunction which is mild in most patients, and thus infectious complications are rare. Routine immunizations are important for the health maintenance of children, but vaccinations for children with CML on TKI therapy should be carefully considered. In general, inactivated vaccines are safe. There was a concern for the safety of live attenuated vaccines, but preliminary experience from a few recent case reports have shown that MMR vaccines could be administered safely. Indications of COVID-19 vaccination for children with CML do not differ from those for the general pediatric population.

Author Contributions: All authors developed the concept of this review, wrote the first draft of the typoscript, critically discussed the content, and approved the final version of the typoscript. All authors have read and agreed to the published version of the manuscript.

Funding: This research received no external funding.

Acknowledgments: The authors thank Bryan Perez for his editorial assistance.

Conflicts of Interest: N.H. is a consultant for Incyte and receives research support from Pfizer. M.S. and A.W.C. declare no conflict of interest to be disclosed with relation to this manuscript.

References

1. Hehlmann, R.; Hochhaus, A.; Baccarani, M.; European, L. Chronic myeloid leukaemia. *Lancet* **2007**, *370*, 342–350. [CrossRef]
2. Surveillance, Epidemiology, and End Results (SEER) Program. Cancer Statistics, Table 3.1: Age-Adjusted Incidence Rates and Number of Cases By Period of Diagnosis for Major Cancer Sites and Subsites. Available online: https://seer.cancer.gov/statistics/nccr/details.html (accessed on 7 September 2021).
3. Smith, D.L.; Burthem, J.; Whetton, A.D. Molecular pathogenesis of chronic myeloid leukaemia. *Expert Rev. Mol. Med.* **2003**, *5*, 1–27. [CrossRef] [PubMed]
4. Hijiya, N.; Suttorp, M. How I treat chronic myeloid leukemia in children and adolescents. *Blood* **2019**, *133*, 2374–2384. [CrossRef] [PubMed]
5. Steegmann, J.L.; Cervantes, F.; le Coutre, P.; Porkka, K.; Saglio, G. Off-target effects of BCR-ABL1 inhibitors and their potential long-term implications in patients with chronic myeloid leukemia. *Leuk. Lymphoma* **2012**, *53*, 2351–2361. [CrossRef]
6. Wolf, D.; Tilg, H.; Rumpold, H.; Gastl, G.; Wolf, A.M. The kinase inhibitor imatinib—An immunosuppressive drug? *Curr. Cancer Drug Targets* **2007**, *7*, 251–258. [CrossRef]
7. Appel, S.; Balabanov, S.; Brummendorf, T.H.; Brossart, P. Effects of imatinib on normal hematopoiesis and immune activation. *Stem Cells* **2005**, *23*, 1082–1088. [CrossRef]

8. Suttorp, M.; Schulze, P.; Glauche, I.; Gohring, G.; von Neuhoff, N.; Metzler, M.; Sedlacek, P.; de Bont, E.; Balduzzi, A.; Lausen, B.; et al. Front-line imatinib treatment in children and adolescents with chronic myeloid leukemia: Results from a phase III trial. *Leukemia* **2018**, *32*, 1657–1669. [CrossRef]
9. Millot, F.; Baruchel, A.; Guilhot, J.; Petit, A.; Leblanc, T.; Bertrand, Y.; Mazingue, F.; Lutz, P.; Verite, C.; Berthou, C.; et al. Imatinib is effective in children with previously untreated chronic myelogenous leukemia in early chronic phase: Results of the French national phase IV trial. *J. Clin. Oncol.* **2011**, *29*, 2827–2832. [CrossRef] [PubMed]
10. Kurosawa, H.; Tanizawa, A.; Muramatsu, H.; Tono, C.; Watanabe, A.; Shima, H.; Ito, M.; Yuza, Y.; Hamamoto, K.; Hotta, N.; et al. Sequential use of second-generation tyrosine kinase inhibitors following imatinib therapy in pediatric chronic myeloid leukemia: A report from the Japanese Pediatric Leukemia/Lymphoma Study Group. *Pediatr Blood Cancer* **2018**, *65*, e27368. [CrossRef]
11. Rohon, P.; Porkka, K.; Mustjoki, S. Immunoprofiling of patients with chronic myeloid leukemia at diagnosis and during tyrosine kinase inhibitor therapy. *Eur. J. Haematol.* **2010**, *85*, 387–398. [CrossRef] [PubMed]
12. Climent, N.; Plana, M. Immunomodulatory Activity of Tyrosine Kinase Inhibitors to Elicit Cytotoxicity against Cancer and Viral Infection. *Front. Pharmacol.* **2019**, *10*, 1232. [CrossRef]
13. Rajala, H.L.M.; Missiry, M.E.; Ruusila, A.; Koskenvesa, P.; Brummendorf, T.H.; Gjertsen, B.T.; Janssen, J.; Lotfi, K.; Markevarn, B.; Olsson-Stromberg, U.; et al. Tyrosine kinase inhibitor therapy-induced changes in humoral immunity in patients with chronic myeloid leukemia. *J. Cancer Res. Clin. Oncol.* **2017**, *143*, 1543–1554. [CrossRef]
14. de Lavallade, H.; Khoder, A.; Hart, M.; Sarvaria, A.; Sekine, T.; Alsuliman, A.; Mielke, S.; Bazeos, A.; Stringaris, K.; Ali, S.; et al. Tyrosine kinase inhibitors impair B-cell immune responses in CML through off-target inhibition of kinases important for cell signaling. *Blood* **2013**, *122*, 227–238. [CrossRef] [PubMed]
15. Totadri, S.; Thipparapu, S.; Aggarwal, R.; Sharma, M.; Naseem, S.; Jain, R.; Trehan, A.; Malhotra, P.; Varma, N.; Bansal, D. Imatinib-Induced Hypogammaglobulinemia in Children and Adolescents with Chronic Myeloid Leukemia. *Pediatr. Hematol. Oncol.* **2020**, *37*, 539–544. [CrossRef] [PubMed]
16. Kin, A.; Schiffer, C.A. Infectious Complications of Tyrosine Kinase Inhibitors in Hematological Malignancies. *Infect. Dis. Clin. N. Am.* **2020**, *34*, 245–256. [CrossRef] [PubMed]
17. Reinwald, M.; Silva, J.T.; Mueller, N.J.; Fortun, J.; Garzoni, C.; de Fijter, J.W.; Fernandez-Ruiz, M.; Grossi, P.; Aguado, J.M. ESCMID Study Group for Infections in Compromised Hosts (ESGICH) Consensus Document on the safety of targeted and biological therapies: An infectious diseases perspective (Intracellular signaling pathways: Tyrosine kinase and mTOR inhibitors). *Clin. Microbiol. Infect.* **2018**, *24* (Suppl. 2), S53–S70. [CrossRef]
18. Yazici, O.; Sendur, M.A.; Aksoy, S. Hepatitis C virus reactivation in cancer patients in the era of targeted therapies. *World J. Gastroenterol.* **2014**, *20*, 6716–6724. [CrossRef] [PubMed]
19. Bhatnagar, V.; Adelakun, A.; Kendall, T.; Holtzman, N.; Farshidpour, M.; Stevenson, B.; Chen, Q.; Emadi, A. Diseases at the crossroads: Chronic myelogenous leukemia and tuberculosis. *Arch. Iran Med.* **2015**, *18*, 65–68.
20. Iqbal, P.; Soliman, A.; De Sanctis, V.; Yassin, M.A. Association of tuberculosis in patients with chronic myeloid leukemia: A treatment proposal based on literature review. *Expert Rev. Hematol.* **2021**, *14*, 211–217. [CrossRef] [PubMed]
21. Orlandi, E.M.; Elena, C.; Bono, E. Risk of hepatitis B reactivation under treatment with tyrosine-kinase inhibitors for chronic myeloid leukemia. *Leuk. Lymphoma* **2017**, *58*, 1764–1766. [CrossRef]
22. Atteya, A.; Ahmad, A.; Daghstani, D.; Mushtaq, K.; Yassin, M.A. Evaluation of Hepatitis B Reactivation among Patients with Chronic Myeloid Leukemia Treated with Tyrosine Kinase Inhibitors. *Cancer Control* **2020**, *27*, 1073274820976594. [CrossRef]
23. Miller, K.; Leake, K.; Sharma, T. Advances in vaccinating immunocompromised children. *Curr. Opin. Pediatr.* **2020**, *32*, 145–150. [CrossRef] [PubMed]
24. Mikulska, M.; Cesaro, S.; de Lavallade, H.; Di Blasi, R.; Einarsdottir, S.; Gallo, G.; Rieger, C.; Engelhard, D.; Lehrnbecher, T.; Ljungman, P.; et al. Vaccination of patients with haematological malignancies who did not have transplantations: Guidelines from the 2017 European Conference on Infections in Leukaemia (ECIL 7). *Lancet Infect Dis.* **2019**, *19*, e188–e199. [CrossRef]
25. de Lavallade, H.; Garland, P.; Sekine, T.; Hoschler, K.; Marin, D.; Stringaris, K.; Loucaides, E.; Howe, K.; Szydlo, R.; Kanfer, E.; et al. Repeated vaccination is required to optimize seroprotection against H1N1 in the immunocompromised host. *Haematologica* **2011**, *96*, 307–314. [CrossRef] [PubMed]
26. Hamarstrom, V.; Pauksen, K.; Svensson, H.; Oberg, G.; Paul, C.; Ljungman, P. Tetanus immunity in patients with hematological malignancies. *Support Care Cancer* **1998**, *6*, 469–472. [CrossRef] [PubMed]
27. Hijiya, N.; Millot, F.; Suttorp, M. Chronic myeloid leukemia in children: Clinical findings, management, and unanswered questions. *Pediatr. Clin. N. Am.* **2015**, *62*, 107–119. [CrossRef] [PubMed]
28. Meral Gunes, A.; Millot, F.; Kalwak, K.; Lausen, B.; Sedlacek, P.; Versluys, A.B.; Dworzak, M.; De Moerloose, B.; Suttorp, M. Features and outcome of chronic myeloid leukemia at very young age: Data from the International Pediatric Chronic Myeloid Leukemia Registry. *Pediatr. Blood Cancer* **2021**, *68*, e28706. [CrossRef]
29. Suttorp, M.; Metzler, M.; Millot, F. Horn of plenty: Value of the international registry for pediatric chronic myeloid leukemia. *World J. Clin. Oncol.* **2020**, *11*, 308–319. [CrossRef]
30. Bettoni da Cunha-Riehm, C.; Hildebrand, V.; Nathrath, M.; Metzler, M.; Suttorp, M. Vaccination with Live Attenuated Vaccines in Four Children With Chronic Myeloid Leukemia While on Imatinib Treatment. *Front. Immunol.* **2020**, *11*, 628. [CrossRef]
31. Huber, F.; Ehrensperger, B.; Hatz, C.; Chappuis, F.; Buhler, S.; Eperon, G. Safety of live vaccines on immunosuppressive or immunomodulatory therapy-a retrospective study in three Swiss Travel Clinics. *J. Travel Med.* **2018**, *25*, tax082. [CrossRef]

32. Mattiuzzi, G.N.; Cortes, J.E.; Talpaz, M.; Reuben, J.; Rios, M.B.; Shan, J.; Kontoyiannis, D.; Giles, F.J.; Raad, I.; Verstovsek, S.; et al. Development of Varicella-Zoster virus infection in patients with chronic myelogenous leukemia treated with imatinib mesylate. *Clin. Cancer Res.* **2003**, *9*, 976–980. [PubMed]
33. Giona, F.; Santopietro, M.; Menna, G.; Putti, M.C.; Micalizzi, C.; Santoro, N.; Ziino, O.; Mura, R.; Ladogana, S.; Iaria, G.; et al. Real-Life Management of Children and Adolescents with Chronic Myeloid Leukemia: The Italian Experience. *Acta Haematol.* **2018**, *140*, 105–111. [CrossRef] [PubMed]
34. Gay, N.J. The theory of measles elimination: Implications for the design of elimination strategies. *J. Infect Dis.* **2004**, *189* (Suppl. 1), S27–S35. [CrossRef]
35. Dabbagh, A.; Laws, R.L.; Steulet, C.; Dumolard, L.; Mulders, M.N.; Kretsinger, K.; Alexander, J.P.; Rota, P.A.; Goodson, J.L. Progress Toward Regional Measles Elimination—Worldwide, 2000–2017. *MMWR Morb. Mortal Wkly. Rep.* **2018**, *67*, 1323–1329. [CrossRef]
36. Strebel, P.M.; Orenstein, W.A. Measles. *N. Engl. J. Med.* **2019**, *381*, 349–357. [CrossRef]
37. Patel, M.K.; Goodson, J.L.; Alexander, J.P., Jr.; Kretsinger, K.; Sodha, S.V.; Steulet, C.; Gacic-Dobo, M.; Rota, P.A.; McFarland, J.; Menning, L.; et al. Progress Toward Regional Measles Elimination—Worldwide, 2000–2019. *MMWR Morb. Mortal Wkly. Rep.* **2020**, *69*, 1700–1705. [CrossRef]
38. Worldwide Measles Deaths Climb 50% from 2016 to 2019 Claiming over 207 500 Lives in 2019. Available online: https://www.who.int/news/item/12-11-2020-worldwide-measles-deaths-climb-50-from-2016-to-2019-claiming-over-207-500-lives-in-2019 (accessed on 13 April 2021).
39. Tanveer, M.; Ahmed, A.; Siddiqui, A.; Gudi, S.K. The mystery of plummeting cases of measles during COVID-19 pandemic in Pakistan: Hidden impact of collateral damage. *J. Med. Virol.* **2021**. [CrossRef]
40. Poethko-Muller, C.; Mankertz, A. Seroprevalence of measles-, mumps- and rubella-specific IgG antibodies in German children and adolescents and predictors for seronegativity. *PLoS ONE* **2012**, *7*, e42867. [CrossRef]
41. Bochennek, K.; Allwinn, R.; Langer, R.; Becker, M.; Keppler, O.T.; Klingebiel, T.; Lehrnbecher, T. Differential loss of humoral immunity against measles, mumps, rubella and varicella-zoster virus in children treated for cancer. *Vaccine* **2014**, *32*, 3357–3361. [CrossRef] [PubMed]
42. Reeves, P.M.; Bommarius, B.; Lebeis, S.; McNulty, S.; Christensen, J.; Swimm, A.; Chahroudi, A.; Chavan, R.; Feinberg, M.B.; Veach, D.; et al. Disabling poxvirus pathogenesis by inhibition of Abl-family tyrosine kinases. *Nat. Med.* **2005**, *11*, 731–739. [CrossRef] [PubMed]
43. Reeves, P.M.; Smith, S.K.; Olson, V.A.; Thorne, S.H.; Bornmann, W.; Damon, I.K.; Kalman, D. Variola and monkeypox viruses utilize conserved mechanisms of virion motility and release that depend on abl and SRC family tyrosine kinases. *J. Virol.* **2011**, *85*, 21–31. [CrossRef]
44. Klitting, R.; Fischer, C.; Drexler, J.F.; Gould, E.A.; Roiz, D.; Paupy, C.; de Lamballerie, X. What Does the Future Hold for Yellow Fever Virus? (II). *Genes* **2018**, *9*, 425. [CrossRef]
45. Wyplosz, B.; Leroy, J.P.; Derradji, O.; Consigny, P.H. No booster dose for yellow fever vaccination: What are the consequences for the activity of vaccination in travel clinics? *J. Travel Med.* **2015**, *22*, 140–141. [CrossRef] [PubMed]
46. Kotton, C.N.; Ryan, E.T.; Fishman, J.A. Prevention of infection in adult travelers after solid organ transplantation. *Am. J. Transplant* **2005**, *5*, 8–14. [CrossRef]
47. Campi-Azevedo, A.C.; Reis, L.R.; Peruhype-Magalhaes, V.; Coelho-Dos-Reis, J.G.; Antonelli, L.R.; Fonseca, C.T.; Costa-Pereira, C.; Souza-Fagundes, E.M.; da Costa-Rocha, I.A.; Mambrini, J.V.M.; et al. Short-Lived Immunity After 17DD Yellow Fever Single Dose Indicates That Booster Vaccination May Be Required to Guarantee Protective Immunity in Children. *Front. Immunol.* **2019**, *10*, 2192. [CrossRef]
48. Burkhard, J.; Ciurea, A.; Gabay, C.; Hasler, P.; Muller, R.; Niedrig, M.; Fehr, J.; Villiger, P.; Visser, L.G.; de Visser, A.W.; et al. Long-term immunogenicity after yellow fever vaccination in immunosuppressed and healthy individuals. *Vaccine* **2020**, *38*, 3610–3617. [CrossRef] [PubMed]
49. Azevedo, L.S.; Lasmar, E.P.; Contieri, F.L.; Boin, I.; Percegona, L.; Saber, L.T.; Selistre, L.S.; Netto, M.V.; Moreira, M.C.; Carvalho, R.M.; et al. Yellow fever vaccination in organ transplanted patients: Is it safe? A multicenter study. *Transpl. Infect Dis.* **2012**, *14*, 237–241. [CrossRef] [PubMed]
50. Lara, A.N.; Miyaji, K.T.; Ibrahim, K.Y.; Lopes, M.H.; Sartori, A.M.C. Adverse events following yellow fever vaccination in immunocompromised persons. *Rev. Inst. Med. Trop. Sao Paulo* **2021**, *63*, e13. [CrossRef] [PubMed]
51. Breccia, M.; Abruzzese, E.; Bocchia, M.; Bonifacio, M.; Castagnetti, F.; Fava, C.; Galimberti, S.; Gozzini, A.; Gugliotta, G.; Iurlo, A.; et al. Chronic myeloid leukemia management at the time of the COVID-19 pandemic in Italy. A campus CML survey. *Leukemia* **2020**, *34*, 2260–2261. [CrossRef] [PubMed]
52. Foa, R.; Bonifacio, M.; Chiaretti, S.; Curti, A.; Candoni, A.; Fava, C.; Ciccone, M.; Pizzolo, G.; Ferrara, F. Philadelphia-positive acute lymphoblastic leukaemia (ALL) in Italy during the COVID-19 pandemic: A Campus ALL study. *Br. J. Haematol.* **2020**, *190*, e3–e5. [CrossRef] [PubMed]
53. Chu, Y.; Chen, Y.; Guo, H.; Li, M.; Wang, B.; Shi, D.; Cheng, X.; Guan, J.; Wang, X.; Xue, C.; et al. SUV39H1 regulates the progression of MLL-AF9-induced acute myeloid leukemia. *Oncogene* **2020**, *39*, 7239–7252. [CrossRef] [PubMed]

54. Coleman, C.M.; Sisk, J.M.; Halasz, G.; Zhong, J.; Beck, S.E.; Matthews, K.L.; Venkataraman, T.; Rajagopalan, S.; Kyratsous, C.A.; Frieman, M.B. CD8+ T Cells and Macrophages Regulate Pathogenesis in a Mouse Model of Middle East Respiratory Syndrome. *J. Virol.* **2017**, *91*, e01825-16. [CrossRef] [PubMed]
55. Sisk, J.M.; Frieman, M.B.; Machamer, C.E. Coronavirus S protein-induced fusion is blocked prior to hemifusion by Abl kinase inhibitors. *J. Gen. Virol.* **2018**, *99*, 619–630. [CrossRef]
56. Bendinelli, M.; Pistello, M.; Maggi, F.; Fornai, C.; Freer, G.; Vatteroni, M.L. Molecular properties, biology, and clinical implications of TT virus, a recently identified widespread infectious agent of humans. *Clin. Microbiol. Rev.* **2001**, *14*, 98–113. [CrossRef]
57. Focosi, D.; Spezia, P.G.; Macera, L.; Salvadori, S.; Navarro, D.; Lanza, M.; Antonelli, G.; Pistello, M.; Maggi, F. Assessment of prevalence and load of torquetenovirus viraemia in a large cohort of healthy blood donors. *Clin. Microbiol. Infect.* **2020**, *26*, 1406–1410. [CrossRef] [PubMed]
58. Galimberti, S.; Petrini, M.; Barate, C.; Ricci, F.; Balducci, S.; Grassi, S.; Guerrini, F.; Ciabatti, E.; Mechelli, S.; Di Paolo, A.; et al. Tyrosine Kinase Inhibitors Play an Antiviral Action in Patients Affected by Chronic Myeloid Leukemia: A Possible Model Supporting Their Use in the Fight Against SARS-CoV-2. *Front. Oncol.* **2020**, *10*, 1428. [CrossRef]
59. COUNTER-COVID—Oral Imatinib to Prevent Pulmonary Vascular Leak in Covid19—A Randomized, Double—Blind, Placebo Controlled, Clinical Trial in Patients with Severe Covid19 Disease'. Effecten van Imatinib bij Patiënten met Longschade Door COVID-19 Infectie. Available online: https://www.clinicaltrialsregister.eu/ctr-search/trial/2020-001236-10/NL (accessed on 2 September 2021).
60. Imatinib in COVID-19 Disease in Aged Patients. Available online: https://clinicaltrials.gov/ct2/show/NCT04357613 (accessed on 2 September 2021).
61. Li, W.; Wang, D.; Guo, J.; Yuan, G.; Yang, Z.; Gale, R.P.; You, Y.; Chen, Z.; Chen, S.; Wan, C.; et al. COVID-19 in persons with chronic myeloid leukaemia. *Leukemia* **2020**, *34*, 1799–1804. [CrossRef]
62. Rea, D.; Mauro, M.J.; Cortes, J.E.; Jiang, Q.; Pagnano, K.B.; Ongondi, M.; Kok, C.H.; Evans, N.; Hughes, T.P.; Foundation, I.C. COVID-19 in patients (pts) with Chronic Myeloid Leukemia (CML): Results from the international CML foundation (iCMLf) CML and COVID-19 (CANDID) study. *Blood* **2020**, *136*, 46–47. [CrossRef]
63. Ector, G.; Huijskens, E.G.W.; Blijlevens, N.M.A.; Westerweel, P.E. Prevalence of COVID-19 diagnosis in Dutch CML patients during the 2020 SARS-CoV2 pandemic. A prospective cohort study. *Leukemia* **2020**, *34*, 2533–2535. [CrossRef]
64. Parri, N.; Lenge, M.; Buonsenso, D.; Coronavirus Infection in Pediatric Emergency Departments Research Group. Children with Covid-19 in Pediatric Emergency Departments in Italy. *N. Engl. J. Med.* **2020**, *383*, 187–190. [CrossRef]
65. Meena, J.P.; Kumar Gupta, A.; Tanwar, P.; Ram Jat, K.; Mohan Pandey, R.; Seth, R. Clinical presentations and outcomes of children with cancer and COVID-19: A systematic review. *Pediatr. Blood Cancer* **2021**, *68*, e29005. [CrossRef] [PubMed]
66. Creech, C.B.; Walker, S.C.; Samuels, R.J. SARS-CoV-2 Vaccines. *JAMA* **2021**, *325*, 1318–1320. [CrossRef] [PubMed]
67. Harrington, P.; Harrison, C.N.; Dillon, R.; Radia, D.H.; Rezvani, K.; Raj, K.; Woodley, C.; Curto-Garcia, N.; O'Sullivan, J.; Saunders, J.; et al. Evidence of robust memory T-cell responses in patients with chronic myeloproliferative neoplasms following infection with severe acute respiratory syndrome coronavirus-2 (SARS-CoV-2). *Br. J. Haematol* **2021**, *193*, 692–696. [CrossRef] [PubMed]
68. Harrington, P.; Doores, K.J.; Radia, D.; O'Reilly, A.; Lam, H.P.J.; Seow, J.; Graham, C.; Lechmere, T.; McLornan, D.; Dillon, R.; et al. Single dose of BNT162b2 mRNA vaccine against severe acute respiratory syndrome coronavirus-2 (SARS-CoV-2) induces neutralising antibody and polyfunctional T-cell responses in patients with chronic myeloid leukaemia. *Br. J. Haematol.* **2021**. [CrossRef] [PubMed]

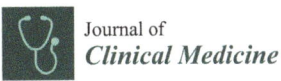

Journal of Clinical Medicine

Review

The Role of Allogeneic Hematopoietic Stem Cell Transplantation in Pediatric Leukemia

Mattia Algeri [1,*], Pietro Merli [1], Franco Locatelli [1,2] and Daria Pagliara [1]

[1] Department of Pediatric Hematology and Oncology, Scientific Institute for Research and Healthcare (IRCCS), Bambino Gesù Childrens' Hospital, 00165 Rome, Italy; pietro.merli@opbg.net (P.M.); franco.locatelli@opbg.net (F.L.); daria.pagliara@opbg.net (D.P.)
[2] Department of Pediatrics, Sapienza University of Rome, 00185 Rome, Italy
* Correspondence: mattia.algeri@opbg.net; Tel.: +39-0668592066

Abstract: Allogeneic hematopoietic stem cell transplantation (HSCT) offers potentially curative treatment for many children with high-risk or relapsed acute leukemia (AL), thanks to the combination of intense preparative radio/chemotherapy and the graft-versus-leukemia (GvL) effect. Over the years, progress in high-resolution donor typing, choice of conditioning regimen, graft-versus-host disease (GvHD) prophylaxis and supportive care measures have continuously improved overall transplant outcome, and recent successes using alternative donors have extended the potential application of allotransplantation to most patients. In addition, the importance of minimal residual disease (MRD) before and after transplantation is being increasingly clarified and MRD-directed interventions may be employed to further ameliorate leukemia-free survival after allogeneic HSCT. These advances have occurred in parallel with continuous refinements in chemotherapy protocols and the development of targeted therapies, which may redefine the indications for HSCT in the coming years. This review discusses the role of HSCT in childhood AL by analysing transplant indications in both acute lymphoblastic and acute myeloid leukemia, together with current and most promising strategies to further improve transplant outcome, including optimization of conditioning regimen and MRD-directed interventions.

Keywords: allogeneic stem cell transplantation; acute lymphoblastic leukemia; acute myeloid leukemia; minimal residual disease; conditioning regimen; alternative donors

1. Introduction

Despite the remarkable achievements obtained with frontline chemotherapy in the treatment of children with acute leukemia (AL), a significant proportion of patients still are treated with allogeneic hematopoietic stem cell transplantation (HSCT), either in first complete remission (CR1) or beyond, to achieve definitive disease eradication [1–5]. Over the years, the outcome of allogeneic HSCT for AL has continuously improved thanks to progress in high-resolution HLA typing, choice of conditioning regimen and supportive care measures. Furthermore, mainly owing to fundamental advances in graft manipulation techniques and graft-versus-host disease (GvHD) prophylaxis, results obtained using alternative donors are no longer inferior to those achieved using HLA-identical siblings and fully matched volunteers [6]. At the same time, successes in the transplant field are constantly paralleled by refinements in chemotherapy protocols, which take advantage of continuous breakthroughs of genomic medicine to achieve better treatment stratification and identify genetic lesions targetable with precision medicine approaches [7,8]. Such targeted approaches may be employed, in their turn, to further improve HSCT outcome by inducing a better remission status before transplant, especially in light of the robust evidence showing that pre- and post-HSCT minimal residual disease (MRD) represents one of the major determinants of subsequent relapse and long-term prognosis in AL [9,10]. This observation is particularly relevant in B-cell acute lymphoblastic leukemia (ALL), owing to the availability of highly effective immunotherapy approaches capable of inducing MRD-negative remissions of otherwise refractory and untreatable diseases [11]. The purpose of this review is to discuss the current role of HSCT in childhood AL by scrutinizing transplant indications in both ALL and acute myeloid leukemia (AML). We also discuss most promising practices to further improve transplant outcome, by analyzing (1) the predictive role of MRD and potential MRD-directed interventions, before and after HSCT; (2) the choice of conditioning regimen and (3) most recent results obtained with the use alternative donors.

2. HSCT Indications in ALL

Since most children with ALL have a good prognosis with current frontline protocols, only a minority of these patients are eligible for HSCT in CR1. On the contrary, most patients who experience a relapse are candidates for HSCT [12]. Despite the criteria used to assess this indication may vary between different cooperative groups, most studies/protocols consider eligible children with an estimated EFS probability lower than 50%, according to response to induction treatment and specific biologic features. Advances in biological characterization, improved MRD measurement capacity and its incorporation in treatment protocols to optimize risk stratification, and the upfront introduction of new biological agents (e.g., blinatumomab in AIEOP-BFM (EUDRACT 2016-001935-12) and COG protocols (AALL1731) and inotuzumab (AALL1732) and tisagenlecleucel (AALL1721/CASSIOPEIA) in COG protocol) have changed (and will continue to shape) the indications for HSCT over time [13]. Current HSCT indications in childhood ALL are summarized in Table 1. For example, criteria that were considered in past studies, such as a high white blood cell (WBC) count at presentation, Philadelphia chromosome positivity (Ph+), or poor-prednisone response, are no longer considered strict indications for transplantation [13]. The strongest criterion for HSCT indication is the response of the disease to induction therapy, this being a surrogate marker of leukemia sensitivity to chemotherapy. Indeed, MRD at selected time points is currently the single most powerful prognostic factor in childhood ALL [14]. Both multiparametric flow cytometry or quantitative PCR for specific rearrangements of immune-receptor genes IgH/TCR are currently used for MRD assessment [15]. The role of MRD for identification of HSCT candidates has been clearly proven by several groups, including The Italian Association of Pediatric Haematology–Oncology (AIEOP)/Berlin–Frankfurt–Muenster (BFM) group [16].

Table 1. HSCT indications in pediatric patients with ALL (adapted from AIEOP-BFM ALL 2017 and IntReALL 2010 protocol).

CR1	TCF3-HLF, irrespective of MRD results
	Positive MRD at TP1 or TP2 (irrespective of MRD value) and: - No CR at d33 - KMT2A-AFF1 - hypodiploidy <44 chr. or DNA index <0.8 - IKZF1plus and intermediate-/high-risk MRD results - T-ALL + poor-prednisone response and/or MFC-MRD d15 >10%
	MRD TP2 $\geq 5 \times 10^{-4}$
	Ph+ positive ALL and MRD $\geq 5 \times 10^{-4}$ at end Induction IB
	Infants (age < 1 year) with KMT2A-rearrangments and: - age < 6 months and initial WBC > 300,000/µL - age < 6 months and Prednisone Poor-Response - No CR at d33 - MRD TP2 $\geq 5 \times 10^{-4}$

Table 1. Cont.

CR2	HR	Very early isolated extramedullary relapse of BCP or T-ALL
		Any bone marrow relapse of T-ALL (irrespectively of the time elapsing between diagnosis and relapse)
		Very early BCP-ALL bone marrow relapse
		Early BCP-ALL bone marrow relapse
		Very early BCP-ALL combined bone marrow relapse
	SR	Late isolated or combined bone marrow relapse of BCP-ALL and poor MRD response at the end of induction therapy *
		Early combined bone marrow relapse and poor MRD response at the end of induction therapy *
		Early isolated extramedullary relapse of BCP or T-ALL
≥CR3		All patients

TCF3-HLF: TCF3-HLF positive acute lymphoblastic leukemia; MRD: minimal residual disease; CR: complete remission; MFC-MRD: flow-citometry MRD; WBC: white blood cells; BCP: B-cell precursor ALL (acute lymphoblastic leukemia). T-ALL: T-cell ALL; TP1: time point 1; TP2: time point 2. Time point of relapse: Very early, <18 months after primary diagnosis; early, ≥18 months after primary diagnosis and <6 after completion of primary; late, ≥6 months after completion of primary therapy. SR: standard risk; HR: high risk. * cut-off is defined by the specific treatment arm.

Additional criteria are employed to identify those patients who would benefit from HSCT in the first CR. Differing from AML, PIF is infrequent in pediatric ALL (being observed in less than 2% of patients); regardless, its occurrence represents a strong indication for HSCT in CR1, as shown by Schrappe and colleagues in a large retrospective study [17]. Hypodiploidy (<44 chromosomes) defines a high-risk group of patients with a poor outcome (the lowest the number of chromosome, the worst the prognosis) [18]. Thus, hypodiplody has been considered a strong indication to HSCT, although two recent retrospective studies, one from COG [19], the other from 16 cooperative groups [20] did not show an advantage for patients transplanted in CR1. Patients carrying the t(17;19)(q22;p13) translocation, resulting into the fusion gene TCF3-HLF (E2A-HLF), have a dismal outcome, irrespectively of MRD clearance [21]. For this reason, these patients are considered eligible for experimental therapies (e.g., BCL-2 inhibitors or anti-CD19-directed immunotherapies) and for HSCT in CR1 [22]. Deletions of Ikaros (IKZF1), a zinc-finger transcription factor required for the development of all lymphoid lineages, have been shown to confer an increased risk of recurrence [23]. In a recent paper, Stanulla and colleagues showed that IKZF1 deletions that co-occurred with deletions in CDKN2A, CDKN2B, PAX5 or PAR1 in the absence of ERG deletion were associated with the worst outcome and were grouped as IKZF1^{plus} [24]. The IKZF1^{plus} prognostic effect differed dramatically according to the MRD levels after induction treatment; in particular, IKZF1^{plus} patients with intermediate and high-risk MRD had a miserable outcome and are now considered candidates to receive HSCT in CR1. Rearrangements involving the KMT2A (MLL) gene on chromosome 11q23 are observed in a large part of infants ALL; on the contrary, in children older than 1 year, they are much less frequent [25]. KMT2A-rearrangments represent a high-risk feature [26] justifying the use of HSCT in CR1, although for children with these abnormalities the indication to HSCT is determined in combination with (i) age less than 6 months and either poor response to steroids or leukocytes $\geq 300 \times 10^9$/L at diagnosis [27] for infant ALL, and (ii) MRD clearance. Intrachromosomal amplification of chromosome 21 is a rare recurrent lesion (found in less than 3% cases of pediatric ALL). The sole use of standard chemotherapy in this population has been associated with an increased risk of relapse [28]. Studies conducted in the UK have reported improved survival with the use of front-line HSCT [29]. Since patients with T-ALL cannot still benefit from immunotherapy approaches (including CAR-T cells and BiTEs), they have a lower chance of being rescued when a relapse occurs. In addition, for this reason, patients with poor MRD clearance at the end of induction are considered candidates for HSCT in CR1.

Indications to HSCT for children with ALL who experience a first relapse are currently based on disease immunophenotype (T/B ALL) time elapsing between diagnosis and recurrence and site of relapse [30–33]. Since persistence of MRD after induction/consolidation therapy has been proven to influence outcome in relapsed children [33–36], MRD measurement has been incorporated in the decision process for treatment stratification and indication to HSCT. In addition, patients with TP53 mutations, t(1;19), t(17;19), hypodiploidy and KMT2A-rearragments have a dismal prognosis regardless of the time elapsing between diagnosis and relapse and should be offered HSCT once a new CR is achieved. Overall, two-thirds of children in CR2 proceed to HSCT. Finally, all patients who have experienced two or more relapses are considered candidates to receive a HSCT, regardless of the type of donor available.

3. HSCT Indications in AML

The use of HSCT as a consolidation strategy for pediatric patients with AML in CR1 has been the subject of much debate [37–39]. Historically, HSCT in CR1 was reserved for those children who had an available, HLA-identical sibling donor. Early studies adopting this Mendelian/genetic randomization strategy reported a reduction in leukemia relapse-rate (RR) in patients receiving transplantation, which was counterbalanced by the occurrence of transplant-related mortality (TRM) [39–41]. The presence of a matched sibling donor as a HSCT indication has been replaced, in most contemporary protocols, by risk assessments based upon disease characteristics and response-related factors. Current HSCT indications in childhood AML are summarized in Table 2. Considering recent improvements in chemotherapy and the potential risk of acute and late toxicities after HSCT, the current practice restricts the use of HSCT in CR1 only to those AML patients with high-risk (HR) features. However, there is no universal agreement on the definition of HR disease and different criteria have been, and continue to be, used by different cooperative groups. There is general consensus that standard-risk patients should not be transplanted in CR1 but only after the first relapse and achievement of a second complete remission. In this regard, the underlying genetic and molecular aberrations represent a major criterion for risk group stratification and allocation to HSCT. In particular, genomic alterations involving core-binding factor (CBF) transcription factors, namely inversion16(p13;1q22), t(16;16)(p13;q22) and t(8;21)(q22;q22), are widely recognized by all study groups as favorable risk group markers. Recently, a further chromosomal aberration involving CBF, t(16;21)(q24;q22), resulting in RUNX1-CBFA2T3 fusion, has been shown to be associated with good prognosis [42]. Noteworthy, a different translocation involving chromosomes 16 and 21, t(16;21)(p11;q22) (FUS-ERG), identifies instead a rare subgroup of AML with extremely poor prognosis, which should be considered for HSCT in CR1 [42]. In patients harboring t(8;21)RUNX1-RUNX1T1, an MRD reduction of less than 2 Log with respect to diagnosis, is associated with a significant higher risk of relapse when compared to patients who reduce MRD more than 3 Log. Although these subjects should be considered candidates for more aggressive therapies, additional studies are needed to determine whether they could benefit from an allogeneic HSCT in CR1 [43]. Less frequent genetic abnormalities, such as biallelic mutations of CEBPα, mutations in nucleophosmin1 (NPM1) with a normal karyotype, are also associated with a favorable prognosis in pediatric AML [44,45]. Patients with acute promyelocytic leukemia (APL) and t(15;17), owing to the advent of ATRA and arsenic trioxide, currently represent a group with an extremely favorable prognosis [46].

Table 2. HSCT indications in childhood AML.

	GENETIC RISK CRITERIA
	Complex karyotype (≥3 aberrations including at least one structural aberration)
	Monosomal karyotype (−7, −5, del 5q)
	11q23/KMT2A rearrangements, involving: - t(10;11)(p12;q23)/KMT2A-AF10 - t(10;11)(p11.2;q23)/KMT2A-ABI1 - t(6;11)(q27;q23)/KMT2A-MLLT4 - t(4;11)(q21;q23.3)/KMT2A-MLLT2
	t(11;12)(p15;p13)/NUP98-KDM5A
	t(7;11)(p15.4;p15)/NUP98-HOXA9
	t(5;11)(q35;p15)/NUP98-NSD1
	t(6;9)(p23;q34)/DEK-NUP214
	t(16;21)(q24;q22)/RUNX1-CBFA2T3
CR1	t(7;12)(q36;p13)/MNX1-ETV6
	t(3;21)(26.2;q22)/RUNX1-MECOM
	t(16;21)(p11.2;q22.2)/FUS-ERG
	FLT3-ITD with AR ≥0.5 without NPM1 mutations
	inv(3)(q21.3q26.2)/t(3;3)(q21.3q26.2)/RPN1-MECOM
	inv(16)(p13.3q24.3)/CBFA2T3-GLIS2
	12p abnormalities
	RESPONSE RISK CRITERIA
	MRD ≥ 1% after the first induction course
	MRD ≥ 0.1% after the second induction course
	Primary Induction Failure [i.e. patients with ≥25% blasts after the first induction course and ≥5% blasts after the second induction course]
	SECONDARY AML
	Therapy-related AML
	AML evolving from myelodysplastic syndrome (MDS)
≥CR2	All patients

HSCT: hematopoietic stem cell transplantation; NPM1: nucleophosmin1.

In the pioneering work from the Medical Research Council (MRC)-AML group, adverse cytogenetic features were originally defined as −5, −7, del(5q), abnormal 3q or complex karyotype [47]. Additional MRC studies focused on childhood AML identified abnormalities of 12p as a new cytogenetic group associated with poor prognosis [48]. Although these alterations cumulatively account for <5% of cases of childhood AML, several groups have demonstrated that their identification correlates with high rates of induction failure and poor survival, and there is general agreement that these patients should be offered allogeneic HSCT in CR1 [3,49–52]. The t(6;9)(p22;q34), which leads to the formation of a leukemia-associated fusion protein DEK-NUP214, occurs infrequently in children (less than 1% of AML cases) and is associated with FLT3 ITD in approximately 40% of cases. AML patients harboring t(6;9) have a high risk of treatment failure, particularly those not proceeding to allogeneic HSCT [48,53,54]. FLT3 internal tandem duplication (FLT3/ITD) occurs in approximately 10% to 20% of pediatric AML cases and conveys a poor prognosis, which is favorably modified by the presence of a low allelic ratio or concomitant NPM1 mutations. By contrast, patients harboring FLT3-ITD with a high allelic ratio and without an NMP1 mutation have a very high risk of relapse and benefit from HSCT in CR1 [55–59]. KMT2A (MLL) rearrangements (which occur in 20% to 24% of all patients with childhood AML) have a different prognostic value depending on the specific fusion partner. Results of a large, retrospective analysis including data from 756 pediatric patients with KMT2A-rearranged AML, showed that the t(4;11)(q21;q23.3)/KMT2A-MLLT2, t(6;11)(q27;q23)/KMT2A-MLLT4, t(10;11)(p12;q23)/KMT2A-AF10 and t(10;11)(p11.2;q23)/KMT2A-ABI1 were associated with a dismal outcome [60]. Patients with such abnormalities are almost unanimously considered candidates for allo-HSCT in CR1 [48,50,61,62]. Cryptic gene fusions, including NUP98-rearrangements (the most common being t(5;11)(q35;p15)/NUP98-NSD1 and t(11;12)(p15;p13)/NUP98-KDM5A) [63–65], CBFA2T3-GLIS2 (resulting from a cryptic inversion of chromosome 16) [65–67] and t(7;12)(q36;p13)/MNX1-ETV6 (occurring virtually exclusively in children younger than 2 years) [50,68] have been shown to predict poor outcome and warrant consolidation with allogeneic HSCT in CR1 [66,68–70]. Finally, the t(8;16)(p11;p13) rearrangement, fusing KAT6A to the CREBBP gene, has an age-dependent impact on prognosis. While in very young children this translocation is associated with spontaneous remission encouraging a watch-and-wait strategy, in older children the prognosis is poor and consolidation with allotransplant in CR1 should be seriously considered [71].

MRD measurement by multiparametric flow cytometry (MFC-MRD) has been recently shown as a strong and independent prognostic marker of relapse in pediatric AML. In a prospective study including 232 children with AML in which MFC-MRD was adopted as risk-stratification criteria together with genetic features, high-level MRD positivity ($\geq 1\%$ leukemic cells) after first induction was associated with a greater cumulative incidence of relapse MRD compared to low-level (<1%) MRD (49.2% $\pm$ 7.4% vs. 16.7% $\pm$ 7.8%, $p < 0.0001$). While the outcome for patients with low levels of MRD after first induction was identical to that of patients with negative MRD, detectable MRD levels below 1% after second induction were associated with a poor outcome [5]. Subsequent studies performed by different cooperative groups have confirmed the strong prognostic relevance of MRD after the first and the second induction course, and MFC-MRD is being increasingly employed to refine the current strategies of disease risk stratification, including identification of candidates for HSCT in CR1 [72–75].

Regardless of the initial risk classification, in relapsed AML allogeneic HSCT offers the best chance of cure, ideally after the achievement of second CR (CR2) [2,62,76]. In subjects who relapse after a previous HSCT, a second transplant can offer remarkable long-term disease-free survival (DFS) probability, even in those cases not obtaining a further remission [77–80]. The proportion of children with refractory AML, defined as failure to achieve a morphological remission after two courses of chemotherapy, is estimated to be as high as 10% [3,81]. Allogeneic HSCT is currently considered as the only curative strategy in these subjects, being capable of producing long-term DFS in up to 50% of cases [82]. Patients below the age of 10 years and those with low leukemia burden or in CR at the time transplant have the highest chance of cure [82,83].

4. The Choice of Conditioning Regimen

Since maximal reduction of leukemia cells is of highest importance for post-HSCT outcome in childhood AL, myeloablative conditioning (MAC) is still considered the gold standard [84].

For what concerns patients affected by ALL, total body irradiation (TBI)-containing regimens are used preferentially over chemotherapy-based ones. This was based on: (i) historical data [85]; (ii) retrospective/registry studies [84,86–89]; (iii) a small randomized controlled trial [90]. Hyperfractionated TBI, combined with cyclophosphamide (CY), was firstly used by investigators at Memorial Sloan Kettering Cancer Center [85]. A number of studies analyzed the effect of different chemotherapy agents in combination with TBI.

Thiotepa (TT) in combination with CY was shown to be safe and effective [91]. In a CIBMTR study, the use of high-dose etoposide in combination with TBI compared favorably with TBI and CY for children with ALL in CR2 [86]. The same conditioning regimen was employed in the ALL-SCT-BFM-2003 study with good efficacy and manageable toxicity, resulting into low incidence of TRM [92]. For this reason, this association was chosen for the prospective randomized FORUM trial (see below). Interestingly, in another retrospective study, melphalan was identified as the best single agent in association with TBI, because of lower relapse incidence as compared with other drug combinations [93]. In view of notable well-known late side effects related to the use of TBI (including growth impairment, gonadal dysfunction, cognitive dysfunction, cataracts and secondary malignancies) [94], an important question is if TBI-based regimens can be replaced by chemotherapy-based conditioning. The combination of TBI and CY resulted into improved OS and leukemia-free survival (LFS) as compared to busulfan (Bu) and CY in a retrospective study on 627 patients [87]. A small, randomized, controlled trial in 43 children with ALL showed higher event-free survival (EFS) when a TBI-based regimen was used as compared to chemotherapy alone [90]. Interestingly, in a recent retrospective registry study on more than 3000 patients conducted by the Pediatric Disease Working Party of EBMT, although TBI was confirmed to be superior to chemotherapy in the whole cohort (for OS, LFS, TRM and relapse), a subgroup analysis showed comparable outcomes of the different type of conditioning regimens for patients in CR1 [84]. In order to obtain a definitive answer on the optimal preparative regimen to be employed in children with ALL, an international, prospective, open-label, randomized, controlled trial to investigate whether chemo-conditioning regimens could replace TBI in pediatric patients with high-risk ALL (For Omitting Radiation Under Majority age (FORUM), NCT01949129) was conducted in 21 countries in patients aged 4–21 years at HSCT, in CR pre-HSCT, and with an HLA-compatible related or unrelated donor [95]. In detail, fractionated 12 Gy TBI combined with etoposide was compared to fludarabine, TT, and either Bu or treosulfan (according to the country preference chosen by national coordinators of the study). The statistical design was a noninferiority study with an 8% margin, with an estimated sample size of 1000 patients randomly assigned in 5 years with 2-year minimum follow-up. However, the trial was terminated early because of application of a stopping rule, since at interim analysis chemo-conditioning resulted significantly inferior to TBI. In particular, 2-year OS (91% versus 75%, $p < 0.0001$) and EFS (86% versus 58%, $p < 0.0001$) were significantly higher for the 212 patients randomly assigned to receive TBI as compared to 201 who were randomized to chemotherapy alone (intention-to-treat analysis). Cumulative incidence of relapse and, more surprisingly, TRM were lower in the TBI group than in the chemotherapy-based preparative regimen. The outcome of children given fludarabine, TT and either Bu or treosulfan was comparable. Notably, in subgroup analyses, TBI remained superior to chemotherapy for almost all the different variables analyzed (including disease status) [95]. Thus, this kind of conditioning is now considered the gold standard for pediatric patients affected by ALL.

In the context of acute myeloid leukemia (AML), TBI and non-TBI regimens have never been compared in a prospective, randomized fashion. The superiority of TBI-based compared to Bu-based regimens, initially reported in older studies present in literature [96–98] has not been confirmed in other reports. A retrospective study from the Japanese Society for Hematopoietic Cell Transplantation comparing TBI/Cy and intravenous Bu/Cy in pediatric AML patients in first or second remission (CR1/CR2) confirmed no significant differences in terms of relapse and TRM, this resulting in a similar 3-year OS (68% and 72% for TBI/Cy and Bu/Cy, respectively) [99]. Similar results have also been reported from the French Group in a retrospective study evaluating TBI/Cy versus Bu/Cy for AML patients in CR1 [100]. Recently, TBI and non-TBI regimens were compared in 624 children transplanted between 2008 and 2016 and reported to CIBMTR registry. Five-year NRM was higher with TBI regimens (22% vs. 11%, $p < 0.0001$), but relapse was lower (23% vs. 37%, $p < 0.0001$) compared to non-TBI conditioning. Consequently, OS (62% vs. 60%, $p = 1.00$)

and LFS (55% vs. 52%, $p = 0.42$) did not differ between treatment groups. TBI regimens were associated with higher incidence of grade II–IV aGVHD and greater 3-year incidence of gonadal failure or growth hormone deficiency while no differences in cGVHD and late pulmonary, cardiac or renal impairment were observed [101].

The first association of Bu and high-dose cyclophosphamide (Cy) (200 mg/kg), reported from Santos et al., resulted into a low relapse rate, but unacceptable transplant related mortality (TRM): for this reason, the Cy dosage was reduced to 120 mg/kg in the subsequent studies, with a lower toxicity and the same efficacy profile [88]. The addition of a third alkylating agent (Melphalan) to a standard Bu/Cy backbone has been shown to be effective with an acceptable toxicity profile, and this conditioning regimen has been adopted by many cooperative groups [61,102]. Results from the Italian protocol AIEOP AML 2001/02, in which 243 patients given either allo- or auto-HSCT after myeloablative regimen including Bu/Cy/Mel were analyzed, showed a 8-year OS and DFS of 75% and 74%, the with cumulative incidence of TRM being of 7% for the allo-HSCT group [61]. Similar results were observed in the AML SCT-BFM 2007 trial [62]. A recent large retrospective study on behalf of the Pediatric Disease Working Party of the EBMT compared the outcomes of pediatric AML patients receiving three different conditioning regimens (TBI/Cy, BU/Cy, BU/Cy and melphalan). Among the three options, Bu/Cy/Mel was associated with a lower incidence of relapse and the higher LFS as compared with the other chemo/radiotherapy combinations [103].

In most recent years, the use of reduced intensity conditioning (RIC) has been explored in pediatric patients with AL as a strategy to maintain a good balance between high antileukemic effect and reduced acute/late chemotherapy toxicity. In this regard, the reduced-intensity approach could offer better outcome and minor toxicity to pediatric patients with AML who are ineligible for myeloablative therapy because of heavy pretreatment, comorbidities or genetic conditions at high-risk of transplant-related toxicities, including Fanconi anemia or Down syndrome [104,105]. Recently, in a large cohort of 180 AML patients, Bitan et al. reported no significant differences in of acute and chronic GvHD and 5-year OS and FFS between patients given or RIC and MAC regimens [106]. Treosulfan-based conditioning regimen appears an interesting alternative to busulfan [107,108]. EBMT data regarding 198 pediatric patients with hematological malignancies including 50 AML conditioned with Treosulfan-based regimens showed an optimal safety profile; the 3-year OS and EFS were 54% and 45%, respectively, with better results if Treosulfan was associated with fludarabine and an alkylating drug such as Tiothepa or Melphalan [108]. In a prospective II phase study evaluating safety and efficacy of a conditioning regimen based on Treosulfan, Fludarabine and Thiotepa in 29 pediatric patients with AML, the 3-year PFS and OS were 79% and 84%, respectively [109]. Results on other RIC or reduced toxicity regimens have been published in smaller cohorts of pediatric patients, reporting promising safety and efficacy results [110–113]. Of note, use of RIC or reduced toxicity regimen was explored in children with relapsed/refractory (R/R) AML in association with Clofarabine. Six patients with R/R AML underwent a reinduction with Clofarabine or high-dose Cytarabine and subsequently received RIC regimen and HSCT; at 21 months after the procedure, 5/6 patients were alive without relapse [114]. More recently, a large study including 103 CR1 AML pediatric patients compared safety and efficacy of Bu/Cy, Bu/Cy/Mel and Clofarabine/Flu/Bu; 5-year LFS was 43%, 59% and 67%, respectively, while 5-year TRM was 14%, 7% and 6%, respectively [115].

Anti-human T-lymphocyte globulin (ATLG) is largely used during the preparation to an allograft from donors other than an HLA-identical sibling to regulate bidirectional alloreactivity; indeed, this type of serotherapy reduces the incidence and severity of the two main immune-mediated complications of the procedure, namely GvHD and graft rejection. Several randomized trials conducted in adults have demonstrated a significant reduction in the incidence of chronic GvHD when ATLG is added to the standard GvHD prophylaxis [116]. Only one randomized controlled trial, comparing different doses of ATLG, has been conducted in children with hematological malignancies transplanted from an unrelated volunteer [117]. This study demonstrated that low-dose ATLG can reduce the incidence of life-threatening infections, without significantly affecting the incidence of acute and chronic GvHD; in addition, a lower dose of ATLG resulted into an improved OS and EFS. Thus, a low-dose ATLG (namely 15 mg/kg of Grafalon®, Neovii Biotech, Rapperswil, Switzerland; formerly ATG Fresenius®), should be regarded as the standard serotherapy regimen for HSCT from UD in pediatric patients with malignant disorders.

5. The Role of Pre-Transplant Minimal Residual Disease: Better Remission for Better HSCT Outcome?

During the last two decades, MRD quantification has emerged as a crucial assessment in the evaluation of early treatment response and in the definition of patient risk stratification in both ALL and AML [5,16,118–120]. At the same time, accumulating evidence has shown that pre-transplant MRD status correlates with the risk of relapse and OS after HSCT. In the late 1990s, Knechtli et al. provided the first demonstration of the key predictive role exerted by pre-transplant PCR-based MRD in a retrospective analysis of 64 pediatric patients undergoing allogeneic HSCT [121]. This observation was confirmed prospectively by the ALL-REZ BFM Study Group in 91 children with relapsed ALL. In this study, children with pre-HSCT PCR-MRD $\geq 10^{-4}$ had a higher cumulative incidence of relapse as compared with patients having PCR-MRD $<10^{-4}$ (57% vs. 13% respectively, $p < 0.001$) [122]. The best cutoff value of pre-transplant PCR-MRD for prognosis prediction in ALL is still a matter of debate. In a large cohort of high-risk relapsed ALL children transplanted in CR2, subjects with PCR-MRD $\geq 10^{-3}$ before HSCT had a significantly worse probability of DFS as compared with patients with PCR-MRD $<10^{-3}$, while no differences were observed between patients with MRD $<10^{-4}$ and those having an MRD within the range of 10^{-4} and 10^{-3} [123]. By contrast, a retrospective analysis of 119 ALL patients, performed by the Italian Association for Paediatric Haematology/Oncology (AIEOP), showed that the level of pre-HSCT MRD positivity has a different impact on EFS according to disease phase at HSCT. Indeed, in patients transplanted in CR1, only an high PCR-MRD level ($\geq 10^{-3}$) was associated with an increased risk of relapse, while in subjects transplanted in CR2, even a low-level MRD positivity ($<10^{-3}$) determined a high relapse rate and poor outcome [124]. In the context of childhood AML, the prognostic value of molecular MRD before HSCT is less defined. In a recent I-BFM-AML collaborative study, the role of PCR-MRD collected within 5 weeks prior to HSCT was evaluated in 108 pediatric AML patients harboring one of the main recurrent AML gene rearrangements (t(8;21)(q22;q22); RUNX1-RUNX1T1, inv(16)(p13.1q22)/t(16;16)(p13.1;q22); CBFB-MYH11, t(9;11)(p22;q23); KMT2A-MLLT3 or FLT3-ITD). In this study, 5-year OS after HSCT was significantly higher in patients with low PCR-MRD (defined as a value below 2.1×10^{-4} calculated by ROC curve analysis with respect to diagnosis or relapse), as compared with subjects having PCR-MRD levels above the cutoff (83% vs. 57%; $p = 0.012$) [125].

The assessment of MRD by means of MFC (MFC-MRD) showed similar results in terms of prognostic value in both ALL and AML. In a cohort of 122 children with very high-risk ALL ($n = 64$) or AML ($N = 58$), Leung and colleagues showed that the 5-year cumulative incidence of relapse after HCT was 40% in the patients with high levels of FCM-MRD ($\geq 0.1\%$ in ALL and $\geq 1.0\%$ in AML), 16% among those with low level of MRD (0.01% to <0.1% in ALL and 0.1% to <1% in AML) and 6% in those with no MRD ($p = 0.0002$). High MRD was also confirmed as an independent adverse prognostic factor for survival in multivariate analysis ($p = 0.0035$) [126]. In a Children's Oncology Group (COG)/Pediatric Bone Marrow Transplant Consortium (PBMTC) multicenter phase III trial evaluating the addition of sirolimus to standard GvHD prophylaxis in children with ALL, patients with MFC-MRD $\geq 0.1\%$ had a higher relapse risk as compared to subjects whose MRD was negative or <0.1% [127]. In the context of AML, detectable MFC-MRD immediately prior to HSCT has been consistently associated with increased risk of post-HSCT relapse and worse OS in both children and adults [10,128,129]. These observations are further supported by a meta-analysis of 19 studies evaluating pre-HSCT MRD (mainly assessed by FCM) in 1431 pediatric and adult AML patients; MRD positivity was associated with decreased DFS,

OS and increased cumulative incidence of relapse [130]. Several groups have also shown the value of next-generation sequencing (NGS) technologies for MRD detection in both ALL and AML [131–134]. When NGS-MRD was compared with MFC-MRD in 56 pediatric B-ALL patients, NGS-MRD predicted relapse and survival more accurately than MFC-MRD ($p < 0.0001$), especially in the MRD negative cohort (2-year relapse probability, 0% vs. 16%; $p = 0.02$; 2-year OS, 96% vs. 77%; $p = 0.003$) [132]. Given the importance of pre-HSCT MRD in determining the probability of cure, modern ALL and AML therapy approaches have focused on strategies to induce MRD-negativity before transplant, especially for patients with high-risk disease features. These approaches are particularly attractive in B-cell ALL (B-ALL) where children may benefit from the tremendous improvements obtained over the past decade owing to the clinical application of different immunotherapy agents. Indeed, before the advent of immunotherapy, strategies to achieve pre-transplant MRD-negative remission in relapsed B-ALL relied on intensive multidrug chemotherapy regimens, which are commonly associated with the occurrence of toxicities that may be fatal or reduce the likelihood of proceeding to allogeneic HSCT [135,136].

In a phase I/II study conducted in children with R/R B-ALL, blinatumomab, a bispecific T-cell engager antibody targeting CD19, was able to induce cytomorphological remission in 39% of subjects, which was MRD-negative in 52% of cases [137]. Higher CR rates were observed in the expanded access study, likely because of the greater proportion of patients with <50% blasts enrolled, these data reflecting the association between lower leukemia burden and clinical response [138]. Recently, the results of two international randomized clinical trials, comparing blinatumomab with conventional chemotherapy as pre-transplant consolidation therapy in children with high-risk first relapse of B-ALL, were published. Randomization was performed after three cycles of chemotherapy in one study and after a single cycle of induction chemotherapy in the other one. In both studies, treatment with blinatumomab resulted in less severe toxicities, higher MRD remission rate, greater probability of proceeding to allogeneic HSCT and improved outcome [139,140].

In the dose-finding part of a phase 1/2 study promoted by the Innovative Therapies for Children With Cancer in Europe (ITCC) consortium, inotuzumab ozogamicin (InO), an antibody–drug conjugate composed of a CD22-directed monoclonal antibody linked to calicheamicin, was able induce a CR/CRi (CR with incomplete hematologic recovery) in 80% of children with relapsed and refractory B-ALL. Among the 19 responders with available MFC-MRD data, 16 (84%) obtained MRD-negativity [141]. Similar results were observed in a retrospective analysis of InO compassionate-use program, which reported a CR rate of 67% with 71% of responders achieving MRD negativity [142]. One possible toxicity concern, regarding the use of InO before HSCT, is related to the risk of sinusoidal obstruction syndrome (SOS), especially in heavily pretreated patients [141,142]. While blinatumomab and InO are mainly recognized as bridge-to-transplant (or, at least, bridge-to-consolidation) strategies in children, the benefit of a consolidative HSCT after chimeric antigen receptor T-cell (CAR T) therapy is currently the object of considerable debate [13]. Anti-CD19 CAR T-cell therapy has produced impressive MRD-negative CR rates, ranging from 56% to 93%. However, durability of response after CAR T is variable and influenced by CAR T-cell expansion, persistence and characteristics of co-stimulatory domains [11,143,144]. Studies with CD28-based anti-CD19 CAR T cells, which are characterized by short persistence after infusion, have a higher tendency of referral to HSCT compared to studies with 41BB-based CAR T cells. In the long-term follow-up study of 50 children and young adults (CAYA) treated with a CD28-based anti-CD19 CAR T, 62.0% patients achieved a CR, which was FCM-MRD negative in 90.3% of cases. Noteworthy, MRD-negative patients proceeding to allo-HSCT had a 5-year EFS of 61.9%, while all MRD-negative subjects who did not proceed to a consolidative HSCT experienced leukemia relapse [143]. In the global phase II trial of tisagenlecleucel in 75 CAYA with R/R B-ALL, only eight patients among those who obtained disease remission underwent allo-HSCT. Despite that, 59% of patients who received tisagenlecleucel remained in remission; the majority of those who relapsed experiencing CD19-negative disease [11]. A benefit from consolidative HSCT after anti-CD19 CAR T cell therapy has also been observed with a different 4-1BB-co-stimulated CAR [144],particularly in patients with rapid loss of B-cell aplasia and those who were not transplanted before CAR-T cells [145]. Consolidation with HSCT was shown to be favorably associated with better EFS ($p = 0.016$) also in a phase I trial evaluating a CD22-targeted/4-1BB CAR T-cell in CAYA with B-ALL [146]. Emerging data suggest that more sensitive NGS-MRD testing may help identify which patients need HSCT consolidation after CAR-T cell therapy [147]. In the near future, the dramatic increase in the number of B-ALL patients who achieve MRD-negative complete remissions owing to immunotherapy approaches, will likely offer the opportunity to re-evaluate the role of HSCT as consolidation strategy in this setting.

For patients with AML and T-cell ALL, the availability of immunotherapy is currently much more limited as compared with B-ALL. In the context of pediatric AML, modest benefit has been observed by the incorporation of CD33-targeted therapy with gemtuzumab ozogamicin (GO) in addition to standard chemotherapy [148]. Despite that, there is evidence that certain subsets of patients, particularly those with FLT3-ITD mutations, KMT2A rearrangements, single-nucleotide polymorphisms in ABCB1 and CD33, and high CD33 expression are more likely to profit from GO administration and GO may be effective at reducing MRD levels before HSCT [5,149–153]. Concerns regarding the risk of increased toxicity of GO in conjunction with HSCT warrant further investigation regarding optimal dosing and timing to improve overall outcomes [151]. Several immunotherapies are in various stages of preclinical and clinical development for AML, including antibody–drug conjugates, bispecific antibodies, cellular therapies and checkpoint inhibitors [154,155]. Currently, most early-phase cellular immunotherapy studies for children with AML are intended as a bridge to transplant in order to achieve more profound remission status. It is too early to speculate whether such approaches will also be able decrease the need for subsequent HSCT [154,155]. Daratumumab, a CD38-targeting monoclonal antibody, is the most promising antibody-based approach in T-ALL treatment [156,157]. Currently, daratumumab in addition to standard chemotherapy is under investigation in a phase II trial for pediatric and young adult patients with R/R T- or B-cell ALL (NCT03384654). Developing CAR-T cell therapies into the setting of T-ALL has been hampered by the risk of fratricide because of the shared expression of target antigens between CAR-T cells and T-leukemia cells, and of severe life-threatening immunodeficiency due to the elimination of normal T lymphocytes [158]. Fratricide-resistant CD7, CD5 and CD1a-targeted CAR-T [159–161], and universal allotolerant off-the-shelf CAR-T cells generated by genome editing [162,163] have been proposed as potential strategies to overcome these limitations.

Although accumulating evidence shows a correlation between the presence of pre-HSCT MRD and the risk or relapse in children with leukemia, merely having a detectable disease prior to HCT does not necessarily indicate an inability to cure the disease [126]. For this reason, especially in settings such as T-ALL and AML where the availability of immunotherapy approaches outside clinical trials is still limited, the benefit of repeated efforts aimed at achieving MRD-negativity before transplant should be carefully weighed against the risks of inducing additional toxicities affecting post-transplant outcome.

6. Post-Transplant Minimal Residual Disease: Is There Room for Intervention?

MRD assessment before transplantation cannot effectively identify all individuals with impending post-transplantation relapse who might benefit for pre-emptive intervention. For this reason, the predictive role of post-transplant MRD has been investigated by several groups, especially in ALL [124,164–166]. In a BFM study evaluating 113 pediatric patients transplanted for relapsed ALL, the level of PCR-MRD was inversely correlated with EFS and positively correlated with the cumulative incidence of relapse at all time points after transplant. In multivariable analysis, MRD $\geq 10^{-4}$ leukemic cells was consistently correlated with inferior EFS [164]. Although high levels of post-transplant MRD are strongly predictive of disease recurrence, low level MRD positivity after transplantation was not invariably associated with relapse, especially if detected early after HSCT [164].

By contrast, this and other studies showed that the further the patient is from HSCT, the more likely even low levels of MRD predict a poor prognosis [124,164–166]. These findings support the assumption that low levels of residual leukemia cells could be controlled by an immunologic GvL effect in the early post-transplant period, before the graft becomes tolerant toward the recipient. In a recent multicenter study, Bader et al. defined the relative risk of pre- and post-HSCT MRD in pediatric ALL, and their relationship with other independent risk factors [9]. When considered individually, however, both pre-HSCT and post-HSCT had significant prognostic value, if the two measures were simultaneously evaluated in a bivariate analysis, pre-HSCT MRD became less important in determining risk compared with the post-HSCT MRD. In this study, both MRD negative or positive patients had an approximately threefold decrease in relapse if they developed aGvHD and patients who had positive MRD recorded post-HSCT and developed aGvHD had relapse rates similar to those who were MRD negative and did not develop aGvHD [9]. The beneficial effect exerted by the occurrence of aGvHD on relapse risk and survival of children with ALL has been documented by several reports. In a COG/PBMTC study, patients with pre-HCT MFC-MRD $\geq 0.1\%$ who did not develop aGvHD compared with those with MFC-MRD $<0.1\%$ who did develop aGvHD had much worse 2-year DFS (18% vs. 71%; $p = 0.001$). Patients with pre-HCT MRD $<0.1\%$ who did not experience aGvHD had higher rates of relapse than those who did develop aGvHD (40% vs. 13%; $p = 0.008$) [166]. Zecca et al. showed that children with hematologic malignancies who developed chronic GvHD (cGvHD) after transplant had a reduced relapse probability (16% $\pm$ 3% vs. 39% $\pm$ 3%, $p = 0.0001$) and a better DFS (68% $\pm$ 4% vs. 54% $\pm$ 3%, $p = 0.01$) compared with children without cGVHD, The anti-leukemic effect of cGvHD was observed mainly in patients with ALL [167]. In patients with B-ALL, post-HSCT NGS-MRD positivity performed better than FCM-MRD for predicting relapse, especially early after HCT. Any post-HSCT NGS positivity resulted in an increase in relapse risk by multivariate analysis (hazard ratio, 7.7; $p = 0.05$) [132]. The role of MRD after transplant in pediatric AML is less defined, although there is evidence that post-HCT positivity of MFC-MRD can predict imminent relapse [129]. Noteworthy, a recent study evaluated the predictive role of NGS-MRD in pediatric and adult AML patients undergoing HSCT. In this study, variant allele frequency (VAF) more than 0.2% on day +21 post-HSCT, was associated with decreased 3-year OS and an increased risk of relapse [133]. Finally, although less sensitive than MRD, close chimerism monitoring on peripheral blood has proven useful for the early detection of impending relapse in both ALL and AML [168–170].

For patients with post-transplant evidence of MRD, additional interventions could influence outcomes by favouring the development of a GvL effect. This goal has been pursued through several strategies, including rapid discontinuation (or abrupt cessation) of immune suppression [168,171–173], administration of cytokines [174] and infusion of donor-derived lymphocytes or cytokine-stimulated immune effector cells [170,175]. Since the benefit derived from GvL may be offset by the increased TRM associated with severe GvHD, caution should be adopted when adopting interventions that stimulate excessive GvHD [9]. In patients with Philadelphia chromosome positive ALL, or FLT3/ITD-positive AML, post-transplant administration of tyrosine kinase inhibitors, such as imatinib and sorafenib or midostaurin, respectively, can improve outcomes, especially for patients showing molecular MRD recurrence after-HSCT [176–178]. In the context of AML, the combination of azacytidine and donor-lymphocyte infusion (DLI) could represent an effective strategy to prevent overt disease recurrence in MRD-positive patients [179]. Recently, Ofran et al. described three patients with T-ALL in whom residual MRD after transplant was eradicated following administration of daratumumab, provided on a compassionate basis, in combination with DLI or rapid tapering of immunosuppression [157]. For patients with B-cell ALL, the availability of highly effective immunotherapy agents, such as blinatumomab and inotuzumab, also makes them attractive strategies to tackle MRD-recurrence in the post-transplant period. Ongoing clinical trials are evaluating these approaches in both children and adults (NCT04785547, NCT04044560, NCT03913559, NCT03104491).

7. Transplantation from Alternative Donors: No Longer a Second Choice?

Eligibility criteria for HSCT in both ALL and AML have been varying over time not only according to disease characteristics and response to treatment, but also depending on type of available donor. The use of HLA-matched related donors is still considered the preferred option [40,92,180,181]. However, more than 70% of children with AL who might benefit from an allograft lack an HLA-identical family donor. With the establishment of donor registries, many patients are able to locate a suitable unrelated donor (UD). Results in children transplanted for either ALL or AML suggest that fully matched UD selected through high-resolution typing of HLA loci offer minimal or possibly no disadvantages in terms of disease outcome compared with HLA-identical siblings [182–187]. In the context of ALL, it has been shown that results obtained using a 9/10 or a 10/10 allelic matched donor, either related or unrelated, are not inferior to those observed after HSCT from an HLA-identical sibling in terms of EFS, OS and CIR [92]. For several years, a wider degree of HLA mismatch has been considered acceptable only in the presence of poor prognostic features indicating an increased risk of leukemia recurrence/progression without HSCT consolidation [92,188], although recent results obtained with different alternative donor approaches strongly suggest that this paradigm could no longer be valid.

UCB transplantation (UCBT) has been largely employed in the past for patients lacking an HLA-matched donor and several reports have demonstrated that unrelated UCBT is able to offer long-term outcomes similar to those observed using an UD in both ALL and AML [189,190]. Eapen et al. compared results observed in 503 children with AL given unrelated UCBT with those of 282 bone marrow transplant (BMT) recipients. DFS was superior in recipients of HLA matched cord blood ($p = 0.040$), while it did not differ between BMT and one or two HLA-disparate UCBTs [190]. The results of UCBT in both childhood ALL and AML have been extensively analyzed by retrospective registry-based studies performed by the Eurocord group. In the context of ALL, a lower risk of relapse (24% vs. 39%; hazard ratio 0.4; $p = 0.01$) and better DFS (54% vs. 29%; hazard ratio 2, $p = 0.003$) were observed in children with negative MRD before UCBT as compared with those with positive MRD [191]. In children given UCBT for AML, the results were particularly promising for children with poor prognostic features, namely secondary leukaemia, high-risk karyotype, or transplanted in CR2 after an early relapse, for whom the DFS and risk of relapse were similar to those of the other patients [192]. Analysis of AML patients who underwent autologous or allogeneic HSCT within the AIEOP AML 2002/01 showed a remarkable DFS overcoming 90% in the subgroup who received UCBT [61]. Subsequent studies have demonstrated that better HLA-matching strategies between donor and recipient (at high-resolution level for HLA-A, -B, -C and -DRB1 loci) may further improve the outcome of patients with AL given a single UCBT [193,194]. Transplantation of two UCB grafts has been proposed to overcome the limitations related to the low cell dose infused; unfortunately, in two prospective randomized studies, the double UCBT strategy did not improve the overall outcome of children and young adults with AL in the presence of a single unit of adequate cell dose, being instead associated with an increased risk of GvHD [195,196]. Despite that, it has been suggested that the double-unit strategy may enhance the GvL effect and be of particular benefit in patients with positive pre-transplant MRD [197,198]. Strategies aimed at expanding the number of UCB progenitors ex vivo and favouring stem-cell-homing in vivo are being developed with encouraging preliminary results, holding the potential to revitalize the field of UCBT in the near future [199–201].

One of the main reasons for the continue decline in the utilization of UCBT observed in the last decade, beyond the intrinsic limitations of the approach (i.e., delayed engraftment, increased risk of TRM), is the emergence of highly effective T-cell depleted and T-cell repleted HLA-haploidentical transplantation platforms [202]. Indeed, HSCT from an HLA-haploidentical relative offers an immediate transplant treatment virtually to any patient lacking a matched donor or a suitable UCB unit and, in addition, easy access to the donor for post-transplant adoptive cell therapies [203,204].

In the setting of T-cell depleted (TCD) haploidentical (haplo) HSCT, a remarkable advance has been obtained through the development of more sophisticated graft manipulation strategies (with respect to the original positive selection of CD34+ cells), based on the selective depletion of CD3+ and CD19+ cells [187,205,206] or, more recently, of TCRα/β+ and CD19+ cells [207]. With the latter approach, in particular, the graft transfers to the recipient not only high numbers of CD34+ cells, but also of mature donor NK cells and TCRγ/δ+ T cells that can display their protective effect against leukemia regrowth and life-threatening infections [208]. By contrast, T cells expressing the αβ chains of the T cell receptor, which are responsible for the development of GvHD, are removed with a median depletion efficiency of 4 Log [209]. Our group has reported the outcome of a cohort of 80 children with AL (ALL, $n = 56$; AML, $n = 24$) transplanted from an haploidentical relative after αβ+ T-cell and CD19+ B-cell depletion [210]. All children received a fully myeloablative preparative regimen and received anti-T-lymphocyte globulin for preventing graft rejection and GvHD; no patient received any post-transplant GVHD prophylaxis. The cumulative incidence of TRM was remarkably low (5%). Nineteen subjects relapsed, the cumulative incidence of recurrence being 24%. The 5-year OS probability was 72% (95% CI, 62–82) for the whole study population. Overall, the 5-year DFS was 71% (95% CI, 61–81), without differences between ALL and AML patients. The cumulative incidence of skin-only, grade I–II acute GvHD (aGvHD) was 30% and no patient developed GvHD with visceral involvement, grade III–IV aGvHD or extensive chronic GvHD. TBI-containing preparative regimen was the only variable favourably influencing relapse incidence and chronic GVHD-free/relapse-free survival (GRFS) [210]. More recently, the results of 98 αβ-TCD haplo-HSCT recipients were compared with those of 127 matched UD (MUD), 118 mismatched UD (MMUD) in a multicenter retrospective analysis. MUD and MMUD-HSCT were characterized by a higher cumulative incidence of grade II–IV and grade III–IV aGvHD (35% vs. 44% and 6% vs. 18%, respectively) compared with 16% and 0% in αβ-TCD haplo-HSCT ($p < 0.001$). Children treated with αβ-TCD haplo-HSCT also had a significantly lower incidence of overall and extensive chronic GVHD ($p < 0.01$). While the GRFS probability of survival of MUD-HSCT and αβhaplo-HSCT recipients was superimposable (61% and 58%, respectively), the choice of MMUD-HSCT had a detrimental effect on this composite end-point (34%; $p < 0.001$) [6]. Noteworthy, although the haploidentical donor was mainly selected privileging NK immunological features [211,212], no favourable influence of NK alloreactivity and of donor KIR B-haplotype was observed in both studies [6,210]. This is in contrast with the observations derived from studies on the infusion of CD34+ cells [213–216], likely because the NK-mediated GVL effect was partially obscured by other cells present in the graft, including γδ T cells [217]. In a retrospective Spanish study performed in children with ALL given ex vivo TCD grafts using different manipulation strategies, the presence of donor–recipient KIR mismatch provided no advantage, while a donor with KIR A haplotype was associated with an increased probability of relapse [218]. Although the benefits of an NK alloreactive asset appear less clear when using refined graft-manipulation strategies, the selection of a donor with favourable NK features continues to be recommended for patients receiving TCD-HSCT [212]. Since preclinical data showed that bisphosphonates can enhance TcRγδ-mediated anti-leukemia activity [219], the administration of zoledronic acid (ZOL) after αβ-TCD haplo-HSCT has been explored as potential strategy for further improving patient outcome, showing encouraging results in terms of better OS, reduced GvHD incidence and lower TRM [220,221]. In addition, TCD haplo-HSCT approaches represent an ideal platform for post-transplant adoptive cell therapies because no (or minimal) immunosuppression is given after HSCT. An intriguing approach to accelerate the recovery of adaptive immunity and to promote anti-tumour activity relies on the administration of suicide gene-modified T cells, which offer the possibility of limiting the risk of uncontrolled GvHD by triggering T-cell apoptosis [222]. In the adult TCD haplo-HSCT setting, post-transplantation infusion of donor T-cells modified with the insertion of the herpes simplex thymidine kinase suicide gene (to achieve in vivo susceptibility to ganciclovir) enabled regulation of GvHD, while promoting immune reconstitution [223,224]. An alternative strategy, developed by the Baylor group, is based on T cells engineered to express the caspase 9 (iC9) suicide gene [225]. Post-transplant infusion of iC9-T cells has been shown to accelerate immune recovery [226,227]. Administration of iC9-T cells after αβ+ TCD-haplo-HSCT was associated with better OS and DFS when compared with an historical cohort of "pure" αβ+ TCD-haplo-HSCT [228]. In order to promote the recovery of pathogen-specific immunity, other groups have investigated the infusion of low-dose memory CD45RA-depleted donor lymphocytes after HSCT with αβ T-cell depletion, with encouraging results [229]. The rationale for this strategy is based on experimental data demonstrating that mouse CD4 memory T-cells, and effector memory CD8 T-cells, are devoid of GvH reactivity [230]. Removal of CD45RA+ *naive* T lymphocytes has been also tested as TCD strategy before haploidentical HSCT. In a recent publication describing the preliminary outcomes of 50 children receiving a CD45RA-depleted haplo-HSCT (of whom 47 having AL), the St. Jude investigators reported moderately high rates of grade III–IV aGvHD (28%) and chronic GvHD (26%). Despite that, GvHD was successfully treated in most patients, and NRM mortality among patients in CR at the time of HCST was 5.6%, the 3-year OS and EFS being 78.9% and 77.7%, respectively [231].

T-cell repleted haplo-HSCT approaches based on the post-transplant administration of cyclophosphamide (PTCy), pioneered by the Johns Hopkins group [232], have been extensively investigated in adult patients [233,234]. In the last few years, accumulating evidence suggests that this strategy may also be successfully employed in children. A recent retrospective analysis compared the outcome of pediatric patients with AL undergoing T-replete haplo-HSCT with PTCy after nonmyeloablative (NMA) conditioning with that of a contemporary cohort of children receiving transplantation from MUD and MMUD. The 5-year OS rates were not different between MUD, MMUD and Haplo patients, while an increased incidence of graft failure was observed in the haplo-group, likely derived from the adoption of an NMA preparative regimen [235]. A full-myeloablative regimen, either busulfan-based or TBI-based, has been employed with success in 29 children and young adults undergoing HLA-haplo-HSCT with PTCy for malignant conditions (of whom 18 with AL), with 3-year OS and EFS of 79% (95% CI, 66, 96) and 69% (95% CI, 54, 88), respectively. In this small cohort, relative high rates of cGvHD were observed (cumulative incidence of cGvHD at 1-year 28% (95% CI, 0.1, 0.4), moderate to severe 14% (95% CI, 0.01, 0.3)), but the limited sample size prevents drawing definitive conclusions [236]. The results of a retrospective analysis of 180 children with ALL who received a HLA-haplo-HSCT with PTCy, were recently reported by Pediatric Disease Working Party (PDWP) of the European Society for Blood and Marrow Transplantation (EBMT). Cumulative incidence of day-100 grade II–IV aGvHD was 28%, and 2-year cGvHD was 21.9%. The 2-year NRM was 19.6% and the estimated 2-year DFS was 65%, 44% and 18.8% for patients transplanted in CR1, CR2 and CR3, respectively. In multivariable analysis for patients in CR1 and CR2, disease status (CR2 (hazard ratio 2.19; $p = 0.04$)), age at HCST greater than 13 years (hazard ratio 2.07; $p = 0.03$) and use of peripheral blood stem cell (PBSC) (hazard ratio 1.98; $p = 0.04$) were independently associated with decreased OS [237]. Recent evidence also suggests that refinements in pharmacological GvHD prophylaxis strategies may improve the outcome of patients receiving unmanipulated HLA-mismatched grafts from UD. In particular, in a prospective multicenter phase II trial, the addition of abatacept, an anti-CTLA-4 monoclonal antibody, to standard calcineurin inhibitor (CNI)/methotrexate (MTX)-based GvHD prophylaxis was able to reduce the incidence of grade III–IV aGvHD in children and adults with haematological malignancies undergoing HSCT from an 8/8 MUD or 7/8 MMUD. Patients receiving abatacept had better severe aGvHD-free survival (SGFS) as compared with controls receiving only CNI/MTX (93.2% vs. 82, $p = 0.05$ in the 8/8 arm; 97.7% vs. 58.7%, $p < 0.001$, in the 7/8 arm) [238]. The impressive results observed in the 7/8 arm are of particular interest for those patients (often belonging to ethnic groups poorly represented in the registries) for whom the possibility of UD-HSCT is mainly restricted to an HLA-mismatched setting [239].

Collectively, most recent transplant results obtained with MUD, MMUD, haploidentical donors and UCB units indicate that all these options are able to offer the chance of transplant to virtually every child with AL in need of an allograft and lacking an HLA-identical sibling, without significant differences in terms of outcome. Each of these strategies has advantages and limitations, but rather than being considered competing alternatives, they should be regarded as complementary options and the final choice should be based on patient's characteristics, clinician/Centre expertise, the urgency of the transplant and specific features of the unrelated/haploidentical donor or UCB unit.

8. Conclusions

Results of HSCT in AL have improved substantially, in particular during the last two decades, and progress using alternative donors has extended the potential application of allotransplantation to most patients. For several years, donor characteristics have played a relevant role in determining eligibility for HSCT, with alternative donors being accepted only in those cases deemed at the highest risk of leukemia relapse. However, current results with alternative donors suggest that this paradigm could no longer be valid and encourage not restricting the indications for HSCT upon availability of a fully matched donor. In this regard, the importance of the specific transplant infrastructure and experience of the team in determining the outcome of HSCT from alternative donors must not be neglected [240]. The importance of MRD before and after transplant is being increasingly clarified and MRD-directed interventions may further improve the outcome of allogeneic HSCT in AL, particularly in view of the growing availability of precision medicine approaches. In addition, incorporation of MRD data in risk stratification models before allo-HSCT may allow better identifying which patients should be offered an allograft and possibly inform how to transplant these subjects [241]. In the last few years, successes obtained by combination chemotherapy and the development of highly effective immunotherapy agents have raised the question of whether HSCT will continue to play a role in modern therapy of childhood AL, particularly in B-ALL [13]. Although the answer to this question should necessarily come from the results of well-designed and randomized clinical trials, the number of variables that may influence transplant outcome and the quantity of innovative approaches that have entered, or are about to enter, into the clinical arena, makes the design and conduct of such studies anything but trivial. For these reasons, determining the appropriate role of HSCT in childhood AL will continue to be a challenging and dynamic process, requiring constant and careful assessment of the likelihood of cure with conventional chemotherapy or novel targeted therapies to identify the subset of children for whom transplant offers a better treatment option. In this regard, close cooperation between chemotherapy cooperative study groups and transplant/cell therapy societies, and monitoring of treatment-related late effects with long-term patient follow-up is crucial.

Author Contributions: Conceptualization, M.A., P.M., F.L. and D.P.; writing—original draft preparation, M.A., P.M. and D.P.; writing—final review, F.L. All authors have read and approved the published version of the manuscript.

Funding: This paper was supported by grants from Accelerator Award – Cancer Research UK/AIRC – INCAR project (F.L.), Associazione Italiana Ricerca per la Ricerca sul Cancro (AIRC)-Special Project 5 × 1000 no. 9962 (F.L.), AIRC IG 2018 id. 21724 (F.L.), Ministero dell'Università e della Ricerca (Grant PRIN 2017 to F.L.); Italian Healthy Ministry project on CAR T RCR-2019-23669115 (Coordinator F.L.).

Institutional Review Board Statement: Not Applicable.

Informed Consent Statement: Not Applicable.

Data Availability Statement: Not Applicable.

Conflicts of Interest: F.L. reports advisory board membership for Amgen, Novartis, Bellicum Pharmaceutical, Neovii, and is on the Speakers' Bureau for Amgen, Novartis, Miltenyi, Medac, Jazz Pharmaceutical, Gilead, Sanofi and Takeda, outside the submitted work.

References

1. Hunger, S.P.; Lu, X.; Devidas, M.; Camitta, B.M.; Gaynon, P.S.; Winick, N.J.; Reaman, G.H.; Carroll, W.L. Improved survival for children and adolescents with acute lymphoblastic leukemia between 1990 and 2005: A report from the children's oncology group. *J. Clin. Oncol.* **2012**, *30*, 1663–1669. [CrossRef] [PubMed]
2. Bunin, N.J.; Davies, S.M.; Aplenc, R.; Camitta, B.M.; DeSantes, K.B.; Goyal, R.K.; Kapoor, N.; Kernan, N.A.; Rosenthal, J.; Smith, F.O.; et al. Unrelated donor bone marrow transplantation for children with acute myeloid leukemia beyond first remission or refractory to chemotherapy. *J. Clin. Oncol.* **2008**, *26*, 4326–4332. [CrossRef] [PubMed]
3. Pession, A.; Masetti, R.; Rizzari, C.; Putti, M.C.; Casale, F.; Fagioli, F.; Luciani, M.; Lo Nigro, L.; Menna, G.; Micalizzi, C.; et al. Results of the AIEOP AML 2002/01 multicenter prospective trial for the treatment of children with acute myeloid leukemia. *Blood* **2013**, *122*, 170–178. [CrossRef]
4. Rasche, M.; Zimmermann, M.; Borschel, L.; Bourquin, J.P.; Dworzak, M.; Klingebiel, T.; Lehrnbecher, T.; Creutzig, U.; Klusmann, J.H.; Reinhardt, D. Successes and challenges in the treatment of pediatric acute myeloid leukemia: A retrospective analysis of the AML-BFM trials from 1987 to 2012. *Leukemia* **2018**, *32*, 2167–2177. [CrossRef] [PubMed]
5. Rubnitz, J.E.; Inaba, H.; Dahl, G.; Ribeiro, R.C.; Bowman, W.P.; Taub, J.; Pounds, S.; Razzouk, B.I.; Lacayo, N.J.; Cao, X.; et al. Minimal residual disease-directed therapy for childhood acute myeloid leukaemia: Results of the AML02 multicentre trial. *Lancet Oncol.* **2010**, *11*, 543–552. [CrossRef]
6. Bertaina, A.; Zecca, M.; Buldini, B.; Sacchi, N.; Algeri, M.; Saglio, F.; Perotti, C.; Gallina, A.M.; Bertaina, V.; Lanino, E.; et al. Unrelated donor vs HLA-haploidentical alpha/beta T-cell- and B-cell-depleted HSCT in children with acute leukemia. *Blood* **2018**, *132*, 2594–2607. [CrossRef]
7. Iacobucci, I.; Mullighan, C.G. Genetic Basis of Acute Lymphoblastic Leukemia. *J. Clin. Oncol.* **2017**, *35*, 975–983. [CrossRef]
8. Iacobucci, I.; Wen, J.; Meggendorfer, M.; Choi, J.K.; Shi, L.; Pounds, S.B.; Carmichael, C.L.; Masih, K.E.; Morris, S.M.; Lindsley, R.C.; et al. Genomic subtyping and therapeutic targeting of acute erythroleukemia. *Nat. Genet.* **2019**, *51*, 694–704. [CrossRef]
9. Bader, P.; Salzmann-Manrique, E.; Balduzzi, A.; Dalle, J.H.; Woolfrey, A.E.; Bar, M.; Verneris, M.R.; Borowitz, M.J.; Shah, N.N.; Gossai, N.; et al. More precisely defining risk peri-HCT in pediatric ALL: Pre- vs. post-MRD measures, serial positivity, and risk modeling. *Blood Adv.* **2019**, *3*, 3393–3405. [CrossRef]
10. Walter, R.B.; Gooley, T.A.; Wood, B.L.; Milano, F.; Fang, M.; Sorror, M.L.; Estey, E.H.; Salter, A.I.; Lansverk, E.; Chien, J.W.; et al. Impact of pretransplantation minimal residual disease, as detected by multiparametric flow cytometry, on outcome of myeloablative hematopoietic cell transplantation for acute myeloid leukemia. *J. Clin. Oncol.* **2011**, *29*, 1190–1197. [CrossRef]
11. Maude, S.L.; Laetsch, T.W.; Buechner, J.; Rives, S.; Boyer, M.; Bittencourt, H.; Bader, P.; Verneris, M.R.; Stefanski, H.E.; Myers, G.D.; et al. Tisagenlecleucel in Children and Young Adults with B-Cell Lymphoblastic Leukemia. *N. Engl. J. Med.* **2018**, *378*, 439–448. [CrossRef]
12. Locatelli, F.; Schrappe, M.; Bernardo, M.E.; Rutella, S. How I treat relapsed childhood acute lymphoblastic leukemia. *Blood* **2012**, *120*, 2807–2816. [CrossRef]
13. Diorio, C.; Maude, S.L. CAR T cells vs. allogeneic HSCT for poor-risk ALL. *Hematol. Am. Soc. Hematol. Educ. Program.* **2020**, *2020*, 501–507. [CrossRef]
14. Borowitz, M.J.; Devidas, M.; Hunger, S.P.; Bowman, W.P.; Carroll, A.J.; Carroll, W.L.; Linda, S.; Martin, P.L.; Pullen, D.J.; Viswanatha, D.; et al. Clinical significance of minimal residual disease in childhood acute lymphoblastic leukemia and its relationship to other prognostic factors: A Children's Oncology Group study. *Blood* **2008**, *111*, 5477–5485. [CrossRef]
15. van Dongen, J.J.; van der Velden, V.H.; Bruggemann, M.; Orfao, A. Minimal residual disease diagnostics in acute lymphoblastic leukemia: Need for sensitive, fast, and standardized technologies. *Blood* **2015**, *125*, 3996–4009. [CrossRef]
16. Conter, V.; Bartram, C.R.; Valsecchi, M.G.; Schrauder, A.; Panzer-Grumayer, R.; Moricke, A.; Arico, M.; Zimmermann, M.; Mann, G.; De Rossi, G.; et al. Molecular response to treatment redefines all prognostic factors in children and adolescents with B-cell precursor acute lymphoblastic leukemia: Results in 3184 patients of the AIEOP-BFM ALL 2000 study. *Blood* **2010**, *115*, 3206–3214. [CrossRef] [PubMed]
17. Schrappe, M.; Hunger, S.P.; Pui, C.H.; Saha, V.; Gaynon, P.S.; Baruchel, A.; Conter, V.; Otten, J.; Ohara, A.; Versluys, A.B.; et al. Outcomes after induction failure in childhood acute lymphoblastic leukemia. *N. Engl. J. Med.* **2012**, *366*, 1371–1381. [CrossRef] [PubMed]
18. Nachman, J.B.; Heerema, N.A.; Sather, H.; Camitta, B.; Forestier, E.; Harrison, C.J.; Dastugue, N.; Schrappe, M.; Pui, C.H.; Basso, G.; et al. Outcome of treatment in children with hypodiploid acute lymphoblastic leukemia. *Blood* **2007**, *110*, 1112–1115. [CrossRef]
19. McNeer, J.L.; Devidas, M.; Dai, Y.; Carroll, A.J.; Heerema, N.A.; Gastier-Foster, J.M.; Kahwash, S.B.; Borowitz, M.J.; Wood, B.L.; Larsen, E.; et al. Hematopoietic Stem-Cell Transplantation Does Not Improve the Poor Outcome of Children with Hypodiploid Acute Lymphoblastic Leukemia: A Report From Children's Oncology Group. *J. Clin. Oncol.* **2019**, *37*, 780–789. [CrossRef]
20. Pui, C.H.; Rebora, P.; Schrappe, M.; Attarbaschi, A.; Baruchel, A.; Basso, G.; Cave, H.; Elitzur, S.; Koh, K.; Liu, H.C.; et al. Outcome of Children with Hypodiploid Acute Lymphoblastic Leukemia: A Retrospective Multinational Study. *J. Clin. Oncol.* **2019**, *37*, 770–779. [CrossRef] [PubMed]
21. Fischer, U.; Forster, M.; Rinaldi, A.; Risch, T.; Sungalee, S.; Warnatz, H.J.; Bornhauser, B.; Gombert, M.; Kratsch, C.; Stutz, A.M.; et al. Genomics and drug profiling of fatal TCF3-HLF-positive acute lymphoblastic leukemia identifies recurrent mutation patterns and therapeutic options. *Nat. Genet.* **2015**, *47*, 1020–1029. [CrossRef] [PubMed]

22. Mouttet, B.; Vinti, L.; Ancliff, P.; Bodmer, N.; Brethon, B.; Cario, G.; Chen-Santel, C.; Elitzur, S.; Hazar, V.; Kunz, J.; et al. Durable remissions in TCF3-HLF positive acute lymphoblastic leukemia with blinatumomab and stem cell transplantation. *Haematologica* **2019**, *104*, e244–e247. [CrossRef] [PubMed]
23. Mullighan, C.G.; Su, X.; Zhang, J.; Radtke, I.; Phillips, L.A.; Miller, C.B.; Ma, J.; Liu, W.; Cheng, C.; Schulman, B.A.; et al. Deletion of IKZF1 and prognosis in acute lymphoblastic leukemia. *N. Engl. J. Med.* **2009**, *360*, 470–480. [CrossRef] [PubMed]
24. Stanulla, M.; Dagdan, E.; Zaliova, M.; Moricke, A.; Palmi, C.; Cazzaniga, G.; Eckert, C.; Te Kronnie, G.; Bourquin, J.P.; Bornhauser, B.; et al. IKZF1(plus) Defines a New Minimal Residual Disease-Dependent Very-Poor Prognostic Profile in Pediatric B-Cell Precursor Acute Lymphoblastic Leukemia. *J. Clin. Oncol.* **2018**, *36*, 1240–1249. [CrossRef] [PubMed]
25. Biondi, A.; Cimino, G.; Pieters, R.; Pui, C.H. Biological and therapeutic aspects of infant leukemia. *Blood* **2000**, *96*, 24–33. [CrossRef]
26. Pieters, R.; Schrappe, M.; De Lorenzo, P.; Hann, I.; De Rossi, G.; Felice, M.; Hovi, L.; LeBlanc, T.; Szczepanski, T.; Ferster, A.; et al. A treatment protocol for infants younger than 1 year with acute lymphoblastic leukaemia (Interfant-99): An observational study and a multicentre randomised trial. *Lancet* **2007**, *370*, 240–250. [CrossRef]
27. Mann, G.; Attarbaschi, A.; Schrappe, M.; De Lorenzo, P.; Peters, C.; Hann, I.; De Rossi, G.; Felice, M.; Lausen, B.; Leblanc, T.; et al. Improved outcome with hematopoietic stem cell transplantation in a poor prognostic subgroup of infants with mixed-lineage-leukemia (MLL)-rearranged acute lymphoblastic leukemia: Results from the Interfant-99 Study. *Blood* **2010**, *116*, 2644–2650. [CrossRef]
28. Heerema, N.A.; Carroll, A.J.; Devidas, M.; Loh, M.L.; Borowitz, M.J.; Gastier-Foster, J.M.; Larsen, E.C.; Mattano, L.A., Jr.; Maloney, K.W.; Willman, C.L.; et al. Intrachromosomal amplification of chromosome 21 is associated with inferior outcomes in children with acute lymphoblastic leukemia treated in contemporary standard-risk children's oncology group studies: A report from the children's oncology group. *J. Clin. Oncol.* **2013**, *31*, 3397–3402. [CrossRef]
29. Moorman, A.V.; Robinson, H.; Schwab, C.; Richards, S.M.; Hancock, J.; Mitchell, C.D.; Goulden, N.; Vora, A.; Harrison, C.J. Risk-directed treatment intensification significantly reduces the risk of relapse among children and adolescents with acute lymphoblastic leukemia and intrachromosomal amplification of chromosome 21: A comparison of the MRC ALL97/99 and UKALL2003 trials. *J. Clin. Oncol.* **2013**, *31*, 3389–3396. [CrossRef]
30. Bailey, L.C.; Lange, B.J.; Rheingold, S.R.; Bunin, N.J. Bone-marrow relapse in paediatric acute lymphoblastic leukaemia. *Lancet Oncol.* **2008**, *9*, 873–883. [CrossRef]
31. Einsiedel, H.G.; von Stackelberg, A.; Hartmann, R.; Fengler, R.; Schrappe, M.; Janka-Schaub, G.; Mann, G.; Hahlen, K.; Gobel, U.; Klingebiel, T.; et al. Long-term outcome in children with relapsed ALL by risk-stratified salvage therapy: Results of trial acute lymphoblastic leukemia-relapse study of the Berlin-Frankfurt-Munster Group 87. *J. Clin. Oncol.* **2005**, *23*, 7942–7950. [CrossRef]
32. Lawson, S.E.; Harrison, G.; Richards, S.; Oakhill, A.; Stevens, R.; Eden, O.B.; Darbyshire, P.J. The UK experience in treating relapsed childhood acute lymphoblastic leukaemia: A report on the medical research council UKALLR1 study. *Br. J. Haematol.* **2000**, *108*, 531–543. [CrossRef]
33. Borgmann, A.; von Stackelberg, A.; Hartmann, R.; Ebell, W.; Klingebiel, T.; Peters, C.; Henze, G.; Berlin-Frankfurt-Munster Relapse Study, G. Unrelated donor stem cell transplantation compared with chemotherapy for children with acute lymphoblastic leukemia in a second remission: A matched-pair analysis. *Blood* **2003**, *101*, 3835–3839. [CrossRef]
34. Parker, C.; Waters, R.; Leighton, C.; Hancock, J.; Sutton, R.; Moorman, A.V.; Ancliff, P.; Morgan, M.; Masurekar, A.; Goulden, N.; et al. Effect of mitoxantrone on outcome of children with first relapse of acute lymphoblastic leukaemia (ALL R3): An open-label randomised trial. *Lancet* **2010**, *376*, 2009–2017. [CrossRef]
35. Eckert, C.; Biondi, A.; Seeger, K.; Cazzaniga, G.; Hartmann, R.; Beyermann, B.; Pogodda, M.; Proba, J.; Henze, G. Prognostic value of minimal residual disease in relapsed childhood acute lymphoblastic leukaemia. *Lancet* **2001**, *358*, 1239–1241. [CrossRef]
36. Coustan-Smith, E.; Gajjar, A.; Hijiya, N.; Razzouk, B.I.; Ribeiro, R.C.; Rivera, G.K.; Rubnitz, J.E.; Sandlund, J.T.; Andreansky, M.; Hancock, M.L.; et al. Clinical significance of minimal residual disease in childhood acute lymphoblastic leukemia after first relapse. *Leukemia* **2004**, *18*, 499–504. [CrossRef]
37. Creutzig, U.; Reinhardt, D. Current controversies: Which patients with acute myeloid leukaemia should receive a bone marrow transplantation? A European view. *Br. J. Haematol.* **2002**, *118*, 365–377. [CrossRef] [PubMed]
38. Chen, A.R.; Alonzo, T.A.; Woods, W.G.; Arceci, R.J. Current controversies: Which patients with acute myeloid leukaemia should receive a bone marrow transplantation? An American view. *Br. J. Haematol.* **2002**, *118*, 378–384. [CrossRef]
39. Hasle, H. A critical review of which children with acute myeloid leukaemia need stem cell procedures. *Br. J. Haematol.* **2014**, *166*, 23–33. [CrossRef]
40. Woods, W.G.; Neudorf, S.; Gold, S.; Sanders, J.; Buckley, J.D.; Barnard, D.R.; Dusenbery, K.; DeSwarte, J.; Arthur, D.C.; Lange, B.J.; et al. A comparison of allogeneic bone marrow transplantation, autologous bone marrow transplantation, and aggressive chemotherapy in children with acute myeloid leukemia in remission. *Blood* **2001**, *97*, 56–62. [CrossRef]
41. Lie, S.O.; Abrahamsson, J.; Clausen, N.; Forestier, E.; Hasle, H.; Hovi, L.; Jonmundsson, G.; Mellander, L.; Gustafsson, G. Treatment stratification based on initial in vivo response in acute myeloid leukaemia in children without Down's syndrome: Results of NOPHO-AML trials. *Br. J. Haematol.* **2003**, *122*, 217–225. [CrossRef]
42. Noort, S.; Zimmermann, M.; Reinhardt, D.; Cuccuini, W.; Pigazzi, M.; Smith, J.; Ries, R.E.; Alonzo, T.A.; Hirsch, B.; Tomizawa, D.; et al. Prognostic impact of t(16;21)(p11;q22) and t(16;21)(q24;q22) in pediatric AML: A retrospective study by the I-BFM Study Group. *Blood* **2018**, *132*, 1584–1592. [CrossRef]

43. Pigazzi, M.; Manara, E.; Buldini, B.; Beqiri, V.; Bisio, V.; Tregnago, C.; Rondelli, R.; Masetti, R.; Putti, M.C.; Fagioli, F.; et al. Minimal residual disease monitored after induction therapy by RQ-PCR can contribute to tailor treatment of patients with t(8;21) RUNX1-RUNX1T1 rearrangement. *Haematologica* **2015**, *100*, e99–e101. [CrossRef]
44. Ho, P.A.; Alonzo, T.A.; Gerbing, R.B.; Pollard, J.; Stirewalt, D.L.; Hurwitz, C.; Heerema, N.A.; Hirsch, B.; Raimondi, S.C.; Lange, B.; et al. Prevalence and prognostic implications of CEBPA mutations in pediatric acute myeloid leukemia (AML): A report from the Children's Oncology Group. *Blood* **2009**, *113*, 6558–6566. [CrossRef]
45. Hollink, I.H.; Zwaan, C.M.; Zimmermann, M.; Arentsen-Peters, T.C.; Pieters, R.; Cloos, J.; Kaspers, G.J.; de Graaf, S.S.; Harbott, J.; Creutzig, U.; et al. Favorable prognostic impact of NPM1 gene mutations in childhood acute myeloid leukemia, with emphasis on cytogenetically normal AML. *Leukemia* **2009**, *23*, 262–270. [CrossRef]
46. Testi, A.M.; Pession, A.; Diverio, D.; Grimwade, D.; Gibson, B.; de Azevedo, A.C.; Moran, L.; Leverger, G.; Elitzur, S.; Hasle, H.; et al. Risk-adapted treatment of acute promyelocytic leukemia: Results from the International Consortium for Childhood APL. *Blood* **2018**, *132*, 405–412. [CrossRef] [PubMed]
47. Grimwade, D.; Walker, H.; Oliver, F.; Wheatley, K.; Harrison, C.; Harrison, G.; Rees, J.; Hann, I.; Stevens, R.; Burnett, A.; et al. The importance of diagnostic cytogenetics on outcome in AML: Analysis of 1612 patients entered into the MRC AML 10 trial. The Medical Research Council Adult and Children's Leukaemia Working Parties. *Blood* **1998**, *92*, 2322–2333. [CrossRef]
48. Harrison, C.J.; Hills, R.K.; Moorman, A.V.; Grimwade, D.J.; Hann, I.; Webb, D.K.; Wheatley, K.; de Graaf, S.S.; van den Berg, E.; Burnett, A.K.; et al. Cytogenetics of childhood acute myeloid leukemia: United Kingdom Medical Research Council Treatment trials AML 10 and 12. *J. Clin. Oncol.* **2010**, *28*, 2674–2681. [CrossRef] [PubMed]
49. Johnston, D.L.; Alonzo, T.A.; Gerbing, R.B.; Hirsch, B.; Heerema, N.A.; Ravindranath, Y.; Woods, W.G.; Lange, B.J.; Gamis, A.S.; Raimondi, S.C. Outcome of pediatric patients with acute myeloid leukemia (AML) and -5/5q- abnormalities from five pediatric AML treatment protocols: A report from the Children's Oncology Group. *Pediatr. Blood Cancer* **2013**, *60*, 2073–2078. [CrossRef]
50. von Neuhoff, C.; Reinhardt, D.; Sander, A.; Zimmermann, M.; Bradtke, J.; Betts, D.R.; Zemanova, Z.; Stary, J.; Bourquin, J.P.; Haas, O.A.; et al. Prognostic impact of specific chromosomal aberrations in a large group of pediatric patients with acute myeloid leukemia treated uniformly according to trial AML-BFM 98. *J. Clin. Oncol.* **2010**, *28*, 2682–2689. [CrossRef]
51. Hasle, H.; Alonzo, T.A.; Auvrignon, A.; Behar, C.; Chang, M.; Creutzig, U.; Fischer, A.; Forestier, E.; Fynn, A.; Haas, O.A.; et al. Monosomy 7 and deletion 7q in children and adolescents with acute myeloid leukemia: An international retrospective study. *Blood* **2007**, *109*, 4641–4647. [CrossRef]
52. Rasche, M.; von Neuhoff, C.; Dworzak, M.; Bourquin, J.P.; Bradtke, J.; Gohring, G.; Escherich, G.; Fleischhack, G.; Graf, N.; Gruhn, B.; et al. Genotype-outcome correlations in pediatric AML: The impact of a monosomal karyotype in trial AML-BFM 2004. *Leukemia* **2017**, *31*, 2807–2814. [CrossRef]
53. Sandahl, J.D.; Coenen, E.A.; Forestier, E.; Harbott, J.; Johansson, B.; Kerndrup, G.; Adachi, S.; Auvrignon, A.; Beverloo, H.B.; Cayuela, J.M.; et al. t(6;9)(p22;q34)/DEK-NUP214-rearranged pediatric myeloid leukemia: An international study of 62 patients. *Haematologica* **2014**, *99*, 865–872. [CrossRef] [PubMed]
54. Tarlock, K.; Alonzo, T.A.; Moraleda, P.P.; Gerbing, R.B.; Raimondi, S.C.; Hirsch, B.A.; Ravindranath, Y.; Lange, B.; Woods, W.G.; Gamis, A.S.; et al. Acute myeloid leukaemia (AML) with t(6;9)(p23;q34) is associated with poor outcome in childhood AML regardless of FLT3-ITD status: A report from the Children's Oncology Group. *Br. J. Haematol.* **2014**, *166*, 254–259. [CrossRef] [PubMed]
55. Meshinchi, S.; Alonzo, T.A.; Stirewalt, D.L.; Zwaan, M.; Zimmerman, M.; Reinhardt, D.; Kaspers, G.J.; Heerema, N.A.; Gerbing, R.; Lange, B.J.; et al. Clinical implications of FLT3 mutations in pediatric AML. *Blood* **2006**, *108*, 3654–3661. [CrossRef] [PubMed]
56. Zwaan, C.M.; Meshinchi, S.; Radich, J.P.; Veerman, A.J.; Huismans, D.R.; Munske, L.; Podleschny, M.; Hahlen, K.; Pieters, R.; Zimmermann, M.; et al. FLT3 internal tandem duplication in 234 children with acute myeloid leukemia: Prognostic significance and relation to cellular drug resistance. *Blood* **2003**, *102*, 2387–2394. [CrossRef]
57. Brunet, S.; Labopin, M.; Esteve, J.; Cornelissen, J.; Socie, G.; Iori, A.P.; Verdonck, L.F.; Volin, L.; Gratwohl, A.; Sierra, J.; et al. Impact of FLT3 internal tandem duplication on the outcome of related and unrelated hematopoietic transplantation for adult acute myeloid leukemia in first remission: A retrospective analysis. *J. Clin. Oncol.* **2012**, *30*, 735–741. [CrossRef]
58. Pratcorona, M.; Brunet, S.; Nomdedeu, J.; Ribera, J.M.; Tormo, M.; Duarte, R.; Escoda, L.; Guardia, R.; Queipo de Llano, M.P.; Salamero, O.; et al. Favorable outcome of patients with acute myeloid leukemia harboring a low-allelic burden FLT3-ITD mutation and concomitant NPM1 mutation: Relevance to post-remission therapy. *Blood* **2013**, *121*, 2734–2738. [CrossRef]
59. DeZern, A.E.; Sung, A.; Kim, S.; Smith, B.D.; Karp, J.E.; Gore, S.D.; Jones, R.J.; Fuchs, E.; Luznik, L.; McDevitt, M.; et al. Role of allogeneic transplantation for FLT3/ITD acute myeloid leukemia: Outcomes from 133 consecutive newly diagnosed patients from a single institution. *Biol Blood Marrow Transpl.* **2011**, *17*, 1404–1409. [CrossRef]
60. Balgobind, B.V.; Raimondi, S.C.; Harbott, J.; Zimmermann, M.; Alonzo, T.A.; Auvrignon, A.; Beverloo, H.B.; Chang, M.; Creutzig, U.; Dworzak, M.N.; et al. Novel prognostic subgroups in childhood 11q23/MLL-rearranged acute myeloid leukemia: Results of an international retrospective study. *Blood* **2009**, *114*, 2489–2496. [CrossRef]
61. Locatelli, F.; Masetti, R.; Rondelli, R.; Zecca, M.; Fagioli, F.; Rovelli, A.; Messina, C.; Lanino, E.; Bertaina, A.; Favre, C.; et al. Outcome of children with high-risk acute myeloid leukemia given autologous or allogeneic hematopoietic cell transplantation in the aieop AML-2002/01 study. *Bone Marrow Transpl.* **2015**, *50*, 181–188. [CrossRef]

62. Sauer, M.G.; Lang, P.J.; Albert, M.H.; Bader, P.; Creutzig, U.; Eyrich, M.; Greil, J.; Gruhn, B.; Holter, W.; Klingebiel, T.; et al. Hematopoietic stem cell transplantation for children with acute myeloid leukemia-results of the AML SCT-BFM 2007 trial. *Leukemia* **2020**, *34*, 613–624. [CrossRef]
63. Struski, S.; Lagarde, S.; Bories, P.; Puiseux, C.; Prade, N.; Cuccuini, W.; Pages, M.P.; Bidet, A.; Gervais, C.; Lafage-Pochitaloff, M.; et al. NUP98 is rearranged in 3.8% of pediatric AML forming a clinical and molecular homogenous group with a poor prognosis. *Leukemia* **2017**, *31*, 565–572. [CrossRef]
64. Bisio, V.; Zampini, M.; Tregnago, C.; Manara, E.; Salsi, V.; Di Meglio, A.; Masetti, R.; Togni, M.; Di Giacomo, D.; Minuzzo, S.; et al. NUP98-fusion transcripts characterize different biological entities within acute myeloid leukemia: A report from the AIEOP-AML group. *Leukemia* **2017**, *31*, 974–977. [CrossRef]
65. de Rooij, J.D.; Branstetter, C.; Ma, J.; Li, Y.; Walsh, M.P.; Cheng, J.; Obulkasim, A.; Dang, J.; Easton, J.; Verboon, L.J.; et al. Pediatric non-Down syndrome acute megakaryoblastic leukemia is characterized by distinct genomic subsets with varying outcomes. *Nat. Genet.* **2017**, *49*, 451–456. [CrossRef]
66. Masetti, R.; Pigazzi, M.; Togni, M.; Astolfi, A.; Indio, V.; Manara, E.; Casadio, R.; Pession, A.; Basso, G.; Locatelli, F. CBFA2T3-GLIS2 fusion transcript is a novel common feature in pediatric, cytogenetically normal AML, not restricted to FAB M7 subtype. *Blood* **2013**, *121*, 3469–3472. [CrossRef]
67. Gruber, T.A.; Larson Gedman, A.; Zhang, J.; Koss, C.S.; Marada, S.; Ta, H.Q.; Chen, S.C.; Su, X.; Ogden, S.K.; Dang, J.; et al. An Inv(16)(p13.3q24.3)-encoded CBFA2T3-GLIS2 fusion protein defines an aggressive subtype of pediatric acute megakaryoblastic leukemia. *Cancer Cell* **2012**, *22*, 683–697. [CrossRef]
68. von Bergh, A.R.; van Drunen, E.; van Wering, E.R.; van Zutven, L.J.; Hainmann, I.; Lonnerholm, G.; Meijerink, J.P.; Pieters, R.; Beverloo, H.B. High incidence of t(7;12)(q36;p13) in infant AML but not in infant ALL, with a dismal outcome and ectopic expression of HLXB9. *Genes Chromosomes Cancer* **2006**, *45*, 731–739. [CrossRef]
69. Shiba, N.; Ichikawa, H.; Taki, T.; Park, M.J.; Jo, A.; Mitani, S.; Kobayashi, T.; Shimada, A.; Sotomatsu, M.; Arakawa, H.; et al. NUP98-NSD1 gene fusion and its related gene expression signature are strongly associated with a poor prognosis in pediatric acute myeloid leukemia. *Genes Chromosomes Cancer* **2013**, *52*, 683–693. [CrossRef]
70. Noort, S.; Wander, P.; Alonzo, T.A.; Smith, J.; Ries, R.E.; Gerbing, R.B.; Dolman, M.E.M.; Locatelli, F.; Reinhardt, D.; Baruchel, A.; et al. The clinical and biological characteristics of NUP98-KDM5A in pediatric acute myeloid leukemia. *Haematologica* **2021**, *106*, 630–634. [CrossRef]
71. Coenen, E.A.; Zwaan, C.M.; Reinhardt, D.; Harrison, C.J.; Haas, O.A.; de Haas, V.; Mihal, V.; De Moerloose, B.; Jeison, M.; Rubnitz, J.E.; et al. Pediatric acute myeloid leukemia with t(8;16)(p11;p13), a distinct clinical and biological entity: A collaborative study by the International-Berlin-Frankfurt-Munster AML-study group. *Blood* **2013**, *122*, 2704–2713. [CrossRef] [PubMed]
72. Tierens, A.; Bjorklund, E.; Siitonen, S.; Marquart, H.V.; Wulff-Juergensen, G.; Pelliniemi, T.T.; Forestier, E.; Hasle, H.; Jahnukainen, K.; Lausen, B.; et al. Residual disease detected by flow cytometry is an independent predictor of survival in childhood acute myeloid leukaemia; Results of the NOPHO-AML 2004 study. *Br. J. Haematol.* **2016**, *174*, 600–609. [CrossRef]
73. Buldini, B.; Rizzati, F.; Masetti, R.; Fagioli, F.; Menna, G.; Micalizzi, C.; Putti, M.C.; Rizzari, C.; Santoro, N.; Zecca, M.; et al. Prognostic significance of flow-cytometry evaluation of minimal residual disease in children with acute myeloid leukaemia treated according to the AIEOP-AML 2002/01 study protocol. *Br. J. Haematol.* **2017**, *177*, 116–126. [CrossRef]
74. Loken, M.R.; Alonzo, T.A.; Pardo, L.; Gerbing, R.B.; Raimondi, S.C.; Hirsch, B.A.; Ho, P.A.; Franklin, J.; Cooper, T.M.; Gamis, A.S.; et al. Residual disease detected by multidimensional flow cytometry signifies high relapse risk in patients with de novo acute myeloid leukemia: A report from Children's Oncology Group. *Blood* **2012**, *120*, 1581–1588. [CrossRef]
75. Inaba, H.; Coustan-Smith, E.; Cao, X.; Pounds, S.B.; Shurtleff, S.A.; Wang, K.Y.; Raimondi, S.C.; Onciu, M.; Jacobsen, J.; Ribeiro, R.C.; et al. Comparative analysis of different approaches to measure treatment response in acute myeloid leukemia. *J. Clin. Oncol.* **2012**, *30*, 3625–3632. [CrossRef]
76. Hoffman, A.E.; Schoonmade, L.J.; Kaspers, G.J. Pediatric relapsed acute myeloid leukemia: A systematic review. *Expert Rev. Anticancer Ther.* **2021**, *21*, 45–52. [CrossRef]
77. Meshinchi, S.; Leisenring, W.M.; Carpenter, P.A.; Woolfrey, A.E.; Sievers, E.L.; Radich, J.P.; Sanders, J.E. Survival after second hematopoietic stem cell transplantation for recurrent pediatric acute myeloid leukemia. *Biol. Blood Marrow Transpl.* **2003**, *9*, 706–713. [CrossRef]
78. Naik, S.; Martinez, C.; Leung, K.; Sasa, G.; Nguyen, N.Y.; Wu, M.F.; Gottschalk, S.; Brenner, M.; Heslop, H.; Krance, R. Outcomes after Second Hematopoietic Stem Cell Transplantations in Pediatric Patients with Relapsed Hematological Malignancies. *Biol. Blood Marrow Transpl.* **2015**, *21*, 1266–1272. [CrossRef]
79. Taga, T.; Murakami, Y.; Tabuchi, K.; Adachi, S.; Tomizawa, D.; Kojima, Y.; Kato, K.; Koike, K.; Koh, K.; Kajiwara, R.; et al. Role of Second Transplantation for Children with Acute Myeloid Leukemia Following Posttransplantation Relapse. *Pediatr. Blood Cancer* **2016**, *63*, 701–705. [CrossRef]
80. Uden, T.; Bertaina, A.; Abrahamsson, J.; Ansari, M.; Balduzzi, A.; Bourquin, J.P.; Gerhardt, C.; Bierings, M.; Hasle, H.; Lankester, A.; et al. Outcome of children relapsing after first allogeneic haematopoietic stem cell transplantation for acute myeloid leukaemia: A retrospective I-BFM analysis of 333 children. *Br. J. Haematol.* **2020**, *189*, 745–750. [CrossRef] [PubMed]
81. Rubnitz, J.E.; Inaba, H. Childhood acute myeloid leukaemia. *Br. J. Haematol.* **2012**, *159*, 259–276. [CrossRef]

82. O'Hare, P.; Lucchini, G.; Cummins, M.; Veys, P.; Potter, M.; Lawson, S.; Vora, A.; Wynn, R.; Peniket, A.; Kirkland, K.; et al. Allogeneic stem cell transplantation for refractory acute myeloid leukemia in pediatric patients: The UK experience. *Bone Marrow Transpl.* **2017**, *52*, 825–831. [CrossRef]
83. Quarello, P.; Fagioli, F.; Basso, G.; Putti, M.C.; Berger, M.; Luciani, M.; Rizzari, C.; Menna, G.; Masetti, R.; Locatelli, F. Outcome of children with acute myeloid leukaemia (AML) experiencing primary induction failure in the AIEOP AML 2002/01 clinical trial. *Br. J. Haematol.* **2015**, *171*, 566–573. [CrossRef] [PubMed]
84. Willasch, A.M.; Peters, C.; Sedlacek, P.; Dalle, J.H.; Kitra-Roussou, V.; Yesilipek, A.; Wachowiak, J.; Lankester, A.; Prete, A.; Hamidieh, A.A.; et al. Myeloablative conditioning for allo-HSCT in pediatric ALL: FTBI or chemotherapy?-A multicenter EBMT-PDWP study. *Bone Marrow Transpl.* **2020**, *55*, 1540–1551. [CrossRef] [PubMed]
85. Brochstein, J.A.; Kernan, N.A.; Groshen, S.; Cirrincione, C.; Shank, B.; Emanuel, D.; Laver, J.; O'Reilly, R.J. Allogeneic bone marrow transplantation after hyperfractionated total-body irradiation and cyclophosphamide in children with acute leukemia. *N. Engl. J. Med.* **1987**, *317*, 1618–1624. [CrossRef]
86. Marks, D.I.; Forman, S.J.; Blume, K.G.; Perez, W.S.; Weisdorf, D.J.; Keating, A.; Gale, R.P.; Cairo, M.S.; Copelan, E.A.; Horan, J.T.; et al. A comparison of cyclophosphamide and total body irradiation with etoposide and total body irradiation as conditioning regimens for patients undergoing sibling allografting for acute lymphoblastic leukemia in first or second complete remission. *Biol. Blood Marrow Transpl.* **2006**, *12*, 438–453. [CrossRef]
87. Davies, S.M.; Ramsay, N.K.; Klein, J.P.; Weisdorf, D.J.; Bolwell, B.; Cahn, J.Y.; Camitta, B.M.; Gale, R.P.; Giralt, S.; Heilmann, C.; et al. Comparison of preparative regimens in transplants for children with acute lymphoblastic leukemia. *J. Clin. Oncol.* **2000**, *18*, 340–347. [CrossRef]
88. Tutschka, P.J.; Copelan, E.A.; Klein, J.P. Bone marrow transplantation for leukemia following a new busulfan and cyclophosphamide regimen. *Blood* **1987**, *70*, 1382–1388. [CrossRef]
89. Tracey, J.; Zhang, M.J.; Thiel, E.; Sobocinski, K.A.; Eapen, M. Transplantation conditioning regimens and outcomes after allogeneic hematopoietic cell transplantation in children and adolescents with acute lymphoblastic leukemia. *Biol. Blood Marrow Transpl.* **2013**, *19*, 255–259. [CrossRef]
90. Bunin, N.; Aplenc, R.; Kamani, N.; Shaw, K.; Cnaan, A.; Simms, S. Randomized trial of busulfan vs. total body irradiation containing conditioning regimens for children with acute lymphoblastic leukemia: A Pediatric Blood and Marrow Transplant Consortium study. *Bone Marrow Transpl.* **2003**, *32*, 543–548. [CrossRef] [PubMed]
91. Zecca, M.; Pession, A.; Messina, C.; Bonetti, F.; Favre, C.; Prete, A.; Cesaro, S.; Porta, F.; Mazzarino, I.; Giorgiani, G.; et al. Total body irradiation, thiotepa, and cyclophosphamide as a conditioning regimen for children with acute lymphoblastic leukemia in first or second remission undergoing bone marrow transplantation with HLA-identical siblings. *J. Clin. Oncol.* **1999**, *17*, 1838–1846. [CrossRef]
92. Peters, C.; Schrappe, M.; von Stackelberg, A.; Schrauder, A.; Bader, P.; Ebell, W.; Lang, P.; Sykora, K.W.; Schrum, J.; Kremens, B.; et al. Stem-cell transplantation in children with acute lymphoblastic leukemia: A prospective international multicenter trial comparing sibling donors with matched unrelated donors-The ALL-SCT-BFM-2003 trial. *J. Clin. Oncol.* **2015**, *33*, 1265–1274. [CrossRef] [PubMed]
93. Kato, M.; Ishida, H.; Koh, K.; Inagaki, J.; Kato, K.; Goto, H.; Kaneko, T.; Cho, Y.; Hashii, Y.; Kurosawa, H.; et al. Comparison of chemotherapeutic agents as a myeloablative conditioning with total body irradiation for pediatric acute lymphoblastic leukemia: A study from the pediatric ALL working group of the Japan Society for Hematopoietic Cell Transplantation. *Pediatr. Blood Cancer* **2015**, *62*, 1844–1850. [CrossRef] [PubMed]
94. Saglio, F.; Zecca, M.; Pagliara, D.; Giorgiani, G.; Balduzzi, A.; Calore, E.; Favre, C.; Faraci, M.; Prete, A.; Tambaro, F.P.; et al. Occurrence of long-term effects after hematopoietic stem cell transplantation in children affected by acute leukemia receiving either busulfan or total body irradiation: Results of an AIEOP (Associazione Italiana Ematologia Oncologia Pediatrica) retrospective study. *Bone Marrow Transpl.* **2020**, *55*, 1918–1927. [CrossRef]
95. Peters, C.; Dalle, J.H.; Locatelli, F.; Poetschger, U.; Sedlacek, P.; Buechner, J.; Shaw, P.J.; Staciuk, R.; Ifversen, M.; Pichler, H.; et al. Total Body Irradiation or Chemotherapy Conditioning in Childhood ALL: A Multinational, Randomized, Noninferiority Phase III Study. *J. Clin. Oncol.* **2021**, *39*, 295–307. [CrossRef] [PubMed]
96. Blaise, D.; Maraninchi, D.; Archimbaud, E.; Reiffers, J.; Devergie, A.; Jouet, J.P.; Milpied, N.; Attal, M.; Michallet, M.; Ifrah, N.; et al. Allogeneic bone marrow transplantation for acute myeloid leukemia in first remission: A randomized trial of a busulfan-Cytoxan versus Cytoxan-total body irradiation as preparative regimen: A report from the Group d'Etudes de la Greffe de Moelle Osseuse. *Blood* **1992**, *79*, 2578–2582. [CrossRef] [PubMed]
97. Gupta, T.; Kannan, S.; Dantkale, V.; Laskar, S. Cyclophosphamide plus total body irradiation compared with busulfan plus cyclophosphamide as a conditioning regimen prior to hematopoietic stem cell transplantation in patients with leukemia: A systematic review and meta-analysis. *Hematol. Oncol. Stem Cell Ther.* **2011**, *4*, 17–29. [CrossRef]
98. Ringden, O.; Ruutu, T.; Remberger, M.; Nikoskelainen, J.; Volin, L.; Vindelov, L.; Parkkali, T.; Lenhoff, S.; Sallerfors, B.; Ljungman, P.; et al. A randomized trial comparing busulfan with total body irradiation as conditioning in allogeneic marrow transplant recipients with leukemia: A report from the Nordic Bone Marrow Transplantation Group. *Blood* **1994**, *83*, 2723–2730. [CrossRef]

99. Ishida, H.; Kato, M.; Kudo, K.; Taga, T.; Tomizawa, D.; Miyamura, T.; Goto, H.; Inagaki, J.; Koh, K.; Terui, K.; et al. Comparison of Outcomes for Pediatric Patients with Acute Myeloid Leukemia in Remission and Undergoing Allogeneic Hematopoietic Cell Transplantation with Myeloablative Conditioning Regimens Based on Either Intravenous Busulfan or Total Body Irradiation: A Report from the Japanese Society for Hematopoietic Cell Transplantation. *Biol. Blood Marrow Transpl.* **2015**, *21*, 2141–2147. [CrossRef]
100. de Berranger, E.; Cousien, A.; Petit, A.; Peffault de Latour, R.; Galambrun, C.; Bertrand, Y.; Salmon, A.; Rialland, F.; Rohrlich, P.S.; Vannier, J.P.; et al. Impact on long-term OS of conditioning regimen in allogeneic BMT for children with AML in first CR: TBI + CY versus BU + CY: A report from the Societe Francaise de Greffe de Moelle et de Therapie Cellulaire. *Bone Marrow Transpl.* **2014**, *49*, 382–388. [CrossRef]
101. Dandoy, C.E.; Davies, S.M.; Woo Ahn, K.; He, Y.; Kolb, A.E.; Levine, J.; Bo-Subait, S.; Abdel-Azim, H.; Bhatt, N.; Chewing, J.; et al. Comparison of total body irradiation versus non-total body irradiation containing regimens for de novo acute myeloid leukemia in children. *Haematologica* **2021**, *106*, 1839–1845. [CrossRef] [PubMed]
102. Phillips, G.L.; Shepherd, J.D.; Barnett, M.J.; Lansdorp, P.M.; Klingemann, H.G.; Spinelli, J.J.; Nevill, T.J.; Chan, K.W.; Reece, D.E. Busulfan, cyclophosphamide, and melphalan conditioning for autologous bone marrow transplantation in hematologic malignancy. *J. Clin. Oncol.* **1991**, *9*, 1880–1888. [CrossRef] [PubMed]
103. Lucchini, G.; Labopin, M.; Beohou, E.; Dalissier, A.; Dalle, J.H.; Cornish, J.; Zecca, M.; Samarasinghe, S.; Gibson, B.; Locatelli, F.; et al. Impact of Conditioning Regimen on Outcomes for Children with Acute Myeloid Leukemia Undergoing Transplantation in First Complete Remission. An Analysis on Behalf of the Pediatric Disease Working Party of the European Group for Blood and Marrow Transplantation. *Biol. Blood Marrow Transpl.* **2017**, *23*, 467–474. [CrossRef]
104. Muramatsu, H.; Sakaguchi, H.; Taga, T.; Tabuchi, K.; Adachi, S.; Inoue, M.; Kitoh, T.; Suminoe, A.; Yabe, H.; Azuma, E.; et al. Reduced intensity conditioning in allogeneic stem cell transplantation for AML with Down syndrome. *Pediatr. Blood Cancer* **2014**, *61*, 925–927. [CrossRef]
105. Giardino, S.; de Latour, R.P.; Aljurf, M.; Eikema, D.J.; Bosman, P.; Bertrand, Y.; Tbakhi, A.; Holter, W.; Bornhauser, M.; Rossig, C.; et al. Outcome of patients with Fanconi anemia developing myelodysplasia and acute leukemia who received allogeneic hematopoietic stem cell transplantation: A retrospective analysis on behalf of EBMT group. *Am. J. Hematol.* **2020**, *95*, 809–816. [CrossRef]
106. Bitan, M.; He, W.; Zhang, M.J.; Abdel-Azim, H.; Ayas, M.F.; Bielorai, B.; Carpenter, P.A.; Cairo, M.S.; Diaz, M.A.; Horan, J.T.; et al. Transplantation for children with acute myeloid leukemia: A comparison of outcomes with reduced intensity and myeloablative regimens. *Blood* **2014**, *123*, 1615–1620. [CrossRef] [PubMed]
107. Strocchio, L.; Zecca, M.; Comoli, P.; Mina, T.; Giorgiani, G.; Giraldi, E.; Vinti, L.; Merli, P.; Regazzi, M.; Locatelli, F. Treosulfan-based conditioning regimen for allogeneic haematopoietic stem cell transplantation in children with sickle cell disease. *Br. J. Haematol.* **2015**, *169*, 726–736. [CrossRef]
108. Boztug, H.; Zecca, M.; Sykora, K.W.; Veys, P.; Lankester, A.; Slatter, M.; Skinner, R.; Wachowiak, J.; Potschger, U.; Glogova, E.; et al. Treosulfan-based conditioning regimens for allogeneic HSCT in children with acute lymphoblastic leukaemia. *Ann. Hematol.* **2015**, *94*, 297–306. [CrossRef]
109. Kalwak, K.; Mielcarek, M.; Patrick, K.; Styczynski, J.; Bader, P.; Corbacioglu, S.; Burkhardt, B.; Sykora, K.W.; Drabko, K.; Gozdzik, J.; et al. Treosulfan-fludarabine-thiotepa-based conditioning treatment before allogeneic hematopoietic stem cell transplantation for pediatric patients with hematological malignancies. *Bone Marrow Transpl.* **2020**, *55*, 1996–2007. [CrossRef]
110. Satwani, P.; Bhatia, M.; Garvin, J.H., Jr.; George, D.; Dela Cruz, F.; Le Gall, J.; Jin, Z.; Schwartz, J.; Duffy, D.; van de Ven, C.; et al. A Phase I study of gemtuzumab ozogamicin (GO) in combination with busulfan and cyclophosphamide (Bu/Cy) and allogeneic stem cell transplantation in children with poor-risk CD33+ AML: A new targeted immunochemotherapy myeloablative conditioning (MAC) regimen. *Biol. Blood Marrow Transpl.* **2012**, *18*, 324–329. [CrossRef]
111. Nemecek, E.R.; Hilger, R.A.; Adams, A.; Shaw, B.E.; Kiefer, D.; Le-Rademacher, J.; Levine, J.E.; Yanik, G.; Leung, W.; Talano, J.A.; et al. Treosulfan, Fludarabine, and Low-Dose Total Body Irradiation for Children and Young Adults with Acute Myeloid Leukemia or Myelodysplastic Syndrome Undergoing Allogeneic Hematopoietic Cell Transplantation: Prospective Phase II Trial of the Pediatric Blood and Marrow Transplant Consortium. *Biol. Blood Marrow Transpl.* **2018**, *24*, 1651–1656. [CrossRef]
112. Oshrine, B.; Adams, L.; Nguyen, A.T.H.; Amankwah, E.; Shyr, D.; Hale, G.; Petrovic, A. Comparison of melphalan- And busulfan-based myeloablative conditioning in children undergoing allogeneic transplantation for acute myeloid leukemia or myelodysplasia. *Pediatr. Transpl.* **2020**, *24*, e13672. [CrossRef] [PubMed]
113. Kato, K.; Yoshida, N.; Matsumoto, K.; Matsuyama, T. Fludarabine, cytarabine, granulocyte colony-stimulating factor and melphalan (FALG with L-PAM) as a reduced toxicity conditioning regimen in children with acute leukemia. *Pediatr. Blood Cancer* **2014**, *61*, 712–716. [CrossRef] [PubMed]
114. Kussman, A.; Shyr, D.; Hale, G.; Oshrine, B.; Petrovic, A. Allogeneic hematopoietic cell transplantation in chemotherapy-induced aplasia in children with high-risk acute myeloid leukemia or myelodysplasia. *Pediatr. Blood Cancer* **2019**, *66*, e27481. [CrossRef]
115. Versluys, A.B.; Boelens, J.J.; Pronk, C.; Lankester, A.; Bordon, V.; Buechner, J.; Ifversen, M.; Jackmann, N.; Sundin, M.; Vettenranta, K.; et al. Hematopoietic cell transplant in pediatric acute myeloid leukemia after similar upfront therapy; a comparison of conditioning regimens. *Bone Marrow Transpl.* **2021**, *56*, 1426–1432. [CrossRef]
116. Locatelli, F.; Merli, P.; Bertaina, A. Rabbit anti-human T-lymphocyte globulin and hematopoietic transplantation. *Oncotarget* **2017**, *8*, 96460–96461. [CrossRef]

117. Locatelli, F.; Bernardo, M.E.; Bertaina, A.; Rognoni, C.; Comoli, P.; Rovelli, A.; Pession, A.; Fagioli, F.; Favre, C.; Lanino, E.; et al. Efficacy of two different doses of rabbit anti-T-lymphocyte globulin to prevent graft-versus-host disease in children with haematological malignancies transplanted from an unrelated donor: A multicentre, randomised, open-label, phase 3 trial. *Lancet Oncol.* **2017**, *18*, 1126–1136. [CrossRef]
118. Schrappe, M.; Valsecchi, M.G.; Bartram, C.R.; Schrauder, A.; Panzer-Grumayer, R.; Moricke, A.; Parasole, R.; Zimmermann, M.; Dworzak, M.; Buldini, B.; et al. Late MRD response determines relapse risk overall and in subsets of childhood T-cell ALL: Results of the AIEOP-BFM-ALL 2000 study. *Blood* **2011**, *118*, 2077–2084. [CrossRef]
119. Vora, A.; Goulden, N.; Mitchell, C.; Hancock, J.; Hough, R.; Rowntree, C.; Moorman, A.V.; Wade, R. Augmented post-remission therapy for a minimal residual disease-defined high-risk subgroup of children and young people with clinical standard-risk and intermediate-risk acute lymphoblastic leukaemia (UKALL 2003): A randomised controlled trial. *Lancet Oncol.* **2014**, *15*, 809–818. [CrossRef]
120. San Miguel, J.F.; Vidriales, M.B.; Lopez-Berges, C.; Diaz-Mediavilla, J.; Gutierrez, N.; Canizo, C.; Ramos, F.; Calmuntia, M.J.; Perez, J.J.; Gonzalez, M.; et al. Early immunophenotypical evaluation of minimal residual disease in acute myeloid leukemia identifies different patient risk groups and may contribute to postinduction treatment stratification. *Blood* **2001**, *98*, 1746–1751. [CrossRef] [PubMed]
121. Knechtli, C.J.; Goulden, N.J.; Hancock, J.P.; Grandage, V.L.; Harris, E.L.; Garland, R.J.; Jones, C.G.; Rowbottom, A.W.; Hunt, L.P.; Green, A.F.; et al. Minimal residual disease status before allogeneic bone marrow transplantation is an important determinant of successful outcome for children and adolescents with acute lymphoblastic leukaemia. *Blood* **1998**, *92*, 4072–4079. [CrossRef] [PubMed]
122. Bader, P.; Kreyenberg, H.; Henze, G.H.; Eckert, C.; Reising, M.; Willasch, A.; Barth, A.; Borkhardt, A.; Peters, C.; Handgretinger, R.; et al. Prognostic value of minimal residual disease quantification before allogeneic stem-cell transplantation in relapsed childhood acute lymphoblastic leukemia: The ALL-REZ BFM Study Group. *J. Clin. Oncol.* **2009**, *27*, 377–384. [CrossRef] [PubMed]
123. Eckert, C.; Hagedorn, N.; Sramkova, L.; Mann, G.; Panzer-Grumayer, R.; Peters, C.; Bourquin, J.P.; Klingebiel, T.; Borkhardt, A.; Cario, G.; et al. Monitoring minimal residual disease in children with high-risk relapses of acute lymphoblastic leukemia: Prognostic relevance of early and late assessment. *Leukemia* **2015**, *29*, 1648–1655. [CrossRef] [PubMed]
124. Lovisa, F.; Zecca, M.; Rossi, B.; Campeggio, M.; Magrin, E.; Giarin, E.; Buldini, B.; Songia, S.; Cazzaniga, G.; Mina, T.; et al. Pre- and post-transplant minimal residual disease predicts relapse occurrence in children with acute lymphoblastic leukaemia. *Br. J. Haematol.* **2018**, *180*, 680–693. [CrossRef] [PubMed]
125. Pigazzi, M.; Benetton, M.; Walter, C.; Hansen, M.; Skou, A.-S.; Da Ros, A.; Marchetti, A.; Polato, K.; Belloni, M.; Tregnago, C.; et al. Impact of Minimal Residual Disease (MRD) Assessed before Transplantation on the Outcome of Children with Acute Myeloid Leukemia Given an Allograft: A Retrospective Study By the I-BFM Study Group. *Blood* **2020**, *136*, 38–39. [CrossRef]
126. Leung, W.; Pui, C.H.; Coustan-Smith, E.; Yang, J.; Pei, D.; Gan, K.; Srinivasan, A.; Hartford, C.; Triplett, B.M.; Dallas, M.; et al. Detectable minimal residual disease before hematopoietic cell transplantation is prognostic but does not preclude cure for children with very-high-risk leukemia. *Blood* **2012**, *120*, 468–472. [CrossRef]
127. Pulsipher, M.A.; Langholz, B.; Wall, D.A.; Schultz, K.R.; Bunin, N.; Carroll, W.L.; Raetz, E.; Gardner, S.; Gastier-Foster, J.M.; Howrie, D.; et al. The addition of sirolimus to tacrolimus/methotrexate GVHD prophylaxis in children with ALL: A phase 3 Children's Oncology Group/Pediatric Blood and Marrow Transplant Consortium trial. *Blood* **2014**, *123*, 2017–2025. [CrossRef]
128. Zhou, Y.; Othus, M.; Araki, D.; Wood, B.L.; Radich, J.P.; Halpern, A.B.; Mielcarek, M.; Estey, E.H.; Appelbaum, F.R.; Walter, R.B. Pre- and post-transplant quantification of measurable ('minimal') residual disease via multiparameter flow cytometry in adult acute myeloid leukemia. *Leukemia* **2016**, *30*, 1456–1464. [CrossRef]
129. Jacobsohn, D.A.; Loken, M.R.; Fei, M.; Adams, A.; Brodersen, L.E.; Logan, B.R.; Ahn, K.W.; Shaw, B.E.; Kletzel, M.; Olszewski, M.; et al. Outcomes of Measurable Residual Disease in Pediatric Acute Myeloid Leukemia before and after Hematopoietic Stem Cell Transplant: Validation of Difference from Normal Flow Cytometry with Chimerism Studies and Wilms Tumor 1 Gene Expression. *Biol. Blood Marrow Transpl.* **2018**, *24*, 2040–2046. [CrossRef]
130. Buckley, S.A.; Wood, B.L.; Othus, M.; Hourigan, C.S.; Ustun, C.; Linden, M.A.; DeFor, T.E.; Malagola, M.; Anthias, C.; Valkova, V.; et al. Minimal residual disease prior to allogeneic hematopoietic cell transplantation in acute myeloid leukemia: A meta-analysis. *Haematologica* **2017**, *102*, 865–873. [CrossRef]
131. Faham, M.; Zheng, J.; Moorhead, M.; Carlton, V.E.; Stow, P.; Coustan-Smith, E.; Pui, C.H.; Campana, D. Deep-sequencing approach for minimal residual disease detection in acute lymphoblastic leukemia. *Blood* **2012**, *120*, 5173–5180. [CrossRef]
132. Pulsipher, M.A.; Carlson, C.; Langholz, B.; Wall, D.A.; Schultz, K.R.; Bunin, N.; Kirsch, I.; Gastier-Foster, J.M.; Borowitz, M.; Desmarais, C.; et al. IgH-V(D)J NGS-MRD measurement pre- and early post-allotransplant defines very low- and very high-risk ALL patients. *Blood* **2015**, *125*, 3501–3508. [CrossRef]
133. Kim, T.; Moon, J.H.; Ahn, J.S.; Kim, Y.K.; Lee, S.S.; Ahn, S.Y.; Jung, S.H.; Yang, D.H.; Lee, J.J.; Choi, S.H.; et al. Next-generation sequencing-based posttransplant monitoring of acute myeloid leukemia identifies patients at high risk of relapse. *Blood* **2018**, *132*, 1604–1613. [CrossRef]
134. Thol, F.; Gabdoulline, R.; Liebich, A.; Klement, P.; Schiller, J.; Kandziora, C.; Hambach, L.; Stadler, M.; Koenecke, C.; Flintrop, M.; et al. Measurable residual disease monitoring by NGS before allogeneic hematopoietic cell transplantation in AML. *Blood* **2018**, *132*, 1703–1713. [CrossRef]

135. Sun, W.; Orgel, E.; Malvar, J.; Sposto, R.; Wilkes, J.J.; Gardner, R.; Tolbert, V.P.; Smith, A.; Hur, M.; Hoffman, J.; et al. Treatment-related adverse events associated with a modified UK ALLR3 induction chemotherapy backbone for childhood relapsed/refractory acute lymphoblastic leukemia. *Pediatr. Blood Cancer* **2016**, *63*, 1943–1948. [CrossRef]
136. Oskarsson, T.; Soderhall, S.; Arvidson, J.; Forestier, E.; Frandsen, T.L.; Hellebostad, M.; Lahteenmaki, P.; Jonsson, O.G.; Myrberg, I.H.; Heyman, M.; et al. Treatment-related mortality in relapsed childhood acute lymphoblastic leukemia. *Pediatr. Blood Cancer* **2018**, *65*. [CrossRef] [PubMed]
137. von Stackelberg, A.; Locatelli, F.; Zugmaier, G.; Handgretinger, R.; Trippett, T.M.; Rizzari, C.; Bader, P.; O'Brien, M.M.; Brethon, B.; Bhojwani, D.; et al. Phase I/Phase II Study of Blinatumomab in Pediatric Patients with Relapsed/Refractory Acute Lymphoblastic Leukemia. *J. Clin. Oncol.* **2016**, *34*, 4381–4389. [CrossRef] [PubMed]
138. Locatelli, F.; Zugmaier, G.; Mergen, N.; Bader, P.; Jeha, S.; Schlegel, P.G.; Bourquin, J.P.; Handgretinger, R.; Brethon, B.; Rossig, C.; et al. Blinatumomab in pediatric patients with relapsed/refractory acute lymphoblastic leukemia: Results of the RIALTO trial, an expanded access study. *Blood Cancer J.* **2020**, *10*, 77. [CrossRef]
139. Locatelli, F.; Zugmaier, G.; Rizzari, C.; Morris, J.D.; Gruhn, B.; Klingebiel, T.; Parasole, R.; Linderkamp, C.; Flotho, C.; Petit, A.; et al. Effect of Blinatumomab vs. Chemotherapy on Event-Free Survival among Children with High-risk First-Relapse B-Cell Acute Lymphoblastic Leukemia: A Randomized Clinical Trial. *JAMA* **2021**, *325*, 843–854. [CrossRef] [PubMed]
140. Brown, P.A.; Ji, L.; Xu, X.; Devidas, M.; Hogan, L.E.; Borowitz, M.J.; Raetz, E.A.; Zugmaier, G.; Sharon, E.; Bernhardt, M.B.; et al. Effect of Postreinduction Therapy Consolidation with Blinatumomab vs. Chemotherapy on Disease-Free Survival in Children, Adolescents, and Young Adults with First Relapse of B-Cell Acute Lymphoblastic Leukemia: A Randomized Clinical Trial. *JAMA* **2021**, *325*, 833–842. [CrossRef]
141. Brivio, E.; Locatelli, F.; Lopez-Yurda, M.; Malone, A.; Diaz-de-Heredia, C.; Bielorai, B.; Rossig, C.; van der Velden, V.H.J.; Ammerlaan, A.C.J.; Thano, A.; et al. A phase 1 study of inotuzumab ozogamicin in pediatric relapsed/refractory acute lymphoblastic leukemia (ITCC-059 study). *Blood* **2021**, *137*, 1582–1590. [CrossRef]
142. Bhojwani, D.; Sposto, R.; Shah, N.N.; Rodriguez, V.; Yuan, C.; Stetler-Stevenson, M.; O'Brien, M.M.; McNeer, J.L.; Quereshi, A.; Cabannes, A.; et al. Inotuzumab ozogamicin in pediatric patients with relapsed/refractory acute lymphoblastic leukemia. *Leukemia* **2019**, *33*, 884–892. [CrossRef] [PubMed]
143. Shah, N.N.; Lee, D.W.; Yates, B.; Yuan, C.M.; Shalabi, H.; Martin, S.; Wolters, P.L.; Steinberg, S.M.; Baker, E.H.; Delbrook, C.P.; et al. Long-Term Follow-Up of CD19-CAR T-Cell Therapy in Children and Young Adults With B-ALL. *J. Clin. Oncol.* **2021**, *39*, 1650–1659. [CrossRef] [PubMed]
144. Gardner, R.A.; Finney, O.; Annesley, C.; Brakke, H.; Summers, C.; Leger, K.; Bleakley, M.; Brown, C.; Mgebroff, S.; Kelly-Spratt, K.S.; et al. Intent-to-treat leukemia remission by CD19 CAR T cells of defined formulation and dose in children and young adults. *Blood* **2017**, *129*, 3322–3331. [CrossRef]
145. Summers, C.; Annesley, C.; Bleakley, M.; Dahlberg, A.; Jensen, M.C.; Gardner, R. Long Term Follow-up after SCRI-CAR19v1 Reveals Late Recurrences as Well as a Survival Advantage to Consolidation with HCT after CAR T Cell Induced Remission. *Blood* **2018**, *132*, 967. [CrossRef]
146. Shah, N.N.; Highfill, S.L.; Shalabi, H.; Yates, B.; Jin, J.; Wolters, P.L.; Ombrello, A.; Steinberg, S.M.; Martin, S.; Delbrook, C.; et al. CD4/CD8 T-Cell Selection Affects Chimeric Antigen Receptor (CAR) T-Cell Potency and Toxicity: Updated Results from a Phase I Anti-CD22 CAR T-Cell Trial. *J. Clin. Oncol.* **2020**, *38*, 1938–1950. [CrossRef] [PubMed]
147. Pulsipher, M.A.; Han, X.; Quigley, M.; Kari, G.; Rives, S.; Laetsch, T.W.; Myers, G.D.; Hiramatsu, H.; Yanik, G.A.; Qayed, M.; et al. Molecular Detection of Minimal Residual Disease Precedes Morphological Relapse and Could be Used to Identify Relapse in Pediatric and Young Adult B-Cell Acute Lymphoblastic Leukemia Patients Treated with Tisagenlecleucel. *Blood* **2018**, *132*, 1551. [CrossRef]
148. Gamis, A.S.; Alonzo, T.A.; Meshinchi, S.; Sung, L.; Gerbing, R.B.; Raimondi, S.C.; Hirsch, B.A.; Kawash, S.B.; Heerema-McKenney, A.; Winter, L.; et al. Gemtuzumab ozogamicin in children and adolescents with de novo acute myeloid leukemia improves event-free survival by reducing relapse risk: Results from the randomized phase III Children's Oncology Group trial AAML0531. *J. Clin. Oncol.* **2014**, *32*, 3021–3032. [CrossRef] [PubMed]
149. Lamba, J.K.; Chauhan, L.; Shin, M.; Loken, M.R.; Pollard, J.A.; Wang, Y.C.; Ries, R.E.; Aplenc, R.; Hirsch, B.A.; Raimondi, S.C.; et al. CD33 Splicing Polymorphism Determines Gemtuzumab Ozogamicin Response in De Novo Acute Myeloid Leukemia: Report from Randomized Phase III Children's Oncology Group Trial AAML0531. *J. Clin. Oncol.* **2017**, *35*, 2674–2682. [CrossRef] [PubMed]
150. Pollard, J.A.; Loken, M.; Gerbing, R.B.; Raimondi, S.C.; Hirsch, B.A.; Aplenc, R.; Bernstein, I.D.; Gamis, A.S.; Alonzo, T.A.; Meshinchi, S. CD33 Expression and Its Association with Gemtuzumab Ozogamicin Response: Results From the Randomized Phase III Children's Oncology Group Trial AAML0531. *J. Clin. Oncol.* **2016**, *34*, 747–755. [CrossRef]
151. Tarlock, K.; Alonzo, T.A.; Gerbing, R.B.; Raimondi, S.C.; Hirsch, B.A.; Sung, L.; Pollard, J.A.; Aplenc, R.; Loken, M.R.; Gamis, A.S.; et al. Gemtuzumab Ozogamicin Reduces Relapse Risk in FLT3/ITD Acute Myeloid Leukemia: A Report from the Children's Oncology Group. *Clin. Cancer Res.* **2016**, *22*, 1951–1957. [CrossRef]
152. Pollard, J.A.; Guest, E.; Alonzo, T.A.; Gerbing, R.B.; Loken, M.R.; Brodersen, L.E.; Kolb, E.A.; Aplenc, R.; Meshinchi, S.; Raimondi, S.C.; et al. Gemtuzumab Ozogamicin Improves Event-Free Survival and Reduces Relapse in Pediatric KMT2A-Rearranged AML: Results from the Phase III Children's Oncology Group Trial AAML0531. *J. Clin. Oncol.* **2021**, JCO2003048. [CrossRef]

153. Rafiee, R.; Chauhan, L.; Alonzo, T.A.; Wang, Y.C.; Elmasry, A.; Loken, M.R.; Pollard, J.; Aplenc, R.; Raimondi, S.; Hirsch, B.A.; et al. ABCB1 SNP predicts outcome in patients with acute myeloid leukemia treated with Gemtuzumab ozogamicin: A report from Children's Oncology Group AAML0531 Trial. *Blood Cancer J.* **2019**, *9*, 51. [CrossRef] [PubMed]
154. Daver, N.; Alotaibi, A.S.; Bucklein, V.; Subklewe, M. T-cell-based immunotherapy of acute myeloid leukemia: Current concepts and future developments. *Leukemia* **2021**, *35*, 1843–1863. [CrossRef]
155. Lamble, A.J.; Tasian, S.K. Opportunities for immunotherapy in childhood acute myeloid leukemia. *Blood Adv.* **2019**, *3*, 3750–3758. [CrossRef]
156. Vogiatzi, F.; Winterberg, D.; Lenk, L.; Buchmann, S.; Cario, G.; Schrappe, M.; Peipp, M.; Richter-Pechanska, P.; Kulozik, A.E.; Lentes, J.; et al. Daratumumab eradicates minimal residual disease in a preclinical model of pediatric T-cell acute lymphoblastic leukemia. *Blood* **2019**, *134*, 713–716. [CrossRef] [PubMed]
157. Ofran, Y.; Ringelstein-Harlev, S.; Slouzkey, I.; Zuckerman, T.; Yehudai-Ofir, D.; Henig, I.; Beyar-Katz, O.; Hayun, M.; Frisch, A. Daratumumab for eradication of minimal residual disease in high-risk advanced relapse of T-cell/CD19/CD22-negative acute lymphoblastic leukemia. *Leukemia* **2020**, *34*, 293–295. [CrossRef] [PubMed]
158. Lamble, A.J.; Gardner, R. CAR T cells for other pediatric non-B-cell hematologic malignancies. *Hematol. Am. Soc. Hematol. Educ. Program* **2020**, *2020*, 494–500. [CrossRef]
159. Gomes-Silva, D.; Srinivasan, M.; Sharma, S.; Lee, C.M.; Wagner, D.L.; Davis, T.H.; Rouce, R.H.; Bao, G.; Brenner, M.K.; Mamonkin, M. CD7-edited T cells expressing a CD7-specific CAR for the therapy of T-cell malignancies. *Blood* **2017**, *130*, 285–296. [CrossRef]
160. Mamonkin, M.; Rouce, R.H.; Tashiro, H.; Brenner, M.K. A T-cell-directed chimeric antigen receptor for the selective treatment of T-cell malignancies. *Blood* **2015**, *126*, 983–992. [CrossRef]
161. Sanchez-Martinez, D.; Baroni, M.L.; Gutierrez-Aguera, F.; Roca-Ho, H.; Blanch-Lombarte, O.; Gonzalez-Garcia, S.; Torrebadell, M.; Junca, J.; Ramirez-Orellana, M.; Velasco-Hernandez, T.; et al. Fratricide-resistant CD1a-specific CAR T cells for the treatment of cortical T-cell acute lymphoblastic leukemia. *Blood* **2019**, *133*, 2291–2304. [CrossRef] [PubMed]
162. Georgiadis, C.; Rasaiyaah, J.; Gkazi, S.A.; Preece, R.; Etuk, A.; Christi, A.; Qasim, W. Base-edited CAR T cells for combinational therapy against T cell malignancies. *Leukemia* **2021**. [CrossRef] [PubMed]
163. Cooper, M.L.; Choi, J.; Staser, K.; Ritchey, J.K.; Devenport, J.M.; Eckardt, K.; Rettig, M.P.; Wang, B.; Eissenberg, L.G.; Ghobadi, A.; et al. An "off-the-shelf" fratricide-resistant CAR-T for the treatment of T cell hematologic malignancies. *Leukemia* **2018**, *32*, 1970–1983. [CrossRef] [PubMed]
164. Bader, P.; Kreyenberg, H.; von Stackelberg, A.; Eckert, C.; Salzmann-Manrique, E.; Meisel, R.; Poetschger, U.; Stachel, D.; Schrappe, M.; Alten, J.; et al. Monitoring of minimal residual disease after allogeneic stem-cell transplantation in relapsed childhood acute lymphoblastic leukemia allows for the identification of impending relapse: Results of the ALL-BFM-SCT 2003 trial. *J. Clin. Oncol.* **2015**, *33*, 1275–1284. [CrossRef]
165. Balduzzi, A.; Di Maio, L.; Silvestri, D.; Songia, S.; Bonanomi, S.; Rovelli, A.; Conter, V.; Biondi, A.; Cazzaniga, G.; Valsecchi, M.G. Minimal residual disease before and after transplantation for childhood acute lymphoblastic leukaemia: Is there any room for intervention? *Br. J. Haematol.* **2014**, *164*, 396–408. [CrossRef] [PubMed]
166. Pulsipher, M.A.; Langholz, B.; Wall, D.A.; Schultz, K.R.; Bunin, N.; Carroll, W.; Raetz, E.; Gardner, S.; Goyal, R.K.; Gastier-Foster, J.; et al. Risk factors and timing of relapse after allogeneic transplantation in pediatric ALL: For whom and when should interventions be tested? *Bone Marrow Transpl.* **2015**, *50*, 1173–1179. [CrossRef]
167. Zecca, M.; Prete, A.; Rondelli, R.; Lanino, E.; Balduzzi, A.; Messina, C.; Fagioli, F.; Porta, F.; Favre, C.; Pession, A.; et al. Chronic graft-versus-host disease in children: Incidence, risk factors, and impact on outcome. *Blood* **2002**, *100*, 1192–1200. [CrossRef]
168. Bader, P.; Kreyenberg, H.; Hoelle, W.; Dueckers, G.; Handgretinger, R.; Lang, P.; Kremens, B.; Dilloo, D.; Sykora, K.W.; Schrappe, M.; et al. Increasing mixed chimerism is an important prognostic factor for unfavorable outcome in children with acute lymphoblastic leukemia after allogeneic stem-cell transplantation: Possible role for pre-emptive immunotherapy? *J. Clin. Oncol.* **2004**, *22*, 1696–1705. [CrossRef]
169. Horn, B.; Petrovic, A.; Wahlstrom, J.; Dvorak, C.C.; Kong, D.; Hwang, J.; Expose-Spencer, J.; Gates, M.; Cowan, M.J. Chimerism-based pre-emptive therapy with fast withdrawal of immunosuppression and donor lymphocyte infusions after allogeneic stem cell transplantation for pediatric hematologic malignancies. *Biol. Blood Marrow Transpl.* **2015**, *21*, 729–737. [CrossRef] [PubMed]
170. Rettinger, E.; Merker, M.; Salzmann-Manrique, E.; Kreyenberg, H.; Krenn, T.; Durken, M.; Faber, J.; Huenecke, S.; Cappel, C.; Bremm, M.; et al. Pre-Emptive Immunotherapy for Clearance of Molecular Disease in Childhood Acute Lymphoblastic Leukemia after Transplantation. *Biol. Blood Marrow Transpl.* **2017**, *23*, 87–95. [CrossRef]
171. Locatelli, F.; Zecca, M.; Rondelli, R.; Bonetti, F.; Dini, G.; Prete, A.; Messina, C.; Uderzo, C.; Ripaldi, M.; Porta, F.; et al. Graft versus host disease prophylaxis with low-dose cyclosporine-A reduces the risk of relapse in children with acute leukemia given HLA-identical sibling bone marrow transplantation: Results of a randomized trial. *Blood* **2000**, *95*, 1572–1579. [CrossRef]
172. Abraham, R.; Szer, J.; Bardy, P.; Grigg, A. Early cyclosporine taper in high-risk sibling allogeneic bone marrow transplants. *Bone Marrow Transpl.* **1997**, *20*, 773–777. [CrossRef] [PubMed]
173. Gandemer, V.; Pochon, C.; Oger, E.; Dalle, J.H.; Michel, G.; Schmitt, C.; de Berranger, E.; Galambrun, C.; Cave, H.; Cayuela, J.M.; et al. Clinical value of pre-transplant minimal residual disease in childhood lymphoblastic leukaemia: The results of the French minimal residual disease-guided protocol. *Br. J. Haematol.* **2014**, *165*, 392–401. [CrossRef] [PubMed]

174. Mehta, J.; Powles, R.; Singhal, S.; Tait, D.; Swansbury, J.; Treleaven, J. Cytokine-mediated immunotherapy with or without donor leukocytes for poor-risk acute myeloid leukemia relapsing after allogeneic bone marrow transplantation. *Bone Marrow Transpl.* **1995**, *16*, 133–137.
175. Rettinger, E.; Huenecke, S.; Bonig, H.; Merker, M.; Jarisch, A.; Soerensen, J.; Willasch, A.; Bug, G.; Schulz, A.; Klingebiel, T.; et al. Interleukin-15-activated cytokine-induced killer cells may sustain remission in leukemia patients after allogeneic stem cell transplantation: Feasibility, safety and first insights on efficacy. *Haematologica* **2016**, *101*, e153–e156. [CrossRef]
176. Carpenter, P.A.; Snyder, D.S.; Flowers, M.E.; Sanders, J.E.; Gooley, T.A.; Martin, P.J.; Appelbaum, F.R.; Radich, J.P. Prophylactic administration of imatinib after hematopoietic cell transplantation for high-risk Philadelphia chromosome-positive leukemia. *Blood* **2007**, *109*, 2791–2793. [CrossRef]
177. Tarlock, K.; Chang, B.; Cooper, T.; Gross, T.; Gupta, S.; Neudorf, S.; Adlard, K.; Ho, P.A.; McGoldrick, S.; Watt, T.; et al. Sorafenib treatment following hematopoietic stem cell transplant in pediatric FLT3/ITD acute myeloid leukemia. *Pediatr. Blood Cancer* **2015**, *62*, 1048–1054. [CrossRef]
178. Gagelmann, N.; Wolschke, C.; Klyuchnikov, E.; Christopeit, M.; Ayuk, F.; Kroger, N. TKI Maintenance After Stem-Cell Transplantation for FLT3-ITD Positive Acute Myeloid Leukemia: A Systematic Review and Meta-Analysis. *Front. Immunol* **2021**, *12*, 630429. [CrossRef] [PubMed]
179. Schroeder, T.; Rachlis, E.; Bug, G.; Stelljes, M.; Klein, S.; Steckel, N.K.; Wolf, D.; Ringhoffer, M.; Czibere, A.; Nachtkamp, K.; et al. Treatment of acute myeloid leukemia or myelodysplastic syndrome relapse after allogeneic stem cell transplantation with azacitidine and donor lymphocyte infusions—A retrospective multicenter analysis from the German Cooperative Transplant Study Group. *Biol. Blood Marrow Transpl.* **2015**, *21*, 653–660. [CrossRef]
180. Barrett, A.J.; Horowitz, M.M.; Pollock, B.H.; Zhang, M.J.; Bortin, M.M.; Buchanan, G.R.; Camitta, B.M.; Ochs, J.; Graham-Pole, J.; Rowlings, P.A.; et al. Bone marrow transplants from HLA-identical siblings as compared with chemotherapy for children with acute lymphoblastic leukemia in a second remission. *N. Engl. J. Med.* **1994**, *331*, 1253–1258. [CrossRef] [PubMed]
181. Horan, J.T.; Alonzo, T.A.; Lyman, G.H.; Gerbing, R.B.; Lange, B.J.; Ravindranath, Y.; Becton, D.; Smith, F.O.; Woods, W.G.; Children's Oncology, G. Impact of disease risk on efficacy of matched related bone marrow transplantation for pediatric acute myeloid leukemia: The Children's Oncology Group. *J. Clin. Oncol.* **2008**, *26*, 5797–5801. [CrossRef]
182. Locatelli, F.; Zecca, M.; Messina, C.; Rondelli, R.; Lanino, E.; Sacchi, N.; Uderzo, C.; Fagioli, F.; Conter, V.; Bonetti, F.; et al. Improvement over time in outcome for children with acute lymphoblastic leukemia in second remission given hematopoietic stem cell transplantation from unrelated donors. *Leukemia* **2002**, *16*, 2228–2237. [CrossRef]
183. Dini, G.; Zecca, M.; Balduzzi, A.; Messina, C.; Masetti, R.; Fagioli, F.; Favre, C.; Rabusin, M.; Porta, F.; Biral, E.; et al. No difference in outcome between children and adolescents transplanted for acute lymphoblastic leukemia in second remission. *Blood* **2011**, *118*, 6683–6690. [CrossRef] [PubMed]
184. Fagioli, F.; Quarello, P.; Zecca, M.; Lanino, E.; Rognoni, C.; Balduzzi, A.; Messina, C.; Favre, C.; Foa, R.; Ripaldi, M.; et al. Hematopoietic stem cell transplantation for children with high-risk acute lymphoblastic leukemia in first complete remission: A report from the AIEOP registry. *Haematologica* **2013**, *98*, 1273–1281. [CrossRef] [PubMed]
185. Saarinen-Pihkala, U.M.; Gustafsson, G.; Ringden, O.; Heilmann, C.; Glomstein, A.; Lonnerholm, G.; Abrahamsson, J.; Bekassy, A.N.; Schroeder, H.; Mellander, L.; et al. No disadvantage in outcome of using matched unrelated donors as compared with matched sibling donors for bone marrow transplantation in children with acute lymphoblastic leukemia in second remission. *J. Clin. Oncol.* **2001**, *19*, 3406–3414. [CrossRef] [PubMed]
186. Shaw, P.J.; Kan, F.; Woo Ahn, K.; Spellman, S.R.; Aljurf, M.; Ayas, M.; Burke, M.; Cairo, M.S.; Chen, A.R.; Davies, S.M.; et al. Outcomes of pediatric bone marrow transplantation for leukemia and myelodysplasia using matched sibling, mismatched related, or matched unrelated donors. *Blood* **2010**, *116*, 4007–4015. [CrossRef] [PubMed]
187. Leung, W.; Campana, D.; Yang, J.; Pei, D.; Coustan-Smith, E.; Gan, K.; Rubnitz, J.E.; Sandlund, J.T.; Ribeiro, R.C.; Srinivasan, A.; et al. High success rate of hematopoietic cell transplantation regardless of donor source in children with very high-risk leukemia. *Blood* **2011**, *118*, 223–230. [CrossRef]
188. Dalle, J.H.; Balduzzi, A.; Bader, P.; Lankester, A.; Yaniv, I.; Wachowiak, J.; Pieczonka, A.; Bierings, M.; Yesilipek, A.; Sedlacek, P.; et al. Allogeneic Stem Cell Transplantation from HLA-Mismatched Donors for Pediatric Patients with Acute Lymphoblastic Leukemia Treated According to the 2003 BFM and 2007 International BFM Studies: Impact of Disease Risk on Outcomes. *Biol. Blood Marrow Transpl.* **2018**, *24*, 1848–1855. [CrossRef]
189. Rocha, V.; Cornish, J.; Sievers, E.L.; Filipovich, A.; Locatelli, F.; Peters, C.; Remberger, M.; Michel, G.; Arcese, W.; Dallorso, S.; et al. Comparison of outcomes of unrelated bone marrow and umbilical cord blood transplants in children with acute leukemia. *Blood* **2001**, *97*, 2962–2971. [CrossRef]
190. Eapen, M.; Rubinstein, P.; Zhang, M.J.; Stevens, C.; Kurtzberg, J.; Scaradavou, A.; Loberiza, F.R.; Champlin, R.E.; Klein, J.P.; Horowitz, M.M.; et al. Outcomes of transplantation of unrelated donor umbilical cord blood and bone marrow in children with acute leukaemia: A comparison study. *Lancet* **2007**, *369*, 1947–1954. [CrossRef]
191. Ruggeri, A.; Michel, G.; Dalle, J.H.; Caniglia, M.; Locatelli, F.; Campos, A.; de Heredia, C.D.; Mohty, M.; Hurtado, J.M.; Bierings, M.; et al. Impact of pretransplant minimal residual disease after cord blood transplantation for childhood acute lymphoblastic leukemia in remission: An Eurocord, PDWP-EBMT analysis. *Leukemia* **2012**, *26*, 2455–2461. [CrossRef]

192. Michel, G.; Rocha, V.; Chevret, S.; Arcese, W.; Chan, K.W.; Filipovich, A.; Takahashi, T.A.; Vowels, M.; Ortega, J.; Bordigoni, P.; et al. Unrelated cord blood transplantation for childhood acute myeloid leukemia: A Eurocord Group analysis. *Blood* **2003**, *102*, 4290–4297. [CrossRef] [PubMed]
193. Eapen, M.; Klein, J.P.; Sanz, G.F.; Spellman, S.; Ruggeri, A.; Anasetti, C.; Brown, M.; Champlin, R.E.; Garcia-Lopez, J.; Hattersely, G.; et al. Effect of donor-recipient HLA matching at HLA A, B, C, and DRB1 on outcomes after umbilical-cord blood transplantation for leukaemia and myelodysplastic syndrome: A retrospective analysis. *Lancet Oncol.* **2011**, *12*, 1214–1221. [CrossRef]
194. Eapen, M.; Klein, J.P.; Ruggeri, A.; Spellman, S.; Lee, S.J.; Anasetti, C.; Arcese, W.; Barker, J.N.; Baxter-Lowe, L.A.; Brown, M.; et al. Impact of allele-level HLA matching on outcomes after myeloablative single unit umbilical cord blood transplantation for hematologic malignancy. *Blood* **2014**, *123*, 133–140. [CrossRef] [PubMed]
195. Wagner, J.E., Jr.; Eapen, M.; Carter, S.; Wang, Y.; Schultz, K.R.; Wall, D.A.; Bunin, N.; Delaney, C.; Haut, P.; Margolis, D.; et al. One-unit versus two-unit cord-blood transplantation for hematologic cancers. *N. Engl. J. Med.* **2014**, *371*, 1685–1694. [CrossRef] [PubMed]
196. Michel, G.; Galambrun, C.; Sirvent, A.; Pochon, C.; Bruno, B.; Jubert, C.; Loundou, A.; Yakoub-Agha, I.; Milpied, N.; Lutz, P.; et al. Single- vs. double-unit cord blood transplantation for children and young adults with acute leukemia or myelodysplastic syndrome. *Blood* **2016**, *127*, 3450–3457. [CrossRef] [PubMed]
197. Milano, F.; Gooley, T.; Wood, B.; Woolfrey, A.; Flowers, M.E.; Doney, K.; Witherspoon, R.; Mielcarek, M.; Deeg, J.H.; Sorror, M.; et al. Cord-Blood Transplantation in Patients with Minimal Residual Disease. *N. Engl. J. Med.* **2016**, *375*, 944–953. [CrossRef] [PubMed]
198. Balligand, L.; Galambrun, C.; Sirvent, A.; Roux, C.; Pochon, C.; Bruno, B.; Jubert, C.; Loundou, A.; Esmiol, S.; Yakoub-Agha, I.; et al. Single-Unit versus Double-Unit Umbilical Cord Blood Transplantation in Children and Young Adults with Residual Leukemic Disease. *Biol. Blood Marrow Transpl.* **2019**, *25*, 734–742. [CrossRef] [PubMed]
199. Algeri, M.; Gaspari, S.; Locatelli, F. Cord blood transplantation for acute leukemia. *Expert Opin. Biol. Ther.* **2020**, *20*, 1223–1236. [CrossRef]
200. Horwitz, M.E.; Wease, S.; Blackwell, B.; Valcarcel, D.; Frassoni, F.; Boelens, J.J.; Nierkens, S.; Jagasia, M.; Wagner, J.E.; Kuball, J.; et al. Phase I/II Study of Stem-Cell Transplantation Using a Single Cord Blood Unit Expanded Ex Vivo with Nicotinamide. *J. Clin. Oncol.* **2019**, *37*, 367–374. [CrossRef]
201. Cohen, S.; Roy, J.; Lachance, S.; Delisle, J.S.; Marinier, A.; Busque, L.; Roy, D.C.; Barabe, F.; Ahmad, I.; Bambace, N.; et al. Hematopoietic stem cell transplantation using single UM171-expanded cord blood: A single-arm, phase 1-2 safety and feasibility study. *Lancet Haematol.* **2020**, *7*, e134–e145. [CrossRef]
202. Passweg, J.R.; Baldomero, H.; Chabannon, C.; Basak, G.W.; de la Camara, R.; Corbacioglu, S.; Dolstra, H.; Duarte, R.; Glass, B.; Greco, R.; et al. Hematopoietic cell transplantation and cellular therapy survey of the EBMT: Monitoring of activities and trends over 30 years. *Bone Marrow Transpl.* **2021**, *56*, 1651–1664. [CrossRef]
203. Dholaria, B.; Savani, B.N.; Labopin, M.; Luznik, L.; Ruggeri, A.; Mielke, S.; Al Malki, M.M.; Kongtim, P.; Fuchs, E.; Huang, X.J.; et al. Clinical applications of donor lymphocyte infusion from an HLA-haploidentical donor: Consensus recommendations from the Acute Leukemia Working Party of the EBMT. *Haematologica* **2020**, *105*, 47–58. [CrossRef]
204. Bertaina, A.; Pitisci, A.; Sinibaldi, M.; Algeri, M. T Cell-Depleted and T Cell-Replete HLA-Haploidentical Stem Cell Transplantation for Non-malignant Disorders. *Curr. Hematol. Malig. Rep.* **2017**, *12*, 68–78. [CrossRef]
205. Handgretinger, R.; Chen, X.; Pfeiffer, M.; Mueller, I.; Feuchtinger, T.; Hale, G.A.; Lang, P. Feasibility and outcome of reduced-intensity conditioning in haploidentical transplantation. *Ann. N. Y. Acad. Sci.* **2007**, *1106*, 279–289. [CrossRef]
206. Lang, P.; Teltschik, H.M.; Feuchtinger, T.; Muller, I.; Pfeiffer, M.; Schumm, M.; Ebinger, M.; Schwarze, C.P.; Gruhn, B.; Schrauder, A.; et al. Transplantation of CD3/CD19 depleted allografts from haploidentical family donors in paediatric leukaemia. *Br. J. Haematol.* **2014**, *165*, 688–698. [CrossRef]
207. Bertaina, A.; Merli, P.; Rutella, S.; Pagliara, D.; Bernardo, M.E.; Masetti, R.; Pende, D.; Falco, M.; Handgretinger, R.; Moretta, F.; et al. HLA-haploidentical stem cell transplantation after removal of alphabeta+ T and B cells in children with nonmalignant disorders. *Blood* **2014**, *124*, 822–826. [CrossRef] [PubMed]
208. Locatelli, F.; Bauquet, A.; Palumbo, G.; Moretta, F.; Bertaina, A. Negative depletion of alpha/beta+ T cells and of CD19+ B lymphocytes: A novel frontier to optimize the effect of innate immunity in HLA-mismatched hematopoietic stem cell transplantation. *Immunol. Lett.* **2013**, *155*, 21–23. [CrossRef] [PubMed]
209. Li Pira, G.; Malaspina, D.; Girolami, E.; Biagini, S.; Cicchetti, E.; Conflitti, G.; Broglia, M.; Ceccarelli, S.; Lazzaro, S.; Pagliara, D.; et al. Selective Depletion of alphabeta T Cells and B Cells for Human Leukocyte Antigen-Haploidentical Hematopoietic Stem Cell Transplantation. A Three-Year Follow-Up of Procedure Efficiency. *Biol. Blood Marrow Transpl.* **2016**, *22*, 2056–2064. [CrossRef] [PubMed]
210. Locatelli, F.; Merli, P.; Pagliara, D.; Li Pira, G.; Falco, M.; Pende, D.; Rondelli, R.; Lucarelli, B.; Brescia, L.P.; Masetti, R.; et al. Outcome of children with acute leukemia given HLA-haploidentical HSCT after alphabeta T-cell and B-cell depletion. *Blood* **2017**, *130*, 677–685. [CrossRef] [PubMed]
211. Moretta, L.; Locatelli, F.; Pende, D.; Marcenaro, E.; Mingari, M.C.; Moretta, A. Killer Ig-like receptor-mediated control of natural killer cell alloreactivity in haploidentical hematopoietic stem cell transplantation. *Blood* **2011**, *117*, 764–771. [CrossRef]

212. Ciurea, S.O.; Al Malki, M.M.; Kongtim, P.; Fuchs, E.J.; Luznik, L.; Huang, X.J.; Ciceri, F.; Locatelli, F.; Aversa, F.; Castagna, L.; et al. The European Society for Blood and Marrow Transplantation (EBMT) consensus recommendations for donor selection in haploidentical hematopoietic cell transplantation. *Bone Marrow Transpl.* **2020**, *55*, 12–24. [CrossRef]
213. Ruggeri, L.; Capanni, M.; Urbani, E.; Perruccio, K.; Shlomchik, W.D.; Tosti, A.; Posati, S.; Rogaia, D.; Frassoni, F.; Aversa, F.; et al. Effectiveness of donor natural killer cell alloreactivity in mismatched hematopoietic transplants. *Science* **2002**, *295*, 2097–2100. [CrossRef] [PubMed]
214. Pende, D.; Marcenaro, S.; Falco, M.; Martini, S.; Bernardo, M.E.; Montagna, D.; Romeo, E.; Cognet, C.; Martinetti, M.; Maccario, R.; et al. Anti-leukemia activity of alloreactive NK cells in KIR ligand-mismatched haploidentical HSCT for pediatric patients: Evaluation of the functional role of activating KIR and redefinition of inhibitory KIR specificity. *Blood* **2009**, *113*, 3119–3129. [CrossRef]
215. Ruggeri, L.; Mancusi, A.; Capanni, M.; Urbani, E.; Carotti, A.; Aloisi, T.; Stern, M.; Pende, D.; Perruccio, K.; Burchielli, E.; et al. Donor natural killer cell allorecognition of missing self in haploidentical hematopoietic transplantation for acute myeloid leukemia: Challenging its predictive value. *Blood* **2007**, *110*, 433–440. [CrossRef]
216. Oevermann, L.; Michaelis, S.U.; Mezger, M.; Lang, P.; Toporski, J.; Bertaina, A.; Zecca, M.; Moretta, L.; Locatelli, F.; Handgretinger, R. KIR B haplotype donors confer a reduced risk for relapse after haploidentical transplantation in children with ALL. *Blood* **2014**, *124*, 2744–2747. [CrossRef] [PubMed]
217. Locatelli, F.; Merli, P.; Rutella, S. At the Bedside: Innate immunity as an immunotherapy tool for hematological malignancies. *J. Leukoc. Biol.* **2013**, *94*, 1141–1157. [CrossRef] [PubMed]
218. Perez-Martinez, A.; Ferreras, C.; Pascual, A.; Gonzalez-Vicent, M.; Alonso, L.; Badell, I.; Fernandez Navarro, J.M.; Regueiro, A.; Plaza, M.; Perez Hurtado, J.M.; et al. Haploidentical transplantation in high-risk pediatric leukemia: A retrospective comparative analysis on behalf of the Spanish working Group for bone marrow transplantation in children (GETMON) and the Spanish Grupo for hematopoietic transplantation (GETH). *Am. J. Hematol.* **2020**, *95*, 28–37. [CrossRef]
219. Airoldi, I.; Bertaina, A.; Prigione, I.; Zorzoli, A.; Pagliara, D.; Cocco, C.; Meazza, R.; Loiacono, F.; Lucarelli, B.; Bernardo, M.E.; et al. gammadelta T-cell reconstitution after HLA-haploidentical hematopoietic transplantation depleted of TCR-alphabeta+/CD19+ lymphocytes. *Blood* **2015**, *125*, 2349–2358. [CrossRef] [PubMed]
220. Bertaina, A.; Zorzoli, A.; Petretto, A.; Barbarito, G.; Inglese, E.; Merli, P.; Lavarello, C.; Brescia, L.P.; De Angelis, B.; Tripodi, G.; et al. Zoledronic acid boosts gammadelta T-cell activity in children receiving alphabeta(+) T and CD19(+) cell-depleted grafts from an HLA-haplo-identical donor. *Oncoimmunology* **2017**, *6*, e1216291. [CrossRef] [PubMed]
221. Merli, P.; Algeri, M.; Galaverna, F.; Milano, G.M.; Bertaina, V.; Biagini, S.; Girolami, E.; Palumbo, G.; Sinibaldi, M.; Becilli, M.; et al. Immune Modulation Properties of Zoledronic Acid on TcRgammadelta T-Lymphocytes After TcRalphabeta/CD19-Depleted Haploidentical Stem Cell Transplantation: An analysis on 46 Pediatric Patients Affected by Acute Leukemia. *Front. Immunol.* **2020**, *11*, 699. [CrossRef]
222. Lucarelli, B.; Merli, P.; Bertaina, V.; Locatelli, F. Strategies to accelerate immune recovery after allogeneic hematopoietic stem cell transplantation. *Expert Rev. Clin. Immunol.* **2016**, *12*, 343–358. [CrossRef]
223. Ciceri, F.; Bonini, C.; Stanghellini, M.T.; Bondanza, A.; Traversari, C.; Salomoni, M.; Turchetto, L.; Colombi, S.; Bernardi, M.; Peccatori, J.; et al. Infusion of suicide-gene-engineered donor lymphocytes after family haploidentical haemopoietic stem-cell transplantation for leukaemia (the TK007 trial): A non-randomised phase I-II study. *Lancet Oncol.* **2009**, *10*, 489–500. [CrossRef]
224. Greco, R.; Oliveira, G.; Stanghellini, M.T.; Vago, L.; Bondanza, A.; Peccatori, J.; Cieri, N.; Marktel, S.; Mastaglio, S.; Bordignon, C.; et al. Improving the safety of cell therapy with the TK-suicide gene. *Front. Pharm.* **2015**, *6*, 95. [CrossRef]
225. Di Stasi, A.; Tey, S.K.; Dotti, G.; Fujita, Y.; Kennedy-Nasser, A.; Martinez, C.; Straathof, K.; Liu, E.; Durett, A.G.; Grilley, B.; et al. Inducible apoptosis as a safety switch for adoptive cell therapy. *N. Engl. J. Med.* **2011**, *365*, 1673–1683. [CrossRef] [PubMed]
226. Zhou, X.; Di Stasi, A.; Tey, S.K.; Krance, R.A.; Martinez, C.; Leung, K.S.; Durett, A.G.; Wu, M.F.; Liu, H.; Leen, A.M.; et al. Long-term outcome after haploidentical stem cell transplant and infusion of T cells expressing the inducible caspase 9 safety transgene. *Blood* **2014**, *123*, 3895–3905. [CrossRef]
227. Locatelli, F.; Ruggeri, A.; Merli, P.; Naik, S.; Agarwal, R.; Aquino, V.; Jacobsohn, D.A.; Qasim, W.; Nemecek, E.R.; Krishnamurti, L.; et al. Administration of BPX-501 Cells Following Aβ T and B-Cell-Depleted HLA Haploidentical HSCT (haplo-HSCT) in Children with Acute Leukemias. *Blood* **2018**, *132*, 307. [CrossRef]
228. Ruggeri, A.; Merli, P.; Algeri, M.; Zecca, M.; Fagioli, F.; Li Pira, G.; Bertaina, V.; Prete, A.; Montanari, M.; Del Bufalo, F.; et al. Comparative Analysis of Alpha-Beta T-Cell and B-Cell Depleted (abTCD) HLA-Haploidentical Hematopoietic Stem Cell Transplantation (haplo-HSCT) Versus Abtcd Haplo-HSCT with T-Cell Add-Back of Rivogenlecleucel Cell [Donor T Cells Transduced with the Inducible Caspase 9 (iC9) Gene Safety Switch] in Children with High-Risk Acute Leukemia (AL) in Remission. *Blood* **2019**, *134*, 145. [CrossRef]
229. Dunaikina, M.; Zhekhovtsova, Z.; Shelikhova, L.; Glushkova, S.; Nikolaev, R.; Blagov, S.; Khismatullina, R.; Balashov, D.; Kurnikova, E.; Pershin, D.; et al. Safety and efficacy of the low-dose memory (CD45RA-depleted) donor lymphocyte infusion in recipients of alphabeta T cell-depleted haploidentical grafts: Results of a prospective randomized trial in high-risk childhood leukemia. *Bone Marrow Transpl.* **2021**, *56*, 1614–1624. [CrossRef]
230. Anderson, B.E.; McNiff, J.; Yan, J.; Doyle, H.; Mamula, M.; Shlomchik, M.J.; Shlomchik, W.D. Memory CD4+ T cells do not induce graft-versus-host disease. *J. Clin. Investig.* **2003**, *112*, 101–108. [CrossRef] [PubMed]

231. Mamcarz, E.; Madden, R.; Qudeimat, A.; Srinivasan, A.; Talleur, A.; Sharma, A.; Suliman, A.; Maron, G.; Sunkara, A.; Kang, G.; et al. Improved survival rate in T-cell depleted haploidentical hematopoietic cell transplantation over the last 15 years at a single institution. *Bone Marrow Transpl.* **2020**, *55*, 929–938. [CrossRef]
232. Luznik, L.; O'Donnell, P.V.; Symons, H.J.; Chen, A.R.; Leffell, M.S.; Zahurak, M.; Gooley, T.A.; Piantadosi, S.; Kaup, M.; Ambinder, R.F.; et al. HLA-haploidentical bone marrow transplantation for hematologic malignancies using nonmyeloablative conditioning and high-dose, posttransplantation cyclophosphamide. *Biol. Blood Marrow Transpl.* **2008**, *14*, 641–650. [CrossRef]
233. Bashey, A.; Zhang, M.J.; McCurdy, S.R.; St. Martin, A.; Argall, T.; Anasetti, C.; Ciurea, S.O.; Fasan, O.; Gaballa, S.; Hamadani, M.; et al. Mobilized Peripheral Blood Stem Cells Versus Unstimulated Bone Marrow as a Graft Source for T-Cell-Replete Haploidentical Donor Transplantation Using Post-Transplant Cyclophosphamide. *J. Clin. Oncol.* **2017**, *35*, 3002–3009. [CrossRef] [PubMed]
234. Lorentino, F.; Labopin, M.; Bernardi, M.; Ciceri, F.; Socie, G.; Cornelissen, J.J.; Esteve, J.; Ruggeri, A.; Volin, L.; Yacoub-Agha, I.; et al. Comparable outcomes of haploidentical, 10/10 and 9/10 unrelated donor transplantation in adverse karyotype AML in first complete remission. *Am. J. Hematol.* **2018**, *93*, 1236–1244. [CrossRef]
235. Saglio, F.; Berger, M.; Spadea, M.; Pessolano, R.; Carraro, F.; Barone, M.; Quarello, P.; Vassallo, E.; Fagioli, F. Haploidentical HSCT with post transplantation cyclophosphamide versus unrelated donor HSCT in pediatric patients affected by acute leukemia. *Bone Marrow Transpl.* **2021**, *56*, 586–595. [CrossRef] [PubMed]
236. Symons, H.J.; Zahurak, M.; Cao, Y.; Chen, A.; Cooke, K.; Gamper, C.; Klein, O.; Llosa, N.; Zambidis, E.T.; Ambinder, R.; et al. Myeloablative haploidentical BMT with posttransplant cyclophosphamide for hematologic malignancies in children and adults. *Blood Adv.* **2020**, *4*, 3913–3925. [CrossRef] [PubMed]
237. Ruggeri, A.; Galimard, J.E.; Paina, O.; Fagioli, F.; Tbakhi, A.; Yesilipek, A.; Navarro, J.M.F.; Faraci, M.; Hamladji, R.M.; Skorobogatova, E.; et al. Outcomes of Unmanipulated Haploidentical Transplantation Using Post-Transplant Cyclophosphamide (PT-Cy) in Pediatric Patients with Acute Lymphoblastic Leukemia. *Transpl. Cell Ther.* **2021**, *27*, 424.e1–424.e9. [CrossRef]
238. Watkins, B.; Qayed, M.; McCracken, C.; Bratrude, B.; Betz, K.; Suessmuth, Y.; Yu, A.; Sinclair, S.; Furlan, S.; Bosinger, S.; et al. Phase II Trial of Costimulation Blockade with Abatacept for Prevention of Acute GVHD. *J. Clin. Oncol.* **2021**, *39*, 1865–1877. [CrossRef] [PubMed]
239. Gragert, L.; Eapen, M.; Williams, E.; Freeman, J.; Spellman, S.; Baitty, R.; Hartzman, R.; Rizzo, J.D.; Horowitz, M.; Confer, D.; et al. HLA match likelihoods for hematopoietic stem-cell grafts in the U.S. registry. *N. Engl. J. Med.* **2014**, *371*, 339–348. [CrossRef]
240. Bakhtiar, S.; Salzmann-Manrique, E.; Hutter, M.; Krenn, T.; Duerken, M.; Faber, J.; Reinhard, H.; Kreyenberg, H.; Huenecke, S.; Cappel, C.; et al. AlloHSCT in paediatric ALL and AML in complete remission: Improvement over time impacted by accreditation? *Bone Marrow Transpl.* **2019**, *54*, 737–745. [CrossRef]
241. Qayed, M.; Ahn, K.W.; Kitko, C.L.; Johnson, M.H.; Shah, N.N.; Dvorak, C.; Mellgren, K.; Friend, B.D.; Verneris, M.R.; Leung, W.; et al. A validated pediatric disease risk index for allogeneic hematopoietic cell transplantation. *Blood* **2021**, *137*, 983–993. [CrossRef] [PubMed]

MDPI
St. Alban-Anlage 66
4052 Basel
Switzerland
Tel. +41 61 683 77 34
Fax +41 61 302 89 18
www.mdpi.com

Journal of Clinical Medicine Editorial Office
E-mail: jcm@mdpi.com
www.mdpi.com/journal/jcm

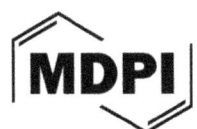

www.ingramcontent.com/pod-product-compliance
Lightning Source LLC
LaVergne TN
LVHW070154100526
838202LV00015B/1940

*9 7 8 3 0 3 6 5 4 1 6 7 9 *